Innovative Perspectives in Oral and Maxillofacial Surgery

Mark R. Stevens • Shohreh Ghasemi
Reza Tabrizi

Editors

Innovative Perspectives in Oral and Maxillofacial Surgery

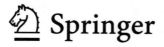

Editors
Mark R. Stevens
Department of Oral and Maxillofacial Surgery
Augusta University
Augusta, GA
USA

Shohreh Ghasemi
Department of Oral and Maxillofacial Surgery
Augusta University
Augusta, GA
USA

Reza Tabrizi
Department of Oral and Maxillofacial Surgery
Dental School, Shahid Beheshti University of
Medical Sciences
Tehran
Iran

ISBN 978-3-030-75752-6   ISBN 978-3-030-75750-2   (eBook)
https://doi.org/10.1007/978-3-030-75750-2

This Springer imprint is published by the registered company Springer Nature Switzerland AG
The registered company address is: Gewerbestrasse 11, 6330 Cham, Switzerland

Preface

This book has assembled a broad spectrum of current topic and exceptional specialists in oral and maxillofacial surgery. Innovation is essential to the lifeline of any profession. This is, especially, true in medicine and dentistry. Technology innovations are rapidly emerging as we move into the twenty-first century, an example of one such advance is in imaging and virtual surgical planning. The purpose of this book is to provide an update on many of the current and new practices in oral and maxillofacial surgery. This book achieves the following:

- Reviews and documents the current predictable practices in oral and maxillofacial surgical techniques
- Exposes the oral and maxillofacial surgeon to new advances in one comprehensive textbook
- Offers an understanding of the recent advances in oral and maxillofacial surgery
- Improves surgical outcomes by dissemination of the latest knowledge
- Provides a "how-to approach and perspective" through examples of common scenarios encountered in the management of oral and maxillofacial surgery

Augusta, GA, USA   Mark R. Stevens
Augusta, GA, USA   Shohreh Ghasemi
Tehran, Iran   Reza Tabrizi

Acknowledgments

We would like to express our sincere appreciation to the many outstanding experts and authors who took their valuable time and effort to give you the latest, state-of-the-art perspectives and concepts in oral and maxillofacial surgery.

Contents

Contributors

Hani Abd-Ul-Salam Faculty of Dentistry, McGill University, Montreal, PQ, Canada
Faculty of Dentistry, University of Sharjah, University City, Sharjah, UAE

Lory Abrahamian Department of Periodontology, Universitat Internacional de Catalunya, Barcelona, Spain

Abdullah Ajili Oral Surgery Department, Universitat Internacional de Catalunya, Barcelona, Spain

Sarah Akbari Department of Dentistry, Dental student of Mazandaran University of Medical Science, Member of the Student Research Committee, Sari, Iran

Jasmine Akbarzadeh Nova Southeastern University, Fort Lauderdale, FL, USA

Vahid Akheshteh Oral and Maxillofacial Radiology Department, Alborz Medical Science University, Karaj, Iran

Pablo Altuna Department of Oral and Maxillofacial Surgery, International University of Catalonia, Barcelona, Spain

Mohammad Hosein Amirzade-Iranaq Universal Network of Interdisciplinary Research in Oral and Maxillofacial Surgery (UNIROMS), Universal Scientific Education and Research Network (USERN), Tehran, Iran

Behrooz Amirzargar Department of Otorhinolaryngology-Head and Neck Surgery, Otorhinolaryngology Research Center, Imam Khomeini Hospital Complex, Tehran University of Medical Sciences, Tehran, Iran

Jessica R. Anderson AU Oral and Maxillofacial Surgery, Augusta, GA, USA

Sina Ayati First year of Dentistry (D1) Dental College of Georgia, Augusta, GA, USA

Mohadeseh Azarsina Private Practice, Tehran, Iran

Shahrokh C. Bagheri Georgia Oral and Facial Reconstructive Surgery, Atlanta, GA, USA

Thomas J. Balshi Prosthodontics Intermedica (Pi Dental Center), Private Implant Mentoring LLC, Fort Washington, PA, USA

Albert Barroso-Panella Department of Oral and Maxillofacial Surgery, International University of Catalonia, Barcelona, Spain

Parsa Behnia Department of Oral and Maxillofacial Surgery, Shahid Beheshti University of Medical Sciences, Tehran, Iran

Justin Bonner Oral and Maxillofacial Surgeon, Private Practice, West, TX, USA

Fargol Mashhadi Akbar Boojar School of Dentistry, Research Committee of Golestan Medical University, Gorgan, Iran

Chara Chatzichalepli Department of Oral and Maxillofacial Surgery, National and Kapodistrian University of Athens, Athens, Greece

Jonathan L. Czerepak Department of Oral and Maxillofacial Surgery, Dwight D. Eisenhower Army Medical Center, Fort Gordon, GA, USA

Alireza Darnahal Tufts University School of Dental Medicine, Boston, MA, USA

Mahmood Dashti Private Practice, Tehran, Iran

Alvaro de la Iglesia Beyme Department of Oral and Maxillofacial Surgery, Faculty of Dentistry – Universitat Internacional de Cataluyna, Barcelona, Spain

Nima Dehghani Department of Oral and Maxillofacial Surgery, Tehran University of Medical Sciences, Tehran, Iran

Alexander B. Faigen Oral and Maxillofacial Surgery, Dental College of Georgia at Augusta University, Augusta, GA, USA

Thomas Farrell IV Department of Oral & Maxillofacial Surgery, Dental College of Georgia at Augusta University, Augusta, GA, USA

Henry Ferguson AU Oral and Maxillofacial Surgery, Augusta, GA, USA

Aaron D. Figueroa Oral and Maxillofacial Surgery, University of Iowa Hospitals and Clinics, Iowa City, IA, USA

Elizabeth Floodeen Department of Oral & Maxillofacial Surgery, Augusta University, Augusta, GA, USA

Pindaros-Georgios Foskolos Department of Prosthodontics, National and Kapodistrian University of Athens, Athens, Greece

Kyle Frazier Augusta University Medical Center, Dental College of Georgia Oral & Maxillofacial Surgery, Augusta, GA, USA

Shohreh Ghasemi Department of Oral and Maxillofacial Surgery, Augusta University, Augusta, GA, USA

Cristina Godoy Clinical Research, College of Dental Medicine, Nova Southeastern University, Fort Lauderdale, FL, USA

Pilar Golmayo Department of Periodontology, Universitat Internacional de Catalunya, Barcelona, Spain

Farnaz Hadaegh Department of Pediatric Dentistry, University of Pittsburgh, School of Dental Medicine, Pittsburgh, PA, USA

Kristopher L. Hasstedt Georgia Oral and Facial Reconstructive Surgery, Atlanta, GA, USA

Ali Heidari Department of Oral and Maxillofacial Surgery, Hamadan University of Medical Sciences, Hamadan, Iran

Reihaneh Heidari Otorhinolaryngology Research Center, Department of Otorhinolaryngology-Head and Neck Surgery, Imam Khomeini Hospital Complex, Tehran University of Medical Sciences, Tehran, Iran

Federico Hernández-Alfaro Department of Oral and Maxillofacial Surgery, International University of Catalonia, Barcelona, Spain

Teknon Medical Center, Barcelona, Spain

Chris Ibrahim Resident of Oral and Maxillofacial Surgery, Dental College of Georgia at Augusta University, Augusta, GA, USA

Yara Ismail Prosthodontics and Esthetic Dentistry Department, Faculty of Dentistry – Saint Joseph University, Beirut, Lebanon

Joseph W. Ivory Oral and Maxillofacial Surgery, Dwight D. Eisenhower Army Medical Center, Fort Gordon, GA, USA

Mohammad Jafarian Department of Oral and Maxillofacial Surgery, School of Dentistry, Shahid Beheshti University of Medical Sciences, Tehran, Iran

Andrew C. Jenzer Department of Oral and Maxillofacial Surgery, Eisenhower Army Medical Center, Augusta, GA, USA

Sindhu Kanikicharla Division of Prosthodontics, University of Maryland School of Dentistry, Baltimore, MD, USA

Ioannis Karoussis Department of Prosthodontics, National and Kapodistrian University of Athens, Athens, Greece

Setare Kazemifard Dental Research Center, Research Institute of Dental Sciences, Shahid Beheshti University of Medical Sciences, Tehran, Iran

Muhammad Taimur Khan Nova Southeastern University College of Dental Medicine, Ft Lauderdale, FL, USA

Reem Kheirallah Faculty of Dentistry, Universitat Internacional de Catalunya, Barcelona, Spain

George Kouveliotis Department of Prosthodontics, National and Kapodistrian University of Athens, Athens, Greece

Department of Oral and Maxillofacial Surgery, International University of Catalonia, Barcelona, Spain

Ghida Lawand Prosthodontics and Esthetic Dentistry Department, Faculty of Dentistry – Saint Joseph University, Beirut, Lebanon

Moosa Mahmoudi Department of OMFS, Kerman University of Medical Sciences, Kerman, Iran

Xaniar Mahmoudi Dental School, Tehran University of Medical Sciences, Tehran, Iran

Reihaneh G. Mauer Mauer Periodontics & Implant Dentistry, LLC, Estero, FL, USA

Roger A. Meyer Department of Surgery, Atlanta, GA, USA

Maxillofacial Consultations, Ltd., Greensboro, GA, USA

Medical College of Georgia, August, GA, USA

Private Practice: Georgia Oral and Facial Reconstructive Surgery, Marietta, GA, USA

Amirhossein Moaddabi Department of Oral and Maxillofacial Surgery, Faculty of Dentistry of Mazandaran University of Medical Science, Member of Dental Research Center, Sari, Iran

Faculty of Dentistry, Mazandaran, University of Medical Sciences, Sari, Iran

Milad Mir Mohammadi Private practice (Iran), Tehran, Iran

Hamidreza Moslemi Department of Oral and Maxillofacial Surgery, School of Dentistry, Shahid Beheshti University of Medical Sciences, Tehran, Iran

Marshall Newman Department of Oral and Maxillofacial Surgery, Dental Collage of Georgia, Augusta University, Augusta, GA, USA

Mahsa Nikaein Department of Operative Dentistry, Shahid Beheshti University of Medical Sciences, Tehran, Iran

Octavi Ortiz-Puigpelat Department of Oral and Maxillofacial Surgery, International University of Catalonia, Barcelona, Spain

Dimitrios Papadopoulos Faculty of Dentistry, International University of Catalonia, Barcelona, Spain

Amir Zahedpasha Oral and Maxillofacial Surgery Department, Babol Medical Science University, Babol, Iran

Pratikkumar Patel Department of Oral and Maxillofacial Surgery, Dental Collage of Georgia, Augusta University, Augusta, GA, USA

J. Bertos Quilez Department of Oral and Maxillofacial Surgery, International University of Catalonia, Barcelona, Spain

Mohit Sachdeva Rajdhani Dental Care Clinic, Dental and Oral Laser Centre, New Delhi, India

Sara Samiei Kerman University of Medical sciences, Kerman, Iran

Francesc Abella Sans Department of Endodontics, Universitat Internacional de Catalunya, Sant Cugat del Vallès, Barcelona, Spain

Saba Sefidabi Private Practice, Tehran, Iran

Ahmed Seyam Department of Endodontics, Universitat Internacional de Catalunya, Sant Cugat del Vallès, Barcelona, Spain

Aida Shadrav Harvard School of Dental Medicine, Boston, MA, USA

Shervin Shafiei Oral and Maxillofacial Surgery Department, Shahid Beheshti University of Medical Sciences, Tehran, Iran

Rishad Shaikh Midwest Oral Maxillofacial Surgery and Implant Center, Saint Louis, MO, USA

Amir Reza Sharifnia Private Practice, Tehran, Iran

Lovleen Sidhu Nova Southeastern University, Ft Lauderdale, FL, USA

Parisa Soltani Department of Oral and Maxillofacial Radiology, Dental Implants Research Center, Dental Research Institute, School of Dentistry, Isfahan University of Medical Sciences, Isfahan, Iran

Danai-Maria Stasinoulia Faculty of Dentistry, International University of Catalonia, Barcelona, Spain

Mark R. Stevens Department of Oral and Maxillofacial Surgery, Augusta University, Augusta, GA, USA

Reza Tabrizi Department of Oral and Maxillofacial Surgery, Dental School, Shahid Beheshti University of Medical Sciences, Tehran, Iran

Theodoros Tasopoulos School of Dentistry, National and Kapodistrian University of Athens, Athens, Greece

Department of Prosthodontics, National and Kapodistrian University of Athens, Athens, Greece

Hani Tohme Removable Prosthodontics Department, Founder and Head of Digital Dentistry Unit, Faculty of Dentistry – Saint Joseph University, Beirut, Lebanon

Zahra Sadat Torabi Department of Oral and Maxillofacial Surgery, School of Dentistry, Shahid Beheshti University of Medical Sciences, Tehran, Iran

Farhad Vahidi Department of Prosthodontics, Newyork University, New York, NY, USA

Adaia Valls-Ontañón Department of Oral and Maxillofacial Surgery, Teknon Medical Center, Barcelona, Spain

Maneli Ardeshir Zadeh Private practice, Irvine, CA, USA

Setareh Zareh Stony Brook University, Stony Brook, NY, USA

Farhad Zeynalzadeh Department of Oral and Maxillofacial Surgery, Faculty of Dentistry-Medical Sciences University, Mashhad, Iran

Heliya Ziaei DDS, Faculty of Dentistry, Tehran University of Medical Sciences, Tehran, Iran

Osteocyte

Jasmine Akbarzadeh and Cristina Godoy

Osteocyte Morphology

The osteocyte is the most abundant cell type in bone and the longest-lived bone cell, being able to survive for up to 25 years within their bone microenvironment [1–3]. As pivotal cells in the biomechanical regulation of bone mass and structure, the osteocytic cell possesses mechanisms used to maintain viability under conditions of stress [3–5]. They are scattered throughout the mineralized bone matrix, comprising more than 90–95% of all bone cells in the adult skeleton, with this percentage increasing with age and size of the bone [1, 6]. Osteocytes lie within the substance of a fully formed bone, while they reside in the lacuna and send their dendritic processes through small channels in ossified bone known as canaliculi, which connect them to cells on the bone surface [6, 7]. However, osteocytic cells do not only communicate with each other on the bone surface, but also within the bone marrow; this is to ensure access of oxygen and nutrients in bone [3, 8].

For many years, osteocytes were thought to be moderately inactive cells, but they are highly active cells that play a key role in multiple physiological processes, both in and out of their microenvironment [2]. Osteocytes react to mechanical strain and send signals of bone formation or resorption to the bone surface to properly adapt to their microenvironment while playing a critical role in systemic and local mineral bone homeostasis [6].

The morphology of an osteocyte fluctuates depending on the type of bone. Specifically, osteocytes that derive from trabecular bone tend to be more rounded compared to ones that come from cortical bone, where they tend to take on a more elongated shape [1]. Mature osteocytes are stellate shaped cells (Fig. 1.1) that are bounded within the lacunar-canalicular network of the bone [3].

Osteocytes as Descendants of Osteoblasts

Osteocytes originate from osteoblasts, known as bone-forming cells, and are fundamentally osteoblasts surrounded by what they secrete. Osteoblasts, derived from mesenchymal stem cells through osteoblast differentiation, are cuboidal cells that can be found along the bone surface that represent 4–6% of the total resident bone cells [1, 9]. In comparison to other cell's responses to mechanical loading and substrate stretching, osteocytes tend to be more sensitive than both fibroblasts and osteoblasts [6, 10].

When an osteoid becomes mineralized and the preosteocytes transform into osteocytes, this osteoblast to osteocyte transition is referred to as osteocytogenesis. Osteocytogenesis has been known to be a passive process where a subpopulation of osteoblasts on the bone surface becomes inactively enclosed in an osteoid that passively mineralizes [1]; the osteoblasts then become "buried alive" below the matrix produced by its neighboring osteoblasts [6, 9, 11, 12]. When the osteoblast undergoes this transformation, the cell has increased three times its own volume in matrix [4, 13]. It has been found that osteocytes can recruit osteoblasts and are able to restore their differentiation by conveying osteoblast stimulating factor-1 (OSF-1) [4, 14]. A key mechanism of osteoblast and osteoclast activity is mechanical strain; the skeleton has the ability to continually adapt to its mechanical environment by adding new bone to resist increased amounts of loading and removing bone as a response to unloading [4, 15, 16].

Osteocytes have many responsibilities in orchestrating bone remodeling by controlling both osteoclast and osteoblast function [6]. These cells regulate bone remodeling by controlling osteoblasts and osteoclasts [8, 17]. However,

J. Akbarzadeh (✉)
Nova Southeastern University, Fort Lauderdale, FL, USA
e-mail: Ja2268@mynsu.nova.edu

C. Godoy
Clinical Research, College of Dental Medicine, Nova Southeastern University, Fort Lauderdale, FL, USA
e-mail: Cristina.godoy@nova.edu

Fig. 1.1 Bone cell structure. (Reproduced with permission from Rezaie 2020)

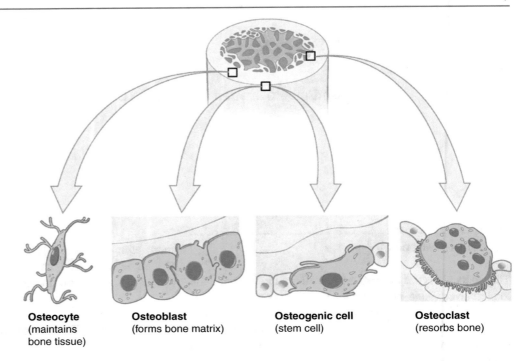

Osteocyte
(maintains
bone tissue)

Osteoblast
(forms bone matrix)

Osteogenic cell
(stem cell)

Osteoclast
(resorbs bone)

they do not only function as mechanosensors and communicators of both bone modeling and remodeling but also as regulators of phosphate and calcium homeostasis and send signals to distant tissues like endocrine cells [4].

Osteocytes as Mechanosensory Cells

Some of the earliest functions attributed to osteocytes were mechanosensation and mechanotransduction [6]. Mechanical loading on bone can result in mechanosensation by osteocytes; mechanosensation can play a role in the process of selection of targeted osteoblasts on the bone surface to become osteocytes [8]. Osteocytic cells are also key mechanotransducers [6]. During mechanotransduction, mechanical loading is necessary in order for bone to develop correctly. Researchers have suggested that mechanical load of an osteocyte can only be sensed through the cell's dendritic processes and have found that the cell body seems to be unaffected by mechanical strain. Studies involving the incorporation of shear stress to the dendrites of MLO-Y4 cells or the cell body have proposed that components of the pericellular matrix, glycocalyx, play a crucial position in mechanotransduction by dendrites while leaving the cell body responsive [4, 18–20].

Osteocytes are known to be a key factor in the network of mechanosensory cells facilitating the effects of mechanical loading in its extensive lacunar-canalicular network [4]. The location in the bone and the dendritic network has led to the idea that the lining cell is a major mechanosensory cell, but little is known about this theory [1, 21–23]. Although there

may not be a singular mechanoreceptor in osteocytes, there are particular events that must occur for mechanosensation and transduction to occur. These events include shear stress along dendritic processes and/or the cell body, cell deformation as a reaction of strain, and primary cilia [8]. Strain-derived flow of interstitial fluid through this absorbency appears to mechanically activate the osteocytes and ensure the passage of cell signaling molecules, nutrients, and waste products [3]. This causes local bone gain and loss and bone remodeling in response to fatigue damage. Signaling can be initiated by calcium channel activation and adenosine triphosphate (ATP), nitric oxide, and prostaglandin release. Signal transfers can be made from gap junctions and hemichannels and the release of signaling molecules into the bone fluid.

Osteocytes can act as mechanosensors to control adaptive responses to mechanical loading of the skeleton as well, and they could be a valuable target cell when it comes to the actions of the parathyroid hormone (PTH) in the bone. Osteocytes have the potential to influence cells and tissues beyond their bone matrix, signaling which occurs between the parathyroid, kidney, cardiac, and skeletal muscle that depict the significance of the osteocyte's endocrine function and the effect of preserving viability could have on other tissues. Although categorizing an osteocyte as an endocrine cell may seem contradictory because of how deeply embedded it is in the bone matrix, the lacunar-canalicular system exposes the cell to hormones within the blood [6].

When a bone is mechanically loaded, there are multiple stimuli that can be identified by the mechanosensory cells including the physical deformation of the osteoid, the load-induced flow of canalicular fluid through the lacunar-canalicular network, which results in fluid flow shear stress, or electrical streaming potentials created from the flow of canalicular fluid past the surfaces of the cell membrane [6]. Furthermore, because both mechanical loading and unloading change the osteocyte gene expression, it further proves how heavy loads may affect osteocyte function [1, 24–27].

Another way that osteocytes signal each other is through gap junctions, which permit the direct cell-to-cell coupling [3, 28]. Gap junction channels are created by connexins, a family of proteins, with Cx43 being the major connexin in bone cells. It has been discovered that these connexins have the ability to function as hemichannels, defined as a connexin channel produced between two cells; these hemichannels are one of the many gaps within the extracellular bone fluid, including calcium, ion, voltage, and mechanosensitive channels. Hence, the gap junctions that are located at the tip of dendrites appear to facilitate a form of intracellular communication, while hemichannels alongside the dendrite facilitate a form of extracellular communication with osteocytes [8].

Osteocytic Remodeling of the Perilacunar Matrix

Osteocytic cells are capable of controlling and conducting bone formation and resorption, regulating all bone remodeling phases, as they play a role as both promoters and inhibitors of mineralization [4, 8]. These cells regulate bone remodeling by regulating osteoclasts and osteoblasts, while functioning as an endocrine cell [1, 8, 17]. However, viable osteocytes are needed to communicate signals of remodeling [8]. The main objective of bone remodeling is to release calcium and growth factors that are found in the bone matrix near the bloodstream, which prompts the regulation of mineral homeostasis. Through bone remodeling, old or damaged bone is replaced with new bone, allowing the skeletal integrity and bone mass to be preserved [2]. In addition, osteocytes induce new bone formation where there is fracture damage by involving mesenchymal cells through the secretion of osteopontin [6]. During bone resorption, the amount of bone loss is matched to the amount added during bone formation [4].

The lacunar-canalicular system is the optimal network allowing the communication of biochemical signals from deeply rooted osteocytes to osteoblasts at the bone surface, enabling osteocytes to influence osteoblast activity [6, 29]. Similar to how osteoclasts and osteoblasts are involved in remodeling of the bone surface, osteocytes are sometimes involved in remodeling the surfaces that they are in contact with; the cell can remodel its surrounding environment, including the canaliculae and lacunae [6, 8].

Numerous concepts regarding osteocytes have disappeared from the literature because investigators seem to lack the proper tools to validate the original observations, specifically how osteocytes are able to not only remove the bone from their perilacunar matrix but add it back. This is referred to as "osteocytic osteolysis," which was originally used to depict the size of lacunae in diagnosed hyperparathyroidism [8, 30–32]. Healthy osteocytes are capable of doing this during processes similar to reproductive function, meaning they could play a function in mineral homeostasis with high calcium demand, like lactation [6].

Early observations support that any modification in the features of perilacunar bone matrix and lacunar size would stimulate fracture risk, while mechanisms that modify the material properties of the matrix would have an effect on mechanosensation [1, 33, 34]. The molecular mechanisms that are responsible for the replacement of the perilacunar matrix are unknown but are thought to be similar to that of the osteoblast [35]. During perilacunar remodeling, osteocytes dynamically resorb and replenish the organic and mineral elements of the extracellular matrix. An aging osteocyte may be forced to undergo hypermineralization of its perilacunar matrix, potentially leading to cell death. In turn, hypermineralization would modify the interactions of bone fluid flow throughout the matrix, drastically influencing both the cell's function and viability [1].

Death Cycle

It is believed that the primary role of osteocytes is to go through cell death, which sends out bone resorption signals [4]. Although osteocytes generally live a long life, bone turnover, where osteoclasts resorb bone and osteoblasts replace it, is what primarily regulates the cell's life span [6]. The osteocyte cell death's occurrence can be associated with pathological conditions, specifically osteoarthritis and osteoporosis, eventually leading to a rise in skeletal fragility [4, 36–38]. There have been multiple conditions that have been shown to have a correlation with osteocyte cell death, like oxygen deprivation, withdrawal of estrogen, and glucocorticoid treatment [8, 37].

When osteoblasts stop developing their new matrix, it can either become an osteocyte or a bone lining cell or can undergo a cell programmed death, called apoptosis [2, 39]. Osteocyte apoptosis can happen where microdamage occurs, and it has been thought that dying osteocytes are utilized for osteoclast removal. Not only microdamage can cause apoptosis, but oxygen deprivation has been seen to promote it, primarily in immobilization. Active protection mechanisms keep some osteocytes from undergoing apoptosis because, although they are damaged, they remain viable osteocytes. Since apoptosis can aid conditions like bone loss, it could be fundamental for both damage repair and skeletal replacement [4].

There is a possibility that osteocyte apoptosis holds responsibility for particular forms of osteonecrosis [8]. Osteonecrosis is "dead bone" made up of empty osteocyte lacunae that is unable to remodel but can remain in the bone for years.

Osteocytes go through a method of self-preservation, known as autophagy, to maintain its viability until advantageous circumstances are present. Autophagy can be defined as a lysosomal degradation process, essential for recovering cellular products. Autophagy can have both favorable and unfavorable consequences; it is able to keep cells from a programmed cell death yet can still terminate cellular mechanisms [1]. Therefore, autophagy can protect osteocytic cells from apoptosis and maintain viability, but if the stress is not relieved, it will result in the cell undergoing apoptosis [4].

Conclusion

The knowledge behind osteocytes continues to expand, playing a key role in bone biology. In the last decade, valuable progress has been made concerning the role that osteocytes play in both bone turnover and metabolism. Studies show that osteocytes contribute to the structural makeup that permit bones to establish the demands for bone enlargement or diminution in regard to mechanical demands [3]. Osteocytes are incredibly important for bone health and may lead to the development of therapeutic products to treat bone diseases.

References

1. Bonewald LF. The amazing osteocyte. J Bone Miner Res. 2011;26(2):229–38.
2. Tresguerres FGF, Torres J, López-Quiles J, Hernández G, Vega JA, Tresguerres IF. The osteocyte: a multifunctional cell within the bone. Ann Anat. 2020;227:151422.
3. Klein-Nulend J, Nijweide PJ, Burger EH. Osteocyte and bone structure. Curr Osteoporos Rep. 2003;1(1):5–10.
4. Bonewald LF. Osteocyte Biology. In: Marcus R, Dempster DW, Luckey M, Cauley JA, editors. Osteoporosis. Fourth Edition: Academic Press; 2013. p. 209–34. https://doi.org/10.1016/B978-0-12-415853-5.00010-8.
5. Xia X, Kar R, Gluhak-Heinrich J, Yao W, Lane NE, Bonewald LF, et al. Glucocorticoid-induced autophagy in osteocytes. J Bone Miner Res. 2010;25(11):2479–88.
6. Dallas SL, Prideaux M, Bonewald LF. The osteocyte: an endocrine cell ... and more. Endocr Rev. 2013;34(5):658–90.
7. Beno T, Yoon YJ, Cowin SC, Fritton SP. Estimation of bone permeability using accurate microstructural measurements. J Biomech. 2006;39(13):2378–87.
8. Bonewald LF. Chapter 4. Osteocytes. In: Primer on the metabolic bone diseases and disorders of mineral metabolism. Washington, D.C.: American Society for Bone and Mineral Research; 2008. p. 22–7.
9. Nefussi JR, Sautier JM, Nicolas V, Forest N. How osteoblasts become osteocytes: a decreasing matrix forming process. J Biol Buccale. 1991;19(1):75–82.
10. Klein-Nulend J, van der Plas A, Semeins CM, Ajubi NE, Frangos JA, Nijweide PJ, et al. Sensitivity of osteocytes to biomechanical stress in vitro. FASEB J. 1995;9(5):441–5.
11. Franz-Odendaal TA, Hall BK, Witten PE. Buried alive: how osteoblasts become osteocytes. Dev Dyn. 2006;235(1):176–90.
12. Palumbo C, Palazzini S, Zaffe D, Marotti G. Osteocyte differentiation in the tibia of newborn rabbit: an ultrastructural study of the formation of cytoplasmic processes. Cells Tissues Organs. 1990;137(4):350–8.
13. Owen M. Cell population kinetics of an osteogenic tissue. I. J Cell Biol. 1963;19(1):19–32.
14. Imai S, Heino TJ, Hienola A, Kurata K, Büki K, Matsusue Y, et al. Osteocyte-derived HB-GAM (pleiotrophin) is associated with bone formation and mechanical loading. Bone. 2009;44(5):785–94.
15. Burr DB, Robling AG, Turner CH. Effects of biomechanical stress on bones in animals. Bone. 2002;30(5):781–6.
16. Ehrlich PJ, Noble BS, Jessop HL, Stevens HY, Mosley JR, Lanyon LE. The effect of in vivo mechanical loading on estrogen receptor alpha expression in rat ulnar osteocytes. J Bone Miner Res. 2002;17(9):1646–55.
17. Rolvien T, Krause M, Jeschke A, Yorgan T, Püschel K, Schinke T, et al. Vitamin D regulates osteocyte survival and perilacunar remodeling in human and murine bone. Bone. 2017;103:78–87.
18. Han Y, Cowin SC, Schaffler MB, Weinbaum S. Mechanotransduction and strain amplification in osteocyte cell processes. Proc Natl Acad Sci U S A. 2004;101(47):16689–94.
19. Adachi T, Aonuma Y, Tanaka M, Hojo M, Takano-Yamamoto T, Kamioka H. Calcium response in single osteocytes to locally applied mechanical stimulus: differences in cell process and cell body. J Biomech. 2009;42(12):1989–95.
20. Burra S, Nicolella DP, Francis WL, Freitas CJ, Mueschke NJ, Poole K, et al. Dendritic processes of osteocytes are mechanotransducers that induce the opening of hemichannels. Proc Natl Acad Sci U S A. 2010;107(31):13648–53.
21. Rubin CT. Skeletal strain and the functional significance of bone architecture. Calcif Tissue Int. 1984;36 Suppl 1:S11–8.
22. Turner CH, Forwood MR, Otter MW. Mechanotransduction in bone: do bone cells act as sensors of fluid flow? FASEB J. 1994;8(11):875–8.
23. Robling AG, Hinant FM, Burr DB, Turner CH. Shorter, more frequent mechanical loading sessions enhance bone mass. Med Sci Sports Exerc. 2002;34(2):196–202.
24. Robling AG, Niziolek PJ, Baldridge LA, Condon KW, Allen MR, Alam I, et al. Mechanical stimulation of bone in vivo reduces osteocyte expression of Sost/sclerostin. J Biol Chem. 2008;283(9):5866–75.
25. Skerry TM, Bitensky L, Chayen J, Lanyon LE. Early strain-related changes in enzyme activity in osteocytes following bone loading in vivo. J Bone Miner Res. 1989;4(5):783–8.
26. Gluhak-Heinrich J, Pavlin D, Yang W, MacDougall M, Harris SE. MEPE expression in osteocytes during orthodontic tooth movement. Arch Oral Biol. 2007;52(7):684–90.
27. Gluhak-Heinrich J, Ye L, Bonewald LF, Feng JQ, MacDougall M, Harris SE, et al. Mechanical loading stimulates dentin matrix protein 1 (DMP1) expression in osteocytes in vivo. J Bone Miner Res. 2003;18(5):807–17.
28. Doty SB. Morphological evidence of gap junctions between bone cells. Calcif Tissue Int. 1981;33(5):509–12.
29. Raheja LF, Genetos DC, Yellowley CE. Hypoxic osteocytes recruit human MSCs through an OPN/CD44-mediated pathway. Biochem Biophys Res Commun. 2008;366(4):1061–6.
30. Bélanger LF. Osteocytic osteolysis. Calcif Tissue Res. 1969;4(1):1–12.

31. Bélanger LF, Bélanger C, Semba T. Technical approaches leading to the concept of osteocytic osteolysis. Clin Orthop Relat Res. 1967;54:187–96.

32. Baylink DJ, Wergedal JE. Bone formation by osteocytes. Am J Phys. 1971;221(3):669–78.

33. Nicolella DP, Feng JQ, Moravits DE, Bonivitch AR, Wang Y, Dusecich V, et al. Effects of nanomechanical bone tissue properties on bone tissue strain: implications for osteocyte mechanotransduction. J Musculoskelet Neuronal Interact. 2008;8(4):330–1.

34. Nicolella DP, Moravits DE, Gale AM, Bonewald LF, Lankford J. Osteocyte lacunae tissue strain in cortical bone. J Biomech. 2006;39(9):1735–43.

35. Qing H, Bonewald LF. Osteocyte remodeling of the perilacunar and pericanalicular matrix. Int J Oral Sci. 2009;1(2):59–65.

36. Dunstan CR, Evans RA, Hills E, Wong SY, Higgs RJ. Bone death in hip fracture in the elderly. Calcif Tissue Int. 1990;47(5):270–5.

37. Weinstein RS, Nicholas RW, Manolagas SC. Apoptosis of osteocytes in glucocorticoid-induced osteonecrosis of the hip. J Clin Endocrinol Metab. 2000;85(8):2907–12.

38. Wong SY, Evans RA, Needs C, Dunstan CR, Hills E, Garvan J. The pathogenesis of osteoarthritis of the hip. Evidence for primary osteocyte death. Clin Orthop Relat Res. 1987;214:305–12.

39. Manolagas SC. Birth and death of bone cells: basic regulatory mechanisms and implications for the pathogenesis and treatment of osteoporosis. Endocr Rev. 2000;21(2):115–37.

Molecular and Cellular Basis of Bone

2

Setare Kazemifard and Mahmood Dashti

Introduction

Human bone marrow has emerged as an organ in evolutionary processes that constitute different cells that originate from a hematopoietic stem cell (HSCs) and mesenchymal stem cells (MSCs). Vital HSC activity is managed through molecular interaction with the niche microenvironment. The development of biomimetic and bioinspired materials has been enhanced due to rapid biotechnology, tissue bioengineering, and regenerative medicine. Moreover, this information is also valuable in creating implants that provide a productive bone/bone marrow healing process after injuries and in the recovery of diseases of various etiologies [1]. Osteoclast research has a stirring history and a testing future. The discovery came 30 years ago that the origin of bone-resorbing osteoclasts is hematopoietic. They are connected to the "basic multicellular unit," where they connect with other cells, including bone-forming osteoblasts. The acknowledgment of the signaling pathways controlling genes appropriate for osteoclast genesis and bone resorption has originated for two decades. It took another 10 years for an approved pharmacologic strategy because of the discovery of hypothesized "osteoclast differentiation." In this study, cathepsin K, a cysteine protease being released by the osteoclast into the resorption compartment, is the primary focus. Genetic deletion and pharmacological blocking of cathepsin K reduce bone resorption. However, this happens with the continuing process of bone formation [2]. Every 10 years, the adult skeleton is remodeled and is renewed. This process of the remodeling continues throughout life. It is approximated that three to four million bone remodeling units (BRUs) are originated every year, and one million out of these are actively involved in bone turnover every time. Remodeling is a four-phased process: first is the activation phase when the osteoclasts are initiated; second is the resorption phase when then osteoclasts resorb bone; third is the reversal phase, where the osteoclasts resorb bone and the osteoblasts are employed; and forth is the formation phase where the osteoblasts set down organic bone matrix that later mineralizes [3]. The process by which two phases of the bone matrix, the mineral and the organic, are dissolved and then degraded is bone resorption. Resorption plays its role in bone modeling, and it is also required for tooth eruption. In the whole life, resorption is essential for bone remodeling and bone formation, formulated by osteoblasts. This procedure is the defensive maintenance of mechanical strength by continuously replacing the tired bone with the new "fresh" bone. The chief reservoir for calcium ions is the bone. The remodeling is crucial for Ca2 fluxes into and from the extracellular fluid for maintaining a suitable level of blood calcium. The exclusive bone resorptive cell is the osteoclast, and the adoption of its morphological features happens accordingly. Moreover, genes are exhibited by the osteoclasts, whose functions are crucial for resorption [4].

Anatomy and Biochemistry of Osteoclast

Osteoclasts are multinucleated cells that originate from hematopoietic progenitors in the bone marrow, producing monocytes in the peripheral blood and other various types of tissue macrophages. The combination of precursor cells stimulates osteoclasts. They perform in bone resorption. They are necessary for normal skeletal development (growth and modeling), perpetuating its dignity throughout life, and calcium metabolism (remodeling). The osteoclasts are fixed with the bone matrix, their cytoskeleton reorganizes, and osteoclasts assume polarized morphology for resorbing bone. They also form ruffled borders to secrete acid and col-

S. Kazemifard
Dental Research Center, Research Institute of Dental Sciences, Shahid Beheshti University of Medical Sciences, Tehran, Iran
e-mail: Setare_kazemi74@yahoo.com

M. Dashti (✉)
Private practice, Tehran, Iran
e-mail: dashti.mahmood72@gmail.com

lagenolytic enzymes and a sealing zone for segregating the resorption site. The considerable progress in the immense understanding of differentiation and the molecular mechanisms' functions has been through recognizing the osteoclast genesis inducer, the receptor activator of nuclear factor-kB ligand (RANKL), its cognate receptor RANK, and its decoy receptor osteoprotegerin (OPG). The large number of analysis which surfaced in the last 10 years depict the advancement discussed above [4].

It is practical to assume that multinucleation enhances resorption efficacy. In other cases, the purpose behind the energy investment needed for the mononuclear precursors' amalgamation to make a large osteoclast would be problematic to comprehend. For example, considering this analogy, one osteoclast resorption with five nuclei is more efficient than five mononuclear osteoclasts' resorption. The multinucleation characterizing the osteoclast is the most pivotal morphological property distinguishing the osteoclast from its precursor. The formation of multinucleated osteoclast from the fusion of mononuclear precursors, the membrane protein, dendritic cell-specific transmembrane protein (DCSTAMP), was discovered to be vital. Interestingly, DCSTAMP – deficient cells, along with failing to fuse – showcase approximate osteoclasts' features, including the formation of actin-ring and ruffled border [4].

Pioneer Work on Osteoclastogenesis

Paget's bone disease serves as a case for osteoclasts containing substantially more nuclei than normal osteoclasts, up to 100 nuclei per cell. This disease is a localized disorder of bone remodeling. The process starts with osteoclast-mediated bone resorption growth with the successive compensatory enhancement in the new bone formation. This results in a disorganized mosaic of woven and lamellar bone at affected skeletal sites [4]. RANKL, whose gene was contemporaneously replicated 15 years ago by four different groups, is also called TNF-related activation-induced cytokine, TRANCE, osteoclast differentiation factor, ODF, and osteoprotegerin ligand, OPGL. It is a type II transmembrane protein belonging to the TNF superfamily [5, 6]. It is found mainly in a membrane-bound form with a short cytoplasmic N-terminal domain and a single transmembrane region. Its soluble existence can be produced through alternative splicing [7]. It can also be generated through cleavage by matrix metalloproteinases and ADAMs (disintegrin and metalloproteinase domain-containing proteins) [8, 9]. RANKL accumulates into homotrimers from conserved and specific residues in the extracellular domain, and trimerization is pivotal for the operation of its cognate receptor RANK [10, 11]. Lately, the determination of the RANKL in complex with its decoy receptor

osteoprotegerin (OPG) has taken place. This discovery showed a different type of interaction: the direct blockage of RANK's availability, which is significant for RANK indication [12, 13]. The RANKL cytokine emerged as a critical finding in the area of osteoimmunology. The first of many and subsequently increasing interconnections between bone and immune systems is highlighted by explaining the signaling pathway of RANKL cytokine. Therapies that focused on blocking this pathway and are designed for diseases with increased bone resorption came into the focus last year. Along with this, the discovery of direct RANKL participation in a rare genetic ailment makes up one of the few cases when a genetic study's conclusion can be converted into a replacement therapy. The combined efforts from various stakeholders, including research centers, clinics, charities, and biotech industries, can be integrated to avoid the safety and regulatory concerns and eventually provide patients with hope and a cure [14].

It is evident that in postmenopausal and older women, the substantial osteoclasts formation has an essential role in osteoporosis. The productive technique for osteoporosis can turn out to be the suppression of extensive osteoclastogenesis and bone resorption. Zoledronic acid (ZOL), which is already used in large clinical trials, plays a critical role in regulating bone mineral density. However, the effects of ZOL on osteoclastogenesis are entirely illustrated. Hence, this analysis focuses on analyzing the effects of ZOL on osteoclastogenesis and examining the corresponding signaling pathways. Through viability assay and in vitro osteoclastogenesis, immunofluorescence, and resorption pit assays, the results become clear that receptor activator of nuclear factor-κB ligand (RANKL)-induced osteoclast differentiation and bone resorptive activity is repressed by the ZOL (0.1–5 μM). Along with this, ZOL hindered the RANKL-induced activation of NF-κB and the phosphorylation of JNK in RAW264.7 cells, which is proven through the western blot analysis and reversed transcription-quantitative PCR. Moreover, ZOL also hampered the expression of osteoclastogenesis-associated genes, including calcitonin receptor, tartrate-resistant acid phosphatase, and dendritic cell-specific transmembrane protein. Furthermore, ZOL suppressed NF-κB and JNK signaling which slowed down the ZOL inhibited osteoclast formation and resorption in vitro. Overall, the results of this study depict that ZOL can be helpful in the cure of osteoclast-associated diseases, including osteoporosis [15].

Throughout life, remodeling keeps renewing the adult skeleton. The process where osteoclasts and osteoblasts work successively in the same bone remodeling unit is bone remodeling. The attainment of peak bone mass results in balanced bone remodeling and stable bone mass for 10–20 years until the age-related bone loss begins. An increase in resorptive activity and reduction in bone formation results in age-related bone loss. With aging, cancellous bone is lost, and remodeling movement is enhanced in both compartments, resulting in the utmost importance of cortical remodeling. When the bones are altered and shaped by osteoblasts' independent action and osteoclasts, the process is known as bone remodeling. The functions of osteoblasts and osteoclasts do not coincide structurally or temporarily. Throughout life, bone modeling continues and shapes skeletal development. Remodeling contributes toward the medullary expansion, which is observed at long bones with aging. Similarly, modeling-based bone formation results in periosteal accumulation. Both modeling and remodeling are affected by the prevailing and forthcoming treatments.

Bone Remodeling Concept

Throughout life, the adult skeleton is updated by remodeling. Bone remodeling is a procedure sequential work of osteoclasts, and osteoblasts take place in the same bone remodeling unit. Bone remodeling is balanced, and bone mass is stable for 10–20 years until the initiation of age-related bone loss after peak bone mass is attained. Enhanced resorptive activity and reduced bone formation result in age-related bone loss. As cancellous cells, bone fades, and remodeling functions increase in both compartment, the relative significance of cortical remodeling is enhanced. The shaping and reshaping of bones through the independent activities of osteoclasts and osteoblasts is bone modeling. The functions of osteoclasts and osteoblasts are not joined naturally or for the time being. For whole life, skeletal development and growth are exhibited by bone modeling. As remodeling-based resorption is critical for the medullary expansion, which is seen with long bones with aging, in the same way, contribution of modeling-based formation takes place in the periosteal expansion. Existing and upcoming treatments affect remodeling and modeling. Teriparatide enhances bone formation, out of which 70% is based on remodeling and 20–30% on modeling. Other than Novo modeling, the sizable majority of modeling highlights overflow from remodeling units. Denosumab is suitable for modeling at the cortex but hinders bone remodeling. Odanacatib hampers bone resorption by reducing cathepsin K activity, whereas modeling-base bone formation is enhanced at periosteal surfaces. The delay of sclerostin enriches the bone formation. Histomorphometric analysis showed that bone formation is mainly modeling based. The way bone mass has responded to the osteoporosis treatments in humans indicates that non-remodeling techniques play their part in this response, and bone modeling is such a technique. This has only been explained for teriparatide; however, rediscover-ing more than a half-century-old phenomenon will significantly affect our analysis and understanding of how updated anti-fracture cure work [16]. On cancellous bone surfaces, bone remodeling becomes notable. Although cancellous bone only constitutes 20% of the bone, 80% of bone remodeling functions occur in the cancellous cells. The separate roles of osteoblasts and osteoclasts result in bone modeling. Their activities possess similarities with the functions in bone remodeling. Therefore, bone modeling maintains the responsibility of shaping the bones and bones' movement through space [16].

References

1. Yurova KA, Khaziakhmatova OG, Melashchenko ES, Malashchenko VV, Shunkin EO, Shupletsova VV, Ivanov PA, Khlusov IA, Litvinova LS. Cellular and molecular basis of osteoblastic and vascular niches in the processes of hematopoiesis and bone remodeling (a short review of modern views). Curr Pharm Des. 2019;25(6):663–9. https://doi.org/10.2174/1381612825666619 0329153626.
2. Gruber R. Molecular and cellular basis of bone resorption. Wien Med Wochenschr. 2015;165(3–4):48–53. https://doi.org/10.1007/s10354-014-0310-0. Epub 2014 Sep 16.
3. Huang XL, Huang LY, Cheng YT, Li F, Zhou Q, Wu C, Shi QH, Guan ZZ, Liao J, Hong W, Hong W, et al. Zoledronic acid inhibits osteoclast differentiation and function through the regulation of NF-κB and JNK signalling pathways. Int J Mol Med. 2019;44:582–92.
4. Bar-Shavit Z. The osteoclast: a multinucleated, hematopoietic-origin, bone-resorbing osteoimmune cell. J Cell Biochem. 2007;102(5):1130–9. https://doi.org/10.1002/jcb.21553. PubMed.
5. Lacey DL, Boyle WJ, Simonet WS, et al. Bench to bedside: elucidation of theOPG-RANK-RANKL pathway and the development of denosumab. Nat Rev Drug Discov. 2012;11(5):401–19.
6. Yasuda H, Shima N, Nakagawa N, et al. Osteoclast differentiation factor is a ligand for osteoprotegerin/osteoclastogenesis inhibitory factor and is identical to TRANCE/RANKL. Proc Natl Acad Sci U S A. 1998;95(7):3597–602.
7. Ikeda T, Kasai M, Utsuyama M, Hirokawa K. Determination of three isoforms of the receptor activator of nuclear factor-κB ligand and their differential expression in bone and thymus. Endocrinology. 2001;142(4):1419–26.
8. Lum L, Wong BR, Josien R, et al. Evidence for a role of a tumor necrosis factor-α (TNF-α)-converting enzyme-like protease in shedding of TRANCE, a TNF family member involved in osteoclastogenesis and dendritic cell survival. J Biol Chem. 1999;274(19):13613–8.
9. Hikita A, Tanaka N, Yamane S, et al. Involvement of a disintegrin and metalloproteinase 10 and 17 in shedding of tumor necrosis factor-α. Biochem Cell Biol. 2009;87(4):81–93.
10. Lam J, Nelson CA, Ross FP, Teitelbaum SL, Fremont DH. Crystal structure of the TRANCE/RANKL cytokine reveals determinants of receptor-ligand specificity. J Clin Investig. 2001;108(7):971–9.
11. Ta HM, Nguyen GTT, Jin HM, et al. Structure based development of a receptor activator of nuclear factor- κB ligand (RANKL) inhibitor peptide and molecular basis for osteopetrosis. Proc Natl Acad Sci U S A. 2010;107(47):20281–6.
12. Luan X, Lu Q, Jiang Y, et al. Crystal structure of human RANKL complexed with its decoy receptor osteoprotegerin. J Immunol. 2012;189(1):245–52.

13. Nelson CA, Warren JT, Wang MW, Teitelbaum SL, Fremont DH. RANKL employs distinct binding modes to engage RANK and the osteoprotegerin decoy receptor. Structure. 2012;20(11):1971–82.

14. Lo Iacono N, Pangrazio A, Abinun M, Bredius R, Zecca M, Blair HC, Vezzoni P, Villa A, Sobacchi C. RANKL cytokine: from pioneer of the osteoimmunology era to cure for a rare disease. Clin Dev Immunol. 2013;2013:412768. https://doi.org/10.1155/2013/412768. Epub 2013 May 15. PMID: 23762088; PMCID: PMC3671266.

15. Huang XL, Huang LY, Cheng YT, Li F, Zhou Q, Wu C, Shi QH, Guan ZZ, Liao J, Hong W. Zoledronic acid inhibits osteoclast differentiation and function through the regulation of NF-κB and JNK signalling pathways. Int J Mol Med. 2019;44(2):582–92. https://doi.org/10.3892/ijmm.2019.4207. Epub 2019 May 23. PMID: 31173157; PMCID: PMC6605660.

16. Langdahl B, Ferrari S, Dempster DW. Bone modeling and remodeling: potential as therapeutic targets for the treatment of osteoporosis. Ther Adv Musculoskelet Dis. 2016;8(6):225–35. https://doi.org/10.1177/1759720X16670154. Epub 2016 Oct 5. PMID: 28255336; PMCID: PMC5322859.

Biomaterial for Osseous Reconstruction

3

Pratikkumar Patel and Marshall Newman

Introduction

A variety of biomaterials for osseous reconstruction are utilized in oral and maxillofacial surgery and orthopedic surgery, among other disciplines. The use of such materials for tissue regeneration has become essential in reconstructing defects of all sizes within the craniomaxillofacial region, and their use often parallels that of spinal fusion surgery. The etiology of craniomaxillofacial bony defects may include trauma, pathology, congenital deformities, or age-related changes. Tissue engineering for regenerative purposes offer the reconstructing practitioner the potential to provide patients an uncompromised osseous reconstruction and avoid the morbidity associated with autogenous bone grafting methods. Historically, autogenous bone grafts have been the gold standard for osseous defect reconstruction [1–4]. However, allografts, xenografts, and alloplasts, as defined below, continue to evolve as engineered alternatives and/or adjunct materials in craniomaxillofacial reconstruction.

Ideal Properties of Grafting Material

Ideal properties of bone grafting materials continue to evolve with advancements in tissue engineering. For the purposes of reconstruction, a given osseous defect may require different graft properties that vary by locations within the defect. Pore size is an essential graft material property as it allows diffusion of bone cells, nutrients, and exchange of waste products [5]. A minimum pore size required to regenerate mineralize bone may be approximately 100 μm [6]; however, pore sizes >300 μm is recommended for allowing vascularization and osteogenesis [7–9]. The surface condition of a chosen grafting material should allow for vascular ingrowth, bone cell attachment, migration, and proliferation. Ideal surface properties relate to a biomaterial's osteoconduction and the formation of bone at the interface of a patient's native bone and the reconstructive material. Mechanical compressive strength and elasticity will influence the biomaterial's overall stability within the reconstructed defect as forces directed on the defect will inevitably change as the patient heals. Biodegradability, which ensures resorption during the tissue remodeling, is an extremely important property of osseous reconstructive materials and can vary widely depending on how a given material is processed [10]. Additionally, the chosen graft material should possess dimensional stability to allow the adaptation of graft material to the defect and facilitate handling of the material by the practitioner.

Autogenous Grafts

Autogenous bone grafts are histocompatible and non-immunogenic and allow the formation of new bone through osteogenesis, osteoinduction, and osteoconduction (Table 3.1). In addition, autologous bone offers the advantage of shorter healing time to formation of viable bone in the maxillofacial region that can then be used for further reconstruction. The favorable bone quality that forms, its potentially lower cost relative to engineered materials, lower risk of disease trans-

Table 3.1 Three general properties of biomaterial

Osteogenesis	Formation and development of new bone by cells contained in the graft
Osteoinduction	Chemical process by which graft material triggers differentiation and stimulation of undifferentiated mesenchymal stem cells of the host to differentiate into osteoblasts, bone-forming cells
Osteoconduction	Characterized by a physical matrix of the graft that serves as a scaffold, which allows osteocompetent cells of the host to penetrate the graft and form new bone

P. Patel (✉) · M. Newman
Department of Oral and Maxillofacial Surgery, Dental Collage of Georgia, Augusta University, Augusta, GA, USA
e-mail: ppatel13@augusta.edu; Marnewman@augusta.edu

M. R. Stevens et al. (eds.), *Innovative Perspectives in Oral and Maxillofacial Surgery*,
https://doi.org/10.1007/978-3-030-75750-2_3

mission or antigenicity, and predictability all make for a reconstructive source that is difficult to replicate [3]. Major drawbacks of autologous bone grafts include the need for a secondary surgical procedure to obtain the graft and a donor site, which may have its own complications, deformity, or scarring [5]. Many donor sites are available to harvest non-vascularized autologous bone both intraorally (mandibular ramus, mandibular symphysis, maxillary tuberosity) and extraorally (iliac crest, tibia, rib, and calvarium) [11]. Harvesting bone from an intraoral site decreases operative time, eliminates the need for hospitalization, and hence reduces overall costs; however, it often does not provide significant quantities of bone for more extensive reconstructions [12]. Although either the anterior or posterior iliac crest can provide a large amount of cortical and cancellous bone relative to other sites, it is associated with donor site morbidity such as chronic donor site pain, sensory disturbances, infection, hematoma/seroma formation, fracture, and hypertrophic scar formations [13, 14]. Dural tears and intracranial hematomas are possible donor site complications associated with calvarial bone grafting [15, 16]. Several techniques for calvarial bone graft harvesting have been suggested to minimize the risk of intracranial complications, such as those from Kellman [17] and modified by Schortinghuis et al. [18]. Many vascularized alternative donor sites for bone graft reconstruction of the craniomaxillofacial region exist, such as the fibula, radial forearm, and scapula, but a detailed discussion of these is beyond the scope of this chapter. Free vascularized tissue transfer can be more technique-sensitive, require additional operative time, prolong hospitalization, and increase postoperative morbidity and mortality [19].

Allogenic Grafts

Allografts are the second most widely used grafting material after autogenous grafts [20]. Allogenic bone graft is harvested from an individual of the same species and processed prior to use. This processing can significantly affect the graft material properties in vivo, such as rate and degree of resorption. Allografts have both osteoinductive and osteoconductive properties but lack osteogenicity because viable cells are removed in the process of sterilization [21]. Graft material is generally harvested from cadavers or from living donors during orthopedic procedures [22]. The risk of disease transmission (HIV, HCV, HBV, malignancy, autoimmune disorders, and toxins) is a potential limitation of allografts despite allogenic material being sterilized by gamma irradiation or ethylene oxide, but is extremely low [23–27].

The three standard form of allogenic bone includes fresh frozen, mineralized freeze-dried, and demineralized freeze-dried. The use of freeze-dried bone allografts (FDBA) and demineralized freeze-dried bone allografts (DFDBA) has reduced the problem of immunogenicity that was associated with fresh frozen bone [28]. Allogenic bone is available in many preparations including cancellous chips, corticocancellous particles or blocks, whole bone segments, and demineralized bone matrices [29]. Wood et al. reported no statistically significant differences in the changes in ridge dimensions after ridge preservation was performed with DFDBA versus FDBA. However, there was a significantly greater percentage of vital bone in sites grafted with DFDBA versus FDBA, and DFDBA sites had significantly fewer residual graft particles [30]. Echoing these findings, Borg TD and Mealey BL found a greater percentage of vital bone at nonmolar extraction sites after ridge preservation that was completed with a combination of demineralized and mineralized freeze-dried bone allografts, compared to the use of only mineralized freeze-dried bone allograft [31].

Xenogenic Grafts

Xenogenic bone graft material is derived from deproteinized cancellous bone from another species, usually bovine or porcine. The graft can be used either alone or in combination with other materials. A concern with bovine-derived products is the potential transmission of zoonotic diseases and prion infections such as bovine spongiform encephalitis (BSE), an immune response of the host tissue after implantation, though this is very rare [32]. The material is subjected to chemical or heat annealing processing to remove organic components, resulting in loss of osteogenic and partly osteoinductive properties [33]. Xenografts processed at higher temperatures, 900–1200 °C as opposed to 250–600 °C, demonstrate a slower resorption time and may lend themselves to particular reconstructive applications depending on site-specific requirements for rate of resorption and replacement with vital bone [10]. This may have site-specific relevance in mandibular ridge augmentation, for example, but all types of xenografts appear to have nearly identical and sufficient clinical utility in sinus augmentation, for example. Comparing xenografts to alloplastic grafting material, a systematic review by Aghaloo et al. of implant survival data following previous bone graft reconstruction indicates that synthetic graft materials are associated with lower dental implant survival rates than xenograft bovine cancellous bone substitutes [34]. Nevertheless, in randomized control clinical trials with a synthetic bone substitute or bovine xenograft, both types of bone grafts presented similar radiographic alveolar bone changes when used for alveolar ridge preservation [35, 36]. This reinforces the dynamic nature of bone graft reconstruction and the possible multitude of ideal property requirements that may be present or vary even within a given reconstruction site.

Alloplastic Grafts

Alloplasts are synthetically derived materials that are readily available for clinical use. An ideal alloplastic material should be biocompatible, induce minimal fibrotic reaction, remodel easily, and possess a strength and elasticity comparable to the natural bone being replaced [37]. Alloplasts include the following: ceramics (hydroxyapatite, biological glasses, tricalcium phosphate, and glass ionomer cements), polymers (polymethyl methacrylate, polylactides/polyglycolides, and copolymers), and cements (calcium phosphate cements). In general, alloplasts tend to be nontoxic and non-inflammatory but often are brittle and may be poorly suited for complex reconstructive sites under stress unless combined with other biomaterials [38].

Hydroxyapatite (HA) Ceramics

Bone tissue is composed of inorganic and organic substituents. The most prevalent inorganic component is hydroxyapatite with citrate, carbonate, and ions such as F^-, K^+, Sr^{2+}, Pb^{2+}, Zn^{2+}, $Cu2+$, and Fe^{2+}. The organic components include type I collagen and non-collagenous proteins. Hardness and resistance of bone are set by the connections between HA and collagen fibers. HA ceramics are nearly chemically identical to natural HA. When HA is used as a bioactive material, it releases free calcium and phosphate ions resulting in a micro-morphological surface anchorage of endosseous implants [22]. In a study by Belouka et al., nanocrystalline and nanoporous HA were found to support bone formation in sinus floor elevation and augmentation procedures by osteoconductivity [39]. These findings support the characteristics of ideal surface properties of hydroxyapatite ceramics despite less than ideal mechanical strength overall.

Calcium Phosphate Ceramics

Calcium phosphate ceramics are synthetic substances that act as a scaffold often applied in reconstructing bony defects. Ceramics in general have the advantage of being biocompatible while being resistant to compression and corrosion. However, these biomaterials have similar disadvantages, such as brittleness and low strength [40]. The most common ceramic biomaterials consist of HA and alpha or beta tricalcium phosphate (α or β TCP) [41]. Synthetic ceramics aid in the formation of osteoid when attached to healthy bone, which subsequently mineralizes to form new vital bone and undergoes further remodeling [22]. Both TCP ceramic and HA are highly biocompatible and act as a scaffold; however, porous TCP is removed from the graft site as bone grows into and replaces the scaffold, while HA is more permanent [22]. ß-TCP undergoes resorption over a 13–20 weeks period and is completely replaced by remodeled bone [42]. ß-TCP are more often used in oral and maxillofacial surgeries given their good biocompatibility, osteoconductive properties, no adverse immunogenic toxic side effects, and resorption times often similar to available xenograft materials [43, 44]. Currently, 3D-printed calcium phosphate ceramic superstructure scaffolds may be utilized alone or to aid in containment and shielding of other reconstructive biomaterials. They are easy to adapt virtually, quickly fixated intraoperatively, help decrease surgery time, and demonstrate good aesthetic results [45].

Bioactive Glasses (Bioglasses)

Bioactive glasses are amorphous silicates that are coupled with minerals naturally found in the body such as Ca, Na_2O, H, and P. When subjected to an aqueous solution or body fluids, the surface of bioglasses converts to a silica-CaO/P_2O_5-rich gel layer that subsequently mineralizes into hydroxycarbonate [42, 46–48]. Bioglasses are biocompatible and osteoconductive and offer interconnective pore system, which enables ingrowth of osseous tissue and may aid in stem-cell recruitment similar to ceramic pores [49–51]. Limitations of bioactive glasses include high brittleness, low mechanical strength, and decreased fracture resistance [49, 52].

Polymers

Polymer-based bone substitutes can be natural or synthetic. Natural polymers mimic the structural and biochemical properties of the natural bone organic matrix. Natural polymers include collagen, fibrinogen, elastin, glycosaminoglycans, cellulose, and amylose. Natural polymers resemble extracellular matrix resulting in possession of osteoinductive properties [5]. Limitations of natural polymers include poor mechanical properties and unpredictable biodegradability compared to synthetic polymers [53, 54].

The following represents some of the most commonly utilized synthetic polymers for bone reconstruction: poly (ε-caprolactone) (PCL), polylactic acid (PLA), polyglycolide (PGA), and the copolymer of poly-(DL-lactic-co-glycolic-acid) (PLGA). Synthetic polymers provide controllability in terms of porosity and physiochemical structure [55, 56]. Synthetic polymers can be further separated into degradable and non-degradable types. Degradable polymers such as polylactic acid and polylactic-co-glycolic acid have also been used in periodontal treatment as standalone devices and combined with hyaluronic acid for guided tissue regeneration [57]. An unfavorable characteristic of degradable synthetic polymers is the change in its microenvironment secondary to the buildup of acidic byproducts from the degradation process [58]. Polymers show great promise in the containment of bone graft materials, guided tissue regeneration, and in their ability to be combined with other biomaterials such as ceramics.

Calcium Phosphate Cements

Calcium phosphate (CP) cements are bioresorbable materials that are approved for the treatment of non-load-bearing bone defects [59]. CP cements consist of a two-part system: calcium phosphate powder mixed with a liquid to form a workable paste. The resulting workable paste can be applied directly to the defect or injected with a syringe. The isothermic curing phase varies from 15 to 80 minutes [60]; this results in formation of nanocrystalline HA, making CP cements osteoconductive [59]. Due to their injectability, bioactivity, and biocompatibility, CP cements are highly promising for a variety of bone tissue engineering applications and are used as scaffolds and carriers to deliver stem cells, drugs, and growth factors [61]. They are commonly used in cranial defect reconstruction or cranial augmentation. Advances in virtual surgical planning have allowed for the manufacturing of reconstructive templates, which can be utilized off the surgical field and aid in minimizing the negative effects of the isothermic curing phase [62].

Composite Biomaterials

Composite biomaterials can now be synthesized by combining various polymers and ceramics scaffolds. These can be integrated with each other or fused to a particular surface of the reconstruction composite. An ideal composite biosynthetic material is synthetized in such a way that it contains one or more components that have osteoconductive, osteogenic, and osteoinductive properties [22]. Composite biomaterials are biocompatible and demonstrate good mechanical strength and load-bearing capabilities making them suitable in tissue engineering [63]. Currently, composite materials are being examined as an alternative to autogenic grafts in fresh human fracture sites to avoid any morbidity and mortality associated with harvesting sites [44]. They show promise in drug delivery and represent the optimization of multiple applications of the above biomaterials [64].

Tissue Engineering

Tissue engineering triad is a new concept in reconstructive surgery. It allows bone regeneration by combining cells from the body, scaffolds, and growth factors. Scaffolds create a three-dimensional structure that not only provides physical support to withstand forces from the overlying soft tissue during the healing phase but also creates a microenvironment that facilitates cellular attachment, proliferation, and differentiation [65]. Biodegradable scaffolds that are currently being utilized as bone replacement materials are synthetic polymers of poly-L-lactic acid and poly-L-glycolic acid [22, 66]. Addition of other materials such as hydroxyapatite, ceramics, and bioactive glass to poly-L-glycolic acid scaffolds has been shown to enhance bone regeneration [66]. A similar concept has been used with the application of Tisseel, a fibrin sealant, for particulate graft stabilization and may aid in prevention of early fibrous ingrowth due to the presence of a protease inhibitor [67].

Growth factors such as bone morphogenetic protein-2 (BMP-2), basic fibroblast growth factor (bFGF), platelet-derived growth factor (PDGF), transforming growth factor-ß (TGF- ß), and vascular endothelial growth factor (VEGF) have essential roles in angiogenesis, bone generation, and regeneration [68–72]. However, growth factors have short half-life; thus, without a carrier, their role is limited [68]. Carriers, such as calcium hydroxyapatite ceramics and synthetic biodegradable polymers, play an essential role in maintaining growth factor concentration at a target site to allow time for chemotaxis, cellular proliferation, and differentiation, ultimately improving clinical efficacy of the growth factors [68, 73–76]. BMPs belong to the TFG- ß superfamily. They are potent regulators of osteoblast differentiation [77]. Recombinant human bone morphogenetic protein-2 (rhBMP-2) has been widely used in continuity defects and sinus augmentations [78–80]. In extraction socket augmentation, a randomized study comparing the placement of rhBMP-2 and an absorbable collagen sponge alone in a human buccal wall defect model demonstrated significantly more bone production in the rhBMP-2 group compared to the control [81]. Vascularization of an osseous reconstructive graft, mediated by growth factors, is essential to its success. Studies have demonstrated that synthetic scaffolds impregnated with adjunctive growth factors such as VEGF and PDGF improve regenerative efforts by promoting angiogenesis and recruitment of osteoblasts and fibroblasts [82, 83].

Conclusion

Numerous bone substitute biomaterials and combinations of materials are available. The difficulty in creating a substitute that demonstrates all the ideal properties of autogenous bone grafts is evident, but significant progress continues to be made. The disadvantages and morbidity of additional surgical sites is real, and patients will appreciate the endeavor to engineer a viable alternative. Not all biomaterials are ready for clinical use, and each osseous reconstruction site

Table 3.2 Summery of materials for osseous reconstruction

	Properties	Advantages	Disadvantages	Clinical application
Autogenous grafts	Osteogenic [3, 5] Osteoinductive Osteoconductive	Biocompatibility Non-immunogenic Short healing time	Harvest site Morbidity Limited bone availability Harvesting requires additional skills and increased operative time [3, 5]	Guided bone regeneration (GBR) Bone defects Ridge augmentation
Allogenic grafts	Osteoinductive Osteoconductive [21]	Many available preparations Good alternative to autografts in patient with poor wound healing	Risk of disease transmission and immune reaction [23–27]	GBR Sinus augmentation Ridge augmentation Bone defects
Xenogenic grafts	Osteoconductive [33]	Slow bio-absorbability preserves augmented bone [10] Easily visible on radiographs volume	Potential transmission of zoonotic diseases [32]	Sinus augmentation Ridge augmentation
Alloplastic				
Hydroxyapatite (HA) [84]	Osteoconductive [39]	Provides structural support	Slow absorption	Bone void filler Bone graft extenders
Ceramics	Osteoconductive [22]	Biocompatible	High brittleness Low ductility [40]	Same as above
Bioglasses	Osteoconductive [49–51]	Biocompatible	Low mechanical strength High brittleness [49, 52]	Same as above
Calcium phosphate Cements	Osteoconductive	Bioabsorbable Excellent moldability [59, 61]	Poor mechanical properties [85]	Same as above

may require the attributes of different materials at different locations with a defect and at different times during hard and soft tissue healing. Table 3.2 highlights general properties and usage of commonly utilized biomaterials. Ultimately, significant research and well-designed studies are needed to ensure that osseous reconstructive results are above all safe and predictable.

References

1. Nyström E, Nilson H, Gunne J, Lundgren S. A 9–14 year follow-up of onlay bone grafting in the atrophic maxilla. Int J Oral Maxillofac Surg. 2009;38(2):111–6.
2. Misch CM. Maxillary autogenous bone grafting. Oral Maxillofac Surg Clin North Am. 2011;23(2):229–38.
3. Misch CM. Autogenous bone: is it still the gold standard? Implant Dent. 2010;19(5):361.
4. Giannoudis PV, Chris Arts JJ, Schmidmaier G, Larsson S. What should be the characteristics of the ideal bone graft substitute? Injury. 2011;42:S1–2.
5. Haugen HJ, Lyngstadaas SP, Rossi F, Perale G. Bone grafts: which is the ideal biomaterial? J Clin Periodontol. 2019;46:92–102.
6. Hulbert SF, Young FA, Mathews RS, Klawitter JJ, Talbert CD, Stelling FH. Potential of ceramic materials as permanently implantable skeletal prostheses. J Biomed Mater Res. 1970;4(3):433–56.
7. Karageorgiou V, Kaplan D. Porosity of 3D biomaterial scaffolds and osteogenesis. Biomaterials. 2005;26(27):5474–91.
8. Murphy CM, Haugh MG, O'Brien FJ. The effect of mean pore size on cell attachment, proliferation and migration in collagen–glycosaminoglycan scaffolds for bone tissue engineering. Biomaterials. 2010;31(3):461–6.
9. Saito E, Saito A, Kuboki Y, Kimura M, Honma Y, Takahashi T, et al. Periodontal repair following implantation of beta-tricalcium phosphate with different pore structures in class III furcation defects in dogs. Dent Mater J. 2012;31(4):681–8.
10. Block MS. The processing of xenografts will result in different clinical responses. J Oral Maxillofac Surg. 2019;77(4):690–7.
11. Zouhary KJ. Bone graft harvesting from distant sites: concepts and techniques. Oral Maxillofac Surg Clin North Am. 2010;22(3):301–16.
12. Bagheri S, Bell B, Khan H. Current therapy in oral and maxillofacial surgery. 1st ed. St. Louis: Elsevier; 2012. p. 19–22.
13. Mertens C, Decker C, Seeberger R, Hoffmann J, Sander A, Freier K. Early bone resorption after vertical bone augmentation - a comparison of calvarial and iliac grafts. Clin Oral Implants Res. 2013;24(7):820–5.
14. Dimitriou R, Mataliotakis GI, Angoules AG, Kanakaris NK, Giannoudis PV. Complications following autologous bone graft harvesting from the iliac crest and using the RIA: a systematic review. Injury. 2011;42:S3–15.
15. Scheerlinck LME, Muradin MSM, van der Bilt A, Meijer GJ, Koole R, Van Cann EMVC. Donor site complications in bone grafting: comparison of iliac crest, calvarial, and mandibular ramus bone. Int J Oral Maxillofac Implants. 2013;28(1):222–7.
16. Kline RM, Wolfe SA. Complications associated with the harvesting of cranial bone grafts. Plast Reconstr Surg. 1995;95(1):5–13.
17. Kellman RM. Safe and dependable harvesting of large outer-table calvarial bone grafts. Arch Otolaryngol Head Neck Surg. 1994;120(8):856–60.
18. Schortinghuis J, Putters TF, Raghoebar GM. Safe harvesting of outer table parietal bone grafts using an oscillating saw and a bone scraper: a refinement of technique for harvesting cortical and "Cancellous"-like calvarial bone. J Oral Maxillofac Surg. 2012;70(4):963–5.
19. Haughey BH, Wilson E, Kluwe L, Piccirillo J, Fredrickson J, Sessions D, et al. Free flap reconstruction of the head and neck: analysis of 241 cases. Otolaryngol Head Neck Surg. 2001;125(1):10–7.
20. Amini AR, Laurencin CT, Nukavarapu SP. Bone tissue engineering: recent advances and challenges. Crit Rev Biomed Eng. 2012;40(5):363–408.
21. Boyan BD, Ranly DM, McMillan J, Sunwoo M, Roche K, Schwartz Z. Osteoinductive ability of human allograft formulations. J Periodontol. 2006;77(9):1555–63.

22. Kolk A, Handschel J, Drescher W, Rothamel D, Kloss F, Blessmann M, et al. Current trends and future perspectives of bone substitute materials – from space holders to innovative biomaterials. J Craniomaxillofac Surg. 2012;40(8):706–18.

23. Bienek C, MacKay L, Scott G, Jones A, Lomas R, Kearney JN, et al. Development of a bacteriophage model system to investigate virus inactivation methods used in the treatment of bone allografts. Cell Tissue Bank. 2007;8(2):115–24.

24. Buck B, Malinin T, Brown M. Bone transplantation and human immunodeficiency virus. An estimate of risk of acquired immunodeficiency syndrome (AIDS). Clin Orthop Relat Res. 1989;(240):129–36.

25. Kappe T, Cakir B, Mattes T, Reichel H, Flören M. Infections after bone allograft surgery: a prospective study by a hospital bone bank using frozen femoral heads from living donors. Cell Tissue Bank. 2010;11(3):253–9.

26. Conrad EU, Gretch DR, Obermeyer KR, Moogk MS, Sayers M, Wilson JJ, et al. Transmission of the hepatitis-C virus by tissue transplantation. J Bone Joint Surg Am. 1995;77(2):214–24.

27. Tomford WW. Transmission of disease through transplantation of musculoskeletal allografts. J Bone Joint Surg Am. 1995;77(11):1742–54.

28. Jamjoom A, Cohen R. Grafts for ridge preservation. J Funct Biomater. 2015;6(3):833–48.

29. Finkemeier CG. Bone-grafting and bone-graft substitutes. J Bone Joint Surg Am. 2002;84(3):454–64.

30. Wood RA, Mealey BL. Histologic comparison of healing after tooth extraction with ridge preservation using mineralized versus demineralized freeze-dried bone allograft. J Periodontol. 2012;83(3):329–36.

31. Borg TD, Mealey BL. Histologic healing following tooth extraction with ridge preservation using mineralized versus combined mineralized-demineralized freeze-dried bone allograft: a randomized controlled clinical trial. J Periodontol. 2015;86(3):348–55.

32. Schroeder JE, Mosheiff R. Tissue engineering approaches for bone repair: concepts and evidence. Injury. 2011;42(6):609–13.

33. Oryan A, Alidadi S, Moshiri A, Maffulli N. Bone regenerative medicine: classic options, novel strategies, and future directions. J Orthop Surg Res. 2014;9(1):18.

34. Aghaloo TL, Moy PK. Which hard tissue augmentation techniques are the most successful in furnishing bony support for implant placement? Int J Oral Maxillofac Implants. 2007;22 Suppl:49–70.

35. Mardas N, Chadha V, Donos N. Alveolar ridge preservation with guided bone regeneration and a synthetic bone substitute or a bovine-derived xenograft: a randomized, controlled clinical trial. Clin Oral Implants Res. 2010;21(7):688–98.

36. Mardas N, D'Aiuto F, Mezzomo L, Arzoumanidi M, Donos N. Radiographic alveolar bone changes following ridge preservation with two different biomaterials. Clin Oral Implants Res. 2011;22(4):416–23.

37. Sukumar S, Drízhal I. Bone grafts in periodontal therapy. Acta Medica (Hradec Kralove). 2008;51(4):203–7.

38. Yoo JS, Ahn J, Patel DS, Hrynewycz NM, Brundage TS, Singh K. An evaluation of biomaterials and osteobiologics for arthrodesis achievement in spine surgery. Ann Transl Med. 2019;7(Suppl 5):S168.

39. Belouka S-M, Strietzel F. Sinus floor elevation and augmentation using synthetic nanocrystalline and nanoporous hydroxyapatite bone substitute materials: preliminary histologic results. Int J Oral Maxillofac Implants. 2016;31(6):1281–91.

40. Kaur G, Pandey OP, Singh K, Homa D, Scott B, Pickrell G. A review of bioactive glasses: their structure, properties, fabrication and apatite formation. J Biomed Mater Res A. 2014;102(1):254–74.

41. Perez JR, Kouroupis D, Li DJ, Best TM, Kaplan L, Correa D. Tissue engineering and cell-based therapies for fractures and bone defects. Front Bioeng Biotechnol. 2018;31:6.

42. Sohn H-S, Oh J-K. Review of bone graft and bone substitutes with an emphasis on fracture surgeries. Biomater Res. 2019;23(1):9.

43. Kao ST, Scott DD. A review of bone substitutes. Oral Maxillofac Surg Clin North Am. 2007;19(4):513–21.

44. Vaccaro AR, Chiba K, Heller JG, Patel TC, Thalgott JS, Truumees E, et al. Bone grafting alternatives in spinal surgery. Spine J. 2002;2(3):206–15.

45. Trombetta R, Inzana JA, Schwarz EM, Kates SL, Awad HA. 3D printing of calcium phosphate ceramics for bone tissue engineering and drug delivery. Ann Biomed Eng. 2017;45(1):23–44.

46. Hench L, Wilson J. Surface-active biomaterials. Science. 1984;226(4675):630–6.

47. Wallace KE, Hill RG, Pembroke JT, Brown CJ, Hatton PV. Influence of sodium oxide content on bioactive glass properties. J Mater Sci Mater Med. 1999;10(12):697–701.

48. Neo M, Nakamura T, Ohtsuki C, Kasai R, Kokubo T, Yamamuro T. Ultrastructural study of the A-W GC-bone interface after long-term implantation in rat and human bone. J Biomed Mater Res. 1994;28(3):365–72.

49. Krishnan V, Lakshmi T. Bioglass: a novel biocompatible innovation. J Adv Pharm Technol Res. 2013;4(2):78.

50. Zhang H, Ye X-J, Li J-S. Preparation and biocompatibility evaluation of apatite/wollastonite-derived porous bioactive glass ceramic scaffolds. Biomed Mater. 2009;4(4):045007.

51. Hollinger JO, Brekke J, Gruskin E, Lee D. Role of bone substitutes. Clin Orthop Relat Res. 1996;324:55–65.

52. Chai F, Raoul G, Wiss A, Ferri J, Hildebrand HF. Bone substitutes: classification and concerns. Rev Stomatol Chir Maxillofac. 2011;112(4):212–21.

53. Mano J, Silva G, Azevedo H, Malafaya P, Sousa R, Silva S, et al. Natural origin biodegradable systems in tissue engineering and regenerative medicine: present status and some moving trends. J R Soc Interface. 2007;4(17):999–1030.

54. Hannink G, Arts JJC. Bioresorbability, porosity and mechanical strength of bone substitutes: what is optimal for bone regeneration? Injury. 2011;42:S22–5.

55. Park JK, Yeom J, Oh EJ, Reddy M, Kim JY, Cho D-W, et al. Guided bone regeneration by poly(lactic-co-glycolic acid) grafted hyaluronic acid bi-layer films for periodontal barrier applications. Acta Biomater. 2009;5(9):3394–403.

56. Fuchs JR, Nasseri BA, Vacanti JP. Tissue engineering: a 21st century solution to surgical reconstruction. Ann Thorac Surg. 2001;72(2):577–91.

57. Kretlow JD, Mikos AG. Review: mineralization of synthetic polymer scaffolds for bone tissue engineering. Tissue Eng. 2007;13(5):927–38.

58. Thrivikraman G, Athirasala A, Twohig C, Boda SK, Bertassoni LE. Biomaterials for craniofacial bone regeneration. Dent Clin N Am. 2017;61(4):835–56.

59. Campana V, Milano G, Pagano E, Barba M, Cicione C, Salonna G, et al. Bone substitutes in orthopaedic surgery: from basic science to clinical practice. J Mater Sci Mater Med. 2014;25(10):2445–61.

60. Burguera EF, Xu HHK, Weir MD. Injectable and rapid-setting calcium phosphate bone cement with dicalcium phosphate dihydrate. J Biomed Mater Res B Appl Biomater. 2006;77B(1):126–34.

61. Xu HH, Wang P, Wang L, Bao C, Chen Q, Weir MD, et al. Calcium phosphate cements for bone engineering and their biological properties. Bone Res. 2017;5:17056.

62. Tel A, Tuniz F, Fabbro S, Sembronio S, Costa F, Robiony M. Computer-guided in-house cranioplasty: establishing a novel standard for cranial reconstruction and proposal of an updated protocol. J Oral Maxillofac Surg. 2020;S0278-2391(20)30982-4.

63. Iaquinta MR, Mazzoni E, Manfrini M, D'Agostino A, Trevisiol L, Nocini R, et al. Innovative biomaterials for bone regrowth. Int J Mol Sci. 2019;20(3):618.

64. Alizadeh-Osgouei M, Li Y, Wen C. A comprehensive review of biodegradable synthetic polymer-ceramic composites and their manufacture for biomedical applications. Bioact Mater. 2018;4(1):22–36.

65. Loh QL, Choong C. Three-dimensional scaffolds for tissue engineering applications: role of porosity and pore size. Tissue Eng Part B Rev. 2013;19(6):485–502.

66. Gentile P, Chiono V, Carmagnola I, Hatton P. An overview of poly(lactic-co-glycolic) acid (PLGA)-based biomaterials for bone tissue engineering. Int J Mol Sci. 2014;15(3):3640–59.

67. Block MS, Zoccolillo M. Use of tisseel, a fibrin sealant, for particulate graft stabilization. J Oral Maxillofac Surg. 2020;78(10): 1674–81.

68. Fischer J, Kolk A, Wolfart S, Pautke C, Warnke PH, Plank C, et al. Future of local bone regeneration – protein versus gene therapy. J Craniomaxillofac Surg. 2011;39(1):54–64.

69. Fujii H, Kitazawa R, Maeda S, Mizuno K, Kitazawa S. Expression of platelet-derived growth factor proteins and their receptor α and β mRNAs during fracture healing in the normal mouse. Histochem Cell Biol. 1999;112(2):131–8.

70. Lee FY-I, Storer S, Hazan EJ, Gebhardt MC, Mankin HJ. Repair of bone allograft fracture using bone morphogenetic protein-2. Clin Orthop Relat Res. 2002;397:119–26.

71. Rundle CH, Miyakoshi N, Ramirez E, Wergedal JE, Lau K-HW, Baylink DJ. Expression of the fibroblast growth factor receptor genes in fracture repair. Clin Orthop Relat Res. 2002;403:253–63.

72. Street J, Bao M, DeGuzman L, Bunting S, Peale FV, Ferrara N, et al. Vascular endothelial growth factor stimulates bone repair by promoting angiogenesis and bone turnover. Proc Natl Acad Sci. 2002;99(15):9656–61.

73. Dai KR, Xu XL, Tang TT, .Zhu ZA, Yu CF, Lou JR, et al. Repairing of goat tibial bone defects with BMP-2 gene–modified tissue-engineered bone. Calcif Tissue Int 2005;77(1):55–61.

74. Kaito T, Myoui A, Takaoka K, Saito N, Nishikawa M, Tamai N, et al. Potentiation of the activity of bone morphogenetic protein-2 in bone regeneration by a PLA–PEG/hydroxyapatite composite. Biomaterials. 2005;26(1):73–9.

75. Seeherman H, Wozney J, Li R. Bone morphogenetic protein delivery systems. Spine (Phila Pa 1976). 2002;27(Supplement):S16–23.

76. Smeets R, Maciejewski O, Gerressen M, Spiekermann H, Hanisch O, Riediger D, et al. Impact of rhBMP-2 on regeneration of buccal alveolar defects during the osseointegration of transgingival inserted implants. Oral Surg Oral Med Oral Pathol Oral Radiol Endod. 2009;108(4):e3–12.

77. Yamaguchi A, Komori T, Suda T. Regulation of osteoblast differentiation mediated by bone morphogenetic proteins, hedgehogs, and Cbfa1. Endocr Rev. 2000;21(4):393–411.

78. Boyne PJ. Application of bone morphogenetic proteins in the treatment of clinical oral and maxillofacial osseous defects. J Bone Joint Surg Am. 2001;83-A Suppl(Pt 2):S146–50.

79. Herford AS, Boyne PJ. Reconstruction of mandibular continuity defects with bone morphogenetic protein-2 (rhBMP-2). J Oral Maxillofac Surg. 2008;66(4):616–24.

80. Boyne PJ, Lilly LC, Marx RE, Moy PK, Nevins M, Spagnoli DB, et al. De novo bone induction by recombinant human bone morphogenetic protein-2 (rhBMP-2) in maxillary sinus floor augmentation. J Oral Maxillofac Surg. 2005;63(12):1693–707.

81. Fiorellini JP, Howell TH, Cochran D, Malmquist J, Lilly LC, Spagnoli D, Toljanic J, Jones A, Nevins M. Randomized study evaluating recombinant human bone morphogenetic protein-2 for extraction socket augmentation. J Periodontol. 2005;76(4):605–13.

82. De la Riva B, Sánchez E, Hernández A, Reyes R, Tamimi F, López-Cabarcos E, et al. Local controlled release of VEGF and PDGF from a combined brushite–chitosan system enhances bone regeneration. J Control Release. 2010;143(1):45–52.

83. Kaigler D, Wang Z, Horger K, Mooney DJ, Krebsbach PH. VEGF scaffolds enhance angiogenesis and bone regeneration in irradiated osseous defects. J Bone Miner Res. 2006;21(5):735–44.

84. Zanotti B, Zingaretti N, Verlicchi A, Robiony M, Alfieri A, Parodi PC. Cranioplasty: review of materials. J Craniofac Surg. 2016;27(8):2061–72.

85. Zhang J, Liu W, Schnitzler V, Tancret F, Bouler JM. Calcium phosphate cements for bone substitution: chemistry, handling and mechanical properties. Acta Biomater. 2014;10(3):1035–49.

Bone Quality

Pindaros-Georgios Foskolos, Danai-Maria Stasinoulia, and Dimitrios Papadopoulos

Introduction

Dental implants are surgical units that attach to maxillary or mandibular bone to support a fixed or a removable dental prosthesis. The foundation of the success of a dental implant lies within the process of osseointegration. Branemark [7] defined the osseointegration as the biomaterial structural and functional anchorage with the existing bone [7]. This process is highly interlinked with the implant itself and the quality of the existing bone that the implant will be anchored on it. Bone with low quality affects the osseointegration fundamentally and, consequently, is a determinant of dental implants' success or failure [1].

According to Buck et al. [8], bone is the entity that assembles the body's skeleton and consists of bone matrix and bone cells. The bone matrix occupies 90% of the total volume, whereas the rest 10% is occupied by bone cells. Those cells are derived from two types of cells, osteoprogenitor cells and osteoclasts. Osteoprogenitor cells are situated in bone canals, endosteum, periosteum, and bone marrow, and they differentiate into osteoblasts and osteocytes which are bone-forming cells [8, 9]. Osteoclasts are larger multinucleated cells, and their primary role is to dissolve bone during the remodeling phase [18].

The Importance of Bone Quality in Osseointegration

Osseointegration has a fundamental role in the success rate and longevity of implants, and it depends on the remodeling of the bone [23, 42]. Higher levels of osseointegration lead to higher success rate of implants [23, 42]. However, low bone quality could affect the inserted implants' primary stability, which will compromise its osseointegration [10, 33]. As a result, in bone with low density, specific methods and techniques should be adopted to ensure the primary stability of the inserted implant [10, 33, 36, 37].

Primary Stability and Bone Density

Primary stability is defined as the strength and rigidity of the union, formed between the implant and the living bone; it is the precursor of osseointegration [10]. The implants' primary stability, which depends on the mechanical anchoring of the implant with the crestal bone, is necessary to attain and maintain optimal osseointegration. After the implant placement, mechanical anchoring starts to deteriorate during the early stages of healing as the bone remodeling process occurs [10, 36]. Investigations have been carried out to examine whether bone density can affect the implant's overall stability. Higher primary stability was observed in bones with higher density than in bones with lower density [36, 37, 43]. The stability of implants and consequently osseointegration was assessed through an electronic device, the Periotest (PTV). Cone beam computed tomography was also utilized to determine bone density and investigate its correlation with implants' primary stability [36, 43].

Influence of Bone Density on the Prognostics of Implants

He et al. demonstrated that bone density is correlated with the success and survival rate of implants. The density of bone was classified according to Lekholm and Zarb, and the success and survival rates were recorded. It was concluded that bone with a higher density leads to a higher survival rate of

P.-G. Foskolos (✉)
Department of Prosthodontics, National and Kapodistrian University of Athens, Athens, Greece
e-mail: pindaros@uic.es

D.-M. Stasinoulia · D. Papadopoulos
Faculty of Dentistry, International University of Catalonia, Barcelona, Spain
e-mail: danae.stasin@gmail.com; dimis572@gmail.com

implants [19, 21]. On the other hand, the failure rate was low, it was attributed mainly to non-successful osseointegration and pre-existing pathologies. Bone density is significantly correlated to the success rate and longevity of implants [21]. The survival rate of implants in bone with a lower quality can be increased through specific methods and surgical techniques [13, 19, 40].

Bone Quality Classification

Lekholm and Zarb (1985) were the first to establish a bone quality classification system, which remains one of the most acknowledged ones. This classification hinges on the amount of trabecular and cortical bone observed in a radiograph [44]. This classification hinges on the amount of trabecular and cortical bone observed in a radiograph [44]. It is divided into four groups. Type I bone quality implies that compact bone occupies the vast majority of the jaw uniformly. In Type II bone quality, we find an area of dense trabecular bone in the center which is enclosed by a thick layer of compact bone. Type III bone quality consists of a central area of dense trabecular bone encapsulated by fragile cortical bone. Type IV bone quality has a low-density trabecular bone in the center and around it presents a thin layer of cortical bone as well [20, 44, 51].

Another classification system of bone quality was proposed by *Misch (1990–2008)*, who formed four density groups according to the morphology of the bone along with the tactile sense that surgeons would experience (clinical hardness of drilling) [44]. D1 bone type has a uniform dense cortical bone and a tactile sense of oak wood. D2 bone type is a merge of dense-to-porous cortical bone on the outside and a trabecular bone on the interior, accompanied by a tactile sense of pine wood. D3 bone type consists of a thin and porous cortical bone on the outside, a fine trabecular bone on the interior, and the sensation of balsa wood. D4 has a thin layer of cortical bone or no cortical bone at all and a trabecular bone with low density as well. It presents a tactile sensation of styrofoam [32, 44].

Radiologic Examination

Intraoral Radiologic Examination

According to the research conducted by Gulsahi [20], periapical radiographs are frequently utilized to assess the condition of adjacent teeth along with the mesiodistal alveolar bone. The vertical height and the quality of the bone can also be evaluated, resulting in the determination of the bone density, the volume of cortical and trabecular bone [20]. However, if a paralleling technique is not adequately applied, the results observed from periapical radiographs are not valid as the image present is foreshortened and elongated. Due to the lack of information provided by periapical radiographs in the buccolingual plane, the use of occlusal radiographs is advised in order to obtain further information in this plane. Another limitation is that occlusal radiographs usually document the widest fraction of the mandible, commonly positioned below the alveolar ridge, making it seem like a more significant amount of bone is present. Moreover, occlusal radiographs are not utilized for the maxilla due to anatomic limitations [20].

Panoramic Radiographs

According to Cjan et al., panoramic radiographs are commonly used as most of the maxillofacial area's main anatomic landmarks can be observed. However, their resolution and sharpness are inferior compared to intraoral radiographs. Moreover, when the patient's head is not appropriately positioned, dimensional alterations of the exposed anatomical components can be observed [11]. Angular measurements are valid, but linear and vertical are not in this type of radiograph. Moreover, these radiographs cannot be correlated to bone density and are usually utilized as a preliminary screening tool for the placement of implants, not as a tool to accurately determine bone quality [20].

Computed Tomography

CT is widely used as there is no superposition of structures, and a high resolution of the image can be achieved. It can detect and differentiate structures with a difference in density of less than 1% [20]. The Voxel is the elementary unit of a CT image, and its value is the Hounsfield unit (HU). This method of radiography can be used to adequately determine bone quality. However, CT induces a higher level of radiation on patients. As a result, it should be thoroughly considered before implementing this method in order to avoid unnecessary high amounts of radiation and toxicity on patients [20, 30].

Cone Beam Computed Tomography (CBCT)

CBCT is extensively used in dentistry as it allows the detection of structures that have high contrast in a high resolution. As a result, it is a modality commonly used to assess bone quality, especially for the planification of surgeries for implant placement. In CBCT, Hounsfield units determine the density of the bone as it sets its ability to attenuate an X-ray beam [20, 38]. However, CBCT has a limitation regarding spatial resolution; in images with bone with a thickness of less than 0.6 mm, the bone cannot be registered. As a result, a lack of bone is perceived in the image. Another limitation is that when a larger field of view (FOV) is used to obtain a more extensive area, the quality is compromised [20].

Pathology of the Bone

A plethora of systemic diseases can affect bone quality and physiology, among which there is osteoporosis [35]. Kanis et al. defined osteoporosis as the clinical state in which a variety of bone fractures can appear due to a reduction in bone mass and density [24]. This disease could be asymptomatic until a trauma occurs leading to a fracture [47]. Osteopenia and cleidocranial dysplasia are among some other pathologies that affect the quality of the bone [16, 25].

There are several studies that examine the effect of osteoporosis and osteopenia on the survival rate of implants. It was concluded that there was no significant correlation between osteoporosis and implant failure [5, 6, 12, 13]. However, further investigation is required [12]. Furthermore, the medication for osteoporosis might be damaging the quality of the bone more than the actual disease [6].

Holahan et al. also demonstrated that patients diagnosed with osteoporosis or osteopenia were not associated with a higher rate of implant failure, and they concluded that should not be a contraindication to dental implant therapy [22].

Methods to Promote Osseointegration of Implants in Low-Quality Bone

Osteotome Technique

Regarding bones with lower quality and especially Type IV bone (Lekholm and Zarb classification) that presents the most significant defect, the surgical technique's significance for the placement of implants is important. During the drilling for the preparation of the implant's bed, a substantial amount of bone is sacrificed [46] .Thus, researchers have tried to find ways that could achieve optimal implant stability with the least sacrifice of native bone. Summers et al. introduced the osteotome technique that leads to the compression of bone in the lateral and apical plane with the use of an osteotome spreader [46, 49]. As a result, the bone quality of the bed of implant is improved, and the primary stability of implants can be higher. For this technique, initially, a small pilot hole is made, followed by the bone's compression in the lateral and apical planes with the use of a spreader or an implant-shaped tool [2, 48].

Undersized Drilling

According to the study conducted by Alghamdi et al., another technique proposed for low quality bone is "undersized drilling" to achieve good stability. The final drill utilized has a smaller diameter than the implant that is decided to be placed [2]. Subsequently, the implant is stabilized from the pressure applied through its placement [2]. This technique primarily intends to enhance bone density on a local level, provide higher insertion torques, and promote primary stability [46]. Moreover, bone fragments were found to be repositioned and relocated on the implant surface, which aided the healing and remodeling of the bone [2].

Modifications of the Surface of the Implants on a Physicochemical Level

Alteration of the implant surface is another feasible way to enhance osseointegration. The process of modifying the surface of implants allows a wider interaction with the organism's fluids and cells and promotes healing of the bone around the implant. Furthermore, this facilitates osseointegration at places where the quality of bone is not sufficient [26]. It seems that micro-roughness of implant's surface promotes osseointegration. Through this modification, a wider area of contact is achieved between bone and implant, which intensifies the anchoring of implants and thus enhances osseointegration between implant and bone [2]. Popularly used techniques to heighten the roughness of the surface of implants are grit-blasting, acid etching, or combinations. Regarding the combination technique, initially, grit blasting is performed, which consists mainly of the projection of particles like silica (sandblasting), titanium oxide, or hydroxyapatite. Usually etching is the next step; hydrofluoric, sulfuric, nitric acid, or a merge are employed. Acid etching is performed in order to discard as much of the particles from grit-blasting from the surface and to make it more homogeneous [27].

Kuroshima et al. [28] demonstrated that the creation of optimally oriented grooves on the neck of implants could significantly affect bone quality. The researchers established that the difference in the grooves' design without mechanical loading did not affect bone quality, but the difference in their angulation and the presence of mechanical loading affected bone quality. When mechanical loading was applied, the density of bone was heightened around implants that had grooves of $+60°$, but surprisingly, the density was not influenced when the implants had $-60°$ grooves [28].

Distinctively from the alterations on implants' physical aspect that aid osseointegration, another modification with a similar outcome is the coating of their surface with bioactive materials [29]. Coatings rich in calcium phosphate (CaP) are nowadays of great interest due to their immense similarity to the tissue of bone. As a result, this escalates the biochemical connection of the bone and implant. Other materials similarly utilized with the same purpose include extracellular matrix proteins (ECM), growth factors, collagen (mostly type I), and some enzymes [2]. According to studies conducted on animals portrayed, this method to stimulate osseointegration could be effective in osteoporotic bone [3]. Overall, surface-treated implants anchored on bone with low quality present a higher survival rate than not treated implants and are indicated for oral rehabilitation [19].

Modifications Through Drugs

It had been proposed through the research that Alghamdi et al. [2] conducted that coating the implants with specific drugs would aid and accelerate the osseointegration and healing of the peri-implant bone. This is quite important in patients who have diseases like osteoporosis where the quality of bone is affected and the osseointegration process altered. Antiresorptive drugs like bisphosphonates and anabolic agents like statins or strontium ranelate could be used [2]. Furthermore, a different study [4] proposed that coated implants with a combination of bisphosphonates along with calcium phosphate nanoparticles (nCaP) showed a significant improvement of the primary stability and thus the osseointegration of implants in bone with a low quality [4].

Conclusion

The quality of bone is correlated to the success of dental implants. There have been various classifications to determine and distinguish bone with low and high quality. To achieve satisfactory results of primary stability of the implant, the peri-implant bone quality is crucial. Subsequently, a good bone quality leads to adequate osseointegration of the implant and a higher success rate of the treatment. There is a plethora of methods and techniques as research has illuminated that promotes implant osseointegration. However, some of these techniques are still quite experimental. Further research is required to obtain higher validity and transparency of the proposed methods and thus be able to adopt these techniques in standard treatments.

Bibliography

1. Albrektsson T, Johansson C. Osteoinduction, osteoconduction and osseointegration. Eur Spine J. 2001;10 Suppl 2(Suppl 2):S96–101. https://doi.org/10.1007/s005860100282. PMID: 11716023; PMCID: PMC3611551.

2. Alghamdi HS. Methods to improve osseointegration of dental implants in low quality (type-IV) bone: an overview. J Funct Biomaterials. 2018;9(1):7.

3. Alghamdi HS, Bosco R, van den Beucken JJ, Walboomers XF, Jansen JA. Osteogenicity of titanium implants coated with calcium phosphate or collagen type-I in osteoporotic rats. Biomaterials. 2013;34:3747–57.

4. Alghamdi HS, Bosco R, Both SK, Iafisco M, Leeuwenburgh SC, Jansen JA, van den Beucken JJ. Synergistic effects of bisphosphonate and calcium phosphate nanoparticles on peri-implant bone responses in osteoporotic rats. Biomaterials. 2014;35:5482–90.

5. Becker W, Hujoel PP, Becker BE, Willingham H. Osteoporosis and implant failure: an exploratory case-control study. J Periodontol. 2000;71(4):625–31. https://doi.org/10.1902/jop.2000.71.4.625. PMID: 10807128.

6. Bornstein MM, Cionca N, Mombelli A. Systemic conditions and treatments as risks for implant therapy. Int J Oral Maxillofac Implants. 2009;24 Suppl:12–27. PMID: 19885432.

7. Branemark PI, Zarb G, Albreksson T. Tissue-integrated prostheses: osseointegration in clinical dentistry. Plast. Reconstr. Surg. 1985;77:496–7.

8. Buck DW 2nd, Dumanian GA. Bone biology and physiology: part I. The fundamentals. Plast Reconstr Surg. 2012;129(6):1314–20. https://doi.org/10.1097/PRS.0b013e31824eca94. PMID: 22634648.

9. Buck DW 2nd, Dumanian GA. Bone biology and physiology: part II. Clinical correlates. Plast Reconstr Surg. 2012;129(6):950e–6e. https://doi.org/10.1097/PRS.0b013e31824ec354. PMID: 22634692.

10. Cehreli MC, Kökat AM, Comert A, Akkocaoğlu M, Tekdemir I, Akça K. Implant stability and bone density: assessment of correlation in fresh cadavers using conventional and osteotome implant sockets. Clin Oral Implants Res. 2009;20(10):1163–9. https://doi.org/10.1111/j.1600-0501.2009.01758.x. Epub 2009 Jul 20. PMID: 19681964.

11. Chan HL, Misch K, Wang HL. Dental imaging in implant treatment planning. Implant Dent. 2010;19(4):288–98.

12. Chen H, Liu N, Xu X, Qu X, Lu E. Smoking, radiotherapy, diabetes and osteoporosis as risk factors for dental implant failure: a meta-analysis. PLoS One. 2013;8(8):e71955. https://doi.org/10.1371/journal.pone.0071955. PMID: 23940794; PMCID: PMC3733795.

13. de Medeiros FCFL, Kudo GAH, Leme BG, Saraiva PP, Verri FR, Honório HM, Pellizzer EP, Santiago Junior JF. Dental implants in patients with osteoporosis: a systematic review with meta-analysis. Int J Oral Maxillofac Surg. 2018;47(4):480–91. https://doi.org/10.1016/j.ijom.2017.05.021. Epub 2017 Jun 23. PMID: 28651805.

14. de Oliveira Nicolau Mantovani AK, de Mattias Sartori IA, Azevedo-Alanis LR, Tiossi R, Fontão FNGK. Influence of cortical bone anchorage on the primary stability of dental implants. Oral Maxillofac Surg. 2018;22(3):297–301. https://doi.org/10.1007/s10006-018-0705-y. Epub 2018 Jun 6. PMID: 29876688.

15. Degidi M, Daprile G, Piattelli A. Influence of underpreparation on primary stability of implants inserted in poor quality bone sites: an in vitro study. J Oral Maxillofac Surg. 2015;73(6):1084–8.

16. Dorotheou D, Gkantidis N, Karamolegkou M, Kalyvas D, Kiliaridis S, Kitraki E. Tooth eruption: altered gene expression in the dental follicle of patients with cleidocranial dysplasia. Orthod Craniofac Res. 2013;16(1):20–7. https://doi.org/10.1111/ocr.12000. Epub 2012 Sep 17. PMID: 23311656.

17. Farrow E, Nicot R, Wiss A, Laborde A, Ferri J. Cleidocranial dysplasia: a review of clinical, radiological, genetic implications and a guidelines proposal. J Craniofac Surg. 2018;29(2):382–9. https://doi.org/10.1097/SCS.0000000000004200. PMID: 29189406.

18. Florencio-Silva R, Sasso GR, Sasso-Cerri E, Simões MJ, Cerri PS. Biology of bone tissue: structure, function, and factors

that influence bone cells. Biomed Res Int. 2015;2015:421746. https://doi.org/10.1155/2015/421746. Epub 2015 Jul 13. PMID: 26247020; PMCID: PMC4515490.

19. Goiato MC, Dos Santos DM, Santiago JJ, Moreno A, Pellizzer EP. Longevity of dental implants in type IV bone: a systematic review. Int J Oral Maxillofac Surg. 2014;43(9):1108–16.

20. Gulsahi A. Bone quality assessment for dental implants. Rijeka: InTech; 2011. p. 437–52.

21. He J, Zhao B, Deng C, Shang D, Zhang C. Assessment of implant cumulative survival rates in sites with different bone density and related prognostic factors: an 8-year retrospective study of 2,684 implants. Int J Oral Maxillofac Implants. 2015;30(2):360–71. https://doi.org/10.11607/jomi.3580. PMID: 25830396.

22. Holahan CM, Koka S, Kennel KA, Weaver AL, Assad DA, Regennitter FJ, Kademani D. Effect of osteoporotic status on the survival of titanium dental implants. Int J Oral Maxillofac Implants. 2008;23(5):905–10. PMID: 19014161.

23. Javed F, Ahmed HB, Crespi R, Romanos GE. Role of primary stability for successful osseointegration of dental implants: factors of influence and evaluation. Interv Med Appl Sci. 2013;5(4):162–7.

24. Kanis JA, Melton LJ 3rd, Christiansen C, Johnston CC, Khaltaev N. The diagnosis of osteoporosis. J Bone Miner Res. 1994;9(8):1137–41. https://doi.org/10.1002/jbmr.5650090802. PMID: 7976495.

25. Karaguzel G, Holick MF. Diagnosis and treatment of osteopenia. Rev Endocr Metab Disord. 2010;11(4):237–51. https://doi.org/10.1007/s11154-010-9154-0. PMID: 21234807.

26. Karl M, Grobecker-Karl T. Effect of bone quality, implant design, and surgical technique on primary implant stability. Quintessence Int. 2018;49(3).

27. Kirmanidou Y, Sidira M, Drosou ME, Bennani V, Bakopoulou A, Tsouknidas A, Michailidis N, Michalakis K. New Ti-alloys and surface modifications to improve the mechanical properties and the biological response to orthopedic and dental implants: a review. Biomed Res Int. 2016;14:2016.

28. Kuroshima S, Nakano T, Ishimoto T, Sasaki M, Inoue M, Yasutake M, Sawase T. Optimally oriented grooves on dental implants improve bone quality around implants under repetitive mechanical loading. Acta Biomater. 2017;48:433–44.

29. Le Guéhennec L, Soueidan A, Layrolle P, Amouriq Y. Surface treatments of titanium dental implants for rapid osseointegration. Dent Mater. 2007;23(7):844–54.

30. Leung CC, Palomo L, Griffith R, Hans MG. Accuracy and reliability of cone-beam computed tomography for measuring alveolar bone height and detecting bony dehiscences and fenestrations. Am J Orthod Dentofac Orthop. 2010;137(4):S109–19.

31. Linetskiy I, Demenko V, Linetska L, Yefremov O. Impact of annual bone loss and different bone quality on dental implant success–a finite element study. Comput Biol Med. 2017;91:318–25.

32. Makary C, Menhall A, Zammarie C, Lombardi T, Lee SY, Stacchi C, Park KB. Primary stability optimization by using fixtures with different thread depth according to bone density: a clinical prospective study on early loaded implants. Materials. 2019;12(15):2398.

33. Merheb J, Temmerman A, Rasmusson L, Kübler A, Thor A, Quirynen M. Influence of skeletal and local bone density on dental implant stability in patients with osteoporosis. Clin Implant Dent Relat Res. 2016;18(2):253–60. https://doi.org/10.1111/cid.12290. Epub 2016 Feb 10. PMID: 26864614.

34. Merheb J, Vercruyssen M, Coucke W, Quirynen M. Relationship of implant stability and bone density derived from computerized tomography images. Clin Implant Dent Relat Res. 2018;20(1):50–7. https://doi.org/10.1111/cid.12579. Epub 2017 Dec 26. PMID: 29277972.

35. Miller PD. Management of severe osteoporosis. Expert Opin Pharmacother. 2016;17(4):473–88. https://doi.org/10.1517/14656566.2016.1124856. Epub 2015 Dec 23. PMID: 26605922.

36. Molly L. Bone density and primary stability in implant therapy. Clin Oral Implants Res. 2006;17(Suppl 2):124–35. https://doi.org/10.1111/j.1600-0501.2006.01356.x. PMID: 16968388.

37. Orlando F, Arosio F, Arosio P, Di Stefano DA. Bone density and implant primary stability. A study on equine bone blocks. Dent J (Basel). 2019;7(3):73. https://doi.org/10.3390/dj7030073. PMID: 31266214; PMCID: PMC6784737.

38. Pauwels R, Jacobs R, Singer SR, Mupparapu M. CBCT-based bone quality assessment: are Hounsfield units applicable? Dentomaxillofac Radiol. 2015;44(1):20140238.

39. Planinić D, Dubravica I, Šarac Z, Poljak-Guberina R, Celebic A, Bago I, Cabov T, Peric B. Comparison of different surgical procedures on the stability of dental implants in posterior maxilla: a randomized clinical study. J Stomatol Oral Maxillofac Surg. 2020:S2468-7855(20)30179-8. https://doi.org/10.1016/j.jormas.2020.08.004. Epub ahead of print. PMID: 32828993.

40. Radi IA, Ibrahim W, Iskandar SMS, AbdelNabi N. Prognosis of dental implants in patients with low bone density: a systematic review and meta-analysis. J Prosthet Dent. 2018;120(5):668–77. https://doi.org/10.1016/j.prosdent.2018.01.019. Epub 2018 Jul 11. PMID: 30006226.

41. Rokn A, Rasouli Ghahroudi AA, Daneshmonfared M, Menasheof R, Shamshiri AR. Tactile sense of the surgeon in determining bone density when placing dental implant. Implant Dent. 2014;23(6):697–703. https://doi.org/10.1097/ID.0000000000000173. PMID: 25347271.

42. Sakka S, Coulthard P. Bone quality: a reality for the process of osseointegration. Implant Dent. 2009;18(6):480–5. https://doi.org/10.1097/ID.0b013e3181bb840d. PMID: 20009601.

43. Sennerby L, Andersson P, Pagliani L, Giani C, Moretti G, Molinari M, Motroni A. Evaluation of a novel cone beam computed tomography scanner for bone density Examinations in Preoperative 3D reconstructions and correlation with primary implant stability. Clin Implant Dent Relat Res. 2015;17(5):844–53. https://doi.org/10.1111/cid.12193. Epub 2013 Dec 27. PMID: 24373386.

44. Lekholm U, Zarb GA. Patient selection and preparation. Tissue integrated prostheses: osseointegration in clinical dentistry. Quintessence Publishing Company, Chicago, USA. 1985:199–209.

45. Shah FA, Thomsen P, Palmquist A. A review of the impact of implant biomaterials on osteocytes. J Dent Res. 2018;97(9):977–86.

46. Shalabi MM, Wolke JG, De Ruijter AJ, Jansen JA. A mechanical evaluation of implants placed with different surgical techniques into the trabecular bone of goats. J Oral Implantol. 2007;33:51–8.

47. Siris ES, Adler R, Bilezikian J, Bolognese M, Dawson-Hughes B, Favus MJ, Harris ST, Jan de Beur SM, Khosla S, Lane NE, Lindsay R, Nana AD, Orwoll ES, Saag K, Silverman S, Watts NB. The clinical diagnosis of osteoporosis: a position statement from the National Bone Health Alliance Working Group. Osteoporos Int. 2014;25(5):1439–43. https://doi.org/10.1007/s00198-014-2655-z. Epub 2014 Feb 28. PMID: 24577348; PMCID: PMC3988515.

48. Strietzel FP, Nowak M, Küchler I, Friedmann A. Peri-implant alveolar bone loss with respect to bone quality after use of the osteotome technique: results of a retrospective study. Clin Oral Implants Res. 2002;13(5):508–13.

49. Tabassum A, Meijer GJ, Wolke JG, Jansen JA. Influence of the surgical technique and surface roughness on the primary stability of an implant in artificial bone with a density equivalent to maxillary bone: a laboratory study. Clin Oral Implants Res. 2009;20:327–32.

50. Turkyilmaz I, McGlumphy EA. Influence of bone density on implant stability parameters and implant success: a retrospective clinical study. BMC Oral Health. 2008;8(1):1–8.

51. Wakimoto M, Matsumura T, Ueno T, Mizukawa N, Yanagi Y, Iida S. Bone quality and quantity of the anterior maxillary trabecular bone in dental implant sites. Clin Oral Implants Res. 2012;23(11):1314–9.

Bone Quantity

5

Sina Ayati and Shohreh Ghasemi

Introduction

Atrophy of the alveolar processes takes place in both horizontal and vertical planes after the loss of teeth. Atrophy's literal meaning means wasting away, specifically diminishing the part, tissue, or organ. The Chronic decay associated with advanced age may lead to tooth loss and necessitate implant and prosthetic treatment for the patient to obtain the function of the tooth. Loss of teeth leads to atrophy of the residual alveolar ridge, that can being chronic and cumulative over the life.

Missing teeth have been a common problem as people rely on dental implants because of their popularity and reliability. A wide range of screw-type implant systems are available today, and the success rate is dependent on the jawbone's quality and quantity. That is why it is essential to precisely measure the alveolar processes to match the proper implant system. Various classifications are suggested according to the atrophy, whether it is partial or complete edentulous jaws.

In 1985, Zarb and Lekholm proposed the classification system of jaw anatomy, which was subsequently used in dental implants. Nonetheless, this system failed in its effectiveness as it only described changes in jaw shapes and was unable to indicate the real measurements.

Dental implant's clinical success depends upon the density, including the bone's quality and quantity. CT, also known as computed tomography, helps get bone's images before dental surgery. It gives three-dimensional anatomic structures and density measurements expressed in HU [1], as it helps provide information on the bone.

Table 5.1 Dental radiology classification: Hounsfield units

D1	HU 1250 and above
D2	HU 850
D3	HU 350–850
D4	HU 150–350

HU or Hounsfield unit originates from computed tomography or CT imaging and they are standard numbers. HU represents a relative value (density) of tissues through a gray-level scale which is based on the amount of water (0 HU), bone density (1000 HU), and air (-1000 HU) [2]. Several studies have also concluded the relative density of bones of jaws in CT imaging, and HU is a useful way to look at bone's density, even though CT imaging is linked with high radiation doses [3, 4] (Table 5.1).

CT is being replaced with cone-beam computed tomography (CBCT) to evaluate mineralized tissues since it gives adequate imaging associated with a lower dose. CBCT also costs lower than CT, and it has a fast scanning time and a smaller number of artifacts [5]. Several researchers and academics have reported CBCT's values as a way to measure bone density [1, 6–10]. Some studies have concluded that values in the form of HU from CBCT and MSCT are not identical [2, 11]. Similarly, there are differences in the methodological aspect of studies regarding of CBCT devices. Isoda et al. [9] has reported that the visibility in panoramic imaging, will be not clear whether the density values measurement could be applied different from one device to another. Nackaerts et al. has also concluded that with five scanner studies demonstrated different value measurements due to different devices.

The implant's success depends on the evaluation of bone density and quantity as it determines the treatment planning. To acquire this information, radiography is used for the examination, and several studies have assessed this evaluation [12, 13]. Initially, this process and analysis of bone density were based on subjectivity [12, 13]. In the later years, studies and research found a correlation between HU and

S. Ayati (✉)
First year of Dentistry (D1) Dental College of Georgia, Augusta, GA, USA
e-mail: sina228ayati@aol.com

S. Ghasemi
Department of Oral and Maxillofacial Surgery, Augusta University, Augusta, GA, USA
e-mail: sghasemi@augusta.edu

Fig. 5.1 Bone quantity
classification

Bone Density Classification (Mish, Judy.1987)

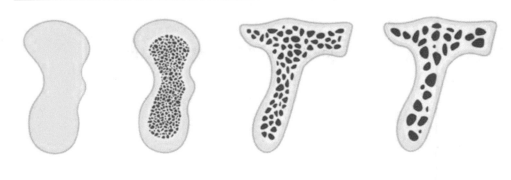

Bone Density Classification (Lekholm & Zarb.1985)

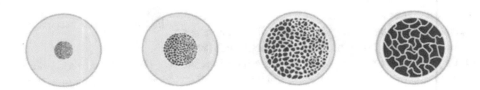

Fig. 5.1 Bone quantity classification

assessment of density, which was objective [3, 4, 14–16]. Similarly, studies have concluded a relation between high density and high implant success [3, 4, 14, 17]. Primary stability of the implants is also related to the high density of bones [9, 18]. We already used MSCT as a gold standard since it is successfully used in the assessment of bone density [2, 3, 14, 17]. Densitometric and histomorphometric evaluations provide accurate bone density, and they are routinely applied in implantology (Fig. 5.1).

Implants replace missing teeth, and all dental implants are considered reliable and successful. The stability of primary implants determines the success rates of these treatments. Primary implant stability is defined as a mechanical engagement between the implant and surrounding bone, whereas bone regernation and remodelling will detemine the biological stability to the implant (secondary stability). It is also dependent upon the quantity and quality of the bone.

Lekholm and Zarb have successfully proposed one of the most popular classification for assessment of bone density, and it has been classified in to four types. The classification is based on morphology and distribution of cancellous and cortical bones. The first one is composed of dense bones, whereas cancellous bone makes up Type 4. Researchers have concluded that there is a correlation between this framework and primary implant stability. The grading and correlation are subjective because they depend upon radiographic sources and the doctor's intuition during osteotomy. That is why accuracy in these classifications can be inaccurate. The classification of bones is as follows: [10, 11, 19]

Type 1 consists of bones that are composed of a single compact bone. Type 2 comprises a core dense trabecular bone that is surrounded by a thick layer of compact bone. Type 3 comprises a core of dense trabecular bone surrounded by a relatively thin cortical bone layer. Type 4 bone consists of a center of low-density trabecular bone, which is surrounded by a thin layer of cortical bone. These classifications are based on the resistance of bones to drilling and their radiographic appearances. The differences can also be categorized based on the upper and lower anatomical structure of the jaws [7, 9, 12].

As compared to maxillas, mandibles are dense in their cortical structure, and upon moving posteriorly, both jaws show decreased thickness and increased trabecular porosity. Several studies have been reported about the lower possibility of success rate with the increase of bone quantity and failed to indicate precise measurements. Statistics have shown that 2% failure rate in type 1, compare to 14% failure rate in type 4 in one group of study, and survival rate of the first group was 98% and 96%, while the survival rate in the second group was 90% in type 1 and 76% in type 4. This data concludes that the quality of bone is essential while replacing bone implants. At the same time, with regard to differences between the results, other factors have also determined the stability. Planning is also crucial because there are four types of bones in the face, and one has to determine the implants based on the types of bones before placing a tooth and crown on it [4–8].

As mentioned earlier, Lekholom and Zarb's (L & Z) method of classification is the most used framework to classify bones. Several studies have tried to equate and relate their frameworks and techniques with L & Z's parameters. It is also argued whether L & Z's radiographic assessment should be used before or after the surgery. Simultaneously, the overall accuracy of this process was considered less accurate, with almost 50% compared to radiography, which may or may not use trabecular bone's images as reference. In one case, the lowest percentage recorded was nearly 28% when the method was applied with trabeculation of the mandible. The trabecular, when seen through the human mandible, was different from L & Z's images. This suggested that this particular feature is not applicable to a well-composed jawbone.

Misch (1990–2008) According to this classification system, four density groups (D1-D4) marked the division of bone types in all jaw areas. This classification was based on the clinician's tactile analogue and descriptive analogy. The data from this classification was also compared with anatomical structures along with radiography scales. The division of the groups of bones is as follows:

- *Division A:* This division has abundant volume in both width and height as its height is above 10 mm, and its width is also above 5 mm. If procedures like modification or grafting are diminished,the result will be less traumatic and the healing period will be reduced.
- *Division B:* This division has less bone volume compared to Division A, it offers sufficient available bone height (at least 10 mm) and reduced bone width (2.5–5 mm). If there is any deficiency in width, it can be made up through the use of narrower implants or even osteoplasty. The favourable treatment plan for such a this case will be ridge expansion. The smaller Diameter implantation induced less bone gain in reconstruction and is less favourable in mechanical stress. The second option is bone augmentation with delayed implant loading will lead to better morphology in soft and hard tissue biotype and correct the emergence of the implant with acceptable subsequent restoration. The third option is osteoplasty, which allows the surgon to insert implant simultaneously, it will lead to reduction of the height of the bone according to the implant placement. Due to the potenitial loss of crestal bone, which lead to the reduction of initial or primary implant stability.
- *Division C:* This division has a lesser height and width. Its height is lower than 10 mm and width is also lesser than 2.5 mm. The most preferred treatment for this division is augmentation or use of grafts before the implant; subperiosteal implant method is also preferred. However, the process of augmentation is more costly and this eventually increases the required skill and time. [10–17]
- *Division D:* severely bone deficiency in height and width. Subperiosteal implant placement, block grafts, extensive

sinus elevation are necessary to achieve the acceptable implant placement [10–18]

UCLA Classification UCLA has classified alveolar bones based on their volume and three-dimensional shape. During implantation, the volume of bone in both vertical and horizontal dimensions was observed by clinical methods [20]. Based on the deficient ridge volume in apical and horizontal patterns, they were divided into eight classes [21]. However, this classification was altered, and a new system of four groups was introduced.

- Type *I* : It has an adequate bone in both horizontal and vertical planes, which lead to an ideal placement for the implant insertion.
- Type *II* : It has sufficient bone volume in the buccal plane.
- Type *III:* It has deficiency in bone volume, but adequte in bone height.
- Type *IV:* has inadequate volume and heights, and all sides are exposed. This is completely opposite to the first type in this group.

D1 type consists of homogeneous dense cortical bone, in this type, there is a sufficient bone in horizontal and vertical dimensions, in this type, the density is due to the cortical lamellar bone, making it ideal for implant placement [8, 9]. Osseointegration is also influenced by high bone contact. At the same, minor blood vessels can obstruct the supply of numerous nutrients, which slows down healing [10, 14, 15].

D2 is thinner and insufficient bone volume on the buccal side, Which we can see at posterior site of the mandible. Good primary stability, good implant interface, healing, and predictable osseointegration is provided by this type of the bone. This type is ideal for an implant and provides sufficient nutrients, which can also allow bleeding during surgical procedures [11, 19, 13].

D3 bone is frequently found in the anterior maxilla and posterior regions of both maxilla and mandible. This type of the bone is weaker than D2 bone. The bone-implant contact is less favourable in this type of bone density classification. This bone is present in the anterior maxilla and is found in the regions of the mouth.

In these divisions, D4 does not have cortical bones, and its trabecular density is the lowest. These bones are rare and are usually present in the posterior region of the maxilla. It is weaker than other types in terms of bone density, and D1 is many times stronger than D4. They also present challenges in bone implants because of their structure and density. Other techniques of bone expansion are used before the final implant, which improves the stability in this type of bones [11, 15, 16].

Type I This type is compared to wood because of its density and hardness. Because of its hard structure, the blood flow is less compared to other types of bones. This is also one of the reasons that this type of bone takes a lot of time to get back into shape after any implant. It takes more than 4 months to integrate after the implant.

Type II This type is compared to pine wood, as it is not much hard. It usually takes lesser time than the first type to integrate with the bone after implant [17–20].

Type III This is compared to balsa wood as its density is lesser than the previously mentioned bone types. It also takes more time after the implant to integrate with the bone. It usually takes more than 5 months, and gradual healing can also improve bone density [20–22].

Type IV This type is compared to foam as it is less dense than all the other types. It also takes more time to integrate with the bones. The time taken for healing is suggested to be more than 7 months, and several implants can be used for any kind of healing [18, 20, 23].

Conclusion

Diagnostic imaging and radiographic assessment is a keyrole for dental implant insertion, in general, accurate preoperative would proceed with panoramic radiograph, but CBCT is the best modality for facilitate the acquisition and classified the bone composition in quality and quantity and post-operative assessment for increase the success rate and diminish the failure rate of a dental implant.

References

1. Aranyarachkul P, Caruso J, Gantes B, Schulz E, Riggs M, Dus I, et al. Bone density assessments of dental implant sites: 2. Quantitative cone-beam computerized tomography. Int J Oral Maxillofac Implants. 2005;20(3):416–24.
2. Nackaerts O, Maes F, Yan H, Couto Souza P, Pauwels R, Jacobs R. Analysis of intensity variability in multislice and cone beam computed tomography. Clin Oral Implants Res. 2011;22(8):873–9.
3. Turkyilmaz I, Tözüm TF, Tumer MC. Bone density assessments of oral implant sites using computerized tomography. J Oral Rehabil. 2007;34(4):267–72.
4. Aksoy U, Eratalay K, Tözüm TF. The possible association among bone density values, resonance frequency measurements, tactile sense, and histomorphometric evaluations of dental implant osteotomy sites: a preliminary study. Implant Dent. 2009;18(4):316–25.
5. Miracle AC, Mukherji SK. Conebeam CT of the head and neck, part 1: physical principles. AJNR Am J Neuroradiol. 2009;30(6):1088–95.
6. Lee S, Gantes B, Riggs M, Crigger M. Bone density assessments of dental implants sites: 3. Bone quality evaluation during osteotomy and implant placement. Int J Oral Maxillofac Implants. 2007;22(2):208–12.
7. Arisan V, Karabuda ZC, Avsever H, Ozdemir T. Conventional multislice computed tomography (CT) and cone-beam CT (CBCT) for computer-assisted implant placement. Part I: Relationship of radiographic gray density and implant stability. Clin Implant Dent Relat Res. 2012. https://doi.org/10.1111/j.1708-8208.2011.00436.x
8. Bland JM, Altman DG. Statistical methods for assessing agreement between two methods of clinical measurement. Lancet. 1986;1(8476):307–10.
9. Lindh C, Nilsson M, Klinge B, Petersson A. Quantitative computed tomography of trabecular bone in the mandible. Dentomaxillofac Radiol. 1996;25(3):146–50.
10. Misch CE. Density of bone: effect on treatment plans, surgical approach, healing, and progressive bone loading. Int J Oral Implantol. 1990;6(2):23–31.
11. Shapurian T, Damoulis PD, Reiser GM, Griffin TJ, Rand WM. Quantitative evaluation of bone density using the Hounsfield index. Int J Oral Maxillofac Implants. 2006;21(2):290–7.
12. Oikarinen K, Raustia AM, Hartikainen M. General and local contraindications for endosseal implants – an epidemiological panoramic radiograph study in 65-year-old subjects. Community Dent Oral Epidemiol. 1995;23(2):114–8.
13. CAtwood DA. Reduction of residual ridges: a major oral disease entity. J Prosthet Dent. 1971;26(3):266–79.
14. Mercier P, Lafontant R. Residual alveolar ridge atrophy: classification and influence of facial morphology. J Prosthet Dent. 1979;41(1):90–100.
15. Seibert JS. Reconstruction of deformed, partially edentulous ridges, using full thickness onlay grafts. Part I. Technique and wound healing. Compend Contin Educ Dent. 1983;4(5):437–53.
16. Allen EP, Gainza CS, Farthing GG, Newbold DA. Improved technique for localized ridge augmentation. A report of 21 cases. J Periodontol. 1985;56(4):195–9.
17. Cawood JI, Howell RA. A classification of the edentulous jaws. Int J Oral Maxillofac Surg. 1988;17(4):232–6.
18. Eufinger H, Gellrich NC, Sandmann D, Dieckmann J. Descriptive and metric classification of jaw atrophy. An evaluation of 104 mandibles and 96 maxillae of dried skulls. Int J Oral Maxillofac Surg. 1997;26(1):23–8.
19. Biological factors contributing to failures of osseointegrated oral implants. (II). Etiopathogenesis. Eur J Oral Sci. 1998;106(3):721–64.
20. Meyer U, Vollmer D, Runte C, Bourauel C, Joos U. Bone loading pattern around implants in average and atrophic edentulous maxillae: a finite-element analysis. J Craniomaxillofac Surg. 2001;29(2):100–5.
21. Tallgren A. The continuing reduction of the residual alveolar ridges in complete denture wearers: a mixed-longitudinal study covering 25 years. J Prosthet Dent. 1972;27(2):120–32.
22. Esposito M, Hirsch JM, Lekholm U, Thomsen P. Biological factors contributing to failures of osseointegrated oral implants. (II). Etiopathogenesis. Eur J Oral Sci. 1998;106(3):721–64.
23. Linck GK, Ferreira GM, De Oliveira RC, Lindh C, Leles CR, Ribeiro-Rotta RF. The influence of tactile perception on classification of bone tissue at dental implant insertion. Clin Implant Dent Relat Res. 2016;18(3):601–8. PMID: 25850635.

Immediate Single Tooth Implant

Pindaros-Georgios Foskolos, Octavi Ortiz-Puigpelat,
Albert Barroso-Panella, Federico Hernández-Alfaro,
and Pablo Altuna

Introduction

Successful implant treatment of edentulism requires an adequate amount and volume of bone and soft tissue [29]. However, after tooth extraction, resorption of hard and soft tissues of the alveolar ridge is noticed [58]. These tissues' reduction appears to be faster during the first 3–6 months, presenting an average decrease of 3.8 mm in width and 1.24 mm in height. Afterward it continues at a slower pace [30, 63]. As a result, implant therapy, in many cases, becomes very difficult.

Many techniques have been proposed in the past decades to overcome the problem of bone deficiencies. A sinus lift, guided bone regeneration, or bone blocks are some of the most used procedures to place simultaneous or delayed implants [13, 22]. These techniques have good survival and success rates, but they increase treatment time, morbidity, treatment's cost, and risks of complications [44].

In order to avoid more invasive procedures, alveolar ridge preservation procedures have been proposed following an atraumatic extraction. They appear to limit the phenomenon of ridge alteration after tooth extraction [37]. However, preservation techniques do not avoid physiological resorption, and in many cases, additional guided bone regeneration or soft tissue procedures would be needed to compensate for the tissue loss [26, 42, 62].

P.-G. Foskolos (✉)
Department of Prosthodontics, National and Kapodistrian
University of Athens, Athens, Greece
e-mail: pindaros@uic.es

O. Ortiz-Puigpelat · A. Barroso-Panella · P. Altuna
Department of Oral and Maxillofacial Surgery, International
University of Catalonia, Barcelona, Spain
e-mail: octavi_ortiz@hotmail.com; albertbarroso@uic.es;
altuna@uic.es

F. Hernández-Alfaro
Department of Oral and Maxillofacial Surgery, International
University of Catalonia, Barcelona, Spain

Teknon Medical Center, Barcelona, Spain
e-mail: h.alfaro@uic.es

Another popular option described in the literature is immediate implant placement (IIP) after the tooth extraction, that can be combined with hard tissue regenerative procedures, soft tissue enhancement, and a provisional crown (often with immediate loading) [9, 16, 23]. A number of publications describe it as a predictable treatment option, that decreases treatment time, the need for additional regenerative procedures, and the patient's morbidity and with high success rates in terms of aesthetics [20].

Diagnosis

Clinical Assessment

The main objectives of implant therapy are biology, function, and aesthetics. However, after tooth extraction and IIP, there could be an alteration of bone and soft tissues that would potentially lead to midfacial recession and aesthetic failure of the treatment [15]. Thus, clinicians should focus on five important diagnosis factors that may affect the predictability of IIP in the esthetic zone [36]:

1. *Relative tooth position/free gingival margin (FGM):*
   (a) Ideally, the restoration over the implant and the soft tissues around it should be in harmony with the relative contralateral structures on the ridge. Therefore, after the tooth extraction, it is expected an approximately 1–2 mm apical migration of free gingival margin (FGM) of the failing tooth, leading to a postoperative disharmony [50]. Consequently, it can be assumed that if the level of FGM of the treated position is 2 mm more coronal than the FGM of the relative tooth on the other side, the predictability of a good aesthetic outcome increases. On the other hand, if the FGM of the treated tooth is more apical, our final results would be less aesthetic.
   (b) Buccolingual position: If the tooth is inclined facially, the buccal bone is usually thinner. In this situation, if

the implant/platform is placed toward the buccal, the chances of midfacial recession increase.

(c) *Mesiodistal position:* A narrower embrasure due to proximity with the neighboring teeth lowers the volume of the interdental papilla and the alveolar bone beneath it. A narrower interdental bone is more prone to resorption while healing, thus increasing the risk of aesthetic failures.

(d) *Mesiodistal inclination:* A mesial inclination of the failing tooth enlarges the interdental space mesially and thickness of the interdental bone beneath this area, lowering the risk for tissues' resorption during the healing period.

2. *Form of periodontium:* There are three types of gingival scallop – high, normal, and flat. The more flat the scallop is, the fewer tissues interfere in the interdental area, and the less are the risks of tissue loss after the tooth extraction.

3. *Phenotype of the periodontium:* The phenotype is characterized as thin or thick. The thicker the tissues are, the higher are the chances to maintain their volume and level postoperatively.

4. *Tooth shape:* There are mainly three tooth shapes – triangular, ovoid, and square. The first shape positions the contact points more coronally, and more tissues cover the interdental space. As a result, the tissue alterations are more evident in the final outcome. On the contrary, ovoid and square shapes are the most preferable. More tooth structure interferes in the embrasure, and the papilla is shorter, leading to less noticeable tissue migration.

5. *Position of the alveolar crest:* The alveolar ridge determines the level of soft tissues. The distance between the bone and the FGM influences the amount of expected tissue resorption after the tooth extraction. In cases where this distance is up to 3 mm, a slight apical repositioning of tissues is expected (up to 1 mm). When it exceeds 4 mm, the post-extraction alterations will be relatively increased. Finally, along with the interproximal space, when the referred relationship overcomes the 4 mm, the risk of fundamental tissues' changes increases.

Radiographic Analysis

Before taking any treatment decision in implant dentistry, a computed tomography or cone beam computed tomography (CBCT) is recommended [31]. For the IIP technique, the clinician should focus on specific aspects of the 3D imaging:

1. *Dimensions and morphology of the existing alveolar ridge.* Elian et al. [21] proposed a simple classification of the post-extraction socket focusing on the level of buccal

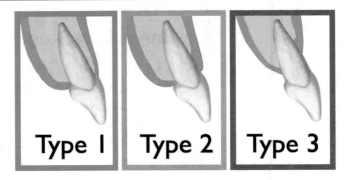

Fig. 6.1 Type I, II, and III socket. (Adapted from Elian et al. [21])

bony aspect and soft tissues (Fig. 6.1). According to this classification:

- On type 1 sockets: "Facial soft tissue and a buccal plate of bone are at normal levels in relation to the cementoenamel junction of the pre-extracted tooth and remain intact post-extraction."
- On type 2 sockets: "Facial soft tissue is present, but the buccal plate is partially missing following extraction of the tooth."
- On type 3 sockets: "The facial soft tissue and the buccal plate of bone are both markedly reduced after tooth extraction."

In type 1 socket, the same authors suggest that the treatment with IIP has the most predictable outcomes when the soft tissue phenotype is thick and the gingiva scallop is flat. In type 3 sockets, it is essential to primarily reconstruct the missing tissues with hard and soft tissues regenerative procedures before the staged implant placement. Concerning type 2 sockets, this article mentions a more complex diagnosis and a high risk of midfacial recession after treatment with IIP [21]. Several articles describe IIP with type 2 sockets with different grafting techniques, obtaining high survival and success rates [17, 47, 57, 60].

Also, the width of the defect should be assessed. Wider defects are more prone to gingival recessions than narrow and short bony defects [35].

2. *Positioning of the root of the failing tooth in the alveolar socket.* Kan et al. classified four main types of socket position in the alveolar ridge [34] (Fig. 6.2):

(a) Class I: "The entire length of the root is in contact with the labial cortical plate, a considerable amount of bone is present on the palatal aspect for implant engagement to attain primary stability during IIP."

(b) Class II: "The root was centered in the middle of the alveolar housing without engaging either the labial or palatal cortical plates at the apical third of the root."

(c) Class III: "The entire length of the root engages the palatal cortical plate; therefore, the stability of the

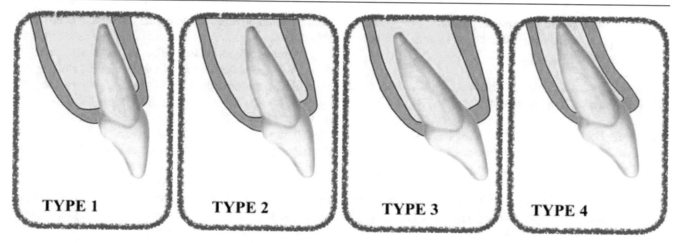

Fig. 6.2 Type I, II, III, and IV sockets. (Adapted from Kan et al. [34])

implant relies on its engagement in the available bone on the labial aspect."

(d) Class IV: "The existing tooth root occupies the majority of the alveolar volume, and the base of the anterior maxilla is often pedunculated."

The Class I sites are considered the most appropriate for IIP. Class II and III are technique sensitive, and, finally, Class IV is a contraindication for IIP [34]

3. *Quality and quantity of the bone:* Enough bone (4–5 mm) is necessary apically (beyond the tooth apex) to anchor the implant in the anterior area [20, 25, 36]. Leckhom and Zarb describe four classifications of bone quality. Type II and III bone quality are the most appropriate for implant insertion [2], while Type IV bone quality is the least favorable for implant therapy success [32].

Implant Design and Selection

Length Fundamental factor for the implant's success is the primary stability, especially when an immediate loading is planned. For this reason, the implant should be long enough so at least 3–5 mm of the implant's apex is inserted in the alveolar bone [20, 46, 52].

Diameter The implant's diameter should be narrow enough so that a gap of at least 2 mm exists between the implant surface and the buccal plate. This space allows biomaterials insertion for bone regeneration of the site. Usually, a narrower selection serves this objective [1, 12, 41].

Type of Connection The choice of abutment should follow the platform switching concept. In contrast with platform matching abutment, the narrower implant platform abutment

decreases the marginal bone loss and provides the space for thicker midfacial soft tissues [38, 54, 55].

Bone Level vs Tissue Level Bone level implants are considered more versatile since they provide a better emergence profile with different abutment heights and diameters and a better aesthetic outcome (higher PES scores) [59, 65].

Shape Tapered shape of the implant can achieve higher primary stability [3].

Abutment Selection and Timing of Placement

Diameter The diameter of the abutment should be chosen according to the platform switching concept. That means that the implant's success should be narrower than the implant's platform diameter [11].

Height Shorter abutments demonstrated higher rates of marginal bone loss. A height of at least 3 mm is necessary to form adequate biological width around the abutment [61].

Timing of Placement The definitive transepithelial abutment placement right after the implant insertion seems to decrease the percentages of marginal bone loss around the implant [10].

Tooth Extraction

The tooth extraction and the whole surgical procedure of IIP should be as atraumatic as possible. The tissues' integrity around the failed tooth and flapless surgery are highly recommended [5, 41]. Some instruments that facilitate this atraumatic concept are the luxator periotome, the powered periotome, the piezosurgery, the Benex system, and others [33, 40, 45, 49].

3D Position of the Implant

The appropriate positioning of the implant in the alveolar bone is essential for protecting the sensitive surrounding tissues. The guidelines for the implant placement are [27]:

(a) *Buccolingually:* The implant should be inserted in the palatal part of the socket so that a gap of at least 2 mm is maintained between the facial bony wall and the implant. This gap, once grafted with a low substitution material, should be sufficient to prevent a future midfacial mucosal recession [51].
(b) *Mesiodistally:* A distance of at least 1.5 mm should be maintained between the tooth structure and the implant surface. If an implant needs to be placed adjacent to another, the respective distance should not be less than 3 mm [24].
(c) *Apicocoronally:* The implant platform should be located 3–4 mm apically from the free gingival margin [24].

Tissues Regeneration

Soft Tissues Thin gingival phenotype is correlated with increased risk of midfacial recession after IIP [39]. Enhancing the gingival thickness of the facial part with a connective tissue graft simultaneous to the implant placement is recommended [6].

Hard Tissues It is suggested that grafting the gap between the implant surface and the buccal wall better preserves the volume in the long term [56]. A low substitution material (xenograft) is recommended [4], with the advantage that it has less morbidity and less resorption than autogenous bone from an intraoral donor site [43, 56]. For the referred purpose, alloplastic biomaterial seems to be an alternative option [7, 8].

Provisionalization and Final Restoration

Immediate aesthetic restoration after the insertion of the IIP lowers the risk of post-healing midfacial recession [16]. It also helps to contain grafting materials, seals the gap, and supports the soft tissues [53]. When immediate loading is not possible, a customized abutment mimicking the emergence profile should be used. If a temporary abutment is not available, then a wide healing abutment should be used [14, 64].

The morphological characteristics of immediate restorations are different for the critical and subcritical contour. The subcritical contour should be as concave as possible [28]. Only the abutment's interproximal emergence profile should be straight and scalloped until it is coronal to the osseous crest. This distance occupies approximately 3 mm [41]. On the contrary, the critical contour should imitate the shape of the relative contralateral tooth. However, it should be reduced approximately 0.5–1 mm on the occlusal aspect, so the restoration is out of occlusion. Furthermore, all the surfaces should be very well polished in order to avoid plaque accumulation around the healing region. Three to four months after the implant insertion, the final restoration can be delivered [28].

Conclusions

IIP is a predictable treatment that presents high success rates in terms of aesthetics, biology, and function in type I sockets of the Elian classification [21]. In type II sockets, some studies suggest IIP is also a successful treatment. However, more studies are needed to investigate the long-term results [18, 19, 47, 48]. There is inadequate evidence that IIP placed in type III sockets can be used on a routine basis.

There is consensus that IIP is a demanding procedure in terms of practitioner's experience. Routine IIP requires an adequate diagnosis to achieve an accurate 3D insertion of the implant in the post-extraction socket, bone grafting in the gap between the implant and buccal wall, soft tissue grafting buccal aspect, and proper design of the abutment and the prosthesis.

References

1. Al-Nawas B, Bragger U, Meijer HJ, Naert I, Persson R, Perucchi A, Quirynen M, Raghoebar GM, Reichert TE, Romeo E, Santing HJ, Schimmel M, Storelli S, Ten Bruggenkate C, Vandekerckhove B, Wagner W, Wismeijer D, Muller F. A double-blind randomized controlled trial (RCT) of Titanium-13Zirconium versus Titanium Grade IV small-diameter bone level implants in edentulous mandibles--results from a 1-year observation period. Clin Implant Dent Relat Res. 2012;14:896–904.
2. Alghamdi HS. Methods to improve osseointegration of dental implants in low quality (type-IV) bone: an overview. J Funct Biomater. 2018;9:7.
3. Alves CC, Neves M. Tapered implants: from indications to advantages. Int J Periodontics Restorative Dent. 2009;29:161–7.
4. Araújo MG, Linder E, Lindhe J. Bio-Oss collagen in the buccal gap at immediate implants: a 6-month study in the dog. Clin Oral Implants Res. 2011;22:1–8.

5. Araújo MG, Lindhe J. Ridge alterations following tooth extraction with and without flap elevation: an experimental study in the dog. Clin Oral Implants Res. 2009;20:545–9.

6. Atieh MA, Alsabeeha NHM. Soft tissue changes after connective tissue grafts around immediately placed and restored dental implants in the esthetic zone: a systematic review and meta-analysis. J Esthet Restor Dent. 2020;32:280–90.

7. Barroso-Panella A, Gargallo-Albiol J, Hérnandez-Alfaro F. Evaluation of bone stability and esthetic results after immediate implant placement using a novel synthetic bone substitute in the anterior zone: results after 12 months. Int J Periodontics Restorative Dent. 2018;38:235–43.

8. Barroso-Panella A, Ortiz-Puigpelat O, Altuna-Fistolera P, Lucas-Taulé E, Hernández-Alfaro F, Gargallo-Albiol J. Evaluation of peri-implant tissue stability and patient satisfaction after immediate implant placement in the esthetic area: a 3-year follow-up of an ongoing prospective study. Int J Periodontics Restorative Dent. 2020;40:731.

9. Bianchi AE, Sanfilippo F. Single-tooth replacement by immediate implant and connective tissue graft: a 1–9-year clinical evaluation. Clin Oral Implants Res. 2004;15:269–77.

10. Borges T, Leitao B, Pereira M, Carvalho A, Galindo-Moreno P. Influence of the abutment height and connection timing in early peri-implant marginal bone changes: a prospective randomized clinical trial. Clin Oral Implants Res. 2018;29:907–14.

11. Canullo L, Fedele GR, Iannello G, Jepsen S. Platform switching and marginal bone-level alterations: the results of a randomized-controlled trial. Clin Oral Implants Res. 2010;21:115–21.

12. Canullo L, Iannello G, Penarocha M, Garcia B. Impact of implant diameter on bone level changes around platform switched implants: preliminary results of 18 months follow-up a prospective randomized match-paired controlled trial. Clin Oral Implants Res. 2012;23:1142–6.

13. Chiapasco M, Casentini P, Zaniboni M. Bone augmentation procedures in implant dentistry. Int J Oral Maxillofac Implants. 2009;24 Suppl:237–59.

14. Chu SJ, Salama MA, Garber DA, Salama H, Sarnachiaro GO, Sarnachiaro E, Gotta SL, Reynolds MA, Saito H, Tarnow DP. Flapless postextraction socket implant placement, part 2: the effects of bone grafting and provisional restoration on peri-implant soft tissue height and thickness- A retrospective study. Int J Periodontics Restorative Dent. 2015;35:803–9.

15. Cosyn J, de Lat L, Seyssens L, Doornewaard R, Deschepper E, Vervaeke S. The effectiveness of immediate implant placement for single tooth replacement compared to delayed implant placement: a systematic review and meta-analysis. J Clin Periodontol. 2019;46(Suppl 21):224–41.

16. Cosyn J, Hooghe N, de Bruyn H. A systematic review on the frequency of advanced recession following single immediate implant treatment. J Clin Periodontol. 2012;39:582–9.

17. da Rosa JC, Rosa AC, da Rosa DM, Zardo CM. Immediate dentoalveolar restoration of compromised sockets: a novel technique. Eur J Esthet Dent. 2013;8:432–43.

18. de Molon RS, de Avila ED, Cirelli JA, Mollo FDA Jr, de Andrade MF, Filho LABB, Barros LAB. A combined approach for the treatment of resorbed fresh sockets allowing immediate implant restoration: a 2-year follow-up. J Oral Implantol. 2015;41:712–8.

19. de Molon RS, de Avila ED, de Barros-Filho LAB, Ricci WA, Tetradis S, Cirelli JA, Borelli de Barros LA. Reconstruction of the alveolar buccal bone plate in compromised fresh socket after immediate implant placement followed by immediate provisionalization. J Esthet Restor Dent. 2015;27:122–35.

20. Ebenezer V, Balakrishnan K, Asir RV, Sragunar B. Immediate placement of endosseous implants into the extraction sockets. J Pharm Bioallied Sci. 2015;7:S234–7.

21. Elian N, Cho SC, Froum S, Smith RB, Tarnow DP. A simplified socket classification and repair technique. Pract Proced Aesthet Dent. 2007;19:99–104; quiz 106.

22. Elnayef B, Monje A, Gargallo-Albiol J, Galindo-Moreno P, Wang HL, Hernandez-Alfaro F. Vertical ridge augmentation in the atrophic mandible: a systematic review and meta-analysis. Int J Oral Maxillofac Implants. 2017;32:291–312.

23. Ferrus J, Cecchinato D, Pjetursson EB, Lang NP, Sanz M, Lindhe J. Factors influencing ridge alterations following immediate implant placement into extraction sockets. Clin Oral Implants Res. 2010;21:22–9.

24. Funato A, Salama MA, Ishikawa T, Garber DA, Salama H. Timing, positioning, and sequential staging in esthetic implant therapy: a four-dimensional perspective. Int J Periodontics Restorative Dent. 2007;27:313–23.

25. Garber DA, Salama MA, Salama H. Immediate total tooth replacement. Compend Contin Educ Dent. 2001;22:210–6, 218.

26. García-González S, Galve-Huertas A, Centenero SA-H, Mareque-Bueno S, Satorres-Nieto M, Hernández-Alfaro F. Volumetric changes in alveolar ridge preservation with a compromised buccal wall: a systematic review and meta-analysis. Med Oral Patol Oral Cir Bucal. 2020;25:e565.

27. Gastaldo JF, Cury PR, Sendyk WR. Effect of the vertical and horizontal distances between adjacent implants and between a tooth and an implant on the incidence of interproximal papilla. J Periodontol. 2004;75:1242–6.

28. Gonzalez-Martin O, Lee E, Weisgold A, Veltri M, Su H. Contour management of implant restorations for optimal emergence profiles: guidelines for immediate and delayed provisional restorations. Int J Periodontics Restorative Dent. 2020;40:61–70.

29. Grunder U, Gracis S, Capelli M. Influence of the 3-D bone-to-implant relationship on esthetics. Int J Periodontics Restorative Dent. 2005;25:113–9.

30. Hammerle CH, Araujo MG, Simion M. Evidence-based knowledge on the biology and treatment of extraction sockets. Clin Oral Implants Res. 2012;23 Suppl 5:80–2.

31. Jacobs R, Salmon B, Codari M, Hassan B, Bornstein MM. Cone beam computed tomography in implant dentistry: recommendations for clinical use. BMC Oral Health. 2018;18:88.

32. Jaffin RA, Berman CL. The excessive loss of Branemark fixtures in type IV bone: a 5-year analysis. J Periodontol. 1991;62:2–4.

33. Jones S. Atraumatic extractions with luxator periotome. Dental Tribune Daily US. 2012;4:7–8.

34. Kan JY, Roe P, Rungcharassaeng K, Patel RD, Waki T, Lozada JL, Zimmerman G. Classification of sagittal root position in relation to the anterior maxillary osseous housing for immediate implant placement: a cone beam computed tomography study. Int J Oral Maxillofac Implants. 2011;26:873–6.

35. Kan JY, Rungcharassaeng K, Sclar A, Lozada JL. Effects of the facial osseous defect morphology on gingival dynamics after immediate tooth replacement and guided bone regeneration: 1-year results. J Oral Maxillofac Surg. 2007;65:13–9.

36. Kois JC. Predictable single tooth peri-implant esthetics: five diagnostic keys. Compend. Contin. Educ. Dent. (Jamesburg, NJ: 1995). 2001;22:199–206; quiz 208.

37. Kubilius M, Kubilius R, Gleiznys A. The preservation of alveolar bone ridge during tooth extraction. Stomatologija. 2012;14:3–11.

38. Lazzara RJ, Porter SS. Platform switching: a new concept in implant dentistry for controlling postrestorative crestal bone levels. Int J Periodontics Restorative Dent. 2006;26:9–17.

39. Lee CT, Sanz-Miralles E, Zhu L, Glick J, Heath A, Stoupel J. Predicting bone and soft tissue alterations of immediate implant sites in the esthetic zone using clinical parameters. Clin Implant Dent Relat Res. 2020;22(3):325–32.

40. Lerner S, Robert C, Handal A. Powered periotome. Google Patents. 2003.

41. Levine RA, Ganeles J, Gonzaga L, Kan JK, Randel H, Evans CD, Chen ST. 10 keys for successful esthetic-zone single immediate implants. Compend Contin Educ Dent. 2017;38:248–60.

42. Lyu C, Shao Z, Zou D, LU, J. Ridge alterations following socket preservation using a collagen membrane in dogs. Biomed Res Int. 2020;2020:1487681.

43. Mendoza-Azpur G, de la Fuente A, Chavez E, Valdivia E, Khouly I. Horizontal ridge augmentation with guided bone regeneration using particulate xenogenic bone substitutes with or without autogenous block grafts: a randomized controlled trial. Clin Implant Dent Relat Res. 2019;21:521–30.

44. Moy PK, Aghaloo T. Risk factors in bone augmentation procedures. Periodontol. 2019;2000(81):76–90.

45. Muska E, Walter C, Knight A, Taneja P, Bulsara Y, Hahn M, Desai M, Dietrich T. Atraumatic vertical tooth extraction: a proof of principle clinical study of a novel system. Oral Surg Oral Med Oral Pathol Oral Radiol. 2013;116:e303–10.

46. Nemcovsky CE, Artzi Z, Moses O. Rotated palatal flap in immediate implant procedures. Clinical evaluation of 26 consecutive cases. Clin Oral Implants Res. 2000;11:83–90.

47. Noelken R, Kunkel M, Wagner W. Immediate implant placement and provisionalization after long-axis root fracture and complete loss of the facial bony lamella. Int J Periodontics Restorative Dent. 2011;31:175.

48. Noelken R, Moergel M, Kunkel M, Wagner W. Immediate and flapless implant insertion and provisionalization using autogenous bone grafts in the esthetic zone: 5-year results. Clin Oral Implants Res. 2018;29:320–7.

49. Papadimitriou DE, Geminiani A, Zahavi T, Ercoli C. Sonosurgery for atraumatic tooth extraction: a clinical report. J Prosthet Dent. 2012;108:339–43.

50. Phillips K, Kois JC. Aesthetic peri-implant site development. The restorative connection. Dent Clin N Am. 1998;42:57–70.

51. Rosa AC, da Rosa JC, Dias Pereira LA, Francischone CE, Sotto-Maior BS. Guidelines for selecting the implant diameter during immediate implant placement of a fresh extraction socket: a case series. Int J Periodontics Restorative Dent. 2016;36:401–7.

52. Rosenquist B, Ahmed M. The immediate replacement of teeth by dental implants using homologous bone membranes to seal the sockets: clinical and radiographic findings. Clin Oral Implants Res. 2000;11:572–82.

53. Saito H, Chu SJ, Reynolds MA, Tarnow DP. Provisional restorations used in immediate implant placement provide a platform to promote peri-implant soft tissue healing: a pilot study. Int J Periodontics Restorative Dent. 2016;36:47–52.

54. Saito H, Chu SJ, Zamzok J, Brown M, Smith R, Sarnachiaro G, Hochman M, Fletcher P, Reynolds MA, Tarnow DP. Flapless postextraction socket implant placement: the effects of a platform switch-designed implant on peri-implant soft tissue thickness-a prospective study. Int J Periodontics Restorative Dent. 2018;38:s9–s15.

55. Santiago JF Jr, Batista VE, Verri FR, Honório HM, de Mello CC, Almeida DA, Pellizzer EP. Platform-switching implants and bone preservation: a systematic review and meta-analysis. Int J Oral Maxillofac Surg. 2016;45:332–45.

56. Sanz M, Lindhe J, Alcaraz J, Sanz-Sanchez I, Cecchinato D. The effect of placing a bone replacement graft in the gap at immediately placed implants: a randomized clinical trial. Clin Oral Implants Res. 2017;28:902–10.

57. Sarnachiaro GO, Chu SJ, Sarnachiaro E, Gotta SL, Tarnow DP. Immediate implant placement into extraction sockets with labial plate dehiscence defects: a clinical case series. Clin Implant Dent Relat Res. 2016;18:821–9.

58. Seibert JS. Treatment of moderate localized alveolar ridge defects. Preventive and reconstructive concepts in therapy. Dent Clin N Am. 1993;37:265–80.

59. Siebert C, Rieder D, Eggert J, Wichmann MG, Heckmann SM. Long-term esthetic outcome of tissue-level and bone-level implants in the anterior maxilla. Int J Oral Maxillofac Implants. 2018;33:905–12.

60. Slagter KW, Meijer HJ, Bakker NA, Vissink A, Raghoebar GM. Immediate single-tooth implant placement in bony defects in the esthetic zone: a 1-year randomized controlled trial. J Periodontol. 2016;87:619–29.

61. Spinato S, Stacchi C, Lombardi T, Bernardello F, Messina M, Zaffe D. Biological width establishment around dental implants is influenced by abutment height irrespective of vertical mucosal thickness: a cluster randomized controlled trial. Clin Oral Implants Res. 2019;30:649–59.

62. Stumbras A, Galindo-Moreno P, Januzis G, Juodzbalys G. Three-dimensional analysis of dimensional changes after alveolar ridge preservation with bone substitutes or plasma rich in growth factors: randomized and controlled clinical trial. Clin Implant Dent Relat Res. 2021;23(1):96–106.

63. Tan WL, Wong TL, Wong MC, Lang NP. A systematic review of post-extractional alveolar hard and soft tissue dimensional changes in humans. Clin Oral Implants Res. 2012;23 Suppl 5:1–21.

64. Tarnow DP, Chu SJ, Salama MA, Stappert CF, Salama H, Garber DA, Sarnachiaro GO, Sarnachiaro E, Gotta SL, Saito H. Flapless postextraction socket implant placement in the esthetic zone: part 1. The effect of bone grafting and/or provisional restoration on facial-palatal ridge dimensional change-a retrospective cohort study. Int J Periodontics Restorative Dent. 2014;34:323–31.

65. Wallner G, Rieder D, Wichmann MG, Heckmann SM. Peri-implant bone loss of tissue-level and bone-level implants in the esthetic zone with gingival biotype analysis. Int J Oral Maxillofac Implants. 2018;33:1119–25.

Reihaneh G. Mauer, Aida Shadrav, and Mahmood Dashti

Introduction

Modern dentistry takes advanced therapeutic measures to prolong the life span of teeth. However, loss of teeth still occurs due to trauma, periodontal disease, caries, developmental defects, and genetic disorders [3, 4]. While the incidence and prevalence of tooth loss has decreased, lack of teeth still impairs quality of life [1, 2]. One option to replace missing teeth is dental implants, which have some advantages over conventional treatment options. Implants replace the root of one or multiple missing teeth to provide anchorage for fixed or removable appliances [5]. The indications for implants are partial edentulism, non-retentive traditional dentures, and preserving the existing current partial dentures [6].

A dental implant is advantageous over fixed partial dentures because implants:

1. Have a 90–95% success over 10 years [7].
2. Have a noticeable effect on residual alveolar ridge preservation [8].
3. Decreased risk of caries [9].

There are four dental implants, including subperiosteal, blade form, ramus frame, and endosseous form [10]. The focus of this chapter will be on endosseous implants. As titanium alloys for excellent biocompatibility and a stable oxide layer [11], endosteal implants are placed into the mandible or the maxilla to replace a tooth root. The mechanical anchorage of the implant to the alveolar bone, also known as osseointegration, determines implant placement [12]. For precise evaluation of implant placement, the clinician should be aware of anatomical landmarks such as the mandibular canal position, maxillary sinus, the width of the cortical bone, and bone density [9].

Although implants have become a top choice of treatment for most dentists, many complications can arise from implant placement [7]. Tricio concluded that age, length of the implant, the implant's diameter, bone quality, and region of implant placement could contribute to dental implant failure.

Alberkson et al. described in 1986 the criteria for implant success [13]:

1. No implant mobility when tested clinically
2. No radiolucency around the implant in the radiograph
3. Bone loss less than 0.2 mm annually after the first year
4. No persistent pain, discomfort, infection, or damage to adjacent teeth
5. Success rate of 90% at the end of 5 years and 85% at the end of 10 years at the time of implant evaluation

These complications can be categorized into the following groups (Fig. 7.1):

1. Patients related factors
2. Practitioner related factors (Iatrogenic)
3. Implant related factors

Patient-Related Factors

Patient's related factors consist of systemic and local factors. Like any other dental treatment, implant treatment plans require a thorough and extensive review of the patient's medical conditions. The medical history should include the latest physical exam results, medication lists, and laboratory works. According to Hwang and Hom-Lay Wang, systemic factors affecting dental implants can be categorized into two

R. G. Mauer (✉)
Mauer Periodontics & Implant Dentistry, LLC,
Estero, FL, USA

A. Shadrav
Harvard School of Dental Medicine, Boston, MA, USA

M. Dashti
Private practice, Tehran, Iran
e-mail: Dashti-mahmood72@gmail.com

M. R. Stevens et al. (eds.), *Innovative Perspectives in Oral and Maxillofacial Surgery*,
https://doi.org/10.1007/978-3-030-75750-2_7

Fig. 7.1 Factors that affect the outcome of dental implant placement

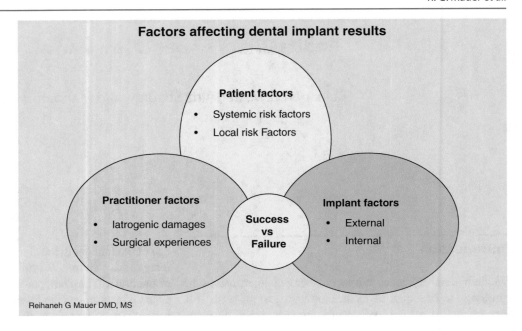

main groups: relative and absolute contraindications. Relative contraindications include adolescence, aging, osteoporosis, smoking, diabetes, positive interleukin-1 genotype, positive human immunodeficiency virus (HIV) antibody, cardiovascular disease, and hypothyroidism. Absolute contraindications include recent myocardial infarction and cerebrovascular accidents, valvular prosthesis surgery, immunosuppression, bleeding issues, active treatment of malignancy, drug abuse, psychiatric illness, current radiotherapy, and intravenous bisphosphonate use [14, 15]. Although the two categories have been discussed in the literature, Bornstein (2009) states that the level of evidence regarding systemic conditions and relative and absolute risks for implant surgeries is low. His study concluded that the controlled trials comparing patients with systemic diseases are scattered [16]. In summary, according to Hom-Lay Wang, implant placement is an elective surgery, "therefore any medical condition that raises the bar for dental implant placement should be reviewed by the patient's physician as well as the dental provider." In the worst possible cases, "noncompliance to the suggested protocol may result in patient mortality" [14, 15].

Patient's Local Factors or Site-Specific Factors

These factors include but may not be limited to oral hygiene habits, occlusal parafunctional habits, anatomical variances, hard and soft tissue quality and quantity, implant location, and restorative implant designs.

Oral Hygiene Habits

Oral hygiene status can be evaluated by plaque index and bleeding on probing. According to Mombelli (2002), the patient's periodontal microbiota may affect implant health status [17]. Schou et al. (2006) stated that the prevalence of peri-implantitis and marginal bone loss around the implant was significantly increased in patients with a history of tooth loss due to periodontitis [18]. Levin (2011) indicated that severe periodontitis and smoking are significant risk factors for late implant failures [19].

Recommendation for the Dental Provider

1. The practitioner should evaluate patients' periodontal status before proceeding with treatment.
2. Patient compliance should be considered to maintain overall oral health.
3. A patient should be aware of any oral habits and their effects on the dental implant outcome. Communication with the patient will strengthen trust with the provider and may increase patient compliance as well.
4. The practitioner should treat periodontal disease and restorative needs before proceeding with implant placement.

Parafunctional Habits

Among the parafunctional habits, bruxism has been counted as the most significant risk factor on implant survival rate [20]. Bruxism may cause mechanical and biological complications, according to Chrcanovic (2017).

Recommendation for the Dental Provider

1. The practitioner should discuss the pros and cons of implant placement with a Bruxer patient before starting the treatment.

2. The practitioner should be aware of restorative reinforcements treatments, including titanium bars, splinting crowns, and occlusal guards, which may increase longevity and survival rate of implant prosthesis [21].

Anatomical Variance

Any practitioner who provides dental implants needs to be equipped with extensive knowledge of anatomic structure. Greenstein et al. evaluated variance of essential structures related to dental implants. They concluded that it is critically important to be familiar with an anatomical variance to reduce any unexpected complications arising during the treatment. An essential diagnostic tool in implant dentistry is computerized tomography (CT) scanning, which evaluates the patient's unique anatomy [22, 23].

Recommendation for the Dental Provider

1. The practitioner should evaluate essential and vital structures related to specific sites before performing any treatment. The vital structures vary based on every individual and may impede dental implant plans. These structures include but are not limited to nerves, incisive canals, maxillary sinuses, and adjacent natural tooth root morphology.
2. The practitioner should consult with a radiologist for a complete evaluation.
3. The practitioner may need to consult with a medical provider if any abnormality is seen in cone beam CT scans.
4. The practitioner should be knowledgeable and capable of controlling unexpected complications such as bleeding due to artery damage, sinus membrane perforations, etc.

Hard Tissues

Similar to every other bone in our body, alveolar bone is a dynamic tissue. Both bone quality and quantity are important factors affecting implant failure [24]. The morphology of the bone, quality, and quantity is varied based on region and ethnic differences, and it is influenced by occlusal forces and skeletal and periodontal phenotype [22]. Zhang et al. also concluded that morphology of bone in the anterior maxilla might be different in patients with periodontitis [22].

Quality of Bone

Lekholm and Zarb classified alveolar bone quality into four groups. Type 1 is an alveolar bone that is largely made of cortical bone. Type 2 is alveolar bone with a dense medullary bone that is surrounded by a thick band of cortical bone. Type 3 is an alveolar bone that is made of thin cortical bone surrounding a dense medullary bone. Finally, type 4 is an alveolar bone that is made of very thin cortical bone surrounding a low-density medullary bone. According to Berman, type 4 alveolar bone showed a higher failure implant rate. Iijima et al. discuss that cortical bone thickness, trabecular bone, and cortical bone mineral density and bone hardness are significantly affected by mean failure force. Misch et al. also classified alveolar bone density in four types (D1 to D4) and related different regions in the jaw to different bone densities, as shown in Fig. 7.2.

Improving the surface of implants has been shown to have improved the survival rates in poor bone density [25].

Bone Quantity

The amount of bone in the implant region will affect implant stability [26]. UCLA has classified bone quantity at the

Fig. 7.2 Depicted bone density classification of jaw sites for different bone density types

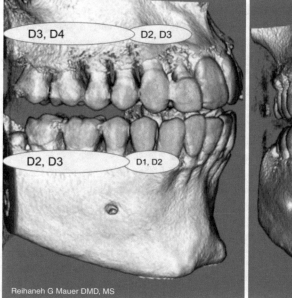
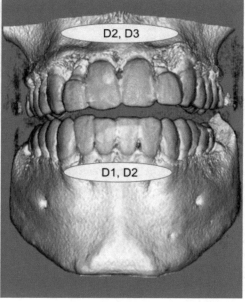

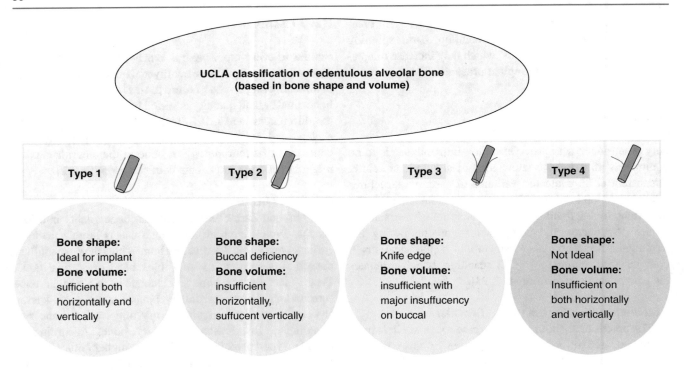

Fig. 7.3 UCLA classification is based on bone shape and volume [27]

implant site into four types, as shown in Fig. 7.3. Type 1 is classified as sufficient bone in horizontal and vertical dimensions, making the site ideal for implant placement. Type 2 is identified as an insufficient bone volume on the buccal side. Type 3 is classified as a knife-shaped alveolar bone, resulting in a significant bone volume deficiency on the buccal side but with sufficient height. Lastly, type 4 is classified as an insufficient alveolar height and width, resulting in implant exposure on all sides [27].

Bone Morphology

As demand for aesthetics increases, the teeth in the maxillary anterior region become a major concern. The alveolar morphology is not static and changes throughout one's life. Factors that should be considered in every implant treatment case include regional morphology and ethnic differences, the pattern of occlusion and occlusal forces, and skeletal and periodontal phenotypes.

Several studies have found thin buccal plates, and the presence of undercuts increase the risk of bone loss around the implant [22]. As mentioned before, CT scans and cone beam CT scans help the practitioner evaluate the sites prior to the treatment and recognize the possible complications.

Recommendation for the Dental Provider

- The practitioner should evaluate the implant site by clinical examination and diagnostic CBCT before the surgical appointment.

- Site preservation after extraction would be recommended as studies show that it preserves ridge dimensions [25].
- Edentulous ridge deficiencies are classified as horizontal, vertical, or combined.[30] The HVC classification method and related recommended treatment modalities by Dr. Hom-Lay Wang is discussed in Fig. 7.4 [29]. Misch et al. provided the treatment options available for ridge augmentation in posterior mandible shown in Table 7.3. In general, surgical procedures that increase vertical or horizontal alveolar bone heights include guided bone regeneration (GBR), ridge split technique, block graft (autogenous, allograft), distraction osteogenesis, sinus lift the maxilla, interpositional osteotomy, and nerve repositioning on the posterior mandible [30]. A practitioner must have extensive knowledge of indications, contraindications, advantages, and disadvantages of every procedure.

Soft Tissues

The need for adequate width and thickness of soft tissue around natural teeth and implants has been mentioned in many studies [31–33].

Width of Attached Keratinized Tissue

Having less than the minimum of 2 mm of keratinized mucosa may result in peri-implant disease [34]. An inadequate kera-

Fig. 7.4 Hom-Lay Wang classification and recommended treatment options [28]. *D.O* distraction osteogenesis, *GBR* guided bone regeneration

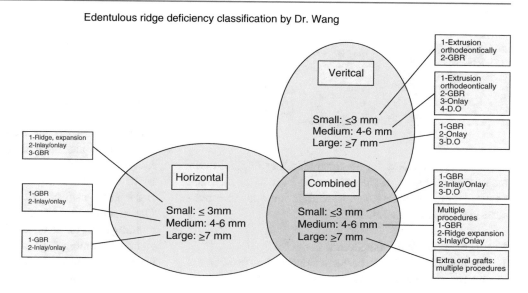

Edentulous ridge deficiency classification by Dr. Wang

tinized tissue and mucosa around the tooth and implant may impede patient oral hygiene and increase inflammation in the surrounding soft tissue. Therefore, it may cause the further mucosal recession and attachment loss [32].

Thickness of Mucosal Connective Tissue

According to the 2nd Osteology Consensus 2017, thickening of connective tissue around implants would increase interproximal bone level around implants compared to non-augmented sites [32].

In summary, increasing keratinized mucosa around the implant mitigates tissue inflammation, plaque index, recession, and attachment loss and increasing oral hygiene effects and vestibular depth [33]. Increasing the thickness of mucosa prevents tissue recession, results in better aesthetic results and less marginal bone loss, and improves adaptation of soft tissue around the implant [32, 33].

Recommendation for the Dental Provider

1. Keratinized soft tissue augmentation in cases with less than 2 mm of keratinized mucosa. Procedures include apically positioned split flaps (vestibulopathy), with or without application of autogenous grafts or collagenous allografts. It can be done any time during implant treatments after the second stage uncovery or final restorations [32].
2. Increasing subepithelial connective tissue in case of a compromised function or aesthetic reason. Surgical procedures include a coronally advanced flap with or without autogenous or allografts, tunneling technique with or without autogenous or allografts, and vestibular incision subepithelial tunnel access technique with or without autogenous or allografts.

Table 7.1 Four functional implant zones were introduced by Tolstunov (2007)

Functional implant zones	Teeth/jaw	Problems
FIZ 1 (traumatic zone)	2 first premolars, 6 anterior teeth/premaxilla	History of trauma and compromised soft tissue and hard tissue, high demand aesthetic zone, thin buccal plates
FIZ 2 (sinus zone)	2 second premolars, molars/posterior maxilla	Sinus pneumatization, vertical bone deficiency, type 3, 4 bone density
FIZ 3 (interforaminal zone)	2 first premolars, 6 anterior teeth/anterior mandible	Thin and narrow alveolar ridge, life-threatening hemorrhage due to damage to sublingual artery branches, highly skilled practitioner
FIZ 4 (ischemic zone)	2 second premolars and molars/behind mental foramen, above IAN canal/posterior mandible	Anatomical limitation, poor blood supply, access difficulties, vertical bone loss

Implant Site and Location

Implant location appears as one of the significant factors affecting the prognosis of the implants [35]. Implant success is influenced by multiple site-specific factors, including quality and quantity of bone in specific zones, history of trauma of the zone, the proximity of anatomical structures, accessibility for surgical procedures, and degree of blood supply and potential healings [35]. Tolstunov (2007) introduced the four functional implant zones, explaining the anatomical structures and what problems dental providers face, shown in Table 7.1. He also compared two functional

Functional implant zone (FIZ)	Main concerns for implant placement	Bone graft needs
FIZ 1	Aesthetic, osseointegration	Increasing width
FIZ 4	Function, osseointegration	Increasing height

implants, zones 1 and 4, and concluded that implant treatment's main challenges in each zone 1 are aesthetics and osseointegration but in zone 4 are function and osseointegration as depicted in Table 7.2.

Recommendation for the Dental Provider

1. The practitioner should perform a comprehensive clinical and radiological examination, in addition to a thorough dental history, to evaluate any deficiency in the area.
2. The practitioner should consider regenerative bone procedures in the early stages before implant placement to prevent complications after placements.
3. The practitioner should treat every patient with a high smile line with the aesthetic needs in mind.
4. Soft tissue augmentation in the anterior area may increase tissue adaptation and prevent further bone loss and recession.
5. A taper implant choice may be more protective of buccal plates, and also platform switching concept may prevent marginal bone loss.
6. The practitioner should consider implant-treated surfaces, which may increase primary stability and improve healing.
7. The practitioner may place a provisional crown to improve healing.
8. The practitioner should give enough time for bone regeneration, which takes approximately 6 months, before fully loading the implants in grafted sites [35].
9. The practitioner should always emphasize oral hygiene instructions, home care, and maintenance.

Implant Restorative Parts

All dental implants should be placed based on comprehensive restorative plans [36]. Unlike teeth, implants lack periodontal ligament and therefore cannot distribute occlusal forces evenly [37]. The restorative problems include but are not limited to unsatisfied aesthetic crown contour, emergence profile, lack of cleanability, ceramic chipping, occlusal screw loosening, abutment loosening, occlusal screw fractures, abutment fracture, and implant fractures [38]. Wittneben et al. (2013) con-

cluded that ceramic chipping had the highest prevalence of complications, and it was higher in implant-supported fixed dental prosthesis than single tooth implants [38]. Thorough treatment planning in advance, including predicting the mechanical forces on the implants in different mouth areas, may prevent biomechanical challenges in the future [32].

Recommendation for the Dental Provider

1. The practitioner should conduct a thorough clinical examination and evaluate the spaces based on restorative needs with special attention to mesiodistal, buccolingual, and interocclusal space.
2. The practitioner should consider regenerative and augmenting procedures in case of any soft or hard tissue deficiency. Planning any additional surgeries to support implant soft and hard tissue in advance will prevent future aesthetic and biomechanical problems.
3. Implant platform should be placed 3–4 mm from the gingival zenith and CEJ of adjacent teeth to provide a natural crown contour, emergence profile, and cleansability [39].
4. The implant should be placed 1.5 mm from the adjacent natural tooth and 3 mm from the adjoining implant and have >1 mm natural bone buccolingually [40].
5. The dental provider should consider interocclusal spaces based on restorative needs, material, and restorative designs, for instance, a range of 8–12 mm for a single tooth implant, a range of 9–16 mm for implant overdenture, and a minimum of 22 mm for double arch hybrid prosthesis between two arches [40, 41].

Iatrogenic Factors

Iatrogenic factors can be divided into surgical miscalculations or restorative mistakes.

Iatrogenic Complications in Surgery

Misplacement of implants may result in failure owing to inflammatory reactions or mechanical problems. Placing an implant too shallow interferes with restorative space needed for excellent crown design and cleanability. On the other hand, placing an implant too deep may cause an inflammatory response and bone resorption. Miscalculations in implant angles, buccolingually or mesiodistally, may violate restorative space needs [38–42]. Research by Trisi et al. concluded that drilling the osteotomy at a speed of 1000 rpm with no irrigation has a negative effect on bone and results in extensive cortical bone loss and implant failure [43].

Iatrogenic Complications in Restorative Dentistry

Restorative crown design and profile is an important factor in implant success.

Restorative Materials

There is no wrong or correct answer to choosing a particular material. Clinicians should consider dental material based on functional and aesthetic needs.

Implant Body Design

The stock or custom abutments should be ordered based on space evaluations to avoid supracrestal attachments violation and food impaction [44]. Similar to natural tooth crown margins, implant crown margins should be placed within 1 mm from the gingival crest to avoid unwanted cement retention and unfavorable inflammatory reactions [44, 45]. The emergence profile is an important factor for aesthetic satisfaction.

Crown/Root Ratio

Schulte (2007) showed that the crown/root ratio of the failed implants was similar to successful ones and concluded that implant crown/root ratio calculations should not follow the same as natural teeth [46].

Recommendation for the Dental Provider

1. The practitioner should avoid the placement of the implant custom or prefabricated margins more than 1 mm below the gingival crest to avoid cement retention [44].
2. The practitioner should take a vertical bitewing after any crown cementation to confirm fit or if any cement remains in the interproximal space when using radiopaque cement.
3. The practitioner should meet patients' aesthetic needs regarding the shade and shape of the crowns.
4. In the case of using cement crowns, screw access should be marked for any retrieval treatment in the future [45].
5. The practitioner should justify irrigation based on the speed of the drill at the time of osteotomy preparation [47].
6. The practitioner should follow the instructions and drill sequences as recommended by each particular implant system. Oversizing of the osteotomy will result in a reduction of primary stability.

Implant Factors

Implant factors include implant size and implant designs categorized as macro-design or micro-design. The macro-design is characterized by the implant body, neck, and apex designs, which have the threads shapes, numbers, and pitches [48, 49]. The micro-design of the implant includes the surface roughness [49]. The screw thread implants are the most popular designs due to their excellent initial retention and optimal stress distribution [50].

Implant Size

The International Team for Implantology (ITI) consensus in 2018 concluded that implants with a short height ≤6 mm are viable options but show decreased survival rates. It was also supposed that implants with a diameter less than 2.5 mm demonstrated a lower survival rate. Furthermore, tapered implants did not show significant differences with non-tapered implants in outcome [51].

Implant Design

Macro-design

Shape

Implant designs include cylindrical, conical, and tapered bodies. Tapered implants increase primary stability by gradually expanding the ridge and reducing the stress at the bone interface [49]. The implant connections are designed as external or internal connections. Esposito (2016) did not find any significant difference regarding implant failure between two types of connections [52].

Threads

Implant threads are categorized based on shape, size, depth, width, and pitch. A study by Ryu (2014) concluded that microthreads at the neck would improve osseointegration. Thread shape includes square, V-shape, trapezius, and buttress. Ryu concluded that square design threads, smaller pitch, and microthread configuration at the neck of the implant provide more stability in immediate loading [48].

Micro-designs

Surface treatment aims to increase the bone-implant contact area to improve the primary stability and further osseointegration. Various methods include surface coating with hydroxyapatite or titanium particles, sandblasting, acid etching, or combining both etching and sandblasting (SLA) [49]. Implants with a smooth neck surface may improve bone integration by reducing the plaque attachments [53]; on the contrary, implants with less body roughness may provoke the formation of fibrous tissue around the implant [54].

Table 7.3 Susan Wingrove (2018) based on AAP/EFP World Workshop on classification of implant health and conditions (2017) [57]

Implant health status	PD	BOP	Bone loss	Exudate (suppuration)	Tissue inflammation
Implant health	3–4 mm	Absent	No, <2.0 mm	Absent	Absent
Peri-implant mucositis	Not increased from baseline	Present	No, <2.0 mm	Maybe present	Present
Peri-implantitis	Increased from baseline	Present	Yes, >2.0 mm	Maybe present	Present

Recommendation for the Dental Provider

1. The practitioner should be familiar with the implant systems and designs as it will affect the treatment's final result.
2. The practitioner should choose every implant's size and design based on different treatment plan scenarios, including immediate or delayed implant placement, immediate or delayed implant loading, and anatomical barriers.
3. The practitioner should educate the patient regarding the importance of periodic maintenance and examinations to diagnose early problems, including screw loosening or biological issues.

Peri-implant Health and Disease

The American Academy of Periodontology (AAP) and the European Federation of Periodontology (EFP) met at World Workshop 2017 to establish a new classification for periodontal status and also peri-implant conditions. The World Workshop classified peri-implant status into four categories including [55]:

1. Peri-implant health
2. Peri-implant mucositis
3. Peri-implantitis
4. Peri-implant soft and hard tissue deficiency

Diagnosis of peri-implant disease is based on the existence or absence of inflammation signs such as changing in gingival color, bleeding on probing, probing depth, suppurations, and bone level at the implant site [56].

Peri-implant Health

The World Workshop 2018 defined implant health as probing depth around implants ranging approximately 3–4 mm and covered by either a keratinized or non-keratinized epithelium.

Peri-implant Mucositis

According to the World Workshop 2018, the primary etiology is based on plaque accumulation moderated by host response. Diabetes, smoking, and radiation may modify this condition [55].

Peri-implantitis

According to World Workshop 2018, peri-implantitis may be linked to remaining cement after restorative appointments and factors affecting plaque retention such as malpositioned implants. In addition, diabetes and smoking are identified as potential risk factors for peri-implantitis. There is a need for more investigations on risk indicators such as the role of peri-implant keratinized mucosa, occlusal overload, titanium particles, bone compression necrosis, overheating, micromotion, and bio-corrosions [55].

Peri-implant Soft and Hard Tissue Deficiencies

Multiple factors are affecting both soft and hard tissue quality and quantity, such as implant malposition, lack of buccal bone, thin, soft tissue, lack of keratinized tissue, the status of attachment of the adjacent teeth, and surgical trauma [55].

Wingrove (2018) discussed the clinical implication of the new World Workshop 2018 classification and provided clinical application [57]. She mentioned that the dental provider should record all the probing depth (PD), bleeding on probing (BOP), soft tissue inflammation, bone loss, and taking radiographs at the time of implant placements, delivery of restoration, and a year after surgical placement. Table 7.3 summarize findings in implant health, peri-implant mucositis, and peri-implantitis status. She also mentioned that in case of absence of baseline information and bone loss of more than 3 mm and presence of recession, pocket depth of more than 6 mm, and exudate/suppuration indicates the peri-implantitis categories.

The cumulative interceptive supportive therapy (CIST) was introduced by Lang (2008), shown in Fig. 7.5. The diagnosis is based on the following [58]:

1. Presence or absence of dental plaque
2. Presence or absence of bleeding on probing
3. Presence or absence of pus and exudate
4. Peri-implant probing depth
5. Evidence of radiographic bone loss

Conclusion

While the incidence and prevalence of tooth loss have decreased, lack of teeth still impairs quality of life [1]. Many practitioners have moved toward using implants over conventional therapies.

Various factors may affect the result of implant surgeries. Therefore, a practitioner should know patient medical and dental history, iatrogenic damages, and implant characteristics. Furthermore, the dental practitioner should perform a

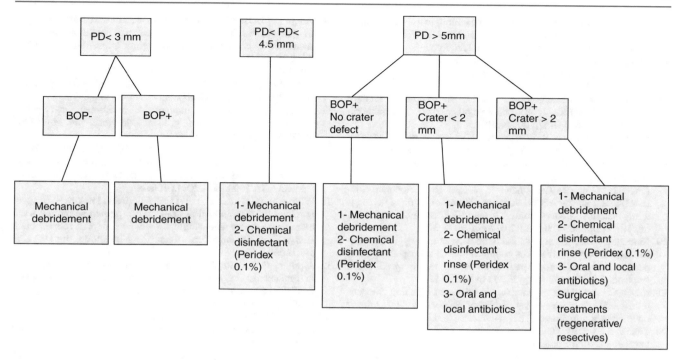

Fig. 7.5 CIST protocol was introduced by Dr. Lang

comprehensive clinical exam before performing any implant surgical procedure. Once the implant is placed, the practitioner should routinely check the status and health of the implant and the tissue surrounding it.

Conflict of Interest The authors of this paper certify that they have no conflict of interest.

References

1. Gerritsen AE, Allen PF, Witter DJ, Bronkhorst EM, Creugers NH. Tooth loss and oral health-related quality of life: a systematic review and meta-analysis. Health Qual Life Outcomes. 2010;8:126. https://doi.org/10.1186/1477-7525-8-126.
2. Saintrain MV, de Souza EH. Impact of tooth loss on the quality of life. Gerodontology. https://doi.org/10.1111/j.1741-2358.2011.00535.x.
3. Zohrabian VM, Sonick M, Hwang D, Abrahams JJ. Dental implants. Semin Ultrasound CT MR. https://doi.org/10.1053/j.sult.2015.09.002.
4. Searson L. Implantology in general dental practice. http://www.quintpub.com/display_detail.php3?psku=B8904#.X3N6iBNKjzI. Accessed 29 Sept 2020.
5. Ihde S, Sipic O. Functional and esthetic indication for dental implant treatment and immediate loading (2) case report and considerations: typical attitudes of dentists (and their unions) toward tooth extractions and the prevention of early, effective, and helpful dental implant treatment in the European Union. Ann Maxillofac Surg. https://doi.org/10.4103/ams.ams_152_19.
6. Grisar K, Sinha D, Schoenaers J, Dormaar T, Politis C. Retrospective analysis of dental implants placed between 2012 and 2014: indi-

cations, risk factors, and early survival. Int J Oral Maxillofac Implants. https://doi.org/10.11607/jomi.5332
7. Tricio J, Laohapand P, van Steenberghe D, Quirynen M, Naert I. Mechanical state assessment of the implant-bone continuum: a better understanding of the Periotest method. Int J Oral Maxillofac Implants. Published February 1995. https://pubmed.ncbi.nlm.nih.gov/7615316/. Accessed 29 Sept 2020.
8. Khalifa AK, Wada M, Ikebe K, Maeda Y. To what extent residual alveolar ridge can be preserved by implant? A systematic review. Int J Implant Dent. 2016;2:22. https://doi.org/10.1186/s40729-016-0057-z.
9. Gupta R, Gupta N, Weber KK. Dental implants. StatPearls Publishing; 2020. https://www.ncbi.nlm.nih.gov/books/NBK470448/. Accessed 29 Sept 2020.
10. Han H. (PDF) Design of new root-form endosseous dental implant and evaluation of fatigue strength using finite element analysis. ResearchGate. https://www.researchgate.net/publication/40721705_Design_of_new_root-form_endosseous_dental_implant_and_evaluation_of_fatigue_strength_using_finite_element_analysis. Accessed 29 Sept 2020.
11. Saini M, Singh Y, Arora P, Arora V, Jain K. Implant biomaterials: a comprehensive review. World J Clin Cases WJCC. 2015;3(1):52–7. https://doi.org/10.12998/wjcc.v3.i1.52.
12. Javed F, Ahmed HB, Crespi R, Romanos GE. Role of primary stability for successful osseointegration of dental implants: factors of influence and evaluation. Interv Med Appl Sci. 2013;5(4):162. https://doi.org/10.1556/IMAS.5.2013.4.3.
13. Albrektsson T, Zarb G, Worthington P, Eriksson AR. The long-term efficacy of currently used dental implants: a review and proposed criteria of success. Int J Oral Maxillofac Implants. Published Summer 1986. https://pubmed.ncbi.nlm.nih.gov/3527955/. Accessed 27 Oct 2020.
14. Hwang D, Wang H-L. Medical contraindications to implant therapy: part I: absolute contraindications. Implant Dent. 2006;15(4):353–60. https://doi.org/10.1097/01.id.0000247855.75691.03.

15. Hwang D, Wang H-L. Medical contraindications to implant therapy: part II: relative contraindications. Implant Dent. 2007;16(1):13–23. https://doi.org/10.1097/ID.0b013e31803276c8.

16. Bornstein MM, Cionca N, Mombelli A. Systemic conditions and treatments as risks for implant therapy. Int J Oral Maxillofac Implants. 2009;24(Suppl):12–27.

17. Mombelli A. Microbiology and antimicrobial therapy of peri-implantitis. Periodontology. 2000. https://doi.org/10.1034/j.1600-0757.2002.280107.x.

18. Schou S, Holmstrup P, Worthington HV, Esposito M. Outcome of implant therapy in patients with previous tooth loss due to periodontitis. Clin Oral Implants Res. https://doi.org/10.1111/j.1600-0501.2006.01347.x.

19. Levin L, Ofec R, Grossmann Y, Anner R. Periodontal disease as a risk for dental implant failure over time: a long-term historical cohort study. J Clin Periodontol. https://doi.org/10.1111/j.1600-051X.2011.01745.x.

20. Chrcanovic BR, Kisch J, Albrektsson T, Wennerberg A. Bruxism and dental implant treatment complications: a retrospective comparative study of 98 bruxer patients and a matched group. Clin Oral Implants Res. https://doi.org/10.1111/clr.12844.

21. Misch C. The effect of bruxism on treatment planning for dental implants. Dentistry today. Published September 2002. https://pubmed.ncbi.nlm.nih.gov/12271847/. Accessed 26 Oct 2020.

22. Zhang X. (PDF) The dimension and morphology of alveolar bone at maxillary anterior teeth in periodontitis: a retrospective analysis—using CBCT. ResearchGate. https://doi.org/10.1038/s41368-019-0071-0.

23. Greenstein G, Cavallaro J, Tarnow D. Practical application of anatomy for the dental implant surgeon. J Periodontol. https://doi.org/10.1902/jop.2008.080086.

24. Iijima M, Takano M, Yasuda Y, et al. Effect of the quantity and quality of cortical bone on the failure force of a miniscrew implant. Eur J Orthod. https://doi.org/10.1093/ejo/cjs066.

25. Avila-Ortiz G, Elangovan S, Kramer KWO, Blanchette D, Dawson DV. Effect of alveolar ridge preservation after tooth extraction: a systematic review and meta-analysis. J Dent Res. 2014;93(10):950. https://doi.org/10.1177/0022034514541127.

26. Themes UFO. Bone density for dental implants. Pocket Dentistry. Published 12 Apr 2015. https://pocketdentistry.com/bone-density-for-dental-implants/. Accessed 27 Oct 2020.

27. Seriwatanachai D. Reference and techniques used in alveolar bone classification. JBR J Interdiscip Med Dent Sci. 2015;03(02). https://doi.org/10.4172/2376-032X.1000172.

28. Wang H-L, Al-Shammari K. HVC ridge deficiency classification: a therapeutically oriented classification. Restor Dent. 2002;22(4):10.

29. Lee Y. A new maxillary anterior ridge classification according to ideal implant restorative position determined by computerized axial tomographic analysis. https://ir.ymlib.yonsei.ac.kr/bitstream/22282913/136061/1/TA01026.pdf. Accessed 26 Oct 2020.

30. Misch CM, Block MS, Pikos MA, Zadeh HM. How consistent are vertical augmentation procedures in anterior versus posterior regions? https://www.aegisdentalnetwork.com/cced/2017/07/how-consistent-are-vertical-augmentation-procedures-in-anterior-versus-posterior-regions. Accessed 26 Oct 2020.

31. Lin G-H, Chan H-L, Wang H-L. The significance of keratinized mucosa on implant health: a systematic review. J Periodontol. 2013;84(12):1755–67. https://doi.org/10.1902/jop.2013.120688.

32. Giannobile W, Jung RE, Schwarz F. Evidence-based knowledge on the aesthetics and maintenance of peri-implant soft tissues: Osteology Foundation Consensus Report Part 1-Effects of soft tissue augmentation procedures on the maintenance of peri-implant soft tissue health. Clin Oral Implants Res. https://doi.org/10.1111/clr.13110.

33. Zucchelli G, Tavelli L, McGuire MK, et al. Autogenous soft tissue grafting for periodontal and peri-implant plastic surgical reconstruction. J Periodontol. 2020;91(1):9–16. https://doi.org/10.1002/JPER.19-0350.

34. Monje A, Blasi G. Significance of keratinized mucosa/gingiva on peri-implant and adjacent periodontal conditions in erratic maintenance compliers. J Periodontol. https://doi.org/10.1002/JPER.18-0471

35. Tolstunov L. Implant zones of the jaws: implant location and related success rate. J Oral Implantol. https://doi.org/10.1563/1548-1336(2007)33[211:IZOTJI]2.0.CO;2.

36. Scherer M. Presurgical implant-site assessment and restoratively driven digital planning. Dent Clin North Am. https://doi.org/10.1016/j.cden.2014.04.002.

37. Kim Y, Oh TJ, Misch CE, Wang HL. Occlusal considerations in implant therapy: clinical guidelines with biomechanical rationale. Clin Oral Implants Res. https://doi.org/10.1111/j.1600-0501.2004.01067.x.

38. Wittneben JG, Buser D, Salvi GE, Bürgin W, Hicklin S, Brägger U. Complication and failure rates with implant-supported fixed dental prostheses and single crowns: a 10-year retrospective study. Clin Implant Dent Relat Res. https://doi.org/10.1111/cid.12066.

39. Aguilera F. Avoiding complications during the restorative phase of implant dentistry. Decisions in Dentistry. https://decisionsindentistry.com/article/avoiding-complications-restorative-implant-dentistry/. Accessed 29 Sept 2020.

40. Shenoy VK. Single tooth implants: pretreatment considerations and pretreatment evaluation. J Interdisc Dent. 2012;2(3):149. https://doi.org/10.4103/2229-5194.113239.

41. Jensen O. The all-on-4 shelf: maxilla. J Oral Maxillofac Surg. 2010;68(10):2520–7. https://doi.org/10.1016/j.joms.2010.05.082.

42. Hanif A, Qureshi S, Sheikh Z, Rashid H. Complications in implant dentistry. Eur J Dent Edu. 2017;11(1):135. https://doi.org/10.4103/ejd.ejd_340_16.

43. Trisi P. New osseodensification implant site preparation method to increase bone density in low-density bone: in vivo evaluation in sheep. - Abstract - Europe PMC. https://europepmc.org/article/pmc/4770273. Accessed 29 Sept 2020.

44. Schoenbaum T. Material selection guidelines for single-unit implant crowns and abutments | Inside Dental Technology. https://www.aegisdentalnetwork.com/idt/2014/07/Material-Selection-Guidelines-for-Single-Unit-Implant-Crowns-and-Abutments. Accessed 17 Oct 2020.

45. Linkevicius T, Vindasiute E, Puisys A, Peciuliene V. The influence of margin location on the amount of undetected cement excess after delivery of cement-retained implant restorations: cement excess around subgingival margins. Clin Oral Implants Res. 2011;22(12):1379–84. https://doi.org/10.1111/j.1600-0501.2010.02119.x.

46. Schulte J, Am F, Weed M. Crown-to-implant ratios of single tooth implant-supported restorations. J Prosthet Dent. 2007;98(1):1–5. https://doi.org/10.1016/s0022-3913(07)60031-6.

47. Pellicer-Chover H, Peñarrocha-Oltra D, Aloy-Prosper A, Sanchis-Gonzalez J-C, Peñarrocha-Diago M, Peñarrocha-Diago M. Comparison of peri-implant bone loss between conventional drilling with irrigation versus low-speed drilling without irrigation. Med Oral Patol Oral Cir Bucal. 2017;22(6):e730. https://doi.org/10.4317/medoral.21694.

48. Ryu H-S, Namgung C, Lee J-H, Lim Y-J. The influence of thread geometry on implant osseointegration under immediate loading: a literature review. J Adv Prosthodont. 2014;6(6):547. https://doi.org/10.4047/jap.2014.6.6.547.

49. Tetè S, Zizzari V, De Carlo A, Sinjari B, Gherlone E. Macroscopic and microscopic evaluation of a new implant design supporting immediately loaded full arch rehabilitation. Ann Stomatol (Roma). 2012;3(2):44–50.

50. Chun H, Cheong S, Han J, et al. Evaluation of design parameters of osseointegrated dental implants using finite element analysis. J Oral Rehabil. https://doi.org/10.1046/j.1365-2842.2002.00891.x.

51. Proceedings of the Sixth ITI Consensus Conference (2018) - Home. https://www.iti.org/academy/publications/proceedings-of-iti-consensus-conferences/proceedings-of-the-sixth-iti-consensus-conference-2018. Accessed 17 Oct 2020.

52. Esposito M, Maghaireh H, Pistilli R, et al. Dental implants with internal versus external connections: 5-year post-loading results from a pragmatic multicenter randomised controlled trial. Eur J Oral Implant. 2016;9 Suppl 1(2):129–41.

53. Heinmann F. Influence of the implant cervical topography on the crestal bone resorption and immediate implant survival. http://www.jpp.krakow.pl/journal/archive/12_09_s8/articles/17_article.html. Accessed 17 Oct 2020.

54. Wennerberg A, Albrektsson T, Andersson B, Krol JJ. A histomorphometric study of screw-shaped and removal torque titanium implants with three different surface topographies. Clin Oral Implants Res. 1995;6(1):24–30. https://doi.org/10.1034/j.1600-0501.1995.060103.x.

55. Berglundh T, Armitage G, Araujo MG, et al. Peri-implant diseases and conditions: consensus report of workgroup 4 of the 2017 World Workshop on the Classification of Periodontal and Peri-Implant Diseases and Conditions. J Periodontol. 2018;89:S313–8. https://doi.org/10.1002/JPER.17-0739.

56. Prathapachandran J, Suresh N. Management of peri-implantitis. Dent Res J. 2012;9(5):516. https://doi.org/10.4103/1735-3327.104867.

57. Wingrove S. Clinical applications for the 2018 classification of peri-implant diseases and conditions. Perio-Implant Advisory. Published 6 Nov 2018. https://www.perioimplantadvisory.com/clinical-tips/hygiene-techniques/article/16412254/clinical-applications-for-the-2018-classification-of-periimplant-diseases-and-conditions. Accessed 4 Oct 2020.

58. Tamim A. Cumulative interceptive supportive therapy (C.I.S.T). ResearchGate. https://doi.org/10.13140/2.1.3208.4488.

Peri-implantitis

Hani Abd-Ul-Salam

Introduction

Dental implants have revolutionized patients' management with missing teeth over the last few decades [1, 2]. As the dental implant market continues to expand globally, and as patients live longer, more implants are placed in partially and completely edentulous and medically compromised patients. Despite the high success of dental implants, the existing biological and mechanical complications should not be underestimated [3, 4]. Maintaining healthy peri-implant tissues is crucial for the long-term success of dental implants. This chapter discusses the peri-implant disease and is divided into two parts: the first part focuses on peri-implant mucositis and peri-implantitis and the second part reviews the peri-apical implant lesions, also known as retrograde peri-implantitis.

Part I: Peri-implant Mucositis and Peri-implantitis

Biological Differences Between Teeth and Implants

Although dental implants are used to replace teeth, biological differences exist between them. Understanding these differences at both the bone and soft tissue levels would help appreciate the pathological process of peri-implant disease etiology.

A dental implant is made up of an intra-osseous component, analogous to the root of a tooth, to which a trans-mucosal component called an abutment is attached. The crown connects to the abutment either via a screw or via a layer of cement. The healing process around the intra-osseous component of a dental implant, in which bone establishes a direct contact and a functional relationship with the implant, is called "osseointegration" [5]. In contrast, a natural tooth connects to the bone indirectly via a periodontal ligament. The absence of a periodontal ligament around an implant contributes to peri-implant disease's potential etiology [6].

A natural tooth is surrounded by gingiva, whereas an implant is surrounded by mucosa. Although both the gingiva and peri-implant mucosa form a barrier around the teeth and implants, respectively, that aid in preventing subgingival plaque formation and bacterial infiltration, microscopic findings show that collagen fibers, around peri-implant mucosa, were oriented parallel to the surface of the abutment [7]. In contrast, around natural teeth, collagen fibers in the periodontal ligament are organized in a more complex fashion. Histologically, the connective tissue attachment around teeth has a complex fiber arrangement that includes transeptal, inter-circular, circular, interpapillary, dento-gingival, and trans-gingival fibers. This fiber arrangement provides a perfect protective architecture [8, 9] compared to a less protective architecture around dental implants. Hence, mucosal tissues around implants tend to be comparatively more fragile and less protective compared to natural teeth, which could be attributed to increased penetration of peroxides from inflammatory cells around peri-implant tissues compared to periodontal tissues [10].

The biologic width is a physiological protective distance that ensures a healthy periodontium's stability around both teeth and dental implants. The biologic width is 2 mm of junctional epithelium and connective tissue attachments with a sulcus depth of 0.7 mm [11]. Similarly, around implants, the biologic width is 2.5 mm with a sulcus depth of 0.5 mm [12]. The biologic width is dynamically stable over time [13], and it is not affected by immediate or early loading [14, 15].

H. Abd-Ul-Salam (✉)
Faculty of Dentistry, McGill University, Montreal, PQ, Canada

Faculty of Dentistry, University of Sharjah, University City, Sharjah, UAE
e-mail: hani.salam@mcgill.ca

Definitions and Classifications

According to the Fifth International Team for Implantology (ITI) consensus conference, peri-implant health was defined as the absence of clinical signs of inflammation. A recent consensus defined peri-implant health as the absence of erythema, bleeding on probing, swelling, and suppuration [16].

The ITI defined peri-implant mucositis as a mucosal inflammatory condition around dental implants clinically evident typically by the presence of clinical signs of soft tissue inflammation such as redness, edema, suppuration, and bleeding on gentle probing without concomitant crestal bone loss. Recently, it was defined as an inflammatory lesion of the soft tissue surrounding an endosseous implant in the absence of loss of supporting bone or continuing marginal bone loss. Bleeding on probing is the primary clinical characteristic [16].

Peri-implantitis, a progressive complication developing at a later stage than peri-implant mucositis, was defined by the ITI as the presence of mucositis in conjunction with radiographic progressive crestal bone loss [17] (Fig. 8.1). Bleeding on probing alone is insufficient to diagnose peri-implantitis. A progressive radiographic bone loss must be demonstrated, as well, to establish a diagnosis of peri-implantitis [18, 19]. It is prudent to distinguish loss of bone peri-implantitis from crestal bone loss associated with clinical signs of inflamma-

tion mentioned earlier. It is also important to differentiate between peri-implantitis that is initiated by bacterial infections and peri-implant mucositis from a failed osseointegrated implant that has been in function for years. In those cases, there is no evidence of any of the inflammatory signs noted in peri-implant mucositis as well as radiographic signs of progressive bone loss. In a recent consensus, peri-implantitis was defined as a plaque-associated pathological condition occurring in tissues around dental implants, characterized by inflammation in the peri-implant mucosa such as bleeding on probing and/or suppuration and subsequent progressive bone loss.

In essence, peri-implant mucositis is comparable to gingivitis around teeth, whereas peri-implantitis is comparable to periodontitis. Depending on the host immune response, the pathogen-induced disease could potentially lead to progressive bone resorption. Therefore, peri-implant mucositis, if untreated, could progress to peri-implantitis [20]. This process is comparable in a way to gingivitis that may lead to alveolar bone loss and periodontitis, potentially resulting in the loss of dentition.

Other classifications of peri-implant disease were based on etiology [21] or prognosis [22]. Recently, a consensus report on the classification of peri-implant disease maintained similar definitions for peri-implant disease [16, 23].

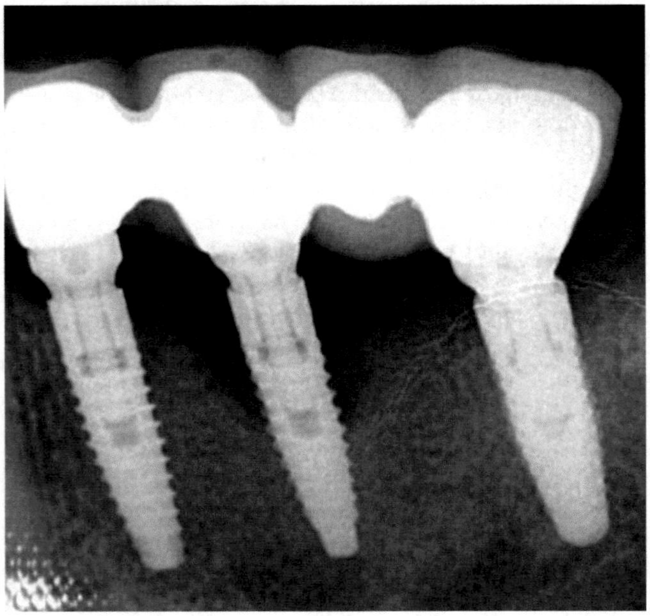

Fig. 8.1 Radiographic image showing peri-implantitis. Radiographic image shows evidence of progressive bone loss around the middle endosseous dental implant. Clinically, erythema and suppuration of mucosal tissues around dental implants were present indicating peri-implantitis. If radiographic examination did not demonstrate progressive bone loss, then the clinical situation is consistent with peri-implant mucositis. (Clinical case report; Dr. Hani Abd-Ul-Salam)

Diagnostic Parameters for Monitoring Peri-implant Health

The third ITI consensus has identified diagnostic parameters for monitoring peri-implant conditions, including the presence of plaque/biofilm, mucosal inflammation, peri-implant probing depth, bleeding on probing, suppuration, and radiographic evaluation. Those diagnostic criteria allow the evaluation of the peri-implant health status and subsequent appropriate therapeutic measures. Despite these measures, occasionally, patients would present with no obvious visible clinical signs of inflammation and/or infection [24].

Prevalence

The prevalence of peri-implant disease ranges from 9% to 50% [25–29]. It is estimated that peri-implant mucositis's mean prevalence is 43% and half of that for peri-implantitis [30]. This extreme variation in the incidence range leads to questions about the basic premise of whether a clear definition or understanding of the disease exists or whether peri-implant disease was confused with the limited crestal bone loss. It was suggested that only 1–2% of the implants show true peri-implantitis over 10 years [31]. In another 10-year study, the prevalence of peri-implantitis was 18% for implants placed in bone-grafted sites compared to 10% in non-grafted sites [32].

Etiology

Various factors affect the health of peri-implant soft and hard tissues. The accumulation of biofilm and plaque, resulting either from prosthetic reconstructions with poor emergence profile or from closed inter-proximal spaces that do not allow adequate cleaning and oral hygiene practices, is the main reason for peri-implant diseases. Other risk factors include excessive cement, exposed rough implant surfaces, lack of keratinized tissues around the implant, and other causes. Chronic periodontitis, smoking, and systemic conditions such as diabetes have all been implicated in the development of peri-implant disease.

Biofilm

It was evident that biofilm is the primary cause and a significant risk factor for both peri-implant mucositis and peri-implantitis [29, 33–35]. In a cross-sectional study among five dental schools in Brazil, 212 non-smoker partially edentulous patients received 578 dental implants and were followed between 6 months and 5 years. The results showed that 65% of patients developed peri-implant mucositis compared to 9% who developed peri-implantitis. Peri-implant mucositis was defined as the presence of peri-implant bleeding on probing, while peri-implantitis was defined as the presence of pocket depth $\geq$ 5 mm in association with peri-implant bleeding on probing and/or suppuration. Patients with poor plaque control are 14 times more likely to develop peri-implantitis compared to controls. Inadequate accessibility to good oral hygiene and plaque control resulted in peri-implantitis in 65% of the implants compared to 18% when good oral hygiene was maintained [36].

Therefore, maintaining good oral hygiene around dental implants is crucial in preventing the risk of developing peri-implantitis [37].

Implant Surfaces

Implant surface characteristics play an important role in peri-implantitis [38, 39]. In a study involving smooth-surface implants, although 3.4% of the implants were lost within the first year of their placement, only 0.3% of the implants were lost between the first and fifth years. However, follow-up periods longer than 5 years demonstrated an increase of implant loss at 0.7%, mainly attributed to peri-implantitis [40]. In a study comparing smooth implant surfaces to rough ones, contradictory results demonstrated that implants with rough surfaces were more prone to plaque accumulation dur-

ing the short-term period. However, long-term results of smooth-surface implants showed higher implant loss compared to rough-surface implants [38].

Nevertheless, the degree of roughness of the implant surface affects peri-implantitis. The average peri-implant bone loss around minimally and moderately rough surfaces is significantly less than around highly rough surfaces leading to peri-implantitis [39, 41], and exposed rough implant surfaces have an increased risk for developing peri-implantitis compared to smooth surfaces [26, 38, 39, 42, 43]. Therefore, it is important to ensure good cleaning if rough surfaces were exposed in the oral cavity. Smoothing or flattening the surface and polishing the surface could be considered, a process known as implantoplasty.

Prosthetic Reconstructions

Prosthetic reconstructions with closed interproximal spaces do not facilitate the use of inter-proximal brushes resulting in inadequate cleaning and the development of peri-implant disease. Therefore, prosthetic reconstructions must be designed to allow proper cleaning. In addition, protheses with a poor emergence profile, over-contoured prostheses, or overhanging ledges lead to food entrapment and disease development [44–46]. Despite that a minimal distance of 3 mm is required between adjacent implants to allow adequate vascularization and nutrition to the surrounding soft and hard tissues, a larger space is still needed to allow proper cleaning using interproximal brushes. Implants placed too close to each other do not allow the use of interproximal brushes and adequate cleanability, thereby increasing the risk of peri-implantitis [47, 48].

In extraction sites exhibiting loss of bone height that was not grafted with bone or bone substitute, deep apical positioning of implants beyond the interproximal bone height level would result in a long clinical crown. These conditions contribute to an increased risk of developing deep pockets, potentially leading eventually to peri-implantitis. Therefore, it is prudent to plan the implant position's apical depth in such a way that the distance between the intra-osseous component of the implant and the trans-mucosal component is at the interproximal bone level [44–46].

Keratinized Mucosa

Around natural teeth, the lack of keratinized gingiva leads to movable unattached gingival margins, facilitating the introduction of microorganisms into gingival crevices resulting in accumulation to subgingival plaque leading to gingivitis and peri-implantitis [49]. A similar concept applies to dental implants [50, 51], where the presence of keratinized mucosa led to a better connective tissue seal around them [52].

Clinical diagnostic and radiographic indicators, including bleeding on probing and bone loss, improved in the presence of keratinized mucosa. This outcome emphasizes the bio-logic width role in protecting the zone of osseointegration from the bacterial accumulation and forms the rationale for augmenting soft tissue prior to abutment connection or non-submerged implant placement when thin mucosal tissues are present. Hence, it is important clinically to ensure that there is enough keratinized mucosa surrounding the implant at the time of implant placement [53, 54]. Better outcomes were achieved with connective tissue grafts compared to xenoge-neic collagen matrix [55].

Excess Cement

Excess cement in cemented implant-supported prostheses is a risk factor for the development of peri-implantitis. Cement penetration is a concern, particularly in immediate loading protocols, because the soft tissue seal is not yet established. Subsequently, the biofilm adheres to excess cement leading to peri-implantitis [56–58].

History of Periodontitis

Several reviews and meta-analyses have documented that a history of periodontitis, depending on the degree of its sever-ity, increases the risk of peri-implantitis [59–63]. A 2- to 6-year study examined the risk of peri-implantitis associated with 513 implants placed in three groups of partially dentate patients who are not susceptible to periodontal disease ver-sus those with a history of chronic periodontitis and aggres-sive periodontitis. The results showed that implant loss in non-susceptible patients and those with treated chronic peri-odontitis were the same at 3%. However, 15% of those with a history of aggressive periodontitis lost their implants [64]. In another study on 70 patients with chronic periodontitis, implant survival was 96% with a follow-up period ranging from 3 to 23 years with an average of 8 years. The authors showed that in patients with chronic periodontitis, and resid-ual pockets ≥5 mm at the end of active treatment, 22% of the implants, and 39% of the patients developed peri-implantitis and implant loss [65]. Therefore, it has been suggested to retain the teeth as long as possible, especially in patients with aggressive periodontal disease, as they present a high risk of developing peri-implantitis.

Smoking

Smoking influenced implant success in patients with aggres-sive periodontitis. The success rates in that group of patients were 63% in smokers and 78% in former smokers who quit more than 5 years earlier compared to 86% in non-smokers. Cessation of smoking prior to surgery is favorable in reduc-ing the risk of peri-implantitis [64, 66–68]. Therefore, cessa-tion of smoking and control of aggressive periodontitis before implant placement are paramount in decreasing the risk of peri-implantitis [69].

Diabetes

Diabetes has been implicated as a risk factor in the develop-ment of peri-implant disease. A systematic review investigat-ing the effect of diabetes on peri-implant mucositis and diabetes suggested that diabetic patients are 3.4 times more likely to develop peri-implantitis than non-diabetics after accounting for smoking a confounding factor [70]. However, marginal, type II diabetes seems to have an increased risk of implant loss compared to non-diabetics [71], even in the case of controlled diabetic disease [72]. In a paradoxical study, there seems to be no difference in implant loss between dia-betic and non-diabetic patients, irrespective of whether they are type I or type II diabetes [73]. Therefore, the substantial scientific evidence for the role of diabetes in peri-implantitis is still inconclusive [51].

Pathogens in Peri-implantitis

It has been suggested that it would take 1 year to eliminate periodontal pathogens in edentulous patients who had chronic periodontitis, dental extractions, and dental implants placed [74]. However, a 10-year follow-up study in patients who had chronic periodontitis who underwent full mouth extraction and dental implants showed persistent high levels of periodontal pathogens, including *Aggregatibacter*, *Porphyromonas*, and *Treponema* species [75]. More often, Candida and Staphylococcus species have also been docu-mented [76–78]. Not only have microbial pathogens been implicated in peri-implantitis, but also the reactive host response to titanium particles could be implicated in bone loss or peri-implantitis [79].

Prevention of Peri-implantitis

Prevention or peri-implantitis could be achieved by placing dental implants after completion of active periodontal ther-apy. Also, adherence to regular supportive periodontal ther-apy has been documented to prevent peri-implantitis and implant loss [80]. Furthermore, therapy for peri-implant mucositis should be considered as a preventive measure for the onset of peri-implantitis [29].

Adult partially edentulous patients with peri-implant muco-sitis but with no history of peri-implantitis whose dental implants were in function over 5 years were divided into two groups: one with supportive periodontal therapy and the other without. The results showed that 18% of patients with support-ive periodontal therapy developed peri-implantitis compared to 44% of those without supportive periodontal therapy [50].

In addition to reinforcing oral hygiene, it is important to identify risk factors that could not allow adequate access to oral hygiene and cleaning. Closed interproximal spaces, overhanging prosthetic reconstructions or those with poor emergence profile, presence of cement, and exposed rough endosseous implant surfaces play a role in the development of peri-implantitis. To facilitate oral hygiene and access to cleaning, opening inter-proximal spaces, adopting a prosthetic restoration with a good emergence profile, removing excess cement remnants, and smoothening the exposed rough surface represent possible solutions in the prevention of the disease. Prosthetic reconstructions must allow adequate space for interproximal cleaning. Although controversial, the lack of keratinized mucosa around the implant could be a contributing factor, necessitating a connective tissue graft.

Treatment

The main goal in treating peri-implant mucositis and peri-implantitis is to control plaque and biofilm formation [4, 81]. Treatment options include non-surgical and surgical interventions. The initial treatment phase for both peri-implant mucositis and peri-implantitis includes a non-surgical approach, which in most cases is very effective in treating peri-implant mucositis. However, in most cases of peri-implantitis, the non-surgical treatment may have to be followed by surgical intervention [82]. The treatment outcome of non-surgical therapy for peri-implantitis is to achieve a pocket probing depth of less than 5 mm, absence of bleeding on probing and/or suppuration, and prevention of additional marginal bone loss. Supportive therapy and maintenance are crucial to controlling the disease. These interventions have been described in protocols and algorithms [4, 22], such as the Cumulative Interceptive Supportive Therapy (CIST) protocols [4, 81]. The protocols developed 20 years ago continue to provide a framework for the maintenance of peri-implant health and management of peri-implant disease. The framework utilizes parameters like bleeding on probing, plaque index, suppuration, peri-implant pocket depth, and radiographic imaging that are assimilated into four protocols that provide the basis of treatment of peri-implant disease.

Non-surgical Therapy

Non-surgical therapy includes cleaning and debridement of peri-implant tissues and decontamination of the implant surface.

Cleaning and debridement of peri-implant tissues are performed using plastic, carbon-fiber-reinforced, titanium alloy and/or gold curettes, and sonic- or ultrasonic-driven plastic tips, titanium brushes, and oscillating chitosan brushes [83–87]. Removing the implant-supported prostheses allow for improved visualization and accessibility to the peri-implant area. Topical antiseptic treatment with chlorhexidine for 4 weeks is recommended during the non-surgical therapeutic phase [88–91]. Compared to natural teeth, non-surgical therapy for implants is more critical than in periodontally involved teeth as the disease's progression is much faster compared to natural teeth [6]. Hence, early intervention is important.

Implant surface decontamination or detoxification could be achieved chemically or mechanically. Chemical implant surface decontamination agents, applied locally, include saline, antiseptics, essential oils, citric acid, chlorhexidine rinses and gels, cetylpyridinium chloride, hydrogen peroxide, sodium hypochlorite, and local antimicrobials like minocycline microspheres or tetracycline. Systemic antimicrobials and probiotics have also been suggested to play a role in the management of peri-implant disease. Each technique has its advantages and disadvantages; however, regardless of which approach is used, they are effective in eliminating inflammation in 40–70% of implants affected by peri-implantitis, yet not one single method leads to a superior clinical outcome [88, 92–107]. Mechanical decontamination is achieved by using hand or powered instruments, air powder abrasive pumice such as glycine powder air polishing, and titanium airbrushes. Those measures, as well as, the use of diode, Nd:YAG and Er:YAG lasers, and photodynamic therapy led to improved clinical indicators [108–120]. Glycine or sodium bicarbonate air abrasion was effective without damaging the surface of implants and could be more effective than the use of chlorhexidine and curettes [119, 121, 122]. Since non-surgical therapy does not lead to complete inflammation resolution, an open flap surgical approach could improve clinical outcomes.

Surgical Therapy

When non-surgical treatment fails to achieve its goals resulting in unsuccessful cleaning or persistence of peri-implant pocket depths more than 6 mm with bleeding on probing or suppuration, surgical intervention is recommended. The surgical intervention's goal is to clean the implant surface, remove granulation tissues, recontour bone in non-accessible areas, and reduce pocket depth via an open flap debridement, resection, or regenerative procedures. A reduction in pocket depths and gain in attachment height have been documented in all three surgical procedures [109].

If patients are presenting with peri-implantitis, non-surgical initial therapy is applied and early re-evaluation within 2 months is recommended. It is then important to consider open surgical debridement and to clean combined with pocket reduction and antibiotics. Recall visits are done quarterly [123]. Peri-implant mucositis is reversible, and adequate biofilm removal is a prerequisite for preventing and managing peri-implantitis [20]. It was suggested that conventional non-surgical mechanical therapy alone could be considered the standard treatment for peri-implant mucositis [124].

Peri-implantitis could be treated via a surgical open flap combined with systematic antibiotics including amoxicillin and metronidazole, removal of granulation tissue, and decontamination of implant surfaces. This protocol showed that >85% of the implants had a mean periodontal pocket depth < 4 mm after 3 months, a result that was stable after a year [125].

The surgical osseous regenerative or reconstructive approach is favorable for peri-implant bone defects whose morphology is conducive for bone regeneration, such as 2, 3, or 4 wall defects. This could be achieved by grafting the peri-implant site with autogenous bone and/or bone substitute or bioactive substance with or without the application of a resorbable membrane. Although reconstructive approaches are successful, the scientific evidence is weak regarding reconstructive therapy when compared to open flap debridement [126]. Submerged healing might reduce the risk of membrane exposure. Re-osseointegration following the regenerative treatment has not been demonstrated in humans, even though radiographs would show bone around the implant [111, 127].

The surgical osseous resection approach includes osseous recontouring or osteoplasty, implant surface modification or implantoplasty, and apical positioning of the flap. It is used in one-wall defects and is associated with improved clinical indicators, including bleeding on probing and maintaining bone levels [109, 128–131]. Implantoplasty, although effective in reducing the biofilm, alters the surface of the implant, and it has been associated with an increased risk of fracture in narrow implants [114].

Failure of non-surgical and surgical measures would lead to the removal of the implant, the last resort given the severity of the infection and being non-responsive to therapy.

In a long-term study on the treatment of peri-implantitis, a group of 24 partially edentulous patients with 36 implants diagnosed with peri-implantitis underwent 4 weeks of non-surgical therapy followed by open flap debridement, including surface decontamination using curettes and saline irrigation, as well as systemic antibiotic therapy. Chlorhexidine 0.2% mouth rinses were used for 4 weeks with a weekly recall visit during the first month. Results showed that after a year, pocket depths were reduced to less than 5 mm, but bleeding on probing was still present at half the sites. Bone levels stabilized at 92% of the affected sites [125]. A systematic review whose aim was to evaluate the success of treatments aimed at the resolution of peri-implantitis. Success was defined as implant survival and a mean probing depth of less than 5 mm, and no further bone loss [132].

Supportive Therapy

Supportive therapy is an essential factor in controlling peri-implant disease. In a systematic review evaluating the suc-cess of anti-infective protocols in preventing peri-implantitis after regular supportive periodontal therapy over 10 years, implant survival ranged from 85% to 99% in patients with regular maintenance. Implant survival and success rates were lower in periodontally compromised patients compared to non-periodontally compromised patients. The importance of being enrolled in regular supportive periodontal therapy and active periodontal treatment prior to dental implants placement could not be overemphasized [123]. Supportive therapy decreased the incidence of peri-implantitis 12-folds in patients with periodontitis. Fifty (50%) of the patients with moderate or severe periodontitis who did not adhere to supportive periodontal therapy lost their implants compared to 4% who adhered to supportive periodontal therapy over 10 years [133]. Therapy of peri-implantitis followed by regular supportive care resulted in improved implant survival and stable peri-implant bone levels in most patients [48]. In a 5-year follow-up study, 18% of patients with peri-implant mucositis who were enrolled in regular preventive maintenance developed peri-implantitis compared to 44% who did not receive preventive maintenance [50]. Treatment of peri-implant mucositis, including plaque control and oral hygiene combined with non-surgical mechanical debridement, was effective in 38% of the implants, thereby not always resulting in complete inflammation resolution [134]. Short-term supportive therapy includes post-operative anti-infective protocol, including chlorhexidine application and systematic antibiotics in case a surgical approach was used. Regular long-term supportive care is recommended every 3–6 months. Supportive therapy following anti-infective surgical treatment for peri-implantitis that included implant surface decontamination with saline and systemic antibiotics was successful in 63% of the cases. Success was defined as the absence of bleeding on probing, suppuration, further bone loss, and peri-implant pocket depth of <5 mm [135].

Summary

Bacterial biofilm, leading to plaque accumulation, is the primary cause of peri-implant mucositis and its progression to peri-implantitis. Therefore, ensuring cleaning and maintaining good oral hygiene are paramount in preventing the disease and its progression. Mucosa around implants, lacking the complex architecture around natural teeth, contributes to the spread of inflammation. Patients presenting with no signs of inflammation could be followed annually, and axial probing at least at one site of each implant for early disease detection is recommended. If there are any signs of peri-implant mucositis, a radiograph should be taken to ensure that there is no progressive bone loss leading to peri-implantitis. The risk of cement remnants accumulating plaque is an early disease occurrence, particularly with immediate restorations.

There is increased risk in patients with a history of periodontal disease, smokers, and diabetics. Therefore, it is important to assess the risks and consider adjunct or alternative treatment options. Although there is no standard of care, non-surgical and surgical treatment options led to favorable clinical outcomes. The current evidence in the literature supports an initial phase to control the risk factors leading to peri-implant disease. Peri-implant mucositis is reversible and is treated using a non-surgical approach including mechanical and chemical debridement. However, complete resolution of inflammation such as bleeding on probing is not predictable, thereby requiring a surgical open flap approach. Progressive disease leading to peri-implantitis requires the use of both non-surgical therapy and additional resection resective or regenerative approaches.

Part II: Peri-apical or Retrograde Peri-implantitis

Definitions

Peri-apical or retrograde peri-implantitis is a disease that occurs at the peri-apical area of a dental implant without affecting the cervical margin. It has been defined as an active symptomatic implant periapical lesion that developed at the apex implant, while the coronal portion of the implant maintains its bone integrity [136, 137]. It has also been defined as localized osteomyelitis secondary to endodontic pathology [138].

Etiology

The etiology of retrograde peri-implantitis has been attributed to bacteria present in a periapical pathology of an extracted tooth [139]. Many implants that developed retrograde peri-implantitis were placed in areas of previously root canal-treated natural teeth or adjacent to a tooth with a periapical pathology [140, 141] or infected sites [142]. Intraoperative factors during dental implant placement, such as contamination or other factors, could also contribute to retrograde peri-implantitis [143–146].

Classifications

Various classifications for retrograde peri-implantitis exist. A type based on clinical and radiographic indicators such as the presence of bleeding, bone loss, mobility, probing depth, proposed treatment, prognosis, and radiographic bone loss has been suggested [147–151]. This classification, however, does not include etiological factors and is complex. Another

classification distributed the disease among four classes. In class 1, an implant placed resulted in the devitalization of an adjacent vital tooth. In class 2, the implant apex is infected by a persistent apical lesion adjacent to a tooth or an implant. In class 3, the implant apex is angulated labially or lingually outside the envelope of bone. In class 4, the apical peri-implant lesion developed due to residual infection at the placement site [143].

Prevalence

Although the prevalence of retrograde peri-implantitis is estimated at 0.26%, it could reach between 8% and 25% when an adjacent tooth next to an implant site has a periapical lesion [152]. The disease affects the maxilla four times more than the mandible [149, 153], which was attributed to the higher frequency of radicular cysts and abundant Malassez cells in the maxilla [137, 154]. There was no increase in the incidence of retrograde peri-implantitis in patients who had apicoectomies [155].

Symptoms

Symptoms of pain, swelling, or a fistula's presence could start as early as the first week after implant placement and could develop over 4 years [149, 153, 156].

Treatment

There is no consensus for the treatment of retrograde peri-implantitis. Any peri-implant radiolucency should be addressed immediately to prevent further loss of osseointegration [157]. Treatment options are similar to the treatment of peri-implantitis, which include implant surface decontamination, antimicrobial therapy, bone grafting using autogenous bone or bone substitutes, guided bone regeneration, low energy laser, photodynamic therapy, root canal treatment, or apicectomy of adjacent teeth RCT (apicoectomy), as well as the possibility of implant apicectomy [129, 144, 158–162].

Other treatment options were based on the classification described earlier. It was suggested that for class 1, non-surgical or surgical root canal treatment of the affected tooth is performed. Depending on the outcome, possible removal of the implant could be considered. In class 2, antibiotic therapy is recommended in addition to non-surgical or surgical root canal treatment of the affected tooth. In class 3, surgical access to an implant, including decontamination and regenerative bone grafting, is recommended. Should this treatment fail, then removal of the implant could be considered. In class 4, surgical debridement, antibiotic therapy,

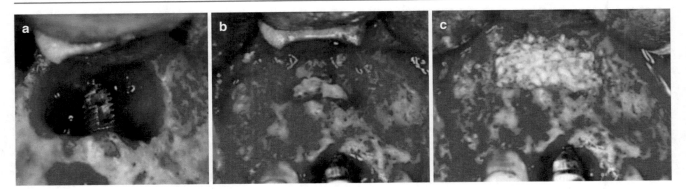

Fig. 8.2 Retrograde or peri-apical peri-implantitis. Clinical images of a patient treated for retrograde peri-implantitis, also known as peri-apical implantitis. The patient presented with erythema, buccal fistula formation, and suppuration. The radiographic examination revealed bone loss limited to the apex of the implant (**a**). Treatment consisted of mechanical and chemical debridement of the implant surface and the surgical site. A regenerative procedure was implemented. A regenerative procedure was implemented. Autogenous bone harvested from adjacent bone was applied around the exposed threads implant surface (**b**) was placed around the exposed threads and a layer of a low substitute material (**c**) was applied as an additional layer. Two collagen membranes were then applied to form two layers, and tension-free closure was achieved. (Clinical case report; Dr. Hani Abd-Ul-Salam)

decontamination, and bone grafting could be considered (Fig. 8.2). Removal of the implant would be the last resort if the treatment failed [143]. Root canal treatment of non-vital teeth adjacent to dental implants resolved retrograde peri-implantitis [163].

Prognosis

The prognosis of retrograde peri-implantitis is good. A retrospective study of 39 implants diagnosed with retrograde peri-implantitis treated with implant apicoectomy had 97.4% success rate after a 5-year follow-up [164]. In a recent study, survival rate was documented at 78% over 7 years [165].

Summary

Retrograde peri-implantitis is a disease that affects the peri-apical implant area without affecting the coronal margin, has multiple etiologies, and there is no consensus on the current treatment modalities. Although controversial, delaying implant placement in an area adjacent to a recent root canal–treated tooth or in an area of an extracted tooth that had a periapical disease should be considered.

References

1. Brånemark PI, Hansson BO, Adell R, Breine U, Lindström J, Hallén O, et al. Osseointegrated implants in the treatment of the edentulous jaw. Experience from a 10-year period. Scand J Plast Reconstr Surg Suppl. 1977;16:1–132.
2. Brånemark PI, Adell R, Breine U, Hansson BO, Lindström J, Ohlsson A. Intra-osseous anchorage of dental prostheses. I. Experimental studies. Scand J Plast Reconstr Surg. 1969;3(2):81–100.
3. Berglundh T, Persson L, Klinge B. A systematic review of the incidence of biological and technical complications in implant dentistry reported in prospective longitudinal studies of at least 5 years. J Clin Periodontol. 2002;29(Suppl 3):197–212; discussion 32–3
4. Lang NP, Wilson TG, Corbet EF. Biological complications with dental implants: their prevention, diagnosis and treatment. Clin Oral Implants Res. 2000;11(Suppl 1):146–55.
5. Branemark P. Introduction to osseointegration. In: Branemark PIZG, Albrektsson T, editors. Tissue-integrated prostheses. Berlin: Quintessence; 1985. p. 11–76.
6. Berglundh T, Zitzmann NU, Donati M. Are peri-implantitis lesions different from periodontitis lesions? J Clin Periodontol. 2011;38(Suppl 11):188–202.
7. Berglundh T, Lindhe J, Ericsson I, Marinello CP, Liljenberg B, Thomsen P. The soft tissue barrier at implants and teeth. Clin Oral Implants Res. 1991;2(2):81–90.
8. Feneis H. Anatomy and physiology of the normal gingiva. Dtsch Zahnarztl Z. 1952;7(8):467–76.
9. Page RC, Ammons WF, Schectman LR, Dillingham LA. Collagen fibre bundles of the normal marginal g-ngiva in the marmoset. Arch Oral Biol. 1974;19(11):1039–43.
10. Ikeda H, Shiraiwa M, Yamaza T, Yoshinari M, Kido MA, Ayukawa Y, et al. Difference in penetration of horseradish peroxidase tracer as a foreign substance into the peri-implant or junctional epithelium of rat gingivae. Clin Oral Implants Res. 2002;13(3):243–51.
11. Gargiulo AW, Wentz FM, Orban B. Mitotic activity of human oral epithelium exposed to 30 per cent hydrogen peroxide. Oral Surg Oral Med Oral Pathol. 1961;14:474–92.
12. Cochran DL, Hermann JS, Schenk RK, Higginbottom FL, Buser D. Biologic width around titanium implants. A histometric analysis of the implanto-gingival junction around unloaded and loaded nonsubmerged implants in the canine mandible. J Periodontol. 1997;68(2):186–98.
13. Hermann JS, Buser D, Schenk RK, Higginbottom FL, Cochran DL. Biologic width around titanium implants. A physiologically formed and stable dimension over time. Clin Oral Implants Res 2000;11(1):1–11.
14. Quinlan P, Nummikoski P, Schenk R, Cagna D, Mellonig J, Higginbottom F, et al. Immediate and early loading of SLA ITI

single-tooth implants: an in vivo study. Int J Oral Maxillofac Implants. 2005;20(3):360–70.

15. Bakaeen L, Quinlan P, Schoolfield J, Lang NP, Cochran DL. The biologic width around titanium implants: histometric analysis of the implantogingival junction around immediately and early loaded implants. Int J Periodontics Restorative Dent. 2009;29(3):297–305.

16. Berglundh T, Armitage G, Araujo MG, Avila-Ortiz G, Blanco J, Camargo PM, et al. Peri-implant diseases and conditions: consensus report of workgroup 4 of the 2017 world workshop on the classification of periodontal and peri-implant diseases and conditions. J Clin Periodontol. 2018;45(Suppl 20):S286–s91.

17. Heitz-Mayfield LJ, Needleman I, Salvi GE, Pjetursson BE. Consensus statements and clinical recommendations for prevention and management of biologic and technical implant complications. Int J Oral Maxillofac Implants. 2014;29(Suppl):346–50.

18. Hashim D, Cionca N, Combescure C, Mombelli A. The diagnosis of peri-implantitis: a systematic review on the predictive value of bleeding on probing. Clin Oral Implants Res. 2018;29(Suppl 16):276–93.

19. Heitz-Mayfield LJ, Aaboe M, Araujo M, Carrión JB, Cavalcanti R, Cionca N, et al. Group 4 ITI consensus report: risks and biologic complications associated with implant dentistry. Clin Oral Implants Res. 2018;29(Suppl 16):351–8.

20. Heitz-Mayfield LJA, Salvi GE. Peri-implant mucositis. J Periodontol. 2018;89(Suppl 1):S257–s66.

21. Tallarico M, Canullo L, Wang HL, Cochran DL, Meloni SM. Classification systems for peri-implantitis: a narrative review with a proposal of a new evidence-based etiology codification. Int J Oral Maxillofac Implants. 2018;33(4):871–9.

22. Nogueira-Filho G, Iacopino AM, Tenenbaum HC. Prognosis in implant dentistry: a system for classifying the degree of peri-implant mucosal inflammation. J Can Dent Assoc. 2011;77:b8.

23. Caton JG, Armitage G, Berglundh T, Chapple ILC, Jepsen S, Kornman KS, et al. A new classification scheme for periodontal and peri-implant diseases and conditions – introduction and key changes from the 1999 classification. J Clin Periodontol. 2018;45(Suppl 20):S1–s8.

24. Salvi GE, Lang NP. Diagnostic parameters for monitoring peri-implant conditions. Int J Oral Maxillofac Implants. 2004;19(Suppl):116–27.

25. Jung RE, Pjetursson BE, Glauser R, Zembic A, Zwahlen M, Lang NP. A systematic review of the 5-year survival and complication rates of implant-supported single crowns. Clin Oral Implants Res. 2008;19(2):119–30.

26. Zitzmann NU, Berglundh T. Definition and prevalence of peri-implant diseases. J Clin Periodontol. 2008;35(8 Suppl):286–91.

27. Cosgarea R, Sculean A, Shibli JA, Salvi GE. Prevalence of peri-implant diseases – a critical review on the current evidence. Braz Oral Res. 2019;33(suppl 1):e063.

28. Lee CT, Huang YW, Zhu L, Weltman R. Prevalences of peri-implantitis and peri-implant mucositis: systematic review and meta-analysis. J Dent. 2017;62:1–12.

29. Salvi GE, Cosgarea R, Sculean A. Prevalence and mechanisms of peri-implant diseases. J Dent Res. 2017;96(1):31–7.

30. Derks J, Tomasi C. Peri-implant health and disease. A systematic review of current epidemiology. J Clin Periodontol. 2015;42(Suppl 16):S158–71.

31. Albrektsson T, Chrcanovic B, Östman PO, Sennerby L. Initial and long-term crestal bone responses to modern dental implants. Periodontol 2000. 2017;73(1):41–50.

32. Salvi GE, Monje A, Tomasi C. Long-term biological complications of dental implants placed either in pristine or in augmented sites: a systematic review and meta-analysis. Clin Oral Implants Res. 2018;29(Suppl 16):294–310.

33. Berglundh T, Jepsen S, Stadlinger B, Terheyden H. Peri-implantitis and its prevention. Clin Oral Implants Res. 2019;30(2):150–5.

34. Lafaurie GI, Sabogal MA, Castillo DM, Rincón MV, Gómez LA, Lesmes YA, et al. Microbiome and microbial biofilm profiles of peri-implantitis: a systematic review. J Periodontol. 2017;88(10):1066–89.

35. Renvert S, Quirynen M. Risk indicators for peri-implantitis. A narrative review. Clinical oral implants research. 2015;26(Suppl 11):15–44.

36. Serino G, Ström C. Peri-implantitis in partially edentulous patients: association with inadequate plaque control. Clin Oral Implants Res. 2009;20(2):169–74.

37. Ferreira SD, Silva GL, Cortelli JR, Costa JE, Costa FO. Prevalence and risk variables for peri-implant disease in Brazilian subjects. J Clin Periodontol. 2006;33(12):929–35.

38. Saulacic N, Schaller B. Prevalence of peri-implantitis in implants with turned and rough surfaces: a systematic review. J Oral Maxillofac Res. 2019;10(1):e1.

39. De Bruyn H, Christiaens V, Doornewaard R, Jacobsson M, Cosyn J, Jacquet W, et al. Implant surface roughness and patient factors on long-term peri-implant bone loss. Periodontol 2000. 2017;73(1):218–27.

40. Roos-Jansåker AM, Lindahl C, Renvert H, Renvert S. Nine- to fourteen-year follow-up of implant treatment. Part I: implant loss and associations to various factors. J Clin Periodontol. 2006;33(4):283–9.

41. Albouy JP, Abrahamsson I, Persson LG, Berglundh T. Spontaneous progression of peri-implantitis at different types of implants. An experimental study in dogs. I: clinical and radiographic observations. Clin Oral Implants Res. 2008;19(10):997–1002.

42. Peixoto CD, Almas K. The implant surface characteristics and peri-implantitis. An evidence-based update. Odontostomatol Trop. 2016;39(153):23–35.

43. Berglundh T, Gotfredsen K, Zitzmann NU, Lang NP, Lindhe J. Spontaneous progression of ligature induced peri-implantitis at implants with different surface roughness: an experimental study in dogs. Clin Oral Implants Res. 2007;18(5):655–61.

44. Dixon DR, London RM. Restorative design and associated risks for peri-implant diseases. Periodontol 2000. 2019;81(1):167–78.

45. Katafuchi M, Weinstein BF, Leroux BG, Chen YW, Daubert DM. Restoration contour is a risk indicator for peri-implantitis: a cross-sectional radiographic analysis. J Clin Periodontol. 2018;45(2):225–32.

46. Yi Y, Koo KT, Schwarz F, Ben Amara H, Heo SJ. Association of prosthetic features and peri-implantitis: a cross-sectional study. J Clin Periodontol. 2020;47(3):392–403.

47. Jung RE, Heitz-Mayfield L, Schwarz F. Evidence-based knowledge on the aesthetics and maintenance of peri-implant soft tissues: osteology foundation consensus report part 3-aesthetics of peri-implant soft tissues. Clin Oral Implants Res. 2018;29(Suppl 15):14–7.

48. Roccuzzo M, Layton DM, Roccuzzo A, Heitz-Mayfield LJ. Clinical outcomes of peri-implantitis treatment and supportive care: a systematic review. Clin Oral Implants Res. 2018;29(Suppl 16):331–50.

49. Lang NP, Löe H. The relationship between the width of keratinized gingiva and gingival health. J Periodontol. 1972;43(10):623–7.

50. Costa FO, Takenaka-Martinez S, Cota LO, Ferreira SD, Silva GL, Costa JE. Peri-implant disease in subjects with and without preventive maintenance: a 5-year follow-up. J Clin Periodontol. 2012;39(2):173–81.

51. Dreyer H, Grischke J, Tiede C, Eberhard J, Schweitzer A, Toikkanen SE, et al. Epidemiology and risk factors of peri-implantitis: a systematic review. J Periodontal Res. 2018;53(5):657–81.

52. Greenstein G, Cavallaro J. The clinical significance of keratinized gingiva around dental implants. Compend Contin Educ Dentistry (Jamesburg, NJ: 1995). 2011;32(8):24–31.

53. Berglundh T, Lindhe J. Dimension of the periimplant mucosa. Biological width revisited. J Clin Periodontol. 1996;23(10):971–3.

54. Brito C, Tenenbaum HC, Wong BK, Schmitt C, Nogueira-Filho G. Is keratinized mucosa indispensable to maintain peri-implant health? A systematic review of the literature. J Biomed Mater Res B Appl Biomater. 2014;102(3):643–50.

55. Cairo F, Barbato L, Selvaggi F, Baielli MG, Piattelli A, Chambrone L. Surgical procedures for soft tissue augmentation at implant sites. A systematic review and meta-analysis of randomized controlled trials. Clin Implant Dent Relat Res. 2019;21(6):1262–70.

56. Jepsen S, Berglundh T, Genco R, Aass AM, Demirel K, Derks J, et al. Primary prevention of peri-implantitis: managing peri-implant mucositis. J Clin Periodontol. 2015;42(Suppl 16):S152–7.

57. Schwarz F, Derks J, Monje A, Wang HL. Peri-implantitis. J Periodontol. 2018;89(Suppl 1):S267–s90.

58. Staubli N, Walter C, Schmidt JC, Weiger R, Zitzmann NU. Excess cement and the risk of peri-implant disease – a systematic review. Clin Oral Implants Res. 2017;28(10):1278–90.

59. Ferreira SD, Martins CC, Amaral SA, Vieira TR, Albuquerque BN, Cota LOM, et al. Periodontitis as a risk factor for peri-implantitis: systematic review and meta-analysis of observational studies. J Dent. 2018;79:1–10.

60. Sousa V, Mardas N, Farias B, Petrie A, Needleman I, Spratt D, et al. A systematic review of implant outcomes in treated periodontitis patients. Clin Oral Implants Res. 2016;27(7):787–844.

61. Sgolastra F, Petrucci A, Severino M, Gatto R, Monaco A. Periodontitis, implant loss and peri-implantitis. A meta-analysis. Clin Oral Implants Res. 2015;26(4):e8–e16.

62. Monje A, Alcoforado G, Padial-Molina M, Suarez F, Lin GH, Wang HL. Generalized aggressive periodontitis as a risk factor for dental implant failure: a systematic review and meta-analysis. J Periodontol. 2014;85(10):1398–407.

63. Ramanauskaite A, Baseviciene N, Wang HL, Tözüm TF. Effect of history of periodontitis on implant success: meta-analysis and systematic review. Implant Dent. 2014;23(6):687–96.

64. De Boever AL, Quirynen M, Coucke W, Theuniers G, De Boever JA. Clinical and radiographic study of implant treatment outcome in periodontally susceptible and non-susceptible patients: a prospective long-term study. Clin Oral Implants Res. 2009;20(12):1341–50.

65. Pjetursson BE, Helbling C, Weber HP, Matuliene G, Salvi GE, Brägger U, et al. Peri-implantitis susceptibility as it relates to periodontal therapy and supportive care. Clin Oral Implants Res. 2012;23(7):888–94.

66. Alqahtani F, Alqhtani N, Divakar DD, Shetty SB, Shetty B, Alkhtani F. Self-rated peri-implant oral symptoms and clinicoradiographic characteristics in Narghile-smokers, cigarette-smokers, and nonsmokers with peri-implantitis. Clin Implant Dent Relat Res. 2019;21(6):1235–40.

67. Mazel A, Belkacemi S, Tavitian P, Stéphan G, Tardivo D, Catherine JH, et al. Peri-implantitis risk factors: a prospective evaluation. J Investig Clin Dent. 2019;10(2):e12398.

68. Sgolastra F, Petrucci A, Severino M, Gatto R, Monaco A. Smoking and the risk of peri-implantitis. A systematic review and meta-analysis. Clin Oral Implants Res. 2015;26(4):e62–e7.

69. Akram Z, Javed F, Vohra F. Effect of waterpipe smoking on peri-implant health: a systematic review and meta-analysis. J Investig Clin Dent. 2019;10(3):e12403.

70. Monje A, Catena A, Borgnakke WS. Association between diabetes mellitus/hyperglycaemia and peri-implant diseases: systematic review and meta-analysis. J Clin Periodontol. 2017;44(6):636–48.

71. Morris HF, Ochi S, Winkler S. Implant survival in patients with type 2 diabetes: placement to 36 months. Ann Periodontol. 2000;5(1):157–65.

72. Lagunov VL, Sun J, George R. Evaluation of biologic implant success parameters in type 2 diabetic glycemic control patients versus health patients: a meta-analysis. J Investig Clin Dent. 2019;10(4):e12478.

73. Moraschini V, Barboza ES, Peixoto GA. The impact of diabetes on dental implant failure: a systematic review and meta-analysis. Int J Oral Maxillofac Surg. 2016;45(10):1237–45.

74. Danser MM, van Winkelhoff AJ, van der Velden U. Periodontal bacteria colonizing oral mucous membranes in edentulous patients wearing dental implants. J Periodontol. 1997;68(3):209–16.

75. Quirynen M, Alsaadi G, Pauwels M, Haffajee A, van Steenberghe D, Naert I. Microbiological and clinical outcomes and patient satisfaction for two treatment options in the edentulous lower jaw after 10 years of function. Clin Oral Implants Res. 2005;16(3):277–87.

76. Harris LG, Meredith DO, Eschbach L, Richards RG. Staphylococcus aureus adhesion to standard micro-rough and electropolished implant materials. J Mater Sci Mater Med. 2007;18(6):1151–6.

77. Kronström M, Svenson B, Hellman M, Persson GR. Early implant failures in patients treated with Brånemark System titanium dental implants: a retrospective study. 2001;16(2):201–7.

78. Rams TE, Feik D, Slots J. Staphylococci in human periodontal diseases. Oral Microbiol Immunol. 1990;5(1):29–32.

79. Albrektsson T, Chrcanovic B, Mölne J, Wennerberg A. Foreign body reactions, marginal bone loss and allergies in relation to titanium implants. Eur J Oral Implantol. 2018;11(Suppl 1):S37–s46.

80. Lin CY, Chen Z, Pan WL, Wang HL. The effect of supportive care in preventing peri-implant diseases and implant loss: a systematic review and meta-analysis. Clin Oral Implants Res. 2019;30(8):714–24.

81. Mombelli A, Lang NP. The diagnosis and treatment of peri-implantitis. Periodontol 2000. 1998;17:63–76.

82. Lang NP, Salvi GE, Sculean A. Nonsurgical therapy for teeth and implants-When and why? Periodontol 2000. 2019;79(1):15–21.

83. Ronay V, Merlini A, Attin T, Schmidlin PR, Sahrmann P. In vitro cleaning potential of three implant debridement methods. Simulation of the non-surgical approach. Clin Oral Implants Res. 2017;28(2):151–5.

84. Schmage P, Kahili F, Nergiz I, Scorziello TM, Platzer U, Pfeiffer P. Cleaning effectiveness of implant prophylaxis instruments. Int J Oral Maxillofac Implants. 2014;29(2):331–7.

85. Schmage P, Thielemann J, Nergiz I, Scorziello TM, Pfeiffer P. Effects of 10 cleaning instruments on four different implant surfaces. Int J Oral Maxillofac Implants. 2012;27(2):308–17.

86. Wohlfahrt JC, Aass AM, Koldsland OC. Treatment of peri-implant mucositis with a chitosan brush-A pilot randomized clinical trial. Int J Dent Hyg. 2019;17(2):170–6.

87. Wohlfahrt JC, Evensen BJ, Zeza B, Jansson H, Pilloni A, Roos-Jansåker AM, et al. A novel non-surgical method for mild peri-implantitis- a multicenter consecutive case series. Int J Implant Dentistry. 2017;3(1):38.

88. de Waal YC, Raghoebar GM, Meijer HJ, Winkel EG, van Winkelhoff AJ. Implant decontamination with 2% chlorhexidine during surgical peri-implantitis treatment: a randomized, double-blind, controlled trial. Clin Oral Implants Res. 2015;26(9):1015–23.

89. Machtei EE, Frankenthal S, Levi G, Elimelech R, Shoshani E, Rosenfeld O, et al. Treatment of peri-implantitis using multiple applications of chlorhexidine chips: a double-blind, randomized multi-centre clinical trial. J Clin Periodontol. 2012;39(12):1198–205.

90. Menezes KM, Fernandes-Costa AN, Silva-Neto RD, Calderon PS, Gurgel BC. Efficacy of 0.12% chlorhexidine gluconate for non-surgical treatment of peri-implant mucositis. J Periodontol. 2016;87(11):1305–13.

91. Pulcini A, Bollaín J, Sanz-Sánchez I, Figuero E, Alonso B, Sanz M, et al. Clinical effects of the adjunctive use of a 0.03% chlorhexidine and 0.05% cetylpyridinium chloride mouth rinse in the management of peri-implant diseases: a randomized clinical trial. J Clin Periodontol. 2019;46(3):342–53.

92. Rokaya D, Srimaneepong V, Wisitrasameewon W, Humagain M, Thunyakitpisal P. Peri-implantitis update: risk indicators, diagnosis, and treatment. Eur J Dent. 2020;14(4):672–82.

93. Kubasiewicz-Ross P, Hadzik J, Gedrange T, Dominiak M, Jurczyszyn K, Pitułaj A, et al. Antimicrobial efficacy of different decontamination methods as tested on dental implants with various types of surfaces. Med Sci Monit. 2020;26:e920513.

94. Kubasiewicz-Ross P, Fleischer M, Pitułaj A, Hadzik J, Nawrot-Hadzik I, Bortkiewicz O, et al. Evaluation of the three methods of bacterial decontamination on implants with three different surfaces. Adv Clin Exp Med. 2020;29(2):177–82.

95. El Chaar E, Almogahwi M, Abdalkader K, Alshehri A, Cruz S, Ricci J. Decontamination of the infected implant surface: a scanning electron microscope study. Int J Periodontics Restorative Dent. 2020;40(3):395–401.

96. Jin SH, Lee EM, Park JB, Kim KK, Ko Y. Decontamination methods to restore the biocompatibility of contaminated titanium surfaces. J Periodontal Implant Sci. 2019;49(3):193–204.

97. Carral C, Muñoz F, Permuy M, Liñares A, Dard M, Blanco J. Mechanical and chemical implant decontamination in surgical peri-implantitis treatment: preclinical "in vivo" study. J Clin Periodontol. 2016;43(8):694–701.

98. Subramani K, Wismeijer D. Decontamination of titanium implant surface and re-osseointegration to treat peri-implantitis: a literature review. Int J Oral Maxillofac Implants. 2012;27(5):1043–54.

99. Cafiero C, Aglietta M, Iorio-Siciliano V, Salvi GE, Blasi A, Matarasso S. Implant surface roughness alterations induced by different prophylactic procedures: an in vitro study. Clin Oral Implants Res. 2017;28(7):e16–20.

100. Schwarz F, Becker K, Bastendorf KD, Cardaropoli D, Chatfield C, Dunn I, et al. Recommendations on the clinical application of air polishing for the management of peri-implant mucositis and peri-implantitis. Quintessence Int (Berlin, Germany: 1985). 2016;47(4):293–6.

101. Bassetti M, Schär D, Wicki B, Eick S, Ramseier CA, Arweiler NB, et al. Anti-infective therapy of peri-implantitis with adjunctive local drug delivery or photodynamic therapy: 12-month outcomes of a randomized controlled clinical trial. Clin Oral Implants Res. 2014;25(3):279–87.

102. Schär D, Ramseier CA, Eick S, Arweiler NB, Sculean A, Salvi GE. Anti-infective therapy of peri-implantitis with adjunctive local drug delivery or photodynamic therapy: six-month outcomes of a prospective randomized clinical trial. Clin Oral Implants Res. 2013;24(1):104–10.

103. Suarez F, Monje A, Galindo-Moreno P, Wang HL. Implant surface detoxification: a comprehensive review. Implant Dent. 2013;22(5):465–73.

104. Felo A, Shibly O, Ciancio SG, Lauciello FR, Ho A. Effects of subgingival chlorhexidine irrigation on peri-implant maintenance. Am J Dent. 1997;10(2):107–10.

105. Riben-Grundstrom C, Norderyd O, André U, Renvert S. Treatment of peri-implant mucositis using a glycine powder air-polishing or ultrasonic device: a randomized clinical trial. J Clin Periodontol. 2015;42(5):462–9.

106. Galofré M, Palao D, Vicario M, Nart J, Violant D. Clinical and microbiological evaluation of the effect of Lactobacillus reuteri in the treatment of mucositis and peri-implantitis: a triple-blind randomized clinical trial. J Periodontal Res. 2018;53(3):378–90.

107. Iorio-Siciliano V, Blasi A, Stratul SI, Ramaglia L, Sculean A, Salvi GE, et al. Anti-infective therapy of peri-implant mucositis with adjunctive delivery of a sodium hypochlorite gel: a 6-month randomized triple-blind controlled clinical trial. Clin Oral Investig. 2020;24(6):1971–9.

108. Figuero E, Graziani F, Sanz I, Herrera D, Sanz M. Management of peri-implant mucositis and peri-implantitis. Periodontol 2000. 2014;66(1):255–73.

109. Khoury F, Keeve PL, Ramanauskaite A, Schwarz F, Koo KT, Sculean A, et al. Surgical treatment of peri-implantitis – consensus report of working group 4. Int Dent J. 2019;69(Suppl 2):18–22.

110. Renvert S, Polyzois I. Treatment of pathologic peri-implant pockets. Periodontol 2000. 2018;76(1):180–90.

111. Schwarz F, Schmucker A, Becker J. Efficacy of alternative or adjunctive measures to conventional treatment of peri-implant mucositis and peri-implantitis: a systematic review and meta-analysis. Int J Implant Dentistry. 2015;1(1):22.

112. Suárez-López Del Amo F, Yu SH, Wang HL. Non-surgical therapy for peri-implant diseases: a systematic review. J Oral Maxillofac Res. 2016;7(3):e13.

113. Chambrone L, Wang HL, Romanos GE. Antimicrobial photodynamic therapy for the treatment of periodontitis and peri-implantitis: an American Academy of Periodontology best evidence review. J Periodontol. 2018;89(7):783–803.

114. Birang E, Talebi Ardekani MR, Rajabzadeh M, Sarmadi G, Birang R, Gutknecht N. Evaluation of effectiveness of photodynamic therapy with low-level diode laser in nonsurgical treatment of peri-implantitis. J Lasers Med Sci. 2017;8(3):136–42.

115. Faggion CM Jr. Laser therapy as an adjunct treatment for peri-implant mucositis and peri-implantitis provides no extra benefit for most clinical outcomes. J Evid Based Dent Pract. 2019;19(2):203–6.

116. Sharab L, Baier R, Ciancio S, Mang T. Influence of Photodynamic Therapy on Bacterial Attachment to Titanium Surface. The Journal of oral implantology. 2020. https://doi.org/10.1563/aaid-joi-D-19-00344

117. Al Deeb M, Alresayes S, Mokeem SA, Alhenaki AM, AlHelal A, Shafqat SS, et al. Clinical and immunological peri-implant parameters among cigarette and electronic smoking patients treated with photochemotherapy: a randomized controlled clinical trial. Photodiagnosis Photodynamic Ther. 2020;31:101800.

118. Al Hafez ASS, Ingle N, Alshayeb AA, Tashery HM, Alqarni AAM, Alshamrani SH. Effectiveness of mechanical debridement with and without adjunct antimicrobial photodynamic for treating peri-implant mucositis among prediabetic cigarette-smokers and non-smokers. Photodiagn Photodyn Ther. 2020;31:101912.

119. Blasi A, Iorio-Siciliano V, Pacenza C, Pomingi F, Matarasso S, Rasperini G. Biofilm removal from implants supported restoration using different instruments: a 6-month comparative multicenter clinical study. Clin Oral Implants Res. 2016;27(2):e68–73.

120. Mettraux GR, Sculean A, Bürgin WB, Salvi GE. Two-year clinical outcomes following non-surgical mechanical therapy of peri-implantitis with adjunctive diode laser application. Clin Oral Implants Res. 2016;27(7):845–9.

121. Moharrami M, Perrotti V, Iaculli F, Love RM, Quaranta A. Effects of air abrasive decontamination on titanium surfaces: a systematic review of in vitro studies. Clin Implant Dent Relat Res. 2019;21(2):398–421.

122. Lupi SM, Granati M, Butera A, Collesano V, Rodriguez YBR. Air-abrasive debridement with glycine powder versus manual debridement and chlorhexidine administration for the maintenance of peri-implant health status: a six-month randomized clinical trial. Int J Dent Hyg. 2017;15(4):287–94.

123. Salvi GE, Zitzmann NU. The effects of anti-infective preventive measures on the occurrence of biologic implant complications and implant loss: a systematic review. Int J Oral Maxillofac Implants. 2014;29(Suppl):292–307.

124. Barootchi S, Ravidà A, Tavelli L, Wang HL. Non-surgical treatment for peri-implant mucositis: a systematic review and meta-analysis. Int J Oral Implantol (Berlin, Germany). 2020;13(2):123–39.

125. Heitz-Mayfield LJA, Salvi GE, Mombelli A, Faddy M, Lang NP. Anti-infective surgical therapy of peri-implantitis. A 12-month prospective clinical study. Clin Oral Implants Res. 2012;23(2):205–10.

126. Tomasi C, Regidor E, Ortiz-Vigón A, Derks J. Efficacy of reconstructive surgical therapy at peri-implantitis-related bone defects. A systematic review and meta-analysis. J Clin Periodontol. 2019;46(Suppl 21):340–56.

127. Schwarz F, Sahm N, Bieling K, Becker J. Surgical regenerative treatment of peri-implantitis lesions using a nanocrystalline hydroxyapatite or a natural bone mineral in combination with a collagen membrane: a four-year clinical follow-up report. J Clin Periodontol. 2009;36(9):807–14.

128. Englezos E, Cosyn J, Koole S, Jacquet W, De Bruyn H. Resective treatment of peri-implantitis: clinical and radiographic outcomes after 2 years. Int J Periodontics Restorative Dent. 2018;38(5):729–35.

129. Chan HL, Lin GH, Suarez F, MacEachern M, Wang HL. Surgical management of peri-implantitis: a systematic review and meta-analysis of treatment outcomes. J Periodontol. 2014;85(8):1027–41.

130. Ramanauskaite A, Daugela P, Faria de Almeida R, Saulacic N. Surgical non-regenerative treatments for peri-implantitis: a systematic review. J Oral Maxillofac Res. 2016;7(3):e14.

131. Romeo E, Ghisolfi M, Murgolo N, Chiapasco M, Lops D, Vogel G. Therapy of peri-implantitis with resective surgery. A 3-year clinical trial on rough screw-shaped oral implants. Part I: clinical outcome. Clin Oral Implants Res. 2005;16(1):9–18.

132. Heitz-Mayfield LJ, Mombelli A. The therapy of peri-implantitis: a systematic review. Int J Oral Maxillofac Implants. 2014;29(Suppl):325–45.

133. Roccuzzo M, De Angelis N, Bonino L, Aglietta M. Ten-year results of a three-arm prospective cohort study on implants in periodontally compromised patients. Part 1: implant loss and radiographic bone loss. Clin Oral Implants Res. 2010;21(5):490–6.

134. Heitz-Mayfield LJ, Salvi GE, Botticelli D, Mombelli A, Faddy M, Lang NP. Anti-infective treatment of peri-implant mucositis: a randomised controlled clinical trial. Clin Oral Implants Res. 2011;22(3):237–41.

135. Heitz-Mayfield LJA, Salvi GE, Mombelli A, Loup PJ, Heitz F, Kruger E, et al. Supportive peri-implant therapy following anti-infective surgical peri-implantitis treatment: 5-year survival and success. Clin Oral Implants Res. 2018;29(1):1–6.

136. Quirynen M, Gijbels F, Jacobs R. An infected jawbone site compromising successful osseointegration. Periodontology 2000. 2003;33(1):129–44.

137. Reiser GM, Nevins M. The implant periapical lesion: etiology, prevention, and treatment. Compend Contin Educ Dent (Jamesburg, NJ : 1995). 1995;16(8):768, 70, 72 passim.

138. Sussman HI, Moss SS. Localized osteomyelitis secondary to endodontic-implant pathosis. A case report. J Periodontol. 1993;64(4):306–10.

139. McAllister BS, Masters D, Meffert RM. Treatment of implants demonstrating periapical radiolucencies. Pract Periodontics Aesthet Dent. 1992;4(9):37–41.

140. Zhou W, Han C, Li D, Li Y, Song Y, Zhao Y. Endodontic treatment of teeth induces retrograde peri-implantitis. Clin Oral Implants Res. 2009;20(12):1326–32.

141. Peñarrocha-Oltra D, Blaya-Tárraga JA, Menéndez-Nieto I, Peñarrocha-Diago M, Peñarrocha-Diago M. Factors associated with early apical peri-implantitis: a retrospective study covering a 20-year period. Int J Oral Implantol (Berlin, Germany). 2020;13(1):65–73.

142. Esposito M, Hirsch JM, Lekholm U, Thomsen P. Biological factors contributing to failures of osseointegrated oral implants. (II). Etiopathogenesis. Eur J Oral Sci. 1998;106(3):721–64.

143. Sarmast ND, Wang HH, Sajadi AS, Angelov N, Dorn SO. Classification and clinical management of retrograde peri-implantitis associated with apical periodontitis: a proposed classification system and case report. J Endod. 2017;43(11):1921–4.

144. Peñarrocha-Diago M, Peñarrocha-Diago M, Blaya-Tárraga J-A. State of the art and clinical recommendations in periapical implant lesions. 9th Mozo-Grau Ticare Conference in Quintanilla, Spain. J Clin Exp Dentistry. 2017;9(3):e471.

145. Quirynen M, Vogels R, Alsaadi G, Naert I, Jacobs R, van Steenberghe D. Predisposing conditions for retrograde peri-implantitis, and treatment suggestions. Clin Oral Implants Res. 2005;16(5):599–608.

146. Marshall G, Canullo L, Logan RM, Rossi-Fedele G. Histopathological and microbiological findings associated with retrograde peri-implantitis of extra-radicular endodontic origin: a systematic and critical review. Int J Oral Maxillofac Surg. 2019;48(11):1475–84.

147. Passi D, Singh M, Dutta SR, Sharma S, Atri M, Ahlawat J, et al. Newer proposed classification of periimplant defects: a critical update. J Oral Biol Craniofacial Res. 2017;7(1):58–61.

148. Shah R, Thomas R, Kumar AB, Mehta DS. A radiographic classification for retrograde peri-implantitis. J Contemp Dent Pract. 2016;17(4):313–21.

149. Ramanauskaite A, Juodzbalys G, Tözüm TF. Apical/retrograde periimplantitis/implant periapical lesion: etiology, risk factors, and treatment options: a systematic review. Implant Dent. 2016;25(5):684–97.

150. Kalyvas D, Tarenidou M, Zorogiannidis G, Tsetsenekou E, Grous A. Deep peri-implantitis: two cases treated with implant apicoectomy with follow-up of at least 7 years. Oral Surg. 2015;8(4):200–7.

151. Dahlin C, Nikfarid H, Alsen B, Kashani H. Apical peri-implantitis: possible predisposing factors, case reports, and surgical treatment suggestions. Clin Implant Dent Relat Res. 2009;11(3):222–7.

152. Lefever D, Assche N, Temmerman A, Teughels W, Quirynen M. Aetiology, microbiology and therapy of periapical lesions around oral implants: a retrospective analysis. J Clin Periodontol. 2013;40(3):296–302.

153. Romanos GE, Froum S, Costa-Martins S, Meitner S, Tarnow DP. Implant periapical lesions: etiology and treatment options. J Oral Implantol. 2011;37(1):53–63.

154. Bhaskar SN. Oral surgery--oral pathology conference No. 17, Walter Reed Army Medical Center. Periapical lesions--types, incidence, and clinical features. Oral Surg Oral Med Oral Pathol. 1966;21(5):657–71.

155. Saleh MHA, Khurshid H, Travan S, Sinjab K, Bushahri A, Wang HL. Incidence of retrograde peri-implantitis in sites with previous apical surgeries: A retrospective study. Journal of Periodontology. 2021; 92(1): 54–61.

156. Tözüm TF, Erdal C, Saygun I. Treatment of periapical dental implant pathology with guided bone regeneration. Turkish J Med Sci. 2006;36(3):191–6.

157. Flanagan D. Apical (retrograde) peri-implantitis: a case report of an active lesion. J Oral Implantol. 2002;28(2):92–6.

158. Mohamed JB, Alam MN, Singh G, Chandrasekaran SC. The management of retrograde peri-implantitis: a case report. J Clin Diagn Res. 2012;6(9):1600–2.

159. Soldatos N, Romanos GE, Michaiel M, Sajadi A, Angelov N, Weltman R. Management of retrograde peri-implantitis using an air-abrasive device, Er,Cr:YSGG laser, and guided bone regeneration. Case Rep Dentistry. 2018;2018:7283240.

160. Nikolaos S, Georgios ER, Michelle M, Ali S, Nikola A, Robin W. Management of retrograde peri-implantitis using an air-abrasive device, Er,Cr:YSGG laser, and guided bone regeneration. Case Rep Dentistry. 2018;2018:1–9.

161. Manfro R, Garcia GF, Bortoluzzi MC, Fabris V, Bacchi A, Elias CN. Apicoectomy and scanning electron microscopy analysis of an implant infected by apical (retrograde) peri-implantitis - a case letter. The Journal of oral implantology. 2018. The Journal of Oral Implantology. 2018; 44 (4): 287–91.

162. Blaya-Tarraga JA, Cervera-Ballester J, Penarrocha-Oltra D, Penarrocha-Diago M. Periapical implant lesion: a systematic review. Medicina Oral Patologia OrAL Y Cirugia Bucal. 2017;22(6):E737–E49.

163. Sarmast ND, Wang HH, Sajadi AS, Munne AM, Angelov N. Nonsurgical endodontic treatment of necrotic teeth resolved apical lesions on adjacent implants with retrograde/apical peri-implantitis: a case series with 2-year follow-up. J Endod. 2019;45(5):645–50.

164. Balshi SF, Wolfinger GJ, Balshi TJ. A retrospective evaluation of a treatment protocol for dental implant periapical lesions: long-term results of 39 implant apicoectomies. Int J Oral Maxillofac Implants. 2007;22(2):267–72.

165. Peñarrocha-Diago MA, Blaya-Tárraga JA, Menéndez-Nieto I, Peñarrocha-Diago M, Peñarrocha-Oltra D. Implant survival after surgical treatment of early apical peri-implantitis: an ambispective cohort study covering a 20-year period. Int J Oral Implantol (Berlin, Germany). 2020;13(2):161–70.

The Art and Science of Guided Bone Regeneration

9

Jonathan L. Czerepak

Introduction

Guided bone regeneration (GBR), derived from guided tissue regeneration (GTR), is one of the foundational ridge augmentation and preservation techniques for the repair of alveolar bone defects. Regeneration of osseous tissue has allowed for the facilitation of prosthetically driven implant site development. The fundamental basis of GBR is exclusion of rapidly growing tissues from an osseous defect allowing adequate time for consolidation of mature lamellar bone by preventing deleterious soft tissue ingrowth [1]. Contemporary guided bone regeneration allows volumetric bone reconstruction in areas with or without simultaneous implant placement [2]. It is generally defined as a technique utilizing either resorbable or non-resorbable membranes, with particulate bone grafts, for the reconstruction of maxillofacial defects [3]. When applying the concepts of GBR, one must be able to recognize the nature of the defect they are attempting to reconstruct, apply the tenets of predictable GBR, and understand the requirements for a prosthetically driven treatment plan (Fig. 9.1).

Historically, the reconstruction of osseous defects has been a daunting clinical problem. Osseous defects filled with autogenous or allogenic bone grafts yielded unpredictable osseous regeneration [4, 5]. Clinicians found that when performing bone grafting procedures, a significant amount of fibrous tissue could be generated within the attempted reconstruction. The development of a periodontal technique for the regeneration of the attachment apparatus of compromised teeth elucidated the possibility of broader regenerative applications, specifically osseous defects.

Guided tissue regeneration (GTR) utilized a barrier membrane to enhance regeneration of the supporting periodontal tissues with attachment defects. Initial experimental models proved adept at producing significantly more periodontal attachment than control groups without barrier membranes [6, 7]. This technique involves the regeneration of multiple tissues types. Creating favorable healing conditions allowed the regenerative capacity of the periodontal ligament to be exploited [8]. GTR, for at least 6–8 weeks, predictably yielded cementum, inserting collagen fibers and bone due to the exclusion of epithelium and connective tissue from the healing defect [8].

Extrapolating from the reported success of GTR, Dahlin et al. [9] hypothesized that a barrier membrane placed over an osseous defect could exclude the rapidly proliferating connective tissue yielding higher quality osseous healing. The investigators were able to regenerate bone at trephine sites in rat mandibles with the aid of a Teflon barrier membrane; this guided regeneration outperformed the control group. Histologically, they observed new immature bone, from 3–6 weeks, in the membrane-protected defects, compared to predominantly connective tissue ingrowth in non-membrane-protected sites even after 22 weeks of observation. The occlusive membrane allowed the relatively slow migration of osteogenic cells into the wound defect preferentially [3].

Guided bone regeneration is elegant in concept, but there are a myriad of techniques and materials that may cause confusion even with the astute clinician. It is imperative that surgeons elucidate the nature of the defect being reconstructed, the ultimate restorative plan, and contraindications to treatment, select appropriate materials/techniques, and understand the general principles necessary to provide predictable patient-specific treatment outcomes.

Principles of Guided Bone Regeneration

Guided bone regeneration is a surgical procedure which utilizes a set of principles or biological requirements, derived from bone wound healing physiology, to allow for predictable bone regeneration [2]. The core therapeutic principles are the

J. L. Czerepak (✉)
Department of Oral and Maxillofacial Surgery, Dwight D. Eisenhower Army Medical Center, Fort Gordon, GA, USA
e-mail: jonathan.l.czerepak.mil@mail.mil

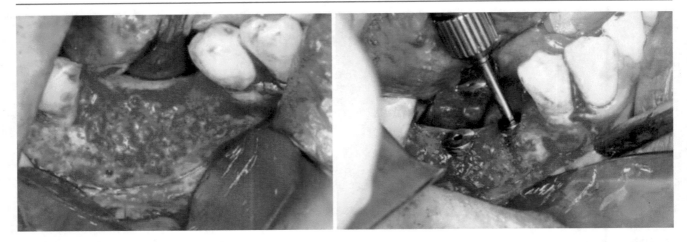

Fig. 9.1 Resultant guided bone regeneration of vertical and horizontal defect, after 6 months, utilizing a non-resorbable barrier membrane and with final implant placement

surgical placement of a cell occlusive membrane and the creation of a nascent space for the migration of osteoprogenitor cells for the regeneration of bone [9]. Wang et al. [2] proposed the "PASS" principles for guided bone regeneration consisting of primary closure, angiogenesis, space creation/maintenance, and stability. Application of these principles results in predictable regeneration.

Creating tension-free primary closure for the site of guided bone regeneration allows for the sequence of healing to occur in the most efficient matter [2]. Wound healing can broadly occur by either primary or secondary intention. When wound healing occurs by primary intention, the wound margins are approximated in order to facilitate efficient clot formation, epithelialization, minimization of collagen/scar formation along the wound margins, and an overall decrease in healing time [2] (see Fig. 9.2). Secondary intention is the disorganized healing that occurs when wound margins are not approximated. Allowing wounds to heal with secondary intention will lead to increase collagen/scar production and delayed healing [2]. While these concepts are elementary, it is apparent why tension-free primary closure of the reconstructed barrier-protected site is desirable. If a wound which has a barrier-protected space is left to heal without primary closure, the wound, graft, and barrier membrane are exposed to the oral environment though it may be acceptable with appropriate membrane selection (see Fig. 9.3). This can lead to bacterial colonization, infection, decreased nutrient perfusion, and decreased angiogenesis within the graft bed, loss of the graft material, and the failure of predictable regeneration [2]. One of the most versatile techniques for advancement of soft tissue to gain primary closure is the use of periosteal scoring with or without vertical releasing incisions; its use should be judicious as not to compromise vascular supply or iatrogenic dehiscence in the soft tissue flap (see Fig. 9.4).

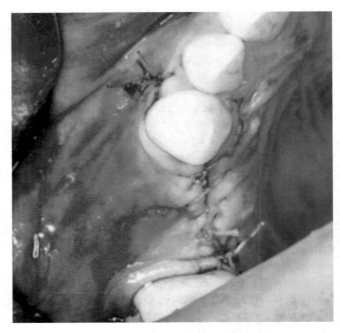

Fig. 9.2 Primary closure of an area that had undergone guided bone regeneration. The wound was closed with a combination of horizontal mattress and interrupted sutures

In order to accomplish osteogenesis, the wound bed requires adequate bloody supply. This is crucial to form the initial blood clot, which then releases cytokines and growth factors, such as interleukin-8 (IL8) and platelet-derived growth factors (PDGF), promoting the healing cascade from vascularly rich granulation tissue to osteoid and eventually mature lamellar bone [1]. This maturation period from stabilized clot to mature bone has been reported between 3–4 and 6–9 month, respectively [1, 2]. The blood supply is primarily

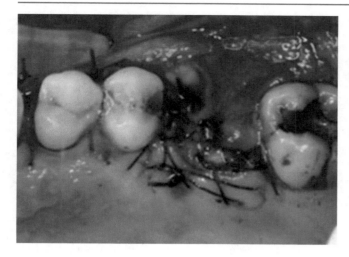

Fig. 9.3 Guided bone regeneration using a resorbable collagen barrier membrane where primary closure was not attained

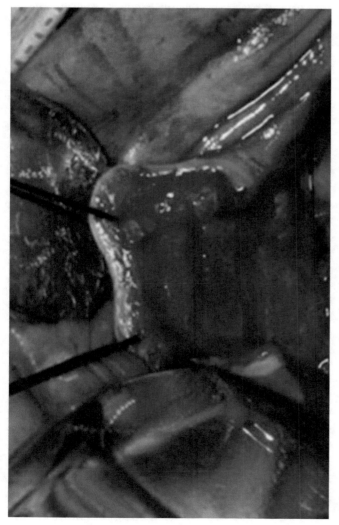

Fig. 9.4 A full-thickness mucoperiosteal flap with periosteal scoring to facilitate primary closure with judicious releasing incisions

from the underlying bone on which the GBR is being attempted. This alveolar bone is cortical in nature. Cortical bone has minimal perforating vessels to supply adequate blood flow to the graft bed. In order to maximize blood supply, initial clot formation, and osteoblast migration from medullary bone, many investigators advocate for cortical perforation or decortication of the graft bed, yet they are not obligatory to predictable osseous regeneration [1–3].

It is in the author's opinion cortical perforations are warranted where dense cortical bone is present to facilitate angiogenesis and migration of osteoblastic precursors from within the medullary bone. Cortical perforations can be omitted in maxillary locations where robust bleeding from the cortical plate is observed. It is necessary to plan any cortical perforations carefully to avoid compromising underlying bone stock necessary for membrane immobilization with either bone screws or tacks.

In order to maintain the blood clot and graft material in the newly created space, it is essential to obtain stability of the barrier membrane. This stability will allow the tenuous process of angiogenesis to proceed into the defect [8]. Angiogenesis is susceptible to shear in its initial phases, and even the slightest micromovement can disrupt it [8]. With disrupted vascular ingrowth in the grafted area, it will be susceptible to fibrous soft tissue ingrowth [10]. The movement will also delay wound healing of the overlying soft tissues due to production of inflammatory mediators and could result in dehiscence of the surgical site, leading to membrane exposure, bacterial colonization, and ultimately graft failure [10].

It is imperative to obtain primary stability on any membrane which is utilized for this technique. There are a myriad of techniques to secure these membranes in place. Sutures can be utilized to secure membranes to the adjacent attached periosteum. Suture fixation can be used in cases where there are multiple walls of the defect that prevent movement of the graft. Typically, membranes are secured with either titanium screws or pins. It is in the author's opinion that titanium screw fixation for non-resorbable reinforced membranes is simpler to use and offers more technical flexibility and reliable fixation. Regardless of the method of fixation used, it is imperative that the membrane is immobilized on both the buccal and lingual aspect of the defect. The principle of stability should also be extended to any implants concurrently placed into areas of GBR [2].

Space Creation and Maintenance

With the final restorative goals in mind, it is necessary to create space under the mucoperiosteal flap for the de novo bone production to occur. If the space is maintained, and a barrier is placed to exclude epithelial tissues, bone formation will result [2]. Typically, with GBR, the space is supported with the inclusion of bone grafting materials. These materials act as a scaffold for new bone formation and space maintainers buttressing the membrane in the appropriate position [10]. Space maintenance can be further aided with the incorporation of dental implants, titanium plates, or tenting screws to prevent membrane from deformation [1]. Recognizing that space maintenance is tenuous, the surgeon should account for patient function encouraging no chew and omission of removable prosthetics for at least 2–3 weeks [10].

Seminal research showed that even without bone grafting material, the isolated defect would fill with bone as long as the primary blood clot was maintained and protected from the pliable soft tissues [9]. Ultimately, the goal of space creation and maintenance is to keep the isolated wound bed in its intended new volume, preventing collapse caused by the epithelial contraction obligatory in wound healing and the patient function generally for 6 months prior to implant placement.

Barrier Membranes

Introduction

Many materials are employed as barrier membranes in GBR. Ideal barrier membrane properties include, biocompatibility, space maintenance, cell occlusiveness, tissue integration, and clinical handling [1,3,8,11]. Barrier membranes are classified as either resorbable or non-resorbable. Non-resorbable barrier membranes can be further subdivided as reinforced or non-reinforced. Porosity of the membrane has been suggested to have a vital role in the diffusion of nutrients, oxygen, fluids, and bioactive substances necessary to promote regeneration [11]. Expanded polytetrafluoroethylene or e-PTFE was utilized for the seminal work on GBR and GTR [11]. Resulting from their preponderance of use, sentiments exist that e-PTFE membranes should be considered the gold standard for comparison of novel barrier membranes [3, 9]. Notwithstanding satisfactory results can be achieved from varying membrane types, and their specific attributes should be considered prior to membrane selection.

Non-resorbable

Non-resorbable membranes offer great flexibility when trying to reconstruct defects. They can be reinforced minimizing deformation when regenerating larger horizontal or vertical defects. Non-resorbable membranes can be maintained in the soft tissues for many months without degradation and offer predictable cellular occlusiveness over those extended periods. Because they are biologically inert, they

have minimal associated immunogenicity and inflammation [11].

The principle difference in available membranes in this class is pore size. E-PTFE has a pore size of 5–20 μm, while high-density polytetrafluoroethylene or d-PTFE has a pore size of less than 0.3 μm [3]. This difference has profound clinical implications. Larger pore sizes found in e-PTFE have been associated with increased bacterial and cellular permeability, while d-PTFE minimizes for bacterial transfer [11]. As a corollary, e-PTFE's increased pore size allows for soft tissue adherence facilitating primary closure and wound healing [11]. Evidence suggests that without signs of infection, it is possible to obtain osseous regeneration using d-PTFE (Fig. 9.5) without primary closure that is a significant benefit in clinical situations where it is not achievable [10].

However, they are not without drawbacks. Both remain susceptible to bacterial surface colonization [11]. Non-resorbable membranes require surgical removal prior to definitive implant placement. They have limited chemotactic function for the facilitation of epithelial wound healing across the surgical wound margin [8]. Without chemotactic properties, flap passivity and primary closure are paramount in their use. They have also shown a tendency for premature exposure, though d-PTFE should be utilized when exposure risk is high or unavoidable due to their decreased bacterial permeability [10]. Should non-resorbable membranes become exposed to the oral cavity during GBR techniques, loss of bone may result, regardless of timeline of exposure [8]. Small early exposure of e-PTFE will continue to enlarge; compromising regeneration and removal is warranted [8].

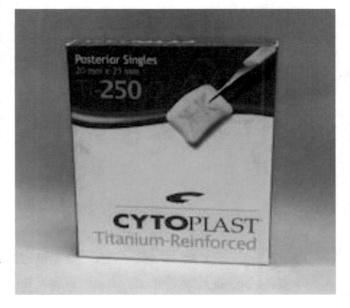

Fig. 9.5 A commercially available reinforced d-PTFE barrier membrane for guided bone regeneration

Resorbable

Resorbable membranes have become used extensively with GBR particularly for smaller defects. Resorbable materials certainly obviate the need for surgical removal. This can be beneficial in situations that do not require future surgical interventions, such as GBR adjacent to a dental implant. They typically are easy to manipulate and can be stabilized with a variety of techniques, including sutures and implant abutments. Resorbable membranes are typically fabricated from copolymers or collagen [1, 8, 11].

Collagen membranes offer the unique ability to aid in hemostasis and platelet aggregation and promote chemotaxis of fibroblast in order to facilitate wound healing [1]. Collagen membranes are manufactured from bovine, human, or porcine sources [1, 10] (Fig. 9.6). While their degradation rates can vary significantly, crosslinking has increased the duration of their occlusive properties [11]. They are broken down in situ by polymorphonucleocytes and macrophages via proteases and collagenases without foreign body reactions [1, 3, 10]. If exposed to the oral cavity, they remain occlusive to bacteria and can facilitate epithelial migration and wound closure, in contrast to e-PTFE [10].

Copolymer membranes include those of polyglycosides (PGAs) and polylactides (PLAs), individually or in combination with plasticizers which are available in sheets or mesh configurations [1, 10]. These membranes undergo hydrolysis and have been associated with increased soft-tissue inflammation and foreign body reactions [1, 10]. Of particular clinical interest is that during their degradation, there can be a precipitous drop in the local soft tissue pH secondary to CO_2 production from hydrolysis. Additionally, when prematurely exposed to the oral environment, these membranes begin

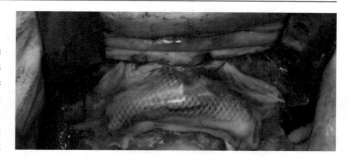

Fig. 9.7 Guided bone regeneration utilizing a resorbable membrane with underlying titanium mesh for added structural rigidity to the anterior maxilla

degradation rapidly, potentially limiting their space-making ability and compromising the underlying regeneration [1].

Resorbable membranes are not without limitations. Their rate of resorption can be unpredictable, though ideal resorbable membranes would last in vivo until re-epithelialization is complete 2–4 weeks [1]. Advancements have been made in crosslinking of collagen to increase the longevity of their cellular occlusiveness. There can be an inflammatory response associated with any resorbable membrane; this inflammation is mild and typically does not interfere with osteogenesis [9]. In locations with questionable soft tissues, this inflammatory response can lead to wound breakdown and loss of nascent bone [9].

It is the experience of the author and supported by literature that well delineated that small to medium defects can be reconstructed with resorbable collagen membranes predictably [8]. They typically lack the rigidity to maintain adequate space for larger horizontal or vertical defects. Their use is not precluded in larger osseous defects but require the introduction of additional supporting structure (Fig. 9.7). Titanium mesh grafting is a separate technique, but it warrants mention that when used in conjunction with a resorbable cross-linked collagen barrier membrane, it harmonizes with the principles of GBR resulting in similar histological and histomorphometric results when compared to non-resorbable titanium-reinforced d-PTFE [12].

Grafting Materials

While the seminal work on GBR was conducted without bone grafting materials, they are routinely used in the contemporary technique. Bone grafts aid in the principle of space maintenance and provide an osteoconductive scaffold for the regeneration of bone. Bone grafts can be classified as autogenous, allogenic, xenogeneic, or alloplastic, each with specific properties which can aid in reconstruction. These graft materials can be used alone or in combination.

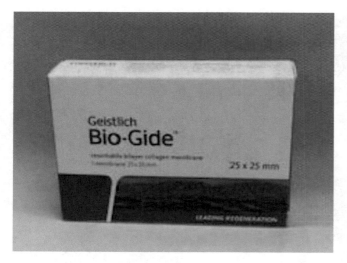

Fig. 9.6 A commercially available resorbable collagen membrane for guided bone regeneration

Autogenous bone grafts, long considered as the gold standard, are sourced from the patient. They are non-immunogenic, and it is possible to transplant viable osteoblasts making it the only osteogenic graft available to clinicians [13]. They can act as a scaffold for osteoconduction and maintain proteins and signaling molecules which allow for osteoinduction. Varying amounts of bone can be harvested from a patient depending on the specific volumetric needs of the reconstruction. Smaller amounts of bone can be harvested intraorally, and for larger defects, distant sites can be harvested.

Allogenic bone grafts are sourced from a human donor. They are treated with various means to reduced immunogenicity and the potential for transfer of pathological entities [13]. Allogenic bone grafts typically function as osteoconductive matrices, though there has been evidence to suggest that when decalcified, sufficient amounts of bone morphogenic protein (BMPs) are exposed to elicit osteoinduction, though significant qualitative variations exist based on donor factors [11].

Xenogeneic bone is animal derived and acts as an osteoconductive scaffold. Xenografts are treated to remove all organic components, eliminating the immunogenicity [13]. Xenografts can have varied resorption and replacement rates which can be used to clinical advantage to maintain graft morphology over extended periods of time.

Additional Considerations

Patients should be comprehensively evaluated as with all surgical interventions. Comorbid medical conditions should be elucidated in order to determine whether a patient is a reasonable candidate for GBR. Special attention should be devoted to the control of long-standing medical conditions. While many clinical disease processes are not absolute contraindications to the procedure, uncontrolled metabolic derangements should be evaluated and assessed. Patients should be deferred from active GBR treatment until those medical conditions are controlled. Smoking is another risk factor for wound breakdown and should be evaluated in all patient prior to undergoing an elective surgical procedure. While smoker's have a high rate of success of dental implant placement [3], they tend to have poorer outcome when undergoing extensive grafting procedures. Patients who have a past history of antiresorptive therapy should be risked assessed for medication-related osteonecrosis of the jaws and treated according to current professional guidelines with possible drug holidays or deferent of active treatment after consultation with their prescribing provider [3, 14].

Defects should be evaluated carefully (Fig. 9.8). GBR has been successful in both horizontal and vertical defects. The larger defects warrant the use of reinforced membranes in order to maintain space and decrease the potential for deformation in the grafting period. Diagnostic wax-ups of the final plan and surgical stent fabrication can be extremely beneficial when planning extensive GBR procedures in order to maximize effort for bone regeneration in the specific areas necessary to support dental implants.

Innovative Perspectives

Guided bone regeneration is a predictable technique, but, as with any procedure, there remains room for innovation and alterations in the therapeutic protocol. Advancements in tissue engineering and regenerative medicine can contribute to

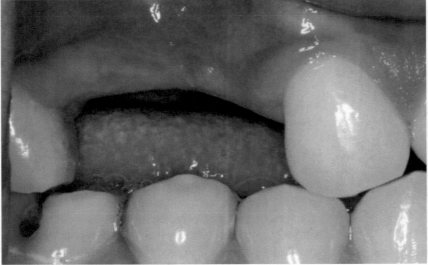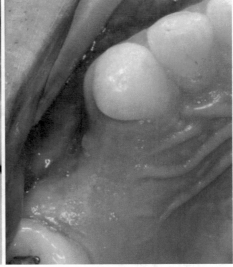

Fig. 9.8 Buccal and occlusal photographs of a combination horizontal and vertical defect amenable to guided bone regeneration prior to definitive implant placement

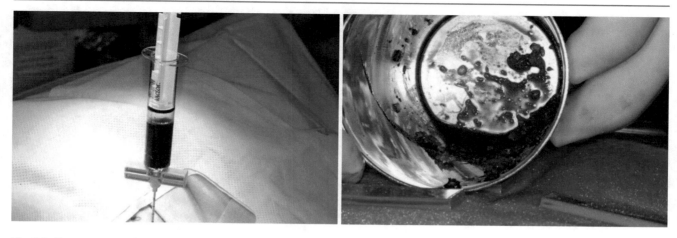

Fig. 9.9 Bone marrow aspirate harvest, after processing combined with bone grafting material for utilization in intraoral bone grafting

the technique. The evolving use of growth factors, membrane technology, and autogenous blood and bone products can contribute biological enhancement making GBR more predictable and yielding higher quality and less morbid results.

Platelet-rich plasma (PRP) has been used in dentistry for some time. Using it concurrently with GBR can introduce additional growth factors to the area of regeneration supporting soft-tissue healing and increasing bone yields. PRP contains platelets, proteins, and numerous growth factors to include platelet-derived growth factor (PDGF), transforming growth factor-B (TGF-B), vascular endothelial growth factor (VEGF), insulin growth factor-1 (IGF-1), and basic fibroblast growth factor (bFGF) [15]. It also contains fibrin, fibronectin, and vitronectin, enhancing cellular adhesion for osteoconduction [15]. The application of cell-based therapies is worth considering when planning GBR. Bone marrow aspirate concentrate or BMAC can be utilized to augment grafting procedures with mesenchymal stem cells and osteoprogenitor cell and may offer many of the benefits of autogenous bone grafting with decreased morbidity from autogenous bone harvesting [16] (Fig. 9.9). Bone morphogenic protein can be utilized to enhance recruitment of stem cells and preosteoblasts into the defect and can be a useful adjunct especially in medium to large defects [16].

References

1. Liu J, Kerns DG. Mechanisms of guided bone regeneration: a review. Open Dent J. 2014;8:56–65.
2. Wang HL, Boyapati L. "PASS" principles for predictable bone regeneration. Implant Dent. 2006;15:8–17.
3. Cucchi A, Chierico A, Fontana F, et al. Statements and recommendations for guided bone regeneration: consensus report of the guided bone regeneration symposium held in Bologna, October 15 to 16, 2016. Implant Dent. 2019;28(4):388–99. https://doi.org/10.1097/ID.0000000000000909.
4. Boyne PJ. Autogenous cancellous bone and marrow transplants. Clin Orthop Relat Res. 1970;73:199–209.
5. Schaberg SJ, Petri WH, Gregory EW, Auclair PL, Jacob E. A comparison of freeze-dried allogeneic and fresh autologous vascularized rib grafts in dog radial discontinuity defects. J Oral Maxillfac Surg [Internet]. 1985;43:932–7. https://doi.org/10.1016/0278-2391(85)90005-9PlumXMetrics.
6. Nyman S, Karring T, Lindhe J, et al. Healing following implantation of periodontitis affected roots into gingival connective tissue. J Clin Periodontol. 1980;7:394–401.
7. Gottlow J, Nyman S, Karring T, Lindhe J. New attachment formation as the result of controlled tissue regeneration. J Clin Periodontol. 1984;11:494–503.
8. Klokkevold P. Localized bone augmentation and implant site development. In: Newman MG, Takei HH, Klokkevold PR, Carranza FA, editors. Newman and carranza's clinical periodontology. 13th ed. Philadelphia: Elsevier; 2019 [cited 7 September 2020]. Chapter 79. p.794.e2-794e.4. Available from: https://www.clinicalkey.com/#!/content/book/3-s2.0-B9780323523004000795?scrollTo=%23hl0000123.
9. Retzepi M, Donos N. Guided bone regeneration: biological principle and therapeutic applications. Clin Oral Impl Res. 2010;21:567–76.
10. Barry KB, Lignelli JLL. Guided tissue regeneration in implant dentistry: techniques for management of localized bone defects. In: Fonseca RJ, editor. Oral and maxillofacial surgery. Philadelphia, PA: Elsevier - Health Sciences Division; 2009. p. 428–57.
11. Elgali I, Omar O, Dahlin C, Thomsen P. Guided bone regeneration: materials and biological mechanisms revisited. Eur J Oral Sci. 2017;125:315–37.
12. Cucchi A, Sartori M, Parrilli A, Aldini NN, Vignudelli E, Corinaldesi G. Histological and histomorphometric analysis of bone tissue after guided bone regeneration with non-resorbable membranes vs resorbable membranes and titanium mesh. Clin Implant Dent Relat Res. 2019;21:693–701. https://doi.org/10.1111/cid.12814.
13. Stevens MR, Emam HA. Dental implant prosthetic rehabilitation: allogenic grafting/bone graft substitutes in implant dentistry. In: Bagheri SC, Bell RB, Khan HA, editors. Current therapy in Oral and maxillofacial surgery. Philadelphia, PA: Elsevier - Health Sciences Division; 2012. p. 157–63.
14. Ruggiero SL, Dodson TB, Fantasia J, et al. American association of oral and maxillofacial surgeons position paper on medication-related osteonecrosis of the jaw 2014 update. J Oral Maxillofac Surg. 2014;72:1938–56.
15. Jimi E, Hirata S, Osawa K, Terashita M, Kitamura C, et al. The current and future therapies of bone regeneration to repair bone defects. Int J Dent. 2012; https://doi.org/10.1155/2012/148261.
16. Marx R, Stevens MR. Atlas of oral and extraoral bone harvesting. Chicago: Quintessence Publishing; 2010.

Direct Sinus Lift

Elizabeth Floodeen

Introduction and History

The direct sinus lift procedure is used to augment a pneumatized sinus with the goal of immediate or delayed endosseous implant placement in the posterior maxilla when there is otherwise insufficient bone. The sinus lifts, now almost exclusively used for pre-prosthetic implant surgery, actually predates the modern implant era. Historically, maxillary sinus augmentations began in the 1960s, almost 20 years prior to Brånemark's presentation of titanium root-form implants [1]. These earliest sinus grafts described by Boyne were to increase the height of the maxillary sinus floor in order to later reduce the alveolar ridge or tuberosity and achieve ideal inter-arch distance for the fabrication of conventional dentures.

Sinus augmentations in the setting of implant placement were first described by Tatum in 1976 and then by Boyne and James in 1980 [2, 3]. With implants as a popular solution for edentulism, sinus augmentation surgery is an essential tool for the surgeon who has a patient presenting with insufficient bone in the posterior maxilla. Over the last several decades, multiple sinus lift techniques have been described and numerous grafting substrates utilized. This chapter will focus on the lateral approach for a direct sinus lift along with indications, surgical variations, potential complications, and management.

Anatomy of the Maxillary Sinus

The maxillary sinus, pyramidal in shape and with an average volume of 12–15 cubic centimeters, is the largest of the paranasal sinuses [4]. Present at birth, the maxillary sinus gradually increases in volume over the first two decades of life, with enlargement generally ceasing around the age of 20. However, continued pneumatization of the sinus during adulthood can occur with tooth loss being the most frequent cause.

The maxillary sinus is bordered on the superior aspect by the orbital floor. The medial aspect borders the nasal cavity, and the antral floor is synchronous with the superior portion of the maxillary alveolus and hard palate. Frequently, root tips of posterior teeth project into the maxillary sinus, creating an irregular floor; these root tips are sometimes covered by only a thin layer of cortical bone. The ostium, or outflow tract, is located at the superior aspect of the medial wall and drains into the nasal cavity via the semilunar hiatus under the middle meatus. This superior location of the ostium is highly beneficial for sinus grafting procedures as obstruction is rare.

The Schneiderian membrane lines the walls of the maxillary sinus, and this membrane consists of multilayered epithelium with ciliated cylindrical cells, basal cells, and mucous-producing goblet cells. It measures approximately 0.13–0.5 mm in thickness and is extremely delicate, making it prone to tearing with excessive manipulation.

The size and shape of maxillary sinuses varies greatly between individuals. Up to 30% of the population may have one or more septa present within the maxillary sinus [5, 6]. These septa are usually located in the premolar region and oriented in a buccal-palatal direction [7]. The surgeon should inspect for septa prior to a sinus lift procedure as their presence increases the risk of membrane perforation [1, 5, 6, 8].

The vascular supply in and around the maxillary sinus is ample, and anatomical awareness of this vasculature will aid the surgeon by reducing the risk of major intraoperative bleeding. The maxillary sinus is supplied by branches of the maxillary artery: the infraorbital artery, the posterior superior alveolar artery, and the posterior lateral nasal artery. When utilizing the lateral window technique for sinus augmentations, the surgeon should be aware of possible intraosseous anastomoses between the infraorbital artery and the posterior superior alveolar artery. Rarely, these anastomoses

E. Floodeen (✉)
Department of Oral & Maxillofacial Surgery, Augusta University, Augusta, GA, USA
e-mail: efloodeen@augusta.edu

can be found extraosseously just medial to the lateral sinus wall; these vessels could be damaged when the Schneiderian membrane is dissected from the sinus walls. Venous outflow is via the facial vein, the sphenopalatine vein, and the pterygoid plexus, which connects with the cavernous sinus. This is significant in the context of infection as a possible tract for spread to the brain, which is why most surgeons recommend antibiotic prophylaxis for any sinus surgery [4].

Indications and Contraindications for Sinus Augmentation Surgery

The indication for a sinus lift procedure is a patient with inadequate bone for implant placement in the posterior maxilla. The minimum amount of bone necessary for standard height implant placement is 10 mm of vertical bone and 4 mm of alveolar ridge width; anything less indicates the need for augmentation [1, 9]. For a severely resorbed ridge with only 1–3 mm of bone remaining, a direct sinus lift with delayed implant placement is recommended. If there are 4–8 mm of alveolar bone, the surgeon should entertain implant placement at the time of direct sinus lift if primary stability can be achieved. For a ridge height of 8–10 mm, where only minimal bone increase is necessary, many surgeons prefer to use the transcrestal or osteotome technique over a direct approach, which will be discussed in future chapters.

Absolute contraindications for sinus augmentation surgery are the presence of sinus pathology, severe chronic sinusitis, or active sinus infection. Surgery may be reconsidered if chronic sinusitis or active infection can be controlled. Sinus pathology should be managed by the surgeon or referred appropriately to obtain a definitive diagnosis and treatment prior to any elective surgery. Relative contraindications include a history of radiation to the maxilla, severe allergic rhinitis, significant smoking, and severely medically compromised patients. In these instances, surgery should proceed on a case-by-case basis, and patients should be informed of an increased risk of complications.

Surgical Procedure

Preoperative Considerations

Typically in a straightforward procedure, most sinus lift surgeries can be performed in the clinical setting on an outpatient basis. Regarding anesthesia, many patients prefer sedation due to case duration and for anxiety management; however, short procedures can certainly be accomplished under local anesthesia. It is important for the surgeon to dis-

cuss with the patient the procedure length and involvement and set proper expectations to ensure selection of appropriate anesthetic modalities. Antibiotic prophylaxis for sinus procedures is recommended with one preoperative dose followed by a postoperative course for 7–10 days. For adequate sinus coverage, the antibiotic of choice is typically amoxicillin-clavulanate, ampicillin, or ciprofloxacin [10]. In an anticoagulated patient, the surgeon may consider holding these medications to minimize bleeding risk; however, holding anticoagulants is not always necessary, and a discussion with the prescribing physician would be prudent. Finally, for any smoker, it is recommended to discontinue smoking for a minimum of 2 weeks prior to surgery to optimize surgical outcome.

Armamentarium

- #15 blade
- Periosteal elevator
- Surgical handpiece or piezoelectric
- Irrigation
- Sinus curette
- Bone graft materials/biologics
- Membrane
- Suture

Surgical Technique

Local anesthesia is achieved via infiltration in conjunction with PSA and/or greater palatine nerve blocks. A #15 blade is used to make an incision down to the bone. The most common flap designs are either a crestal incision with a vertical release on the mesial and distal aspects or a semilunar incision. Next, a full-thickness flap is raised to provide direct access to the buccal cortex of the maxilla.

There are several variations to window preparation in order to gain direct access to the maxillary sinus. Traditionally, a large cortical window is created and either removed in its entirety or intentionally left attached at the superior aspect and then pushed into the sinus so as to create the new "floor" of the elevated sinus as pictured in Fig. 10.1. If a large access to the sinus is not required, some surgeons prefer to simply "bur away" a small oval window of cortical bone measuring less than a centimeter in diameter. Regardless of window technique, the surgeon should leave a paper-thin layer of bone to protect the Schneiderian membrane and break this thin bone with a hand instrument to avoid membrane perforation. There are numerous types of burs available. Many surgeons prefer a round diamond bur as it is less likely to tear the Schneiderian membrane as compared to a carbide.

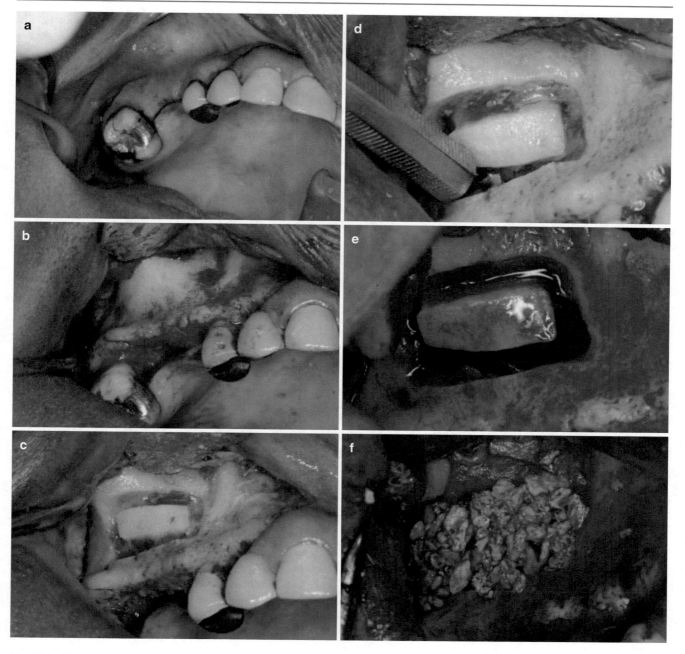

Fig. 10.1 Direct sinus lift "trap door" technique. (**a**) Incision design, (**b**) full-thickness flap reflection, (**c**) outline of lateral window with gray outline of sinus membrane just visible, (**d**) pushing lateral window through into sinus, (**e**) elevation of lateral window to create "trap door" serving as new sinus floor, (**f**) after particulate graft placement just prior to membrane placement

However, other providers prefer the cutting efficiency of an egg-shaped bone bur used with great caution.

The use of piezoelectric over the traditional rotary instruments has been proposed for making the lateral window with the argument it reduces risk of tearing the membrane. Rickert et al. performed a split mouth trial evaluating the use of piezoelectric vs. rotary instruments in direct sinus lifts and found no major advantage in regard to membrane damage; however, the piezoelectric did take significantly longer to

make the osteotomy than the traditional rotary instrument [11]. Ultimately it remains at the surgeon's discretion which instrument to use for osteotomy creation.

Once the cortical window is fashioned and access to the maxillary sinus is achieved, the Schneiderian membrane must be elevated in order to create space for the bone graft. The surgeon should elevate the sinus membrane with the utmost care as this paper-thin tissue is prone to tearing. It is recommended that initially 5 mm of circumferential membrane is loosened around the window in order to prevent tearing [9]. Once this tissue adjacent to the window is relaxed, the sinus membrane elevation may then continue along the floor and the medial wall of the sinus. The bone graft is then placed under the elevated sinus membrane, beginning with the anterior and medial locations first to prevent any voids [9]. When grafting, it is important to remain inferior of the ostium at the superior medial portion of the sinus to avoid obstruction of the outflow tract.

Many providers prefer to place a membrane over the graft to cover the lateral window, and surgeons debate as to whether this step is necessary. Those in favor of membrane placement argue that it aids in containment of particulate grafts, prevents possible soft tissue invasion of the graft, and increases bone formation. Others contend there is benefit from the additional blood supply offered by the adjacent soft tissue and prefer to not use a covering membrane. In a randomized clinical trial evaluating the difference in overall bone formation and the histological differences between sinus grafts with and without membrane use, it was discovered those grafts without membrane had slight increases in connective tissue present in histologic bone samples; however, there was no difference in the amount of total bone formation, ridge height, or the overall success of the graft and subsequent implants [4]. Once grafting is complete, it is recommended a minimum of 4–6 months healing time prior to implant placement if performing a delayed implant procedure [9].

Often, implants are placed simultaneously at the time of the sinus augmentation. Typically, 4–5 mm of alveolar bone height is required to obtain primary implant stability, although this may vary depending on the quality of bone [1, 12]. The order of operations when performing a combined procedure involves first making the lateral window with membrane elevation. Next the implant osteotomy is created taking care to protect the sinus membrane, usually with a sinus curette or small retractor inserted through the lateral window. Bone graft material should then be placed starting in the anterior and medial aspects, followed by implant placement, and then bone graft can be packed around the apex of the implant prior to flap closure [9].

With the increasing popularity of computer-aided implant planning and guided implant placement surgery, some surgeons have expanded this technology to include sinus augmentation procedures [13]. After obtaining a 3D scan, the exact location of implant placement is digitally planned and the desired amount of sinus elevation determined. Then a surgical guide is fabricated indicating both the position of implants and the location of lateral access to the sinus. The use of 3D technology with guided surgery may assist with evaluation of critical structures and aid the surgeon in ideal placement of both the lateral window and implants. The main disadvantage of this adjunct is the additional cost of planning software and guide fabrication and time spent planning surgery.

Another modification when placing implants at the time of sinus augmentation is to perform a "graftless" sinus lift procedure. It has been demonstrated with this technique that the apical portion of the implants are able to elevate or "tent-up" the sinus membrane and the space created under will fill with blood and subsequently mature to form new bone. Several authors have evaluated this technique and shown implant survival well above 90% [12, 14–16]. In 2016, Silva et al. performed a systematic review comparing implant success with and without bone graft and found implant survival was 99.6% when a bone graft was used and 96% when graftless procedure was performed [14]. The most significant benefits of performing a graftless procedure is no autogenous donor site morbidity, no risk of disease transmission with allograft or xenograft, and reduced cost to the surgeon.

Postoperative Instructions

The surgeon should always inform patients of expected postoperative findings including mild to moderate edema, possible epistaxis and ecchymosis, sinus congestion, and mild to moderate pain. Postoperative instructions include cold pack application for 24–48 hours, a soft food diet for 7–10 days, avoiding tooth-brushing in the surgical area for several days, and sinus precautions for 2 weeks (no nose-blowing, avoid plane travel, sneeze with open mouth, etc.) [10]. Prescription medications should include appropriate analgesics along with postoperative antibiotics; some providers may choose to prescribe nasal decongestants. Patients who smoke should be counseled to abstain for 6 weeks postoperatively and educated on the increased risk of postoperative complications and possible graft failure if they choose to smoke during the perioperative period.

Graft Materials, Biologics, and Expected Bone Gain

Numerous grafting substrates are available to the surgeon as outlined in Table 10.1. Autogenous bone has always been considered the gold standard for any grafting procedure due to its osteoconductive, osteoinductive, and osteogenic properties. However, depending on the volume of graft needed, it may be difficult to obtain sufficient quantities from an oral site such as the mental, ramus, or tuberosity areas, which may necessitate turning to an extraoral site such as the iliac

Table 10.1 Possible grafting materials and biologics

Material	Osteoconductive	Osteogenic	Osteoinductive	Advantages	Disadvantages
Autogenous	Yes	Yes	Yes	Osteogenic and osteoinductive, no risk of disease transmission	Donor site morbidity, increased surgical time
Allograft	Yes	No	Yes	No donor site morbidity	Requires sterilization, small risk of disease transmission
Xenograft	Yes	No	No	No donor site morbidity	Osteoconductive only
BMP with collagen sponge	Yes	No	Yes	No donor site morbidity	Cost, postoperative edema

crest or tibial bone. The greatest disadvantages of autogenous bone are donor site morbidity and additional time of surgery for bone harvest. For these reasons, many practitioners prefer to use either allograft or xenograft in order to avoid donor site morbidity. The main disadvantage of using allograft or xenograft is the additional cost of these materials.

Many have also explored the use of bone inductor materials such as bone morphogenic protein (BMP) with sinus augmentation procedures. One study found a 1.5 mg/mL concentration of BMP on an absorbable collagen sponge which showed a similar volume and density of bone as compared with autogenous graft for sinus lift procedures [17]. A 2014 Cochrane Review searched the available literature regarding what type of graft material and/or biologics would prove best for maxillary sinus augmentations and found "there was insufficient evidence to claim a benefit for any of these techniques for the primary outcomes of prosthesis and implant failure" [18].

The amount of bone gain with a lateral window technique can be substantial. Figure 10.2 shows radiographic bone increase of 11 mm immediately after an augmentation procedure of the left maxillary sinus using a mixture of demineralized allograft and xenograft. This type of bone mixture provides the osteoinductive benefits of the allograft with the radiopaque benefit of the xenograft to allow for immediate postoperative radiographic evaluation. As the graft matures, some resorption may occur. One study showed volume decreases of up to 65% when using only autogenous bone in maxillary sinus augmentation grafts in an animal model [19]. Other studies indicate this resorption decreases proportional to the addition of allograft and xenograft, indicating yet another potential benefit for the inclusion of these materials [16, 19].

Regardless of the grafting substrate selected, host factors inevitably play a critical role regarding healing progresses and ultimate graft success. The volume of the original defect in addition to the quality of the native bone and the ability of the host system to generate new bone is a significant factor in overall success. As the surgeon cannot control these patient variables, proper patient education is essential along with setting appropriate expectations.

Complications and Considerations

Table 10.2 outlines the possible complications of sinus augmentation surgery both during the procedure and postoperatively. We will discuss some of the more common complications and management strategies.

Membrane Perforation

The most common complication during sinus lift procedures is membrane perforation, which has been reported to occur in 7–35% of cases [20]. Risk factors that may increase the chance of membrane perforation include patients with an irregular sinus floor, presence of scar tissue from prior surgery, an acute angle between the medial and lateral walls of the sinus, and the presence of chronic sinus disease that results in membrane inflammation [4, 9, 21]. The presence of septa, which occur in approximately 30% of the population, also increases the risk for membrane perforation. It is recommended to obtain a cone beam computed tomography (CBCT) scan prior to surgery in order to evaluate the presence of sinus irregularities and septa. If a septum is present, the surgeon should modify the lateral access either by creating a larger window to span both sides of the septum or conversely create two small windows on either side of the septum to make appropriate access to the membrane for elevation and reduce the risk of damage [21].

If membrane perforation does occur, it needs to be managed appropriately to avoid risk of graft loss or infection. Small membrane perforations can be dealt with by placing a resorbable membrane over the perforation prior to graft placement. Larger perforations may necessitate abandonment of the procedure and allow for 6 months of healing prior to re-attempting an augmentation procedure.

Bleeding

Intraoperative bleeding during sinus surgery, while rarely dangerous, can make augmentation surgery difficult or impossible due to visual field obstruction. Arterial bleeding

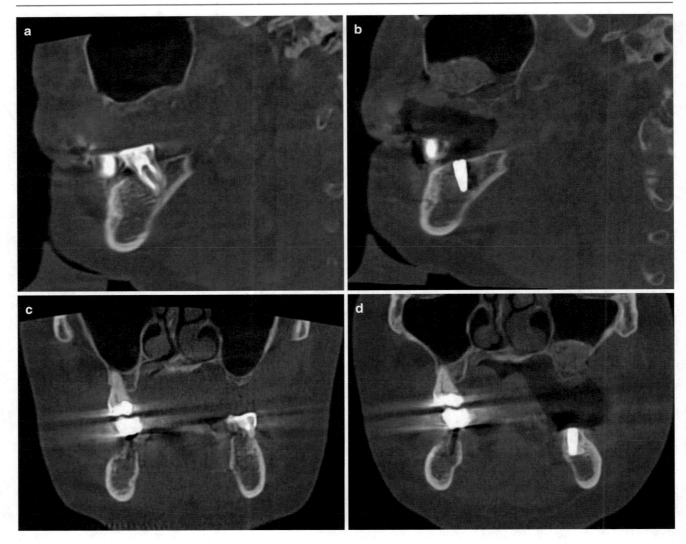

Fig. 10.2 Radiographic bone gain. (**a**) Sagittal view of left maxillary sinus prior to bone graft, (**b**) sagittal view of left maxillary sinus immediately after bone graft, (**c**) coronal view of maxillary sinuses prior to bone graft, (**d**) coronal view of maxillary sinuses immediately after bone graft to left sinus

Table 10.2 Potential complications of direct sinus lift

Intraoperative	Early	Late
Membrane perforation	Infection (acute)	Infection (chronic)
Bleeding	Implant failure	Implant failure
Alveolar ridge fracture	Graft loss	Chronic sinus disease
	Ostium obstruction	Implant migration
	OA fistula	

is typically from the intraosseous artery of the posterior superior alveolar artery which is usually found 16–19 mm from the alveolar ridge [9]. Occasionally, the posterior lateral nasal artery may be encountered and damaged with forceful curettage/elevation of the posterior-lateral aspect of the sinus, and therefore care should be taken if elevation in this region is required. A CBCT may be helpful in evaluating for any large arterial branches in the surgical area.

If heavy intraoperative bleeding is encountered, tools for management include head elevation, application of direct pressure, and addition of local vasoconstrictors. If direct pressure is insufficient to cease bleeding after a few minutes, then bone burnishing, electrocautery, or vessel ligation may be considered. Electrocautery should be used with caution in proximity to the sinus as in may result in membrane perforation.

Infection

While some maxillary sinuses are sterile, up to 75% of sinuses do contain bacteria, usually analogous to normal oral flora [22]. A biogram of sinus bacteria demonstrated the majority are streptococcus 45% (usually viridans) and staphylococcus

25%, but *Haemophilus* and *Enterobacteriaceae* species are found as well [10]. Infection can occur early or late in the postoperative period. To prevent the risk of infection, it is recommended to provide prophylaxis to the patient and continue a 7–10 days postoperative course. For appropriate coverage, amoxicillin-clavulanate, ampicillin, or ciprofloxacin are recommended [10].

Implant Failure and Migration

Implant success in the setting of sinus augmentation procedures is typically greater than 95%. However, implant failure can and does occur. In the event an implant fails, it should be removed and the site allowed to heal for several months prior to replacement. Additional grafting may be necessary if concurrent bone loss is present.

While highly unusual, migration of an implant into the maxillary sinus has been reported on multiple occasions. Displacement typically occurs at the time of implant placement or within 1–2 weeks, before osteointegration begins [20, 23]. However, there have been reports of implant displacement months or even years after the implant was placed. Some patients will develop chronic sinusitis, while others will be completely asymptomatic. Removal of the displaced implant is recommended either via intraoral approach/Caldwell-Luc or transnasal approach via functional endoscopic sinus surgery [24]. Sinus lift procedures do not appear to increase the instance of implant displacement, but rather lack of primary implant stability is the culprit [23]. Therefore, if performing implant placement at the time of sinus lift procedure, primary stability is essential for implant survival.

Conclusion

The lateral window approach for a direct sinus lift has been utilized for decades in order to augment an edentulous maxillary ridge with inadequate bone volume for implant placement. While many providers prefer an indirect sinus lift technique when only 1–3 mm of bone gain is necessary, the direct lateral window approach remains the standard when substantial grafting is required for a moderately to severely resorbed ridge. Evidence has shown overall excellent bone gain and long-term implant survival with the direct sinus lift technique. Over the years, the choice of grafting material has broadened from autologous bone to allograft and xenograft, to including BMP, and even graftless surgery with immediate implant placement. 3D imaging has also improved the surgical process by allowing for a more thorough preoperative evaluation of the sinus and move to a fully digital workflow

with precise cutting guides if the surgeon so chooses. With the popularity of implants as the primary choice for tooth replacement, the direct sinus lift is a necessary skill for all oral and maxillofacial surgeons.

References

1. Jensen O, editor. The sinus bone graft. 1st: Quintessence Publishing Co; 1999.
2. Tatum H Jr. Maxillary and sinus implant reconstructions. Dent Clin N Am. 1986;30:207–29.
3. Boyne PJ, James R. Grafting of the maxillary sinus floor with autogenous marrow and bone. J Oral Surg (Chic). 1980;38:613–6.
4. Danesh-Sani SA, Loomer PM, Wallace SS. A comprehensive clinical review of maxillary sinus floor elevation: anatomy, techniques, biomaterials and complications. Br J Oral Maxillofac Surg. 2016;54:724–30.
5. Danesh-Sani SA, Loomer PM, Wallace SS. A comprehensive clinical review of maxillary sinus floor elevation: anatomy, techniques, biomaterials and complications. Br J Oral Maxillofac Surg. 2016;54:724–30.
6. Park YB, Jeon HS, Shim JS, Lee KW, Moon HS. Analysis of the anatomy of the maxillary sinus septum using 3-dimensional computed tomography. J Oral Maxillofac Surg. 2011;69:1070–8.
7. Underwood AS. An inquiry into the anatomy and pathology of the maxillary sinus. J Anat Physiol. 1910;44:354–69.
8. Qian L, Tian XM, Zeng L, Gong Y, Wei B. Analysis of the morphology of maxillary sinus septa on reconstructed cone-beam computed tomography images. J Oral Maxillofac Surg. 2016;74:729–37.
9. Choi C, Misek DJ. Sinus lift grafting. First Ed Atlas Oper Oral Maxillofac Surg. 2015; https://doi.org/10.1002/9781118993729.ch6.
10. Carreño Carreño J, Gómez-Moreno G, Aguilar-Salvatierra A, Martínez Corriá R, Menéndez López-Mateos ML, Menéndez-Núñez M. The antibiotic of choice determined by antibiogram in maxillary sinus elevation surgery: a clinical study. Clin Oral Implants Res. 2018;29:1070–6.
11. Rickert D, Vissink A, Slater JJRH, Meijer HJA, Raghoebar GM. Comparison between conventional and piezoelectric surgical tools for maxillary sinus floor elevation. A randomized controlled clinical trial. Clin Implant Dent Relat Res. 2013;15:297–302.
12. Falah M, Sohn DS, Srouji S. Graftless sinus augmentation with simultaneous dental implant placement: clinical results and biological perspectives. Int J Oral Maxillofac Surg. 2016;45:1147–53.
13. Strbac GD, Giannis K, Schnappauf A, Bertl K, Stavropoulos A, Ulm C. Guided lateral sinus lift procedure using 3-dimensionally printed templates for a safe surgical approach: a proof-of-concept case report. J Oral Maxillofac Surg. 2020;78:1529–37.
14. de Silva LF, de Lima VN, Faverani LP, de Mendonça MR, Okamoto R, Pellizzer EP. Maxillary sinus lift surgery—with or without graft material? A systematic review. Int J Oral Maxillofac Surg. 2016;45:1570–6.
15. Nasr S, Slot DE, Bahaa S, Dörfer CE, Fawzy El-Sayed KM. Dental implants combined with sinus augmentation: what is the merit of bone grafting? A systematic review. J Cranio-Maxillofacial Surg. 2016;44:1607–17.
16. Starch-Jensen T, Jensen JD. Maxillary sinus floor augmentation: a review of selected treatment modalities. J Oral Maxillofac Res. 2017;8:1–13.
17. Triplett RG, Nevins M, Marx RE, Spagnoli DB, Oates TW, Moy PK, Boyne PJ. Pivotal, randomized, parallel evaluation of recom-

binant human bone morphogenetic Protein-2/absorbable collagen sponge and autogenous bone graft for maxillary sinus floor augmentation. J Oral Maxillofac Surg. 2009;67:1947–60.

18. Esposito M, Felice P, Hv W, Esposito M, Felice P, Hv W. Interventions for replacing missing teeth: augmentation procedures of the maxillary sinus (review). Cochrane Libr Syst Rev. 2014; https://doi.org/10.1002/14651858.CD008397.pub2.www.cochranelibrary.com.

19. Jensen T, Schou S, Svendsen PA, Forman JL, Gundersen HJG, Terheyden H, Holmstrup P. Volumetric changes of the graft after maxillary sinus floor augmentation with bio-Oss and autogenous bone in different ratios: a radiographic study in minipigs. Clin Oral Implants Res. 2012;23:902–10.

20. Schwartz-Arad D, Herzberg R, Dolev E. The prevalence of surgical complications of the sinus graft procedure and their impact on implant survival. J Periodontol. 2004;75:511–6.

21. Testori T, Weinstein T, Taschieri S. Wallace SS (2019) risk factors in lateral window sinus elevation surgery. Periodontol. 2000;81:91–123.

22. Peleg O, Blinder D, Yudovich K, Yakirevitch A. Microflora of normal maxillary sinuses: does it justify perioperative antibiotic treatment in sinus augmentation procedures. Clin Oral Investig. 2019;23:2173–7.

23. Jeong KI, Kim SG, Oh JS, You JS. Implants displaced into the maxillary sinus: a systematic review. Implant Dent. 2016;25:547–51.

24. Chiapasco M, Felisati G, Maccari A, Borloni R, Gatti F, Di Leo F. The management of complications following displacement of oral implants in the paranasal sinuses: a multicenter clinical report and proposed treatment protocols. Int J Oral Maxillofac Surg. 2009;38:1273–8.

Conservative Technique for Sinus Elevation

Milad Mir Mohammadi and Shohreh Ghasemi

Introduction

The standard sinus window method (Caldwell-Luc) was a highly invasive bone augmentation surgery that was to be bettered by the osteotome sinus lift system and was initially founded as a lower invasive method, such that the implants could be attached into the rear end of the maxillary region with a minimal bone height. Summers originally defined it as the procedure to enlarge the maxillary sinus and affix implants in regions where there was 6 mm or an increase in the area of the native bone. The repositioning of the apical of the Schneiderian membrane was carried out along with the bone grafting substances, comprising autogenous bone, utilizing osteotomes. Simultaneously implant placement reduces the mandatory surgical revisits [1, 2].

The explanation in this manuscript is about the process of traditional osteotome augmentation surgery. This surgery is not that stressful. It needs minimum bone height (below 5 mm) and utilizes non-autogenous substances in the graft with calcium-sulfate to speed up bone development. There is no need to infracture the bone, and it comprises a bone-level platform switching. The validation of cone beam computed tomography (CBCT) is also included.

Steps and Safety Measures in the Osteotome Structure

A regular and a full-thickness flap with a crestal slit can be undertaken to ensure entry to the bony ridge. The lap can be raised to study the palatal and facial contours of the bone in two procedures relating to the surgical access [3].

M. M. Mohammadi (✉)
Private Practice (Iran), Tehran, Iran
e-mail: miladmirmohammadi1367@yahoo.com

S. Ghasemi
Department of Oral and Maxillofacial Surgery, Augusta University, Augusta, GA, USA

The gingival punch process is another choice for easy entry. A tiny opening can be created where the center of the punch will be utilized along with a small portion of *gutta-percha* which is attached within this tiny slit to help in the placement of the punch. The placement can be validated by radiography. This punch method is ideal for utilizing a tiny scalar or chisel following the punch's formation and expelling the tissue to loosen the circumferential tissue inside eventually. To operate a 3.75 mm implant, a 5.75 mm thick ridge is the least mandatory measurement [4]. (An implant consisting of titanium alloy within this diameter is suggested, as the alloy is more solid than the commercially unmixed titanium.) Usually, with implant attachment, the primary phase is the employment of a round bur to initiate the osteotomy. To obtain the validation of the placement, as mentioned above, a tiny portion of gutta-percha can be fixed within this small osteotomy, including the use of the radiography and the expulsion of the *gutta-percha*. The subjection of the Schneiderian membrane is the next critical stage. A tool measuring a 2 mm twist drill is worked at a maximum speed of 250 rpm, with a very gentle contact. As the maxillary posterior is predominantly known for inferior bone quality, it's mostly simple to detect the breaking through the medullary bone and the point of access of the dense cortical bone of the floor of the sinus. It is suggested that, before the surgery, the cortical plate of the floor relating to the sinus is to be cautiously assessed with periapical radiography. However, it's mostly approximately 1 mm thick. The highly critical stage that is also reliant on great dexterity is breaking through the bone's cortical plate, lining the sinus to prevent any tear of the sinus membrane. The lessening of the subantral bone area by efficient supervision, a strong finger rest, the least drilling pressure, copious irrigation, and a steady pace of drilling, which is the result of post-extraction ridge resorption and secondary pneumatization of the maxillary sinus, can be expected to be enlarged by numerous sinus floor elevation (SFE) methods, by implementing a parallel or slower method, regarding implant attachment or various graft substances [3, 5, 6].

A minor "give" happens due to very low drilling pressure, steady control, presence of a strong finger rest, and the low pace of a drilling copious irrigation, thereby, the result being breaking through this plate. The membrane can get torn if the complete width of the twist drill ruptures the sinus floor. A late-ended implant probe can be applied by sliding it into the osteotomy and experiencing the minor "give" or motion of the membrane if there is any uncertainty regarding the membrane's subjection. A radiographic marker can be applied if the surgeon is uncertain regarding the membrane's subjection [7, 8]. The use of the radiograph marker must be avoided if the membrane is greatly exposed, as it can eventually cause the membrane significant damage. The patient must be informed about the marker when the radiograph is in operation because on biting it, the membrane can tear. If required, the missing membrane can be recovered and should be affixed to the marker. On baring a part of the membrane, the osteotomy is expanded to 2.8 mm with a very low pressure, again not above 250 rpm as it must cease at the lift of the conventional membrane (membrane must be tiny); a portion of the collagen membrane can be fixed on the inner region of the membrane. Later, the continuation of the regular bone packing process is executed [9]. The lap can also be stitched as another choice at the correct position. The patient is to be intimated that the process will continue in around 6–8 weeks. Then the tender tissue within the osteotomy can be utilized to raise the sinus membrane by an acute dissection of the lap of that part that is above the osteotomy. The Schneiderian membrane, thereby elevating the lap, doesn't suffer any damage. However, a coronally placed lap should be affixed and elevated to conceal the osteotomy to prevent the development of a postoperative sinus – antral slit [10], if a flapless technique was carried out.

An osteotome-mediated technique offers benefits like the potential to fill the implants in the least period; it's mostly traditional surgical access, a lower magnitude of postoperative morbidity, and the sinus is mostly enlarged in a restrained manner (Fugazzotto, 2001) [2].

The present guidelines for the maximum application of the maxillary sinus floor elevation are to accomplish the objectives of lower morbidity, greater success rates of implants, lessen the duration of the cure, and encourage concurrent implant fixation is a never-ending hurdle for surgeons. The flapless surgery is less invasive; hence, it reduces postoperative trauma and complications to a great extent than the traditional open-flap operation [11, 12].

The implanted osteotomy area implements the sinus membrane elevation and the transcrestal osteotomy in the absence of a tactile or visual guide in the case of the flapless crestal sinus augmentation procedure [13].

There are usual drawbacks in the cure of edentulous maxilla in terms of the presence of bone in the posterior region. In such situations, the sinus elevation methods are highly apt for an efficient cure.

Various substances like homograft, xenograft can load the sub-Schneiderian region, and autograft, etc [14].

There are drawbacks regarding the autograft application as it depends on the requirement of the donor site (more morbidity and complexity). This graft can have extraoral sources, in tricky conditions, or intraoral sources, if the requirement for the reconstruction is minimal [15].

Setting Up the Transalveolar Technique: Osteotome Process

Table 11.1 (tools comprise the osteotome surgery process)

The concave tips and the continuous taper are the primary Summers' osteotomes. The concave structure can grip and cumulate and help propel the bone graft substances in front of the developing osteotome (Fig. 11.1).

A concave tip is a common feature of osteotomes that is present to slit and cumulate the bone. Thus, making the vertical compression of the bone possible. The movement of the bone at the apical is gathered by the osteotome that will result in the lift of the Schneiderian membrane and the sinus floor.

A surgical mallet is applied to develop the osteotome (Fig. 11.2). The tactile sensitivity variation may help the clinician notice the cortical floor of the sinus cavity when malleting the osteotome – another pitch of tapping [16].

Table 11.1 Osteotome tool kit

Nylon cap mallet
Straight sinus elevation concave osteotome
Angled sinus elevation concave osteotome
Bone carrier
Bone bowl

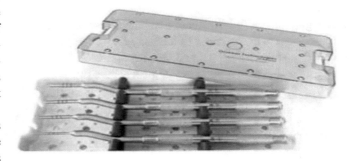

Fig. 11.1 The osteotome kit for sinus elevation

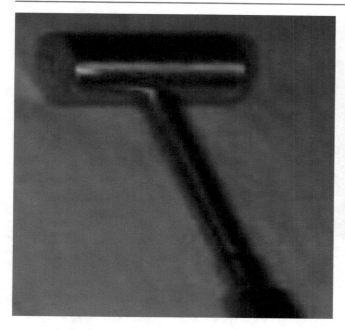

Fig. 11.2 Surgical mallet

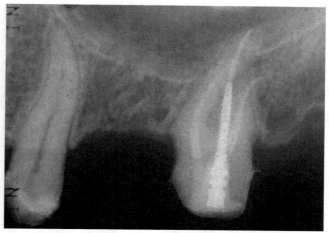

Fig. 11.3 A periapical radiograph has been taken to confirm the cortex of sub-sinus and planification of implant position

Incision Structure

The lateral window system is comparatively modern to the transalveolar technique's flap structure, with the flap reflection usually restricted to the crestal region. The vascular reserve of the lateral wall of the sinus thereby has a lesser occurrence of injury. The employment of a surgical mallet to compress the alveolar bone by an osteotome is the crestal technique's procedure. A broader ever-growing series of osteotomes are pierced in an apical direction near the sinus floor to set up the osteotomy and infracture the cortical plates according to the bone density [17].

First Stage

(a) The sterile surgical area and the operative area are separated.
(b) Perioral antisepsis including 2% chlorhexidine.
(c) Regional infiltration local anesthesia including 2% mepivacaine with adrenaline in the ratio of 1:100,000.
(d) Intraoral antisepsis including 0.12% chlorhexidine.

The option to elevate the flap or not is the principal step of the crest method. A flapless procedure can be administered if there is a sufficient proportion of keratinized gingival at the alveolar ridge and the buccal area in the absence of undercuts. The gingival is eliminated by a tissue punch equal to the diameter of the fitted implant in the preset implant region. The bare minimum subjection of the bone will suffice on elevating a flap. An opening at the crestal is executed, which is entirely thick, and the use of osteotomes can meet the region's whole constitution. On the contrary, a mix of osteotomes and drills are essential regarding dense bones [1, 2].

The alveolar crest is revealed by the flap reflection. Tiny vertical releasing slits are carried out if there is tightness at the flap.

The flapless procedure and the region around the bur in the twin flaps can be utilized to mark the recommended area of the implant (Fig. 11.3a).

Second Stage

(a) Raising the completely thick flap.
(b) The use of a No. 15 blades for mucoperiosteal slit at the crest of the bone ridge and mesial and distal relieving slits far from the space of the surgery.
(c) Ascertaining the osteotomy location by using a surgical yardstick. The implant spot is set to a depth of 1 mm lower than the sinus floor by a 2 mm cylindrical bur. The precautionary measures of fixing the 1 mm gap are to avoid the tip of the drill from damaging the Schneiderian membrane (Fig. 11.4).

Third Stage

The 2 mm guide pin in the position is used for the periapical radiography. This is implemented to assure the solidarity of the sub-sinus cortex and to validate the gap and the placement of the implant from the apex of the osteotomy until the sinus floor (Fig. 11.5).

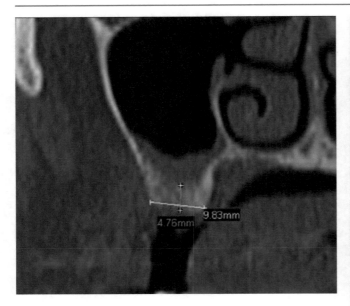

Fig. 11.4 CBCT analysis for measurement of vertical and horizontal bone before osteotome technique

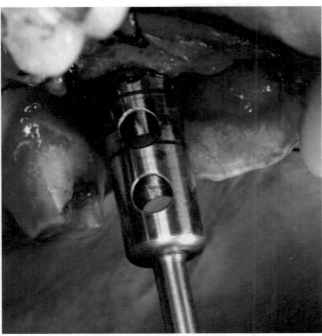

Fig. 11.6 Enlarge the osteotomy with a larger diameter; the sequence is adding graft with tapping the osteotome for the demand of amount of sinus lift

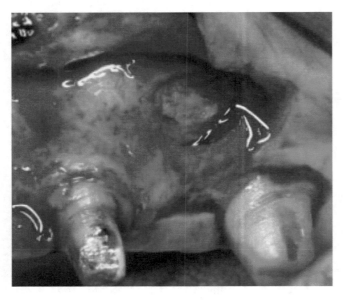

Fig. 11.5 Illustration of the distance from the apex of the osteotomy to the sinus floor

Fourth Stage

The osteotomy augmentation is carried out with a 3 mm cylindrical drill till the appropriate depth and should continue to be 1 mm lower than the sinus floor (Fig. 11.6).

Fifth Stage

The graft substance is mixed in the osteotomy before striving to raise the sinus floor. The space of the substance must be within 2–3 mm in height. The accidental perforation of the sinus membrane is a remote possibility of mixing this substance (Fig. 11.7).

Sixth Stage

The piezoelectric procedure with an osteotomy (Piezotome®-Satelec) is performed with a diamond-coated tip below the saline irrigation. The next step is formation of an elliptical lateral window, where the upper perimeter was fixed at 15 mm higher than the alveolar crest; the anterior edge was 3 mm behind the anterior perimeter of the maxillary sinus; the bottom edge was 3 mm higher than the sinus floor, and the posterior perimeter as per the positioning of the total implants.

The window measurements were 12 mm in mesiodistal width and 10 mm in height. A 3 mm osteotome is developed with light malleting and placed inside the osteotomy.

Ascertaining the piercing force is challenging as the rest of the bone quantity, and quality varies for multiple patients and surgeries. But, if the osteotome struggles to move or the magnitude of the struggle is too much, you could work with a tiny diameter around bur or piezo surgical tools to gently puncture a dense area of the apical bone (Fig. 11.8).

Seventh Stage

The osteotomy will be continued until the depth of the sinus floor, by infracturing the cortical bone, the rest of the bone is

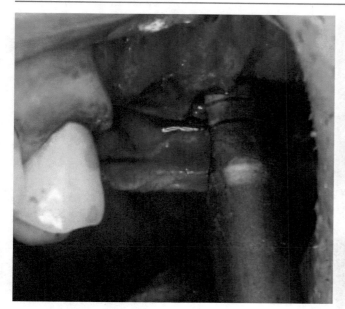

Fig. 11.7 The implant site is prepared to a 1 mm depth below the sinus; use piezo surgical instruments for adjustment

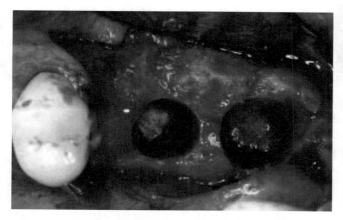

Fig. 11.8 The osteotomy of implant placement in osteotome technique

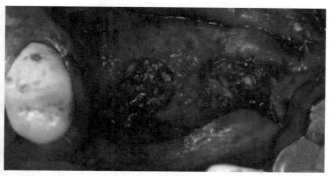

Fig. 11.9 Bone graft added to lift the sinus membrane

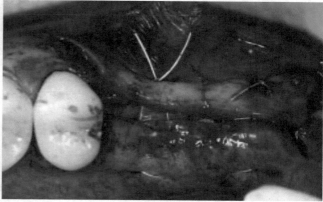

Fig. 11.10 Suturing after sinus elevation by osteotome technique

fitted apically into the sinus cavity, thereby lifting the sinus membrane. The tool's movement is then feasible around 2 mm deeper than the depth of the infracture for every operation. On every progression, the bone graft substance must be mixed inside the osteotomy. The tip of the osteotome should never enter the sinus or come in contact with the Schneiderian membrane (Fig. 11.9).

Eighth Stage

The osteotomy is broadened by a higher diameter osteotome, like 3.5 mm, after the tip has attained the necessary height. The piercing of the osteotome at the preset depth in this pattern after mixing the graft substance is sustained until the complete accomplishment of the required proportion of lifting [16, 17] (Fig. 11.10).

Tip: A stop to control the apical progression may be fixed to prevent the accidental entry and the perforation of the membrane.

Tip: The last osteotome diameter should be lower than the implants' needed width, mostly lower in the range of 0.5–1.2 mm. The constriction of the osteotome during the implant attachment can be performed by shortening the osteotomy, specifically in Type IV bone. For example, the last osteotome for a 5 mm implant is 4.2 mm, and for a 4 mm implant, a 3.5 mm would be the final osteotome.

Ninth Stage

The sliding of the final osteotome or guide pin as per the needed length is the concluding phase of the osteotome surgery.

Tenth Stage

Before fixing the implant, extra graft substance should be mixed into the osteotomy (Fig. 11.11).

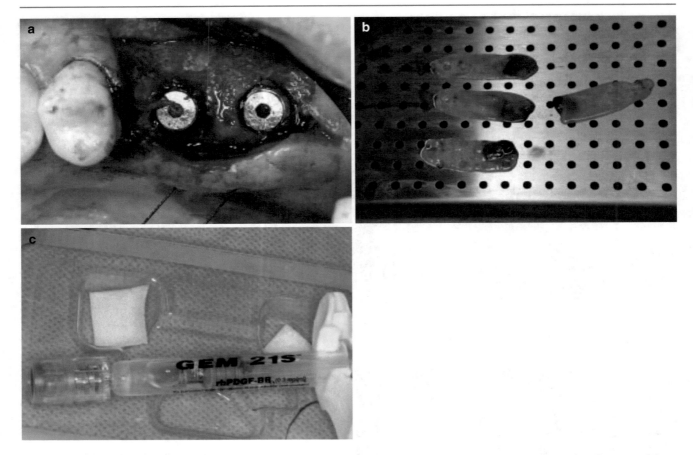

Fig. 11.11 The sequence of adding graft material and tapping the osteotome to the predetermined depth continues for the needed amount of elevation. (**a**) Ostetome approach combined with xenograft and PRF. (**b**) Osteotome approach and Prf Graft in the delayed approach (**c**) Synthetic bone graft material containing growth factor

The substance will move more apical and lateral by the definite sliding of the implants; henceforth, the Schneiderian membrane is expanded even more (Fig. 11.11a). The 2–3 mm of the bone graft substance enclosing the implant's apex may strengthen the implant's main durability (Fig 11.11b).

Extraction can also be integrated with the osteotome procedure. A suitable diameter cylinder drill in the premolar condition can be operated to get to 1 mm from the sinus membrane. Execute the earlier stages until accomplishing the right proportion of the tented height. The rest of the alveolar bone quality in this specific condition and the bone graft resistance is ideal for a concurrent dental implant procedure [15, 18].

The osteotome in the deferred technique is positioned in the right implant attachment area in the future, and gentle malleting starts to break through the crest. If the alveolar bone is hard to advance and is dense, a trephine bur is eventually chosen to slit 1.2 mm from the sinus floor. The osteotome is loaded with graft substance, and the osteotome is administered to infringe the bone cylinder by some millimeters and to force through the substance [16–19]. The intrusion is carried out three or four times till the accomplishment of the targeted lift of the membrane and the sinus floor. The

main concealment is accomplished by the stitching of the flap. The maxillary molar removal with the deferred method can be implemented simultaneously. A trephine bur is utilized to make the cylinder of the alveolar bone progress, succeeding the tooth removal as per this combined procedure, which will therefore enclose the septal region. The next phases of mixing the graft substance and to raise the segment are carried out until attaining the preset proportion of the alveolar height. To succeed in the principal closure is quite challenging when the osteotome sinus lift is implemented with the molar uprooting, which may affect the proportion of the real procurement of the alveolar bone [19, 20]. The study includes the complete phases with radiography of the pre- (Fig. 11.12) and postop cure of the osteotome procedure (Fig. 11.13).

Complication

The first and common failure is the lack of stability, infection, and occlusal trauma due to the habitual parafunction or wears in the denture; if the implant site is unprepared, it results in necrosis, delay in osteointegration, and develop-

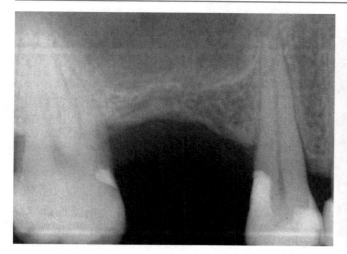

Fig. 11.12 First periapical graft with pneumatization of maxillary sinus

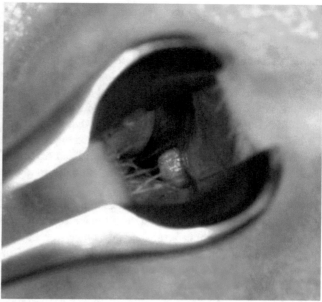

Fig. 11.14 An unusual complication in sinus elevation procedure

the sinus, after Vlassi and Fugazzoto, because of the presence of perforations in the Schneiderian membrane. The sub-Schneiderian region was occupied with DBBM as per the dimension of the fragment assigned in the draw; there was no attachment of the collagen membrane concealing the antrostomy. The region was filled up with a 4–0 silk stitch (Ethicon®), [20, 22, 24].

Postoperative Guidelines

The use of ice (crushed), including taking the necessary anti-inflammatory drugs and antibiotics, is mandatory to reduce ache and swelling by taking turns after 15–20 minutes and pressing the ice on the face of the affected region and "on" and "away" from the operated area too. After the surgery, this should extend for the first 24 hours. We advise the patient to recover, rest, and stay at home after the sinus augmentation surgery. The patient can resume work if they're comfortable; on the contrary, it's best not to perform vigorous workouts. The patient should be given guidance as mentioned regarding the usual occurrence of swelling in terms of the proper application of ice on the affected part of the face [25].

A few chips, too, maybe affixed in the surgical portion for a while to aid in any agony soothing. The patient can use a warm compress or a heating pad if the swelling persists after the third day of the surgery [26]. Additionally, the individual should be told not to sleep on the side of the face of the operated tooth. And, there shouldn't be any situation of raising the pressure on the intraoral region. Hence, the patient should be advised concerning coughing, drinking via a straw, or sneezing to safeguard the operated tooth. Bleeding within

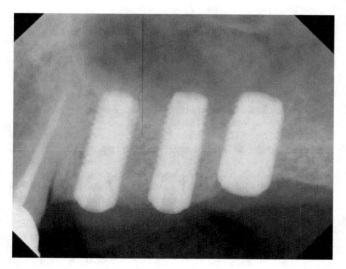

Fig. 11.13 Dental implant insertion with osteotome technique

ment of mucogingival defect. Infection is so common. It can be ruled out by a preoperative CT scan. On the other hand, it can happen due to contamination of graft material, development of peri-implantitis, and non-integration of the implant.

Improper bone height and bone quality are two causes of primary stability; gaining primary stability can be handled by larger diameter implant and graft material at the same time of insertion. If the bone preparation was not done adequately, it could lead to oro-antral fistula and complications [20–25] (Fig. 11.14).

On the detection of perforations of the Schneiderian membrane while performing the osteotomy, the Valsalva maneuver and, visually, Biomet3I® sinus curettes can be applied to disjoin the sinus membrane. The detachment outcome led to the detection of membrane perforations as per what was discovered in the item. A Bio-Gide resorbable collagen membrane was affixed ® (Geistlich) before loading

the first day after the surgery is expected and usual. The patient must be ready and not worry about noticing their saliva looking red and thereby should be briefed about it. The patient can enforce some pressure, precisely on the surgical region, if bleeding continues with a tea bag or gauze pads for 15–20 minutes. The patient must diligently take their medicines as advised as they may have to endure some discomfort. On being instructed to use ibuprofen, this drug should be had with a light supper or milk to reduce any expected G.I.-related affliction. Patients must refrain from driving if prescribed a narcotic pain reliever like codeine or avoid drinking altogether too.

The instruction to consume antibiotics must be carried out until its supply is entirely exhausted. If the antibiotics cause itching, rashes, breathing issues, or any other side effects, they must stop having it and get in touch with the doctor. The mouth rinsing should be replaced by just using gravity to wash the mouth by slanting the head from left to right and then letting the water drain out from the mouth for 3–4 days post-surgery. The use of pressure to rinse can affect the operated region and eventually cause harm [20, 22, 26].

The patient, excluding the operated area, must be told to clean, brush, and revive every other part as a routine. The individual can gently wash and clean the sutures twice with a cotton swab regularly using chlorhexidine 0.12%. On the first day post-surgery, it's advised to consume many fluids every 2 hours (no alcoholic or carbonated beverages) [27]. The individual can eat a balanced diet. However, the food must not damage the stitches. It's better to chew food on the opposing side of the operated tooth and also only limit yourself to easy-to-chew foods, and a liquid supplement like Ensure, Sego, or Boost may be consumed to not be devoid of any of the essential nutrients [27–30].

Conclusion

For implant attachment in the maxillary bone, the osteotome procedure is an effective and reliable method. It will lead to an advancement near the sinus and in the tuberosity at the time of the standard office-related methodology. This surgery doesn't produce heat, is not that strenuous, has an accessible bone for moving the implant to different areas, and it aids in facilitating the implant procedure by lessening the surgical expenses, duration, and post-surgery distress.

References

1. Summers RB. Staged osteotomies in sinus areas: preparing for implant placement. Dent Implantol Updat. 1996;7:93–5.
2. Fugazzotto PA. The modified trephine/osteotome sinus augmentation technique: technical considerations and discussion of indications. Implant Dent. 2001;10:259–64.
3. Fornell J, Johansson LA, Bolin A, Isaksson S, Sennerby L. Flapless, CBCT-guided osteotome sinus floor elevation with simultaneous implant installation. I: radiographic examination and surgical technique. A prospective 1-year follow-up. Clin Oral Implants Res. 2012;23:28–34.
4. Barone A, Cornelini R, Ciaglia R, Covani U. Implant placement in fresh extraction sockets and simultaneous osteotome sinus floor elevation: a case series. Int J Periodontics Restorative Dent. 2008;28:283–9.
5. Crespi R, Cappare P, Gherlone E. Osteotome sinus floor elevation and simultaneous implant placement in grafted biomaterial sockets: 3 years of follow-up. J Periodontol. 2010;81:344–9.
6. Kolhatkar S, Bhola M, Thompson-Sloan TN. Sinus floor elevation via the maxillary premolar extraction socket with immediate implant placement: a case series. J Periodontol. 2011;82:820–8.
7. Bruschi GB, Crespi R, Cappare P, Bravi F, Bruschi E, Gherlone E. Localized management of sinus floor technique for implant placement in fresh molar sockets. Clin Implant Dent Relat Res. 2013;15:243–50.
8. Summers RB. A new concept in maxillary implant surgery: the osteotome technique. Compendium. 1994;15:152, 154–6, 158.
9. Summers RB. Staged osteotomies in sinus areas: preparing for implant placement. Dent Implantol Update. 1996;7:93–5.
10. Summers RB. Sinus floor elevation with osteotomes. J Esthet Dent. 1998;10:164–71.
11. Tatum H. Maxillary implants. Florida Dent J. 1989;60:23–7.
12. Davarpanah M, Martinez H, Tecucianu JF, Hage G, Lazzara R. The modified osteotome technique. Int J Periodontics Restorative Dent. 2001;21:599–607.
13. Vitkov L, Gellrich NC, Hannig M. Sinus floor elevation via hydraulic detachment and elevation of the Schneiderian membrane. Clin Oral Implants Res. 2005;16:615–21.
14. Tan WC, Lang NP, Zwahlen M, Pjetursson BE. A systematic review of the success of sinus floor elevation and survival of implants inserted in combination with sinus floor elevation. Part II: transalveolar technique. J Clin Periodontol. 2008;35:241–54.
15. Di Girolamo M, Napolitano B, Arullani CA, Bruno E, Di Girolamo S. Paroxysmal positional vertigo as a complication of osteotome sinus floor elevation. Eur Arch Otorhinolaryngol. 2005;262:631–3.
16. Penarrocha M, Perez H, Garcia A, Guarinos J. Benign paroxysmal positional vertigo as a complication of osteotome expansion of the maxillary alveolar ridge. J Oral Maxillofac Surg. 2001;59:106–7.
17. Chiarella G, Leopardi G, De Fazio L, Chiarella R, Cassandro E. Benign paroxysmal positional vertigo after dental surgery. Eur Arch Otorhinolaryngol. 2008;265:119–22.
18. Saker M, Ogle O. Benign paroxysmal positional vertigo subsequent to sinus lift via closed technique. J Oral Maxillofac Surg. 2005;63:1385–7.
19. Penarrocha M, Garcia A. Benign paroxysmal positional vertigo as a complication of interventions with osteotome and mallet. J Oral Maxillofac Surg. 2006;64:1324. author reply 1324.
20. Chen L, Cha J. An 8-year retrospective study: 1,100 patients receiving 1,557 implants using the minimally invasive hydraulic sinus condensing technique. J Periodontol. 2005;76:482–91.
21. Sotirakis EG, Gonshor A. Elevation of the maxillary sinus floor with hydraulic pressure. J Oral Implantol. 2005;31:197–204.
22. Chiapasco M, Zaniboni M, Rimondini L. Dental implants placed in grafted maxillary sinuses: a retrospective analysis of clinical outcome according to the initial clinical situation and a proposal of defect classification. Clin Oral Implants Res. 2008;19:416–28.
23. Wallace SS, Froum SJ. Effect of maxillary sinus augmentation on the survival of endosseous dental implants: a systematic review. Ann Periodontol. 2003;8:328–43.
24. Pjetursson BE, Tan WC, Zwahlen M, Lang NP. A systematic review of the success of sinus floor elevation and survival of implants inserted in combination with sinus floor elevation. J Clin Periodontol. 2008;35:216–40.

25. Emmerich D, Att W, Stappert C. Sinus floor elevation using osteotomes: a systematic review and meta-analysis. J Periodontol. 2005;76:1237–51.

26. Tan WC, Lang NP, Zwahlen M, Pjetursson BE. A systematic review of the success of sinus floor elevation and survival of implants inserted in combination with sinus floor elevation. Part II: transalveolar technique. J Clin Periodontol. 2008;35:241–2.

27. Sigurdsson TJ, Lee MB, Kubota K, Turek TJ, Wozney JM, Wikesjo UM. Periodontal repair in dogs: recombinant human bone morphogenetic protein-2 significantly enhances periodontal regeneration. J Periodontol. 1995;66:131–8.

28. Kinoshita A, Oda S, Takahashi K, Yokota S, Ishikawa I. Periodontal regeneration by Application of recombinant human bone morphogenetic protein-2 to horizontal Circumferential defects created by experimental periodontitis in beagle dogs. J Periodontol. 1997;31:103–9.

29. Boyne PJ, Marx RE, Nevins M, et al. A feasibility study evaluating rhBMP-2/absorbable collagen sponge for maxillary sinus augmentation. Int J Periodontics Restorative Dent. 1997;16:400–11.

30. Boyne PJ, Lilly LC, Marx RE, Moy PK, Nevins M, Spagnoli DB, Triplett RG. De novo bone induction by recombinant human bone morphogenetic protein-2 (rhBMP-2) in maxillary sinus floor augmentation. J Oral Maxillofac Surg. 2005;63:1693–707.

Ultra-short Implant Outcome in Poor Bone Quality

12

Mohammad Hosein Amirzade-Iranaq and Fargol Mashha di Akbar Boojar

Introduction

The dental implant world was dramatically changed in 1982 when Branemark presented his research and long-term findings at an invitational conference in Toronto [1, 2]. Shortly after the Branemark implant system was brought to the US market, this most significant dentistry innovation for oral rehabilitation expanded worldwide. Various implant companies began to design and manufacture shorter implants in those early days, but the length of dental implants (traditional implant design) was relatively long (13–16 mm). Even introducing shorter dental implants in the early 1980s with 10–11 mm length did not stop the research on shorter designs. When major companies were focused on the development of the market and use, smaller companies such as 7br, MegaGen, Bicon, Jeneric, and BTI developed the short implant design with only 8–10 mm length. However, the race continues by introducing short implants by larger companies like Nobel, Astra, and Straumann [1, 3, 4]. Hence, the "big question" in implant dentistry formed: Do these short implants have long-term success, and how much can be shortened? The journey to find the answer lead to the development of the "ultra-short" dental implant. With a 5–6 mm length, these ultra-short implants overcome the limitation of implant insertion in low-height and poor-bone ridges without the need for extensive grafting, which seems impossible 10–15 years ago. Considering the controversy in practitioners' opinion toward ultra-short implants, recent research evidence has revealed a non-significant difference in success rate compared to short (8–10 mm) and traditional (above 10 mm) length implants. The current chapter aims to review the high-quality scientific literature to determine the success rate and application of ultra-short implants. It should have been noticed that due to similar properties and lack of specific catagorizations majority of determinants of "short" and "ultra-short" dental implants are impartible.

Short Implant Vs. Traditional Implant

Over the years, various strategies have been proposed to overcome the dimensional limitations of the bone available for implant placement. Some surgical mediators for bone augmentation are bone grafting, guided bone regeneration, distraction osteogenesis, transposition of the mandibular nerve, zygomatic implant or tilted implants, and sinus floor elevation. These techniques have relative success rates, although there is inadequate information for their predictability [5–9].

Short implants have been proposed for atrophic alveolar ridges' prosthetic treatment, which may provide surgical advantages, including reducing morbidity, treatment time, and costs. However, several reasons are making long implants more reliable: (1) achievement of larger surface area for osseointegration, (2) reduction of occlusal forces, and (3) crown to implant ratio improvement [6, 10, 11].

Many studies aimed to compare short and traditional implants, followed by many systematic reviews to appraise these studies and conclude this comparison critically. Table 12.1 demonstrates the summary of some systematic reviews.

Short Implant and Ultra-short Implant

Nowadays, there is no consensus about the definition of short implants. According to Striezel and Reichart, an implant length of ≤11 mm is considered short [25], while Talleman

M. H. Amirzade-Iranaq (✉)
Universal Network of Interdisciplinary Research in Oral and Maxillofacial Surgery (UNIROMS), Universal Scientific Education and Research Network (USERN), Tehran, Iran
e-mail: h.amirzade@gmail.com

F. M. A. Boojar
School of Dentistry, Research Committee of Golestan Medical University, Gorgan, Iran

© The Author(s), under exclusive license to Springer Nature Switzerland AG 2021
M. R. Stevens et al. (eds.), *Innovative Perspectives in Oral and Maxillofacial Surgery*,
https://doi.org/10.1007/978-3-030-75750-2_12

Table 12.1 Summary of some systematic reviews aiming to compare traditional, short, and ultra-short implant outcomes

Study	Comparing	Included records for review	Key findings
Atieh et al. (2012) [12]	Traditional vs. ≤ 8.5 mm implants	Total number of 33 studies	The initial survival rate for short implants for posterior partial edentulism is high and not related to implant surface, design, or width. Short implants may constitute a viable alternative to longer implants, which may often require additional augmentation procedures
Neldam et al. (2010) [13]	Traditional vs. ≤ 8 mm implants	Total number of 27 studies	Data on 6 mm implants were few and the most frequently represented was manufactured Straumann implants Short implant length was not related to observation time; installment region, failures, and dropouts were not specified; subsequently a meta-analysis was not possible to perform
Hualing Sun et al. (2011) [14]	Traditional vs. ≤ 10 mm implants	Total number of 35 studies	There was no statistically significant difference between the failure rates of short dental implants and standard implants Among the risk factors examined, most failures of short implants can be attributed to poor bone quality in the maxilla and a machined surface. Although short implants in atrophied jaws can achieve similar long-term prognoses as standard dental implants with a reasonable prosthetic design
Telleman et al. (2011) [15]	Traditional vs. ≤ 10 mm implants	Total number of 29 studies	There is fair evidence that short implants can be placed successfully in the partially edentulous patient, although with a tendency toward an increasing survival rate per implant length, and the prognosis may be better in the mandible of non-smoking patients
Annibali et al. (2012) [5]	Traditional vs. ≤ 10 mm implants	Total number of 16 studies	The provision of short implant-supported prostheses in patients with atrophic alveolar ridges appears to be a successful treatment option in the short term More scientific evidence is needed for the long term
Ravida et al. (2019) [16]	Traditional vs. ≤ 6 mm implants	Total number of 19 studies	Extra-short implants are a viable treatment alternative in ridges exhibiting atrophy, demonstrating a satisfactory survival rate, and a low rate of prosthetic and biologic complications across a 5-year follow-up Splinting extra-short implants is associated with fewer prosthetic complications and lower implant failure rate compared with non-splinted implants
Tengfei Fan et al. (2016) [17]	Traditional vs. ≤ 8 mm implants	Total number of 7 studies	There is no difference between the survival rates of short implants (5–8 mm) and long implants (>8 mm) Complications in short implants are lower than that in long implants However, further studies are required to substantiate our findings
Monje et al. (2013) [18]	Traditional vs. ≤ 10 mm implants	Total number of 5 studies	It could be concluded that short dental implants (<10 mm) had similar peri-implant MBL as standard implants (≥10 mm) for implant-supported fixed prostheses
Kotsovilis et al. (2009) [19]	Traditional vs. ≤ 10 mm implants	Total number of 37 studies	The placement of short rough-surface implants is not a less efficacious treatment modality compared to the placement of conventional rough-surface implants for the replacement of missing teeth in either totally or partially edentulous patients
Srinivasan et al. (2012) [20]	Traditional vs. ≤ 6 mm implants	Total number of 12 studies	Micro-rough 6-mm-short dental implants are a predictable treatment option, providing favorable survival rates. The failures encountered with 6-mm-short implants were predominantly early, and their survival in the mandible was slightly superior
Lemos et al. (2016) [21]	Traditional vs. ≤ 8 mm implants	Total number of 13 studies	Short implants with length less than 8 mm present greater risk to failures
Papaspyridakos et al. (2017) [22]	Traditional vs. ≤ 6 mm implants	Total number of 10 studies	Short implants (≤6 mm) were found to have higher variability and lower predictability in survival rates compared to longer implants (>6 mm) after periods of 1–5 years in function Short implants with ≤6 mm length should be carefully selected because they may present a greater risk for failure compared to implants longer than 6 mm
Rivida et al. (2019) [23]	Traditional vs. ≤ 6 mm implants	Total number of 12 studies	The placement of short implants is a predictable option in treating patients with maxillary atrophy up to a 3-year follow-up Studies with a longer observational period are needed to study the long-term performance of these implants
Nielsen et al. (2018) [24]	Traditional vs. ≤ 8 mm implants	Total number of 3 studies	Short implants seem to be a suitable alternative to standard length implants in conjunction with maxillary sinus floor augmentation Further randomized controlled trials with larger patient samples and an observation period of more than 3 years are needed before one treatment modality might be considered superior to the other

and Monje et al. considered <10 mm implants as short [15, 18]. However, the literature is not clear in defining short implants. Most of the articles consider short implants below 8 mm and ultra-short implants below 6 mm [20, 22, 23].

Reduced bone height in posterior areas, especially in the mandible, is the major criterion for ultra-short implants (5-6 mm). In a study, Peñarrocha et al. revealed that short implants with onlay autogenous block bone graft in the posterior of mandibles have a better outcome than traditional implants. They suggested that when residual bone height over the mandibular canal is between 7 and 8 mm, short implants (with 5.5 mm intra-bony length) might be a preferable treatment option over vertical augmentation, reducing chair time, expense, and morbidity [26].

Anitua et al. analyzed the relationship between the effect of crown height space, crown-to-implant ratio, and offset placement of the prosthesis on the implant survival and bone loss around ultra-short implants. They found a statistically significant increase of bone loss for implants opposing a partial denture and lower implants opposing a natural dentition or a complete denture. Analysis of marginal bone loss and the factors crown-to-implant ratio, crown height space, and offset placement according to antagonist dentition indicated a significant positive correlation between bone loss and crown height space [27].

With various categorizations, generally, dental implants up to 8 mm and 6 mm of length are categorized as "Short" and "Ultra-short" dental implants, respectively. Although, this categorization does not reflect the mechanical properties and prognosis. The logic of different modifications in design and their effect on the function of a sample implant system (Bicon System) is demonstrated in Table 12.2.

Indications and Contraindications

Indications and contraindications for the short and ultra-short implant are nearly the same as traditional length implants. A literature review shows considerable indications for implant usage for both traditional lengths, short and ultra-short implants. It is very much recorded that traditional length implants helped mandibular denture retention [1].

The indications could be divided into mutual and specific indications. Edentulism, missed-tooth replacements, and implant-supported over-denture are considered mutual indications for both traditional and short or ultra-short dental implants. Also, lack of sufficiency and quality of bone is the main indication for short and ultra-short dental implants, which is considered a contraindication for traditional ones.

The controversy is in contraindications which are divided into absolute and relative. Tobacco usage (mostly mentioned by smoking) was previously considered an absolute contraindication. Recently literature demonstrated a non-significant

difference in dental implant success rate between smokers compared to non-smoking cases. These results were originated from original works, such as Ewers et al. in 2005, that revealed a high success rate in a mixed sample, including smokers [1–3]. Branemark implants were recommended for bicortical placement with a minimum of 10 and 13 mm bone heights in the mandible and maxilla, respectively. As a result, lower bone amounts were considered a contraindication for dental implant insertion. In contrast, evaluation of 4641 Branemark dental implants by Friberg et al. [29] revealed no difference in success rates of traditional "long" dental implants and 7-mm "short" ones. The failure rates were 7.1% and 3.1% for 7-mm dental implants in maxillary and mandibular edentulism, respectively.

With demonstrations of relatively equal success rates in these "short-implants" in research articles and progress in augmentation and grafting techniques, the bone amount was not considered a limitation for dental implants. This achievement leads to a maximum reduction in implant diameter and introducing the "ultra-short" dental implant, which is considered a reliable treatment option [1, 30].

With updates in research, only progressive systemic conditions and severe medical problems causing failure in

Table 12.2 Advantages of different design and modalities of dental implants [28]

Properties	Advantages
Plateaued and tapered microgeometry	Fast secondary stability/osseointegration
Sloping shoulder	This specificity provides extended vitality for marginal alveolar bone and gingiva regeneration
Bacterial seal	Perfect implant-abutment connection prevents bacterial colonization of the implant surface
Short length	Minimally invasive, thus allowing limited augmentation or no augmentation at all
Narrow width	Minimally invasive often requiring no augmentation or orthodontic movement
Slow drilling	Minimally invasive and preserves the vitality of adjacent tissues while allowing bone to be collected
Spherical biomechanics	Gives support for bone gain induction through load transfer
The locking-taper implant to abutment connection	Secure abutment in place without the use of internal screws. It entirely avoids the additional concern of the technical failure of the screw
Precise and delicate osteotomy	Allows intramembranous-like healing/osseointegration
Osteotomy technique (especially hand reamers)	Allows complete collection of autologous bone chips for additional immediate alveolar bone augmentation
Age limitation	Complementation of 3D skeletal changes in adolescents with the help of step-by-step abutments and/or prosthetic supra-structures modification instead of implant replantations

osseointegration and soft-tissue healing are considered abso- lute contraindications for dental implant placement. Uncontrolled diabetes, treatment with bisphosphonate- related medications, massive radiation exposure in the sur- rounding implant area, and severe immuno-suppressive diseases are considered absolute contraindications.

"Short" and "ultra-short" dental implants had overcome some relative contraindications. Conditions such as heavy smoking, poor oral hygiene, low bone quantity or quality, and several systemic diseases were considered contraindica- tions for traditional "long" dental implants [1].

Also, adolescent and age limitation is mentioned as a rela- tive contraindication for traditional dental implants, which is frequently described as postponing the implant insertion until the end of growth in individuals. This issue had been solved with short and ultra-short dental implants, which were reported to be successfully placed in 8–9 years old cases. Minimum insertion in bone (subcrestal placement ability), which is the critical properties of diameter-reduced dental implants, allows jaws to continue their growth in ado- lescents. The other factor concerns the restorative ability, which the implant design allows for periodic restorative adjustments for esthetic concerns [31].

Inadequate interdental space leads to another contraindi- cation for traditional dental implants. This lack of space needs implants narrower than 4.0 mm, without encroaching on other structures and maintaining mechanical properties. The application of short and ultra-short dental implants in these cases, such as congenital missed lateral incisors or angled adjacent roots, is considered as an alternative to solve this "often-difficult" problem [1, 32]. The short and ultra- short dental implants also changed some "old-fashioned" paradigms in dental implantology, such as minimum space required between the implant and adjacent roots. Scientific literature with long-term follow-ups mentioned that the con- tact with adjacent roots did not affect the success rate in short and ultra-short dental implants [5, 9, 33].

For complex cases, either with atrophic jaws or proximity of anatomical structure such as incisive canal, the treatment choice is short and ultra-short implants [4, 34]. A compre- hensive review by de Mello et al. [9] with meta-analyzing 10 out of 238 clinical articles revealed that 91 implants placed in the incisal foramen had 84.6 up to 100% success rate.

In severe atrophic jaws, short and ultra-short dental implants overcome the space limitations that were once considered to treat only with excessive augmentation and traditional "long" dental implants. Short and ultra-short dental implants could successfully be inserted proximate to anatomical structres such as incisal foramen with similar success rates.

Briefly, the indications and contraindications for short and ultra-short implants are similar to traditional length implants. Also, short and ultra-short implants revealed a similar success rate compared to traditional dental implants [1, 35]. However,

as described previously, specific optimal designs of these implants overcome the limitations of the traditional "long" implants and make them preferable alternatives.

Cleft Patients

Cleft cases represent a comprehensive interdisciplinary issue in oral and maxillofacial rehabilitation. They have the central issue of not only the function but also the facial esthetics. In terms of oral and maxillofacial treatment, the planned result can be accomplished by long-term controlled therapy con- sisting of orthodontics, craniomaxillofacial surgery, and oral surgery, restorative dentistry, and long-term follow-up [10, 28]. As described by Poruban et al. The goals and outlines of treatment steps are demonstrated in Table 12.3.

While there is a slightly higher implant failure in all cleft patients with compromised tissue conditions, this should not prevent the use of short and ultra-short implants early in the complex cleft patient's therapy. The extension and time con- sumption of three-wall bone regeneration techniques with short and ultra-short implants often result in the same or bet- ter functional and aesthetic result than traditional "long" dental implants.

Sinus Lift

Posterior maxillary edentulism, due to trauma, progressive periodontitis, or simply extractions, lead to bone atrophy in the maxillary ridge and pneumatization of the maxillary

Table 12.3 Practical goal of different disciplines concerning cleft patients' treatment [10, 28]

Discipline	Practical goal
Orthodontics	The jaw and dental arch's size and position and proper tooth position regardless of the opposite jaw/arch. In cases of craniomaxillofacial procedures, it is essential to adhere to postoperative sequential therapy
Craniomaxillofacial surgery	The correction of the intermaxillary relation usually by bimaxillary orthographic procedures after growth is finished. Aesthetic results of a patient with similar combined intermaxillary and aesthetic discrepancies. Oro-nasal fistulas can be closed in the age range of 10–14 years
Oral surgery	The reconstruction of the alveolar ridge within the cleft and soft tissue coverage using guided tissue regeneration techniques (GTR), followed by dental implant placement and dental restorations
Prosthodontics	The prosthetic reconstruction of the dental arches, including the use of dental implants
All including dentistry	To sustain the treatment results and prevent any possible complications

sinus. These conditions need augmentations procedures, first introduced by Tatum in 1974 as sinus lift with a lateral approach. Interestingly the procedure by Tatum was performed without any grafting materials. In contrast application of grafts was demonstrated by Boyne and James in 1980. Further investigations lead to the acceptance of lateral approach and grafting materials as a standard routine procedure [36–39]. Long-term follow-up research of the Ewers [40] in 2005 and also recommendations of the American Association of Oral and Maxillofacial Surgeons and the Academy of Osseointegration promoted the lateral approach for sinus lift as a successful procedure with predictable results [41–43]. Evaluation of surgical procedures aimed to perform minimal-invasive interventions to reduce post-surgical complications and consequences. By this means, the lateral approach and cortical window access to maxillary sinus were considered an aggressive procedure, leading to introducing the indirect "close" sinus lift technique by Summers in 1994 [41–43]. The evaluation and research towards more minimal techniques continued, and nowadays, indirect "close" sinus lift proved reduction of procedure time, patient's discomfort, and post-surgical complications [41, 44, 45].

With stablishments of minimal-invasive surgery concepts, the old gold rule towards implant length indicates "The longer; The better" seems impractical. As a primary concern of sinus lift procedures, sinus membrane perforation has a high risk of occurrence, especially in an indirect "close" crestal approach due to lack of visualization, making further management tortures [46]. The traditional "long" dental implants increase the risk of this perforation. In addition, more augmentation may be needed to provide an adequate bone amount for implant insertion. Short and ultra-short dental implants with reduced implant length are optimal alternatives for direct or indirect sinus lift procedures. The risk of sinus perforation is reduced with a reduction of implant length and avoid further complications. These are all consistent with concepts of minimal-invasive surgery, so it could be concluded that the application of short and ultra-short dental implants is inevitable to reach the ultimate goal in the "minimal-invasive sinus lift" procedure [47]. Based on the original work of Cawood and Howell in 1988, a new classification was introduced by Marincola et al., categorizing the type of sinus graft based on residual bone height. Summarized and adapted from Tomasetti and Ewers, this classification demonstrated in Table 12.4 [6, 41, 48].

In cases with 3–7 residual bone heights, application of short and ultra-short dental implants leads to a minimum need for grafting materials and augmentation. Also, the application of ultra-short implants may avoid the need for grafting materials. However, there is a controversy about the need for grafting materials to predict implant success rate. As mentioned previously, Tatum performed sinus lift without

Table 12.4 Type of sinus graft based upon the residual bone height [41, 48]

Amount of residual bone height	Approach
Traditional implants	
Less than 1 mm	A horizontal horseshoe LeFort I osteotomy with an interpositional iliac crest bone graft
1–5 mm	Staged procedures with lateral approach sinus lift and graft followed by implant placement approximately 6 months later
5–8 mm	Lateral approach sinus lift with simultaneous implant placement
8 mm or more	A sinus floor intrusion through the implant osteotomy along with simultaneous implant placement
Short and ultra-short implants	
Less than 1 mm	A horizontal horseshoe LeFort I osteotomy with an interpositional iliac crest bone graft. One can also consider a lateral sinus lift and graft or a crestal sinus lift/graft
Less than 3 mm	Either a lateral sinus lift/graft or a crestal lift/graft
3–7 mm	A sinus floor intrusion through the implant osteotomy with immediate placement of a short or ultra-short implant
7 mm or more	Normal implant placement using short or ultra-short implants

any grafting materials, which contrasted with Summer's recommendation to use grafting materials for sinus lift procedure. Recent evidence indicated that bone gain does not depend on grafting materials. A study by Nedir et al. [49] revealed no significant difference in the success rate of internal sinus lift with or without grafting materials. In addition, Rammelsberg et al. [50] observed bone gain in internal "close" sinus lift cases with no grafting material uses. Their study indicated that more minor invasive procedures and maintaining crestal bone are more valuable predictors for implant success and survival through long-term follow-ups [51].

Platform switching is considered the key to successful treatment [52]. There are some concerns about length-reduced dental implant stability leading to the question: Are this amount of insertion and surrounding bone enough for the long-term stability of dental implant? The concept of "platform switching" aimed to increase crestal bone gain in the implant insertion area and served other aesthetic zone benefits. The primary mechanism of platform switching is to decrease mechanical stress leading to improved tension-free angiogenesis and vascularization, which is beneficial for surrounding bone and tissues.

Once the pilot drilling has been completed, the osteotomy is widened using a series of latch reamers without irrigation. This allows the surgeon to collect bone from the osteotomy site. This bone will be used combined with the previously collected blood and graft material for insertion into the graft site. It is recommended that a radiograph of the site be taken with the 2.5 mm latch reamer in place in order to determine the final drilling length. The osteotomy is gradually widened to the desired size using 0.5 mm, increasing latch reamers and hand reamers [6].

When the desired diameter is reached, a hand reamer is used to perform a comminuted fracture of the sinus floor's cortical bone. Using a reamer with a smaller diameter than the osteotomy site allows the reamer's sharp tip to be placed at four different points at the apex of the site. The reamer is gently tapped to fracture the thin cortical layer of the sinus floor at the distal aspect of the osteotomy site and then the buccal and mesial areas, followed by the palatal area. The second and fourth fracture points are always the buccal and palatal because of the higher sinus pneumatization in these areas. The 3.5 mm osteotome is then gently tapped, pushing the material against the fractured sinus floor and Schneiderian membrane, thus elevating the sinus floor [6].

A 5-year follow-up of a crestal sinus lift shows the bone transformation and remodeling, according to Wolff's law [53]. The bone transforms from resorbable TCP augmentation material into well-mineralized bone. The described method leads to minimal-invasive "close" sinus lift, which, alongside the application of short or ultra-short dental implants, presents a successful alternative in complex cases. Although, this method is not entirely complication-free. Complications associated with a surgical procedure such as hemorrhage, infection, and chronic sinusitis may occur. The aim is to minimize the complecations and provide a treatment option for complex cases that were once considered contraindications for implant insertion.

In conjunction with the precautionary, short and ultra-short implants reduce the need for an extensive osteotomy via a lateral approach. While the short and ultra-short implants can be used with the conventional lateral approach, they are more attuned to the minimally invasive precautionary. The procedure is less traumatic, and the patient has less swelling and pain. In many cases, the procedure is also less costly to the patient.

Conclusion

Short implants gained a relatively stable position in current implant dentistry. On the other hand, the present chapter demonstrated that ultra-short implant needs more studies with extended follow-ups. However, due to our current knowledge, ultra-short implants are safe and predictable for implant therapy in the atrophic maxilla as a treatment option. The survival rate of implants is high, according to the literature. Also, biological complications are frequent but mainly associated with traditional implants in the augmented sinus.

In comparison, outcomes are in favor of ultra-short implants. With the higher number of biological complications, increasing morbidity, costs, and surgical time of longer dental implants (traditional and short implants) in bone deficiency, ultra-short implants may represent the favorable treatment alternative. There is a strong need for follow-up patients included in future well-designed studies to determine the long-term outcomes.

References

1. Tomasetti BJ, Ewers R. Short implants: indications and contraindications. In: Short implants. Springer; 2020. p. 9–23.
2. Branemark PI. Osseointegrated implants in the treatment of the edentulous jaw. Experience from a 10-year period. Scand J Plast Reconstr Surg Suppl. 1977;16.
3. Zarb GA. Proceedings of the Toronto conference on osseointegration in clinical dentistry. Mosby; 1984.
4. Allard R, De Vries K, Van der Kwast W. Persisting bilateral nasopalatine ducts: a developmental anomaly: report of a case. Oral Surg Oral Med Oral Pathol. 1982;53(1):24–6.
5. Annibali S, Cristalli M, Dell'Aquila D, Bignozzi I, La Monaca G, Pilloni A. Short dental implants: a systematic review. J Dent Res. 2012;91(1):25–32.
6. Tomasetti BJ, Ewers R. Short implants. Springer; 2020.
7. Oh J-h. Recent advances in dental implants. Maxillofac Plast Reconstr Surg. 2017;39(1):33.
8. Ali Al-Hashedi A, Bai Taiyeb Ali T, Yunus N. Short dental implants: an emerging concept in implant treatment. Quintessence Inter. 2014;45(6).
9. de Mello J, Faot F, Correa G, Júnior OC. Success rate and complications associated with dental implants in the incisive canal region: a systematic review. Int J Oral Maxillofac Surg. 2017;46(12):1584–91.
10. Nisand D, Renouard F. Short implant in limited bone volume. Periodontology 2000. 2014;66(1):72–96.
11. Akça K, Iplikçioğlu H. Finite element stress analysis of the effect of short implant usage in place of cantilever extensions in mandibular posterior edentulism. J Oral Rehabil. 2002;29(4):350–6.
12. Atieh MA, Zadeh H, Stanford CM, Cooper LF. Survival of short dental implants for treatment of posterior partial edentulism: a systematic review. Inter J Oral Maxillofac Implants. 2012;27(6).
13. Neldam CA, Pinholt EM. State of the art of short dental implants: a systematic review of the literature. Clin Implant Dent Relat Res. 2012;14(4):622–32.
14. Sun HL, Wu YR, Huang C, Shi B. Failure rates of short (≤ 10 mm) dental implants and factors influencing their failure: a systematic review. Inter J Oral Maxillofac Implants. 2011;26(4).
15. Telleman G, Raghoebar GM, Vissink A, Den Hartog L, Huddleston Slater JJ, Meijer HJ. A systematic review of the prognosis of short (< 10 mm) dental implants placed in the partially edentulous patient. J Clin Periodontol. 2011;38(7):667–76.
16. Ravidà A, Barootchi S, Askar H, del Amo FS-L, Tavelli L, Wang H-L. Long-Term Effectiveness of Extra-Short (≤ 6 mm) Dental Implants: A Systematic Review. Inter J Oral Maxillofac Implants. 2019;34(1).
17. Fan T, Li Y, Deng WW, Wu T, Zhang W. Short implants (5 to 8 mm) versus longer implants (> 8 mm) with sinus lifting in atrophic posterior maxilla: a meta-analysis of RCTs. Clin Implant Dent Relat Res. 2017;19(1):207–15.
18. Monje A, Suarez F, Galindo-Moreno P, García-Nogales A, Fu JH, Wang HL. A systematic review on marginal bone loss around short

dental implants (< 10 mm) for implant-supported fixed prostheses. Clin Oral Implants Res. 2014;25(10):1119–24.
19. Kotsovilis S, Fourmousis I, Karoussis IK, Bamia C. A systematic review and meta-analysis on the effect of implant length on the survival of rough-surface dental implants. J Periodontol. 2009;80(11):1700–18.
20. Srinivasan M, Vazquez L, Rieder P, Moraguez O, Bernard JP, Belser UC. Survival rates of short (6 mm) micro-rough surface implants: a review of literature and meta-analysis. Clin Oral Implants Res. 2014;25(5):539–45.
21. Lemos CAA, Ferro-Alves ML, Okamoto R, Mendonça MR, Pellizzer EP. Short dental implants versus standard dental implants placed in the posterior jaws: a systematic review and meta-analysis. J Dent. 2016;47:8–17.
22. Papaspyridakos P, De Souza A, Vazouras K, Gholami H, Pagni S, Weber HP. Survival rates of short dental implants (≤ 6 mm) compared with implants longer than 6 mm in posterior jaw areas: a meta-analysis. Clin Oral Implants Res. 2018;29:8–20.
23. Ravidà A, Wang I-C, Sammartino G, Barootchi S, Tattan M, Troiano G, et al. Prosthetic rehabilitation of the posterior atrophic maxilla, short (≤ 6 mm) or long (≥ 10 mm) dental implants? A systematic review, meta-analysis, and trial sequential analysis: Naples consensus report working group a. Implant Dent. 2019;28(6):590–602.
24. Nielsen H, Schou S, Isidor F, Christensen A-E, Starch-Jensen T. Short implants (≤ 8 mm) compared to standard length implants (> 8 mm) in conjunction with maxillary sinus floor augmentation: a systematic review and meta-analysis. Int J Oral Maxillofac Surg. 2019;48(2):239–49.
25. Strietzel FP, Reichart PA. Oral rehabilitation using Camlog® screw–cylinder implants with a particle-blasted and acid-etched microstructured surface. Results from a prospective study with special consideration of short implants. Clin Oral Implants Res. 2007;18(5):591–600.
26. Peñarrocha-Oltra D, Aloy-Prósper A, Cervera-Ballester J, Peñarrocha-Diago M, Canullo L, Peñarrocha-Diago M. Implant treatment in atrophic posterior mandibles: vertical regeneration with block bone grafts versus implants with 5.5-mm intrabony length. Inter J Oral Maxillofac Implants. 2014;29(3).
27. Anitua E, Alkhraist MH, Piñas L, Begoña L, Orive G. Implant survival and crestal bone loss around extra-short implants supporting a fixed denture: the effect of crown height space, crown-to-implant ratio, and offset placement of the prosthesis. Inter J Oral Maxillofac Implants. 2014;29(3).
28. Poruban D, Slavik R, Stebel A. Short implant in cleft cases. In: Short implants. Springer; 2020. p. 125–42.
29. Friberg BJT. Early failures in 4641 consecutively placed Branemark dental implants: a study from stage 1 surgery to the connection of completed prosthesis. Int J Oral Maxillofac Implants. 1991;142(6)
30. Neugebauer J, Nickenig H, Zöller J, editors. Update on short, angulated and diameter-reduced implants. In: Proceedings of the 11th European Consensus Conference (EuCC'16); 2016.
31. Mankani N, Chowdhary R, Patil BA, Nagaraj E, Madalli P. Osseointegrated dental implants in growing children: a literature review. J Oral Implantol. 2014;40(5):627–31.
32. Kendrick S, Wong D. Vertical and horizontal dimensions of implant dentistry: numbers every dentist should know. Inside Dent. 2009;4287:2–5.
33. Romeo E, Bivio A, Mosca D, Scanferla M, Ghisolfi M, Storelli S. The use of short dental implants in clinical practice: literature review. Minerva Stomatol. 2010;59(1–2):23.
34. Friedrich RE, Laumann F, Zrnc T, Assaf AT. The nasopalatine canal in adults on cone beam computed tomograms–A clinical study and Review of the literature in vivo. 2015;29(4):467–86.
35. Lombardo G, Pighi J, Marincola M, Corrocher G, Simancas-Pallares M, Nocini PF. Cumulative success rate of short and ultrashort implants supporting single crowns in the posterior maxilla: a 3-year retrospective study. Inter J Dentistry. 2017;2017.
36. Wagner F, Dvorak G, Nemec S, Pietschmann P, Figl M, Seemann R. A principal components analysis: how pneumatization and edentulism contribute to maxillary atrophy. Oral Dis. 2017;23(1):55–61.
37. Tatum O. Lecture presented to the Alabama implant congress. Alabama Implant Congress; 1976.
38. Mellonig JT, Bowers GM, Bailey RC. Comparison of bone graft materials: part I. new bone formation with autografts and allografts determined by Strontium-85. J Periodontol. 1981;52(6):291–6.
39. Tatum H Jr. Maxillary and sinus implant reconstructions. Dent Clin N Am. 1986;30(2):207–29.
40. Ewers R. Maxilla sinus grafting with marine algae derived bone forming material: a clinical report of long-term results. J Oral Maxillofac Surg. 2005;63(12):1712–23.
41. Marincola M, Ewers R, Tomasetti BJ. Minimally invasive sinus lift using short implants. In: Short implants. Springer; 2020. p. 161–76.
42. Jensen O, Block MS, Iacono V. Guest editorial: 1996 sinus consensus conference revisited in 2016. Inter J Oral Maxillofac Implants. 2016;31(3).
43. Summers RB. A new concept in maxillary implant surgery: the osteotome technique. Compendium (Newtown, PA). 1994;15(2):152, 4–6, 8 passim; quiz 62.
44. Summers RB. The osteotome technique: Part 3--Less invasive methods of elevating the sinus floor. Compendium (Newtown, Pa). 1994;15(6):698, 700, 2–4 passim; quiz 10.
45. Ali SA, Karthigeyan S, Deivanai M, Kumar A. Implant rehabilitation for atrophic maxilla: a review. J Indian Prosthodont Soc. 2014;14(3):196–207.
46. Hernández-Alfaro F, Torradeflot MM, Marti C. Prevalence and management of Schneiderian membrane perforations during sinus-lift procedures. Clin Oral Implants Res. 2008;19(1):91–8.
47. Felice P, Checchi L, Barausse C, Pistilli R, Sammartino G, Masi I, et al. Posterior jaws rehabilitated with partial prostheses supported by 4.0 x 4.0 mm or by longer implants: one-year post-loading results from a multicenter randomised controlled trial. Eur J Oral Implantol. 2016;9(1):35–45.
48. Cawood J, Howell R. A classification of the edentulous jaws. Int J Oral Maxillofac Surg. 1988;17(4):232–6.
49. Nedir R, Nurdin N, Khoury P, Bischof M. Short implants placed with or without grafting in atrophic sinuses: the 3-year results of a prospective randomized controlled study. Clin Implant Dent Relat Res. 2016;18(1):10–8.
50. Rammelsberg P, Mahabadi J, Eiffler C, Koob A, Kappel S, Gabbert O. Radiographic monitoring of changes in bone height after implant placement in combination with an internal sinus lift without graft material. Clin Implant Dent Relat Res. 2015;17:e267–e74.
51. Ghensi P, Tonetto G, Soldini C, Bettio E, Mortellaro C, Soldini C. Dental implants with a platform-switched Morse taper connection and an Osteo growth induction surface. J Craniofac Surg. 2019;30(4):1049–54.
52. Lago L, da Silva L, Martinez-Silva I, Rilo B. Radiographic Assessment of Crestal Bone Loss in Tissue-Level Implants Restored by Platform Matching Compared with Bone-Level Implants Restored by Platform Switching: A Randomized, Controlled, Split-Mouth Trial with 3-year Follow-up. Inter J Oral Maxillofac Implants. 2019;34(1).
53. Wolff J. Das gesetz der transformation der knochen. DMW-Deutsche Medizinische Wochenschrift. 1893;19(47):1222–4.

Options or Alternatives to Sinus Elevation

Mahmood Dashti and Mahsa Nikaein

Introduction

Implant-supported prostheses is impossible in patients without adequate bone volume. This scenario is observed at the posterior region and specifically underneath the maxillary sinuses [1]. The full restoration of edentulous patients with implant is difficult due to the restricted area of the bone at hand and the pneumatization of the maxillary sinus or both [2].

To successfully place an implant, the bone height of at least 2 mm and 5 mm between the pneumatized sinus floor and the alveolar crest should be accessible [3–5]. In cases of less severe bone atrophy, osteotomes are also utilized as a less-invasive method to accomplish a partial elevation of the maxillary sinus by the transalveolar entry [6–9].

Sinus lift operations may lead to complications or be contraindicated in spite of success rates as given below:

1. The perforation of the sinus membrane is the most common complication reported in the surgeries.
2. This issue may cause infection and the threat of graft loss or resorption, peri-implantitis, and chronic or acute sinusitis [10–13].
3. Though not that high, the postoperative existence of acute and/or chronic sinusitis has been associated with patients with a history of the disease, despite the supervision prior to the surgery.

The high probability of intervention in sinuses must be discussed with these patients; therefore they need attentive follow-ups and immediate treatment if the symptoms of sinusitis reappear [14].

M. Dashti
Private Practice, Tehran, Iran

M. Nikaein (✉)
Department of Operative Dentistry, Shahid Beheshti University of Medical Sciences, Tehran, Iran
e-mail: Msa_nik@yahoo.com

In patients with extreme posterior maxilla atrophy, fixed prosthesis can only be implemented using dental implants following sinus lift surgeries [15], zygomatic implants [16], and, occasionally, pterygoid implants or tilted implants [1].

The optimum care for patients having an "intermediate" bone area is debatable even today [1].

There are normally three major issues that exist regarding bone augmentation surgeries:

1. The success rates are not that precise.
2. The time and expenses of the treatment [15, 17].
3. Patient morbidity is higher.

In the case of the utilization of the autogenous bone, the lateral window sinus lift method is one of the highest standard implemented augmentation surgeries and is also regarded as one of the most dependable surgical methods [18, 19].

Crestal Sinus Elevation

An alternative to elevate the sinus is the crestal approach in which is done directly from the implanted region to further reduce the patient's discomfort [1].

Tatum [20] in 1986 was the first to document this method and was later revised by Summers in 1994 [21].

The leading contrast to the lateral window method is that the sinus membrane is elevated via the crestal bone with the osteotomes, and the implants are directly placed in the region provided with the osteotomes [22].

The few probable shortcomings linked with this method are:

1. The needed area of bone height is 3 mm to stabilize the implants during placement [23].

2. The acquired bone area, by the crestal method, is less than the bone area achieved with the lateral window technique.

Hydrodynamic Ultrasonic Sinus Floor Elevation

This elevation method is utilized as a different procedure for the sinus floor lifts of any dimension and volume with just a 3 mm diameter transcrestal method [24]. The hydrodynamic ultrasonic cavitational sinus lift (HUCSL) was invented to lift the sinus membrane in the absence of any tearing forces on the sinus membrane by applying the Acteon Piezotome I (Acteon, Bordeaux, France).

The outcomes of late have revealed that the standard pressure to elevate the sinus membrane in the sheep model is quite less if the pneumatic pressure is replaced with the hydraulic pressure [24].

Short Implants

A less invasive alternative to sinus lift is the implementation of short implants, in the existence of 4 mm to 7 mm of residual bone height at the maxillary sinus [1]. Short implants are classed as being 10 mm or less [25–27]. They are beneficial due to the certainty of being inserted within a restricted bone height, hence preventing nerve repositioning, sinus elevation, or onlay grafts [27].

The earlier outcomes of inserting short implants were quite discouraging with failure rates in the range of 17% to 25% [28–31]. This was caused by the inferior bone quality of the posterior region [32]. The advent of the satisfactorily rough implants improved the rates of survival from 95.1% to 100% [26, 33, 34].

There are multiple randomized controlled trials conducted comparing short implants against longer implants in elevated sinuses [35–40]. They displayed impressive short-term outcomes with both techniques [1].

The study on the success of the short (5 mm or 6 mm long) dental implants compared to the longer or 10 mm implants inserted into the crestally elevated sinuses exhibited remarkable outcomes in the both methods with no signs of any variations between the prostheses supported by one to two implants 5 mm to 6 mm-long or 10 mm-long for 1–3 years following loading. Hence, the clinicians choose this method to be implemented despite the requirement of longer follow-ups [1, 41].

Angulated Implants

Dr. Paulo Malo in 1993 favored the angulated insertion of implants and defined the concept as "All on Four" where two vertical implants are placed in the posterior at an angulation of 35–40 degrees and two vertical implants are also fixed in the anterior region, respectively [2].

Benefits of tilting implants:

1. Remarkable clinical outcomes [2].
2. The longer implants can be applied at the minimum bone area with the bone-to-implant junction and to minimize the requirement of a vertical bone augmentation validating the strength even at the least bone area [2].
3. Patients having multiple systemic contraindicated for bone grafting.
4. The requirement for bone grafting is ruled out as it's invasive with uncertain results [42].
5. The positioning due to angulation avoids anatomical structures [43].
6. The application of tilted distal implants over distal cantilever units has a biomechanical benefit [44].
7. The length of cantilevers is to be lessened in the absence of executing sinus lifting or bone grafting [45].
8. It's a reliable and efficient choice than the maxillary sinus floor augmentation surgery [46] and the pneumatized maxillary sinus [47].
9. Distally tilted implants produce an improved loading transmission versus vertical implants [48].
10. Excellent prognosis for short and moderate durations [49] also for longer durations [50].

Limitations of Tilting Implants

1. The procedure is extremely technique sensitive.
2. A computerized surgical stent is essential for the implants to be placed in the appropriate angulation.
3. The operation is highly reliant on the great technical abilities of the surgeon.
4. Lack of long-term research documentation.
5. A minor variation in angulation can create issues for the clinician and the patient [2].

This procedure greatly relies on surgical skills, useful in the patients having resorbed ridges; however, there is a need for long-term research to determine its effectiveness regarding load dispersal, prosthesis survival, and marginal bone loss; however, patients are being operated on at present by a lot of clinicians applying this technique with resounding success [2].

In the maxilla, the posterior implants were inserted close and parallel with the sinus walls and were angulated posteriorly/anteriorly in the range of 30 to 35 degrees [51].

Wide-Body Implants

The wide-body implants with dimensions of 7 to 9 mm length and 8 to 9 mm wide had a survival rate of 96.5% on an average follow-up around 15 months; hence, the grafting surgeries can be prevented by replacing it with a wide-body implant.

This is possibly associated with the increased implant surface area and acceptable primary stability [52].

Sinus Augmentation by Orthodontic Development

The insertion of short implants (5 mm) in a maxilla with a residual bone height of 4 to 6 mm might have an unknown long-term prognosis [53]. Hence, a bone height of at least 7.0 mm is suggested for implant placed in the absence of a maxilla sinus elevation [54–56].

The surgical sinus elevation method has its contraindications and limitations; not highlighting an outright contraindication to the method, some studies have documented greater failure rates in patients that smoke [57, 58].

Baig and Rajan [59] documented that when the implants were placed in patients having sinus elevation operation, the non-smoking patients had a double success rate than the patients that smoked who received the same treatment. Kan et al. [60] reported a success rate of just 65.3% in patients that smoke, when the implants were inserted following the maxillary sinus elevation, and Levin and Schwartz-Arad [61] explained that the reason for the greater failure rates of implants and grafts in the maxillary sinus is due to the release of heat and poisonous byproducts of cigarettes like hydrogen cyanide, carbon monoxide, and nicotine.

An orthodontic procedure can be implemented to reduce complications and prevent surgical maxillary sinus elevation and bone graft.

This method was first utilized in case of missing maxillary right first molar with a slight mesial displacement of the maxillary right second and third molars and the successive lessening of the initial space of the maxillary right first molar, that was removed 24 years before, because of a carious lesion.

The objective was to change the position of the maxillary right second premolar distally to occupy the remaining area of the maxillary right first molar, which had been lowered by the mesial development of the maxillary right second and the third molars.

This development would clear the region for the placement of an implant at the area of the maxillary right second premolar, apart from the lessening of the augmented sinus area by constricting its anterior wall that eradicates the requirement for a surgical intervention and sinus grafting [62].

The tissue preserved its earlier thickness and height in the region of the bone from where the tooth was moved. The foundation of a modern histophysiology and the practical requirement in the field regarding the preservation of the bone height are hinted by the placing of an implant in the area that was earlier taken up by a tooth.

The distal displacement of the tooth and the gradual bone remodeling is due to the mild and moderate forces that steadily take up the pneumatized region. The cortical bone shifts the maxillary sinus floor throughout the bone and periodontal remodeling process induced due to the orthodontic movement.

The sinus mucosa accompanies the cortical bone in this movement, along with the underlying periosteum. Therefore, the placement of an endosseous implant can be used if the orthodontic movement is the choice as an alternative to lessen the pneumatized maxillary sinus regions in the alveolar bone.

The overall duration of the treatment including orthodontics, implant insertion, and crown delivery is similar to the regular surgery with the surgical sinus elevation method as the orthodontic procedure needs half a year and the implant healing takes 4 months before the crown delivery.

A recovery time of 6 months (at least), which is also dependent to the grafting material, is advised before the implant insertion if the surgical sinus method is carried out [62].

Conclusion

Numerous prevailing methods with lower invasion can be applied to rectify the maxillary sinus pneumatization in the maxillary posterior area despite the success rate of standard sinus elevation to treat the edentulous patients. However, extended follow-ups are essential to examine the advantages and limitations of modern techniques.

References

1. Felice P, Pistilli R, Barausse C, Bruno V, Trullenque-Eriksson A, Esposito M. Short implants as an alternative to crestal sinus lift: a 1-year multicentre randomised controlled trial. Eur J Oral Implantol. 2015;8(4):375–84.
2. Asawa N, Bulbule N, Kakade D, Shah R. Angulated implants: an alternative to bone augmentation and sinus lift procedure: systematic review. J Clin Diagn Res. 2015;9(3):ZE10.

3. Fenner M, Vairaktaris E, Fischer K, Schlegel KA, Neukam FW, Nkenke E. Influence of residual alveolar bone height on osseointegration of implants in the maxilla: a pilot study. Clin Oral Implants Res. 2009;20(6):555–9.

4. Fenner M, Vairaktaris E, Stockmann P, Schlegel KA, Neukam FW, Nkenke E. Influence of residual alveolar bone height on implant stability in the maxilla: an experimental animal study. Clin Oral Implants Res. 2009;20(8):751–5.

5. Sivolella S, Bressan E, Gnocco E, Berengo M, Favero GA. Maxillary sinus augmentation with bovine bone and simultaneous dental implant placement in conditions of severe alveolar atrophy: a retrospective analysis of a consecutively treated case series. Quintessence Inter. 2011;42(10).

6. Toffler M. Osteotome-mediated sinus floor elevation: a clinical report. Inter J Oral Maxillofac Implants. 2004;19(2).

7. Engelke W, Schwarzwäller W, Behnsen A, Jacobs HG. Subantroscopic laterobasal sinus floor augmentation (SALSA): an up-to-5-year clinical study. Inter J Oral Maxillofac Implants. 2003;18(1).

8. Pontes F, Zuza E, de Toledo B. Summers' technique modification for sinus floor elevation using a connective tissue graft. A case report. J Inter Acad Periodontol. 2010;12(1):27.

9. Fermergård R, Åstrand P. Osteotome sinus floor elevation without bone grafts–a 3-year retrospective study with Astra tech implants. Clin Implant Dent Relat Res. 2012;14(2):198–205.

10. Biglioli F, Pedrazzoli M, Colletti G. Repair of a perforated sinus membrane with a palatal fibromucosal graft: a case report. Minerva Stomatol. 2010;59(5):299–302.

11. Kim Y-K, Hwang J-W, Yun P-Y. Closure of large perforation of sinus membrane using pedicled buccal fat pad graft: a case report. Inter J Oral Maxillofac Implants. 2008;23(6).

12. Hong S-B, Kim J-S, Shin S-I, Han J-Y, Herr Y, Chung J-H. Clinical treatment of postoperative infection following sinus augmentation. J Periodontal Implant Sci. 2010;40(3):144–9.

13. Sohn D-S, Lee J-K, Shin H-I, Choi B-J, An K-M. Fungal infection as a complication of sinus bone grafting and implants: a case report. Oral Surg Oral Med Oral Pathol Oral Radiol Endodontol. 2009;107(3):375–80.

14. Manor Y, Mardinger O, Bietlitum I, Nashef A, Nissan J, Chaushu G. Late signs and symptoms of maxillary sinusitis after sinus augmentation. Oral Surg Oral Med Oral Pathol Oral Radiol Endodontol. 2010;110(1):e1–4.

15. Esposito M, Felice P, Worthington HV. Interventions for replacing missing teeth: augmentation procedures of the maxillary sinus. Cochrane Database Syst Rev. 2014;5.

16. Esposito M, Worthington HV, Coulthard P. Interventions for replacing missing teeth: dental implants in zygomatic bone for the rehabilitation of the severely deficient edentulous maxilla. Cochrane Database Syst Rev. 2005;4.

17. Coulthard P, Esposito M, Jokstad A, Worthington H. Interventions for replacing missing teeth: horizontal and vertical bone augmentation techniques for dental implant treatment. Cochrane Database Syst Rev. 2009;3:1–13.

18. Wallace SS, Froum SJ. Effect of maxillary sinus augmentation on the survival of endosseous dental implants. A systematic review. Ann Periodontol. 2003;8(1):328–43.

19. Del Fabbro M, Testori T, Francetti L, Weinstein R. Systematic review of survival rates for implants placed in the grafted maxillary sinus. Inter J Periodont Restorat Dentistry. 2004;24(6).

20. Tatum JH. Maxillary and sinus implant reconstructions. Dent Clin N Am. 1986;30(2):207–29.

21. Summers RB. A new concept in maxillary implant surgery: the osteotome technique. Compendium (Newtown, Pa). 1994;15(2):152, 4–6, 8 passim; quiz 62.

22. Emmerich D, Att W, Stappert C. Sinus floor elevation using osteotomes: a systematic review and meta-analysis. J Periodontol. 2005;76(8):1237–51.

23. Cosci F, Luccioli M. A new sinus lift technique in conjunction with placement of 265 implants: a 6-year retrospective study. Implant Dent. 2000;9(4):363–8.

24. Troedhan AC, Kurrek A, Wainwright M, Jank S. Hydrodynamic ultrasonic sinus floor elevation—an experimental study in sheep. J Oral Maxillofac Surg. 2010;68(5):1125–30.

25. Feldman S, Boitel N, Weng D, Kohles SS, Stach RM. Five-year survival distributions of short-length (10 mm or less) machined-surfaced and Osseotite® implants. Clin Implant Dent Relat Res. 2004;6(1):16–23.

26. Griffin TJ, Cheung WS. The use of short, wide implants in posterior areas with reduced bone height: a retrospective investigation. J Prosthet Dent. 2004;92(2):139–44.

27. Morand M, Irinakis T. The challenge of implant therapy in the posterior maxilla: providing a rationale for the use of short implants. J Oral Implantol. 2007;33(5):257–66.

28. Bahat O. Brånemark system implants in the posterior maxilla: clinical study of 660 implants followed for 5 to 12 years. Inter J Oral Maxillofac Implants. 2000;15(5).

29. Jemt T, Lekholm U. Implant treatment in edentulous maxillae: a 5-year follow-up report on patients with different degrees of jaw resorption. Inter J Oral Maxillofac Implants. 1995;10(3).

30. Naert I, Koutsikakis G, Duyck J, Quirynen M, Jacobs R, Van Steenberghe D. Biologic outcome of implant-supported restorations in the treatment of partial edentulism: part 1: a longitudinal clinical evaluation. Clin Oral Implants Res. 2002;13(4):381–9.

31. Wyatt CC, Zarb GA. Treatment outcomes of patients with implant-supported fixed partial prostheses. International J Oral Maxillofac Implants. 1998;13(2).

32. Levin L, Laviv A, Schwartz-Arad D. Long-term success of implants replacing a single molar. J Periodontol. 2006;77(9):1528–32.

33. Nedir R, Bischof M, Briaux JM, Beyer S, Szmukler-Moncler S, Bernard JP. A 7-year life table analysis from a prospective study on ITI implants with special emphasis on the use of short implants: results from a private practice. Clin Oral Implants Res. 2004;15(2):150–7.

34. Bischof M, Nedir R, Abi Najm S, Szmukler-Moncler S, Samson J. A five-year life-table analysis on wide neck ITI implants with prosthetic evaluation and radiographic analysis: results from a private practice. Clin Oral Implants Res. 2006;17(5):512–20.

35. Esposito M, Barausse C, Pistilli R, Sammartino G, Grandi G, Felice P. Short implants versus bone augmentation for placing longer implants in atrophic maxillae: one-year post-loading results of a pilot randomised controlled trial. Eur J Oral Implantol. 2015;8(3):257–68.

36. Felice P, Barausse C, Pistilli R, Ippolito DR, Esposito M. Five-year results from a randomised controlled trial comparing prostheses supported by 5-mm long implants or by longer implants in augmented bone in posterior atrophic edentulous jaws. Int J oral Implant. 2019;12:25–37.

37. Gastaldi G, Felice P, Pistilli V, Barausse C, Ippolito DR, Esposito M. Posterior atrophic jaws rehabilitated with prostheses supported by 5× 5 mm implants with a nanostructured calcium-incorporated titanium surface or by longer implants in augmented bone. 3-year results from a randomised controlled trial. Eur J Oral Implantol. 2018;11(1):49–61.

38. Guljé FL, Raghoebar GM, Vissink A, Meijer H. Single crowns in the resorbed posterior maxilla supported by either 6-mm implants or by 11-mm implants combined with sinus floor elevation surgery: a 1-year randomised controlled trial. Eur J Oral Implantol. 2014;7(3):247–55.

39. Pistilli R, Felice P, Cannizzaro G, Piattelli M, Corvino V, Barausse C, et al. Posterior atrophic jaws rehabilitated with prostheses supported by 6 mm long 4 mm wide implants or by longer implants in augmented bone. One-year post-loading results from a pilot randomised controlled trial. Eur J Oral Implantol. 2013;6(4).

40. Thoma DS, Haas R, Tutak M, Garcia A, Schincaglia GP, Hämmerle CH. Randomized controlled multicentre study comparing short dental implants (6 mm) versus longer dental implants (11–15 mm) in combination with sinus floor elevation procedures. Part 1: demographics and patient-reported outcomes at 1 year of loading. J Clin Periodontol. 2015;42(1):72–80.

41. Gastaldi G, Felice P, Pistilli R, Barausse C, Trullenque-Eriksson A, Esposito M. Short implants as an alternative to crestal sinus lift: a 3-year multicentre randomised controlled trial. Eur J Oral Implantol. 2017;10(4):391–400.

42. Bilhan H. An alternative method to treat a case with severe maxillary atrophy by the use of angled implants instead of complicated augmentation procedures: a case report. J Oral Implantol. 2008;34(1):47–51.

43. Christopher B, Ho C, Hons B. Implant rehabilitation in the edentulous jaw: the "All-on-4" immediate function concept. Australasian Dent Pract. 2012:138–48.

44. Zampelis A, Rangert B, Heijl L. Tilting of splinted implants for improved prosthodontic support: a two-dimensional finite element analysis. J Prosthet Dent. 2007;97(6):S35–43.

45. Iglesia MA. Anteriorly tilted implants in maxillary tuberosity: avoiding the maxillary sinus. CPOI. 2012;3(1):6–16.

46. Aparicio C, Perales P, Rangert B. Tilted implants as an alternative to maxillary sinus grafting: a clinical, radiologic, and periotest study. Clin Implant Dent Relat Res. 2001;3(1):39–49.

47. Lim TJ, Csillag A, Irinakis T, Nokiani A, Wiebe CB. Intentional angulation of an implant to avoid a pneumatized maxillary sinus: a case report. J Can Dent Assoc. 2004;70(3):164–9.

48. Baggi L, Pastore S, Di Girolamo M, Vairo G. Implant-bone load transfer mechanisms in complete-arch prostheses supported by four implants: a three-dimensional finite element approach. J Prosthet Dent. 2013;109(1):9–21.

49. Del Fabbro M, Bellini CM, Romeo D, Francetti L. Tilted implants for the rehabilitation of edentulous jaws: a systematic review. Clin Implant Dent Relat Res. 2012;14(4):612–21.

50. Rosén A, Gynther G. Implant treatment without bone grafting in edentulous severely resorbed maxillas: a long-term follow-up study. J Oral Maxillofac Surg. 2007;65(5):1010–6.

51. Krekmanov L, Kahn M, Rangert B, Lindström H. Tilting of posterior mandibular and maxillary implants for improved prosthesis support. Inter J Oral Maxillofac Implants. 2000;15(3).

52. Vandeweghe S, De Ferrerre R, Tschakaloff A, De Bruyn H. A wide-body implant as an alternative for sinus lift or bone grafting. J Oral Maxillofac Surg. 2011;69(6):e67–74.

53. Esposito M, Grusovin MG, Rees J, Karasoulos D, Felice P, Alissa R, et al. Effectiveness of sinus lift procedures for dental implant rehabilitation: a Cochrane systematic. Eur J Oral Implantol. 2010;3(1):7–26.

54. Pommer B, Frantal S, Willer J, Posch M, Watzek G, Tepper G. Impact of dental implant length on early failure rates: a meta-analysis of observational studies. J Clin Periodontol. 2011;38(9):856–63.

55. Karthikeyan I, Desai SR, Singh R. Short implants: a systematic review. J Indian Soc Periodontol. 2012;16(3):302.

56. De Santis D, Cucchi A, Longhi C, Vincenzo B. Short threaded implants with an oxidized surface to restore posterior teeth: 1-to 3-year results of a prospective study. Inter J Oral Maxillofac Implants. 2011;26(2).

57. Kahnberg KE, Vannas-Löfqvist L. Sinus lift procedure using a 2-stage surgical technique: I. Clinical and radiographic report up to 5 years. Inter J Oral Maxillofac Implants. 2008;23(5).

58. Anzalone JV, Vastardis S. Oroantral communication as an osteotome sinus elevation complication. J Oral Implantol. 2010;36(3):231–7.

59. Baig MR, Rajan M. Effects of smoking on the outcome of implant treatment: a literature review. Indian J Dent Res. 2007;18(4):190.

60. Kan JY, Rungcharassaeng K, Lozada JL, Goodacre CJ. Effects of smoking on implant success in grafted maxillary sinuses. J Prosthet Dent. 1999;82(3):307–11.

61. Levin L, Schwartz-Arad D. The effect of cigarette smoking on dental implants and related surgery. Implant Dent. 2005;14(4):357–63.

62. de Carvalho RS, Consolaro A, Francischone CE Jr, de Macedo Carvalho APR. Sinus augmentation by orthodontic movement as an alternative to a surgical sinus lift: a clinical report. J Prosthet Dent. 2014;112(4):723–6.

Alveolar Ridge Splitting Technique

14

Jessica R. Anderson and Henry Ferguson

There is a universal unanimity in dental implant surgery that a minimum amount of bone is crucial at the time of placement in order to create a predictable treatment outcome. The presence of a bone width of at least 1–1.5 mm is required on both the buccal and palatal/lingual sides of the implant [1]. Subsequently, this means that for placement of an implant of 3.5–4 mm diameter, a ridge of at least 6 mm is required for predictable placement; additionally, more bone would be needed for wider diameter implants. Unfortunately, ridge resorption can occur exceedingly fast, particularly in the edentulous mandible. In fact, over a period of 12 months, this can equal an unbelievable 6.1 mm of alveolar ridge dimension loss in a buccolingual direction after a single tooth extraction [2]. Horizontal bone loss occurs faster and to a greater extent than vertical bone loss [3]. This bone loss can be associated with many etiologies, including trauma, periodontal disease, infection, neoplasms, malformation, or atrophy [4, 5]. Many of our patients, particularly in the academic setting, go substantially longer than 12 months in preparation for a single implant because of various reasons including finances, fear, lack of a GP to restore the implant, or simply being lost to follow-up.

Despite the difficulty that can potentially accompany replacement of edentulous spaces with implant-retained prostheses, it is associated with greater increases in patient satisfaction, general health, oral health, and social interaction-related quality of life compared to conventional dentures [6, 7]. Because of this, it is important to develop a repertoire of techniques to combat this bone loss while maintaining the high level of implant success rate that occurs in the pristine native bone.

In guided bone regeneration, or GBR, resorbable membranes can be used in combination with particulate autologous bone or a mixture of autologous bone chips and xenogenic bone material, autogenous block onlay grafts harvest intraorally, or from the hip, or distraction osteogenesis [8–11]. Although these procedures do augment the ridge, they are associated with increased treatment time and costs, have risk of dehiscence and infections, and negatively affect patients' morbidity [12]. In comparison, an advantage of methods such as alveolar ridge splitting is that implants can be inserted at the same time as the bone is widened, which reduces morbidity and treatment costs and time [13].

In the past two decades, several surgical techniques have been established to manage an extremely atrophic alveolar ridge [7]. Of note, several ridge-splitting techniques have been developed, including split crest osteotomy, ridge expansion osteotomy, and various other modifications [14]. The concept for this novel technique was introduced first by Tatum in 1986 [15]. This was described as a split by means of osteotomes with gradually increasing dimensions. In 1982, Simeon described a surgical technique involving a longitudinal alveolar ridge splitting in two parts, provoking a greenstick fracture using small chisels [16].

Unfortunately, in both techniques described above, it was necessary that it only be performed in bone of soft quality (types 3 and 4). The operator was, however, able to perform the osteotomy and place the implant at the same time, which shortened the time of procedure. Procedure time is a known factor in likelihood of morbidity of a procedure [17].

With the introduction of microsaw devices or piezoelectric devices for cutting hard alveolar bone under adequate control, the alveolar ridge splitting/expansion technique (ARST) can be used regardless of the bone quality [18, 19]. Currently, ridge splitting is a procedure that may be performed with many different instruments including the aforementioned chisel and mallet, scalpel blades, spatula, osteotomes, and newer options including piezoelectrical surgical systems, lasers, and ultrafine fissure burs. It still stands that among the various instruments used for ridge expansion, osteotomes are the most popular [20]. In a systematic review by Jha et al., it was noted that 65% of individuals in the study used osteotomes, 18% of practitioners used motorized

J. R. Anderson (✉) · H. Ferguson
AU Oral and Maxillofacial Surgery, Augusta, GA, USA
e-mail: janderson4@augusta.edu; hferguson@augusta.edu

© The Author(s), under exclusive license to Springer Nature Switzerland AG 2021
M. R. Stevens et al. (eds.), *Innovative Perspectives in Oral and Maxillofacial Surgery*,
https://doi.org/10.1007/978-3-030-75750-2_14

expanders, and 17% used other devices (extension crest devices, piezosurgery devices, threaded bone expanders, etc.).

It should be noted, however, that piezoelectric devices have been found to be the most effective [14]. With this device, selective cutting of the bone without affecting the soft tissue (nerves and blood vessels) may be carried out; further, an oscillating tip with an irrigating fluid provides a cleaner working area and greater visibility (cavitation effect) at the surgical site without causing bone heating compared to conventional devices [21, 22].

Jha et al. stated that while using an osteotome is cost-effective and simple to use and allows excellent manual control with adequate determination of the implant axis, piezoelectric and other modern devices should be used more in the future because they are more suitable to present any trauma to the vulnerable structures like mucosa, blood vessels, and nerves and results in less trauma to the bone. This in turn allows for patient satisfaction increases associated with faster healing.

Requirements of the Technique

Ridge splitting techniques have multiple requirements in order to ensure favorability and survivability of the procedure. According to Jha et al., successful implantation using alveolar ridge split requires a minimum alveolar bone width of 3 mm to ensure sufficient trabecular bone substrate, as well as cortical and cancellous bone on both sides of the split ridge [14]. Bassetti et al. in 2013 compiled the following four anatomical parameters for successful implementation of alveolar ridge splitting technique with successful implant placement (Fig. 14.1).

Procedure

Among the various techniques introduced for the expansion of alveolar ridges with a horizontal bone deficit, alveolar ridge split technique has proved to have a 98% to 100% survival rate following the contextual insertion of implants [23]. Although many providers may have their own surgical tech-

nique, a common technique for the use of piezoelectric devices proposed by Moro et al. [24] will be described in this part of the chapter.

After local anesthesia, a crestal incision can be performed on the atrophic edentulous ridge. This incision should be followed by two vertical releasing incisions beyond the muco-gingival line to avoid trauma to the tissue. The bone should be exposed utilizing a full-thickness mucoperiosteal flap. Once the flap is raised, the bone is adequately exposed, and the planned osteotomies should be outlined with a piezo tip at low power to obtain a cut depth of around 1 mm. The lower power setting assists in avoiding oscillation of the piezosurgical tip.

The first osteotomy should be carried out at the center of the occlusal aspect of the ridge and subsequently traced and extended in an anteroposterior direction for the desired and previously planned length. Successively, the vertical osteotomies should be performed on the proximal and distal ends of the crestal incision.

In this proposed technique, the vertical osteotomies should be convergent and oblique so that the distance between the two vertical osteotomies is greater on the outer side than on the inner side of the vestibular cortical plate. The length of the vertical osteotomies should ideally be determined by the extension of the atrophic ridge.

As the procedure is continued, the osteotomy lines can continue to be deepened using longer piezo tips and higher power level progressively. Because the grooves will become retentive once deepened, the oscillation of the higher power should not affect the cut, and the subsequent depths should occur more aggressively and quicker for the operator.

Once the desired depth is achieved, the caudal ends of the vertical osteotomies are connected by a horizontal incision. The last incision should be a partial-thickness osteotomy. The greenstick fracture is then made using chisels.

The bone graft is then placed between the vestibular and lingual or palatal cortex. In order to obtain supracrestal regeneration, the bone graft can be fixed at a higher level in order to let it protrude from the occlusal aspect of the two bone plates and act as a vertical support.

At this time, the grafted site can be covered by a resorbable collagen membrane and closed with sutures. The surgical site should be allowed to heal for 6–9 months.

Fig. 14.1 Four anatomical requirements for the accomplishment of ARST according to Bassetti et al.

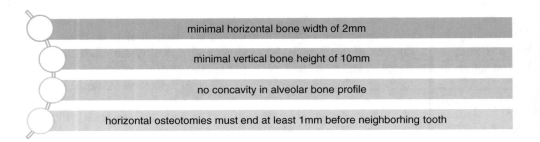

minimal horizontal bone width of 2mm

minimal vertical bone height of 10mm

no concavity in alveolar bone profile

horizontal osteotomies must end at least 1mm before neighborhing tooth

Complications and Disadvantages Associated with ARST

Despite the successes noted in the literature, alveolar ridge splitting technique does have several disadvantages. It is an operator-dependent technique with a learning curve as are most surgical techniques. In addition, single tooth areas present with greater challenges as compared to multi tooth edentulous spaces or entire arches. The bone in these smaller areas will have lack of bone elasticity, and difficulty is increased in smaller work areas as a general principle.

In addition, one must be careful to avoid complications during the execution of this technique including clinical infections and fractures in the medullar bone tissue between the two cortical plates, and implant failure is of course a risk as in any implant placement technique.

The most common complications associated with ridge expansion procedures is bone fracture [14]. The mandibular bone has a thicker cortical plate and is less flexible than the maxilla; hence, the rate of bone fracture during ridge expansion is more for the mandibular regions. To prevent bone fracture, Holtzclaw et al. used a modified technique whereby apical hinge cuts were used, which were not fully in the buccal plate so that some mobilization of the buccal plate could be achieved.

References

1. Scipioni A, Bruschi GB, Calesini G. The edentulous ridge expansion technique: a five-year study. Int J Periodontics Restorative Dent. 1994;14(5):451–9.
2. Schropp L, Wenzel A, Kostopoulos L, Karring T. Bone healing and soft tissue contour changes following single-tooth extraction: A clinical and radiographic 12- month prospective study. Int J Periodontics Restorative Dent. 2003;23:313–23.
3. Gurler G, Delilbasi C, Garip H, Tufekcioglu S. Comparison of alveolar ridge splitting and autogenous onlay bone grafting to enable implant placement in patients with atrophic jaw bones. Saudi Med J. 2017;38(12):1207–12. https://doi.org/10.15537/smj.2017.12.21462.
4. Sakkas A, Schramm A, Karsten W, Gellrich N, Wilde F. A clinical study of the outcomes and complications associated with zygomatic buttress block bone graft for limited preimplant augmentation procedures. J Cranio-Maxillofac Surg. 2016;44(3):249–56. https://doi.org/10.1016/j.jcms.2015.12.003.
5. Chiapasco M, Zaniboni M, Boisco M. Augmentation procedures for the rehabilitation of deficient edentulous ridges with oral implants. Clin Oral Implants Res. 2006;17(S2):136–59. https://doi.org/10.1111/j.1600-0501.2006.01357.x.
6. Emami E, Thomason JM. In individuals with complete tooth loss, the mandibular implant-retained overdenture increases patient satisfaction and oral health related quality of life compared to conventional dentures. J Evid Based Dent Pract. 2013;13:94–6. https://doi.org/10.1016/j.jebdp.2013.02.003.
7. Berger S, Hakl P, Sutter W, Meier M, Roland H, Bandura P, Turhani D. Interantral alveolar ridge splitting for maxillary horizontal expansion and simultaneous dental implant insertion: a case report. Ann Med Surg. 2019;48:83–7. https://doi.org/10.1016/j.amsu.2019.10.018.
8. Buser D, Bragger U, Lang NP, Nyman S. Regeneration and enlargement of jaw bone using guided tissue regeneration. Clin Oral Implants Res. 1990;1:22–32.
9. Urban LA, Nagursky H, Lozada JL. Horizontal ridge augmentation with a resorbable membrane and particulated autogenous bone with or without anorganic bovine bone-derived mineral: a prospective case series in 22 patients. Inter J Oral Maxillofac Implants. 2011;26:404–14.
10. Felice P, Pistilli R, Lizio G, Pellegrino G, Nisii, a. & Marchetti, C. Inlay versus onlay iliac bone grafting in atrophic posterior mandible: a prospective controlled clinical trial for the comparison of two techniques. Clin Implant Dent Relat Res. 2009;11:69–82.
11. Takahashi T, Funaki K, Shintani H, Haruoka T. Use of horizontal alveolar distraction osteogenesis for implant placement in a narrow alveolar ridge: a case report. Inter J Oral Maxillofac Implants. 2004;19:291–414.
12. Laurie SW, Kaban LB, Mulliken JB, Murray JE. Donor-site morbidity after harvesting rib and iliac bone. Plast Reconstr Surg. 1984.
13. Bassetti MA, Bassetti RG, Bosshardt DD. The alveolar ridge splitting/expansion technique: a systematic review. Clin Oral Implants Res. 2015;27(3):310–24. https://doi.org/10.1111/clr.12537.
14. Jha N, Choi EH, Kaushik NK, Ryu JJ. Types of devices used in ridge split procedure for alveolar bone expansion: a systematic review. PLoS One. 2017;12(7) https://doi.org/10.1371/journal.pone.0180342.
15. Tatum H Jr. Maxillary and sinus implant reconstructions. Dent Clin N Am. 1986;30:207–29.
16. Simeon M, Baldoni M, Zaffe D. Jawbone enlargement using immediate implant placement associated with a split-crest technique and guided tissue regeneration. Int J Periodontics Restorative Dent. 1992;12:462–73.
17. Scott CF Jr. Length of operation and morbidity: is there a relationships? Plast Reconstr Surg. 1982;69(6):1017–21. https://doi.org/10.1097/00006534-198206000-00024.
18. Suh JJ, Shelemay A, Choi SH, Chai JK. Alveolar ridge splitting: a new microsaw technique. Int J Periodontics Restorative Dent. 2005;25:165–71.
19. Vercolletti T. Piezoelectric surgery in implantology: a case report-a new piezoelectric ridge expansion technique. Int J Periodontics Restorative Dent. 2000;20:358–65.
20. Gonzalez-Garcia R, Monje F, Moreno C. Alveolar split osteotomy for the treatment of the severe narrow ridge maxillary atrophy: a modified technique. Int J Oral Maxillofac Surg. 2011;40:57–64.
21. Holtzclaw DJ, Toscano NJ, Rosen PS. Reconstruction of posterior mandibular alveolar ridge deficiencies with the piezoelectric hinge-assisted ridge split technique: a retrospective observational report. J Periodontal. 2010;81(11):1580–6.
22. Sohn DS, Lee HJ, Heo JU, Moon JW, Park IS, Romanos GE. Immediate and delayed lateral ridge expansion technique in the atrophic posterior mandibular ridge. J Oral Maxillofac Surg. 2010;68(9):2283–90.
23. Engelke WGH, Diederichs CG, Jacobs HG, Deckwer I. Alveolar reconstruction with splitting osteotomy and microfixation of implants. Int J Oral Maxillofac Implants. 1997;12(3):310–8.
24. Moro A, Gasparini G, Foresta E, Saponaro G, Falchi M, Cardarelli L, De Angelis P, Forcione M, Garagiola U, D'Amato G, Pelo S. Alveolar ridge split technique using piezosurgery with specially designed tips. Biomed Res Int. 2017;2017:4530378. https://doi.org/10.1155/2017/4530378. Epub 2017 Jan 29. PMID: 28246596; PMCID: PMC5303585.

Outcomes of Short Implants in Bone Deficiency

15

Thomas Farrell IV

Introduction

In many clinical situations, insufficient bone volume is a critical limiting factor for dental implant rehabilitation. Tooth loss rapidly results in alveolar ridge remodeling which can lead to an average of 40 to 60% decrease in the horizontal and vertical dimensions of the alveolar ridge during the first 2 years of post-extraction [1, 2]. This often leads to compromised edentulous sites that traditionally necessitated procedures in order to increase bone volume for traditional dental implant placement. Procedures such as maxillary sinus augmentation, nerve lateralization, and guided bone regeneration for horizontal and vertical augmentation are designed to replace the lost alveolar bone. These procedures are technique sensitive and involve prolonged treatment time, higher morbidity, and increased cost. This has led to the application of short dental implants (SDIs) as a therapeutic option that reduces the need for augmentation therapy in compromised edentulous sites (Fig. 15.1).

The true definition of SDIs is still controversial, with studies lacking consensus about its definition, with disagreement over the length between short and standard dental implants. Some authors considered "short" implants as those with a length of 7–10 mm [3], whereas others consider "short" as those implants with a designated intra-bony length (DIL) of less than or equal to 8 mm [4]. The DIL is the length of implant intended to engage and remain in contact with bone once the implant becomes functional [5]. The DIL does not include the length of the implant collar segment which is meant to accommodate the peri-implant soft tissues. In this chapter, we define dental implants with a DIL of 8 mm or less as short based on the available data in the current literature.

Recently, there have been several improvements that have increased the predictability of SDIs. These include innovations in dental implant design, modifications in prosthetic connections, and alterations in the surgical technique of placement, all aimed to increase the usefulness of SDIs. In this chapter, we discuss these innovations and present a protocol for the dental implant surgeon to maximize the successful application of SDIs.

Rethinking Occlusal Force

Historically, the use of SDIs was not recommended by some clinicians because it was believed that occlusal forces must be dissipated over a large implant area in order for the bone to be preserved [6]. Recently, finite element analysis (FEA) has been utilized to understand the effect of load distributions on dental implant surfaces. These studies have revealed that the highest strains to a bone stimulant occur in the crestal region of an implant and that little stress is transferred to the apical portion. This means that the occlusal forces are primarily distributed to the crestal bone rather than throughout the entire implant-bone interface. Pierrisnard and colleagues [7] by means of three-dimensional FEA of machine turned implants lengths from 6 to 12 mm and found that the magnitude in distribution of stress to the bone was constant and independent of implant length. They also showed that short implants subjected to lateral forces tended to move within the bone, whereas longer implants have a tendency to fold under similar stress [8]. Anitua et al. [9] conducted FEA of the influence of implant length, diameter, and geometry on implant surface stress distribution. The authors also found that maximum stress was concentrated around the neck of the implant and that the stress was localized on the bone adjacent to the first six implant threads, independent of implant length. This evidence has been reinforced by other biomechanical studies suggesting that maximum bone stress is independent of implant length and that there is no distinct

T. Farrell IV (✉)
Department of Oral & Maxillofacial Surgery, Dental College of Georgia at Augusta University, Augusta, GA, USA
e-mail: tfarrell@augusta.edu

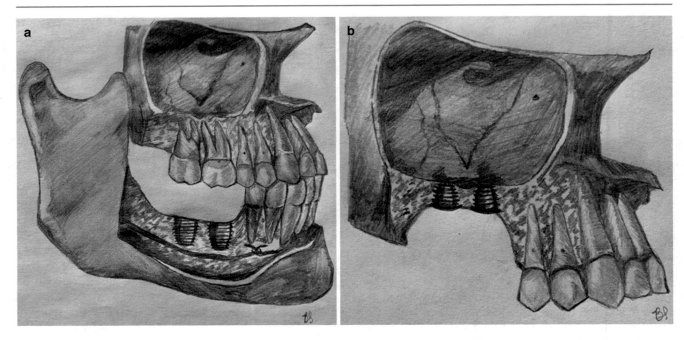

Fig. 15.1 (**a**, **b**) Schematic drawing of the application of short dental implants in patients with insufficient residual alveolar bone volume due to mandible alveolar atrophy (**a**) or a combination of maxillary alveolar atrophy and sinus pneumatization (**b**). (Courtesy of Brooke Stevens)

linear relationship between dental implant length and survival rate. Recent systematic reviews have reported that SDIs have similar long-term prognosis as traditional implants [10, 11, 12, 13, 14, 15]; thus, the early preference for longer implants seems to have been misguided. SDIs can offer a clear advantages for the clinician when trying to restore atrophic sites where patient factors, financial or anatomic, may preclude bone augmentation.

Short dental implant success is achieved by the synergistic combination of numerous biomechanical features, which include the following:

1. Implant microdesign
2. Implant macrodesign
3. Platform switching
4. Progressive early loading protocols
5. Crown to implant (C/I) ratio
6. Splinting to adjacent implants
7. Surgical preparation of the osteotomy

We will now discuss these factors that help SDIs achieve success.

Implant Microdesign: Surface Topography

Implant microdesign consists of the implant material and surface treatment and morphology. One of the factors that affects the performance of dental implants is their surface roughness, which is categorized by their Sa value (average

height deviation in a given surface). Traditionally, dental implant surface topography has been classified as smooth (Sa < 0.5 μm), minimally rough (Sa 0.5–1.0 μm), moderately rough (1.0–2.0 μm), and rough (Sa >2.0 μm). The advantages of rougher implant surfaces are that it increases surface area and subsequent bone-to-implant contact (BIC), as well as promoting faster and stronger osseointegration compared to smooth surface implants. The disadvantage of rougher surfaced implants is that they increase bacterial plaque retention if they become exposed above bone, promoting peri-implantitis. Various surface roughening techniques have been introduced over the years and they can be classified as additive or subtractive (or reductive). Examples of additive roughening techniques include hydroxyapatite coatings, titanium plasma spray, and nanoparticle deposition. Examples of subtractive roughening techniques include electropolishing, mechanical polishing, titanium oxide blasting, acid etching, laser etching, and grit blasting (or a combination of two or more). Wennerberg and Albrektsson [16] determined that surface roughness influences bone response at the micrometer level.

The early failures of SDIs are thought to be primarily due to the fact that they had machine-turned (smooth to minimally rough) surfaces and thus did not supply adequate surface area for ideal BIC. In a systematic review with a meta-analysis, Pommer et al. [17] reported higher failure rates with machine-turned implant surfaces compared to rough implant surfaces. As stated earlier, truly rough implant surfaces (Sa >2.0 μm) are susceptible to bacterial plaque accumulation and subsequent progressive bone loss and are thus not recommended for SDIs. Moderately rough dental implants (Sa 1.0–2.0 μm) have become the most commonly utilized surface topography for SDIs because they balance the need for increased BIC with slightly less risk of bacterial plaque retention. This shift in short implant surface design from smooth to moderately rough has greatly increased the success rates for short dental implants. Fugazzotto et al. [18] reviewed 979 short implants with rough or moderately rough surfaces placed in the posterior maxilla and reported a cumulative success rate of 95.1%. Lai et al. [19] reported a similar cumulative survival rate of 98% for short, moderately rough threaded implants placed in posterior sites.

Another innovation in implant surface design has been the creation of sintered porous-surfaced (SPS) press-fit implants. These implants have a unique surface structure that permits faster osseointegration than smooth surface implants [20, 21]. The sintered surface provides three-dimensional mechanical interlock via bone ingrowth into their macroporous surface layer and has been noted to increase BIC by three to four times, when compared to smooth surface implants [22]. In a prospective study by Deporter et al. [23], non-splinted SPS implants were used for mandibular overdentures. Four separate implant lengths were studied ranging from 7 to 10 mm, and after 10 years, the shortest implant group (7 mm, with a 2 mm transgingival machined collar, making a DIL of 5 mm) performed the best. This remained the case after 20 years as well [22].

Implant Macrodesign: Thread Geometry

Implant macrodesign includes thread geometry and body shape. There have been several innovations in implant body design and thread geometry in order to provide SDIs with improved initial stability and greater success in poor bone quality. Implant thread geometry can be described in terms of thread pitch, thread width, thread depth, and thread shape [24] (Fig. 15.2). Thread pitch is defined as the distance between adjacent threads, measured on the same side of the axis. A smaller thread pitch (i.e., more threads on the implant body) results in a greater surface area per unit length and is noted to positively influence implant stability [25]. Thread width is the distance in the same axial plane between the coronal most and the apical most parts at the tip of a single thread [26]. Thread depth is the distance from the outermost tip to the innermost body of the thread, also described as the distance between the major and minor diameters of the thread [26]. Deeper threads increase surface area and are better suited for softer bone [25], and shallow threads allow for easier placement of the implant in hard bone. Thread shapes

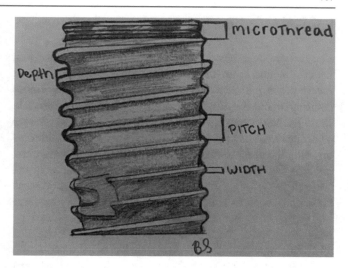

Fig. 15.2 Diagram depicting implant thread depth, thread pitch, and thread width. (Courtesy of Brooke Stevens)

available for endosteal implants include square-shape, V-shape, buttress, and reverse buttress, which are defined by the thread thickness and face angle [27]. Misch et al. [28] reported that smaller thread pitch and greater thread depth are vital for the success of short dental implants in posterior regions of the mouth with reduced bone density.

Implant Macrodesign: Increased Implant Diameter

There has been a recent trend to increase the diameter of SDIs to improve their performance. Recent literature has shown that the effect of implant diameter on stress distribution in bone is more significant than the effect of implant length [9, 29]. Baggi et al. [30] through 3D FEA of five different implant systems found that increasing implant diameter reduced stress values and concentration areas for cortical bone. Reducing stress on the crestal bone will reduce the incidence of microfractures and subsequent crestal bone resorption. Increasing diameter will also make up for the lost implant surface area of shortening implant length. Esposito et al. [31] in a split mouth study comparing short implants to standard length implants found that short, wide implants had significantly less mean crestal bone loss. Several other studies have shown predictable success rates employing large diameters (>5 mm) on short and ultrashort implants [21, 32, 33]. As with any implant application, success requires adequate interproximal and bucco-lingual bone volume. A minimum of 1–1.5 mm of bone should be maintained circumferentially around the implant to avoid crestal bone loss and soft-tissue recession.

Implant Macrodesign: Implant Crest Module

The crest module of an implant body is the transosteal region, which extends from the implant body where the implant meets the soft tissue and changes from a virtually sterile environment to the hostile oral cavity [26]. The crest module should provide features that seal the osteotomy and provide a barrier to prevent the ingress of bacteria or soft tissue from invading the threads of the implant body. Originally the crest module was always smooth and polished, but recently the concept of adding microthreads in the crestal portion has been introduced to maintain crestal bone levels by preserving the peri-implant connective tissue attachment and by providing a lower physiologic stress on the crestal bone. The term "biologic width" was based on the work of Gargiulo et al. [34] who described the dimensions and relationship of dentogingival junction in human cadavers. It has been hypothesized that a similar relationship exists between the bone and the soft tissues around dental implants, generally at the level of the implant to abutment interface or "microgap." Unlike the natural dentition, the gingival connective tissue fibers typically do not attach directly to the implant surfaces but take the form of a fibrous capsule with collagen fibers oriented circumferentially. In the early days of dental implants, clinicians utilized dental implants with smooth necks in order to prevent bacterial plaque accumulation [35], but this led to the connective tissue to dental implant relationship as just described. Recently, there have been modifications in the surface topography of the implant crest module that can allow for a more tooth-like gingival attachment. Laser surface treatments of the implant neck and abutment can create microgrooves that have been shown to have directional effects on the orientation of bone cells, fibroblasts, and epithelial cells [36] (Fig. 15.3). This has been shown to create a connective tissue attachment similar to that of the cementum layer of a natural tooth root surface [37]. This type of peri-implant soft tissue attachment to the implant collar appears to limit crestal bone loss and reduce the likelihood of soft tissue inflammation. Nevins et al. [38] studied laser-ablated surfaces on implant abutments using a canine model. Their study had four cohorts, using a combination of resorbable blast textured implants with or without a coronal machine turned collar; used in conjunction with a laser-ablated microgrooved or full machine turned healing abutment. The study showed that the groups that utilized the laser-ablated microgrooves had perpendicularly oriented fibers that attached to the abutment microgrooves. This in turn prevented the apical migration of the junctional epithelium and thus protected the microgaps from microbial plaque contamination. In a human study comparing implants with laser-ablated surfaces on their collar segments to control implants (with 2 mm machined-turned collars), Pecora et al.

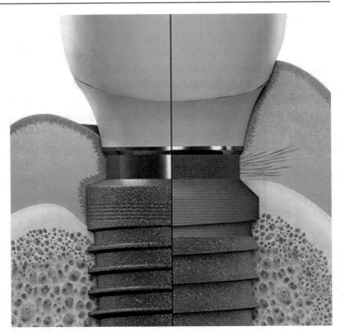

Fig. 15.3 Diagram depicting the parallel connective tissue attachment to the Laser-Lok® surface of the BioHorizons implant (BioHorizons, Birmingham, AL), thus preventing apical migration of epithelium and preserving crestal bone levels. (Reproduction with permission from BioHorizons)

[39] found that the laser-ablated collar implants had significantly less crestal bone loss at 7 months (0.59 mm versus 1.94 mm) (Figs. 15.4 and 15.5).

As stated before, recent FEA studies have demonstrated that the peak stress occurs around the crestal bone, and many have speculated that crestal bone loss around smooth implant collars can be attributed to the lack of effective mechanical stress distribution. Alexander et al. [40] used FEA to compare axial and side loading on implants with laser-treated versus machine turned collars. They found significantly lower maximum crestal bone distortional stress with the laser-treated implants (22.6 MPa compared to 91.9 MPa for control group for 80 N load), which they suggest that the diminished stress overload will preserve crestal bone levels. Hansson [41] on review of implants with smooth versus retention elements on the implant neck found a positive correlation between surface roughness and interfacial shear strength. He suggested that implant neck retention elements may counteract marginal bone resorption and also increase the axial load an implant can support. There have been several studies in the literature that suggest that microgrooved implant collars maintain stable marginal bone levels. Zuffetti et al. [42] reported a 97.2% success rate for short implants with a laser-microgrooved collar (≤7.5 mm) in posterior areas. Shin et al. [35] compared crestal bone loss among three different threaded implants with different neck designs.

Fig. 15.4 Implant design features of Bicon Short® Implants (Bicon Corp., Boston, MA) include a wide-diameter threaded design with a locking taper that has an inherent platform switch mechanism. (Reproduction with permission from Bicon Dental Implants)

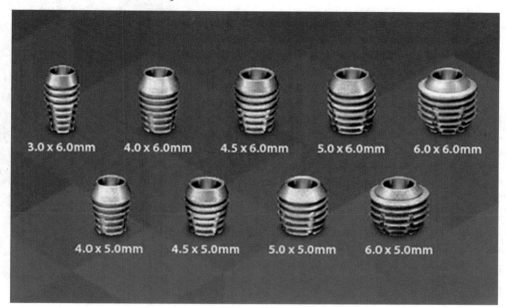

Bicon SHORT® Implants

3.0 x 6.0mm 4.0 x 6.0mm 4.5 x 6.0mm 5.0 x 6.0mm 6.0 x 6.0mm

4.0 x 5.0mm 4.5 x 5.0mm 5.0 x 5.0mm 6.0 x 5.0mm

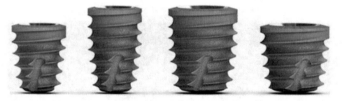

Fig. 15.5 Implant design features of BioHorizons Tapered Short® Implant (BioHorizons, Birmingham, AL) include an aggressive thread profile, platform switching features, and an implant collar with laser-ablated dual-affinity microgrooves (Laser-Lok®) for crestal bone retention and connective tissue attachment. (Reproduction with permission from BioHorizons)

One cohort had a machined neck, one with a rough-surfaced neck, and one with a rough surface with microthreads. After 12 months, there was a significant difference in the amount of alveolar bone recorded for the three groups, with the rough surface with microthreads at the implant neck the most effective at preserving crestal bone levels (mean crestal bone loss of 0.18 mm compared to 1.32 mm for machined neck).

Platform Switching

As stated earlier, the mucosal barrier surrounding dental implants is referred to as the peri-implant biologic width, a term borrowed from the natural dentition [34]. It has been well described that a prosthetic design that violates biologic width will result in crestal bone loss until the space needed for the connective tissue component of the biologic width is reestablished. After the connection of dental implants to abutments and exposure to the oral environment, a predictable loss of approximately 1.5–2.0 mm of vertical bone has been documented to occur. With traditional dental implants, 2 mm of crestal bone loss is of little consequence, but for SDIs, this can significantly reduce the total implant-to-bone interface and thus greatly affect treatment outcomes. The concept of platform switching as a means of reducing crestal bone loss around dental implants was first described by Lazzara and Porter [5, 43] and has since been employed as an effective strategy to mitigate post-restorative peri-implant bone loss. In platform-switched implants, the diameter of the prosthetic abutment is less than the diameter of the implant collar, resulting in a circumferential and horizontal offset at the top of the implant. This will reduce the vertical length of the implant surface needed to establish biologic width. This offset also separates the crestal bone and connective tissue from the bacteria-inhabited microgap. This separation prevents soft tissue inflammation mediated crestal bone loss. It is also postulated that platform switching reduces the stress directed to the crestal bone-implant interface by directing the loading forces down the long axis of the implant. These theories were tested in two clinical trials by Telleman et al. [44, 45], evaluating platform-switched connections to platform-matched connections in short dental implants (8.5 mm in length). In both studies, the marginal bone loss around short platform-switched implants was significantly smaller than the marginal bone loss around short platform-matched implants. These results have been confirmed by a meta-analysis by Aslam [46], which found significantly less mean marginal bone loss around platform-switched implants when compared to platform-matched implants.

Progressive Early Implant Loading

When SDIs were first introduced, a staged approach was suggested, believing that submerging the implants would protect from early implant failures due to micromovement or implant surface contamination. Recently, several clinicians have advocated for the use of provisional prostheses or healing abutments to introduce gradual loading in order to produce a reactive increase in the bone density at the implant-bone interface [47]. Wolff's law states that "the bone in a healthy person will adapt to the loads under which it is placed. If loading on a particular bone increases, the bone will remodel itself over time to become stronger to resist that sort of loading [41]." This would imply that increased stresses act as a stimulus to new bone formation. And conversely, lack of stresses or "stress shielding" can lead to bone atrophy. Esposito et al. [31] performed a split mouth study comparing 5 mm long implants of 6 mm diameter without augmentation to longer implants placed in vertically augmented bone. Implants were initially submerged. After 4 months, a provisional prosthesis was placed slightly in occlusion, followed by definitive prosthesis at 8 months. They found that 5mm short implants achieved similar, if not better, results than longer implants placed in augmented bone. Felice et al. [48] performed a similar study with the same loading protocol and similar results. Cannizzaro et al. [49] studied the outcomes of short dental implants (7 mm) that were immediately and early loaded. He found survival rates above 96% for both groups after 9 months of loading.

Crown to Implant (C/I) Ratio

The placement of SDIs in vertically compromised edentulous sites regularly increases the crown to implant (C/I) ratio (sometimes referred to as C/R, for crown to implant root ratio) (Fig. 15.6). Some clinicians have considered the greater crown height to be a vertical cantilever that could increase the peri-implant bone stress and eventually result in crestal bone loss, implant failures, or prosthetic complications. This reasoning has been inferred from the known impact crown to root ratios have on natural teeth. An ideal crown to root ratio for natural teeth is 0.5 (1 length crown: 2 lengths root). However, the current evidence seems to show that integrated dental implants do not behave in this way. In a review of partially edentulous patients treated with SPS short implants, Rokni [50] reported that C/R had no significant effect on steady-state crestal bone levels. The mean C/R ratio for the implants studied was 1.5. Schincaglia et al. [51] investigated the use of SDIs in the posterior maxilla compared with longer implants placed in combination with a lateral window sinus augmentation. The investigators found no correlation between the unfavorable C/I ratio in the short implant cohort and marginal bone loss. Anitua et al. [52] also

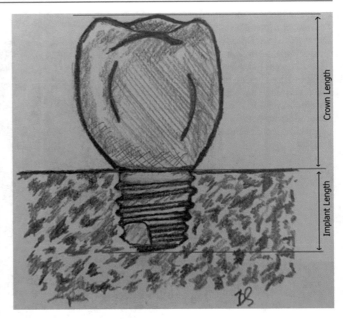

Fig. 15.6 Diagram representing crown-to-implant (C/I) ratio. This would be an example of a C/I of 2.0 (two crown lengths, per implant length). (Courtesy of Brook Stevens)

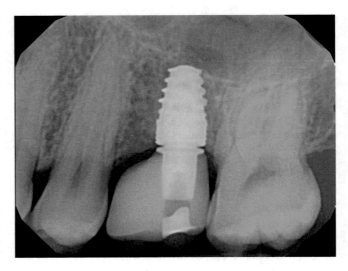

Fig. 15.7 A 5.0 × 8.0 mm Nobel Active® implant placed at the left maxillary first molar site. This implant was both immediately placed and immediately restored with a provisional restoration. (Source: Dr. Ian Mackenzie Farnham, Jacksonville, FL. Reproduced with permission of Dr. Farnham)

found that C/I ratio had no significant effect on marginal bone loss in short and extra-short implants placed in the posterior sites. In a study by Tawil et al. [53], C/I ratios as high as 3.0 did not seem to represent a biomechanical risk factor in cases of favorable force orientation and load distribution. Consequently, Hingsammer and Pommer [54] in a study of splinted short implants found that C/I ratios greater than 1.7 can lead to early marginal bone loss (Figs. 15.7, 15.8, 15.9, 15.10, and 15.11) .

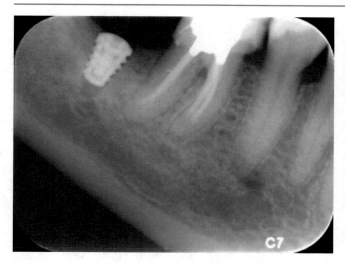

Fig. 15.8 A 4.7 × 6.0 mm BioHorizons Tapered Short® Implant placed at a right mandibular second molar site which had compromised vertical bone height due to failure of a previously placed traditional length implant. The radiograph shows the implant immediately after placement. (Source: Dr. Thomas Farrell IV, Augusta, GA)

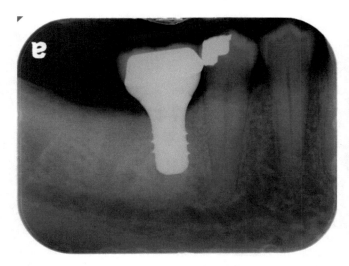

Fig. 15.9 A 4.8 × 8 mm (with 2.8 mm polished neck) Straumann SLActive® tissue level implant restoring a right mandibular first molar site. The radiograph shows the implant after 3 years in function. (Source: Dr. Jeremy Oakley, Hilo, HI. Reproduced with permission from Dr. Oakley)

Splinting

The question on whether to splint adjacent SDI crowns is still up for debate. The perceived risks associated with an unfavorable C/I ratio and greater occlusal forces on SDI posterior restorations may be offset by increasing the implant number to support the prosthesis [28]. In the past, splinting was advised for SDIs in order to decrease the lateral forces on the prosthesis and reduce stress directed on the crestal aspect of the dental implant [55]. Yilmaz et al. [56] studied

the strain generated by splinted and non-splinted short implant crowns and concluded that splinting provides a more even strain distribution during functional loading. A meta-analysis performed by Vazouras [57] looking at SDI failure rates over time in function found implant-supported fixed partial dentures on short implants with >3 years in function had superior outcomes compared to single crowns supported by short implants.

Although splinting implant crowns is known to provide a more uniform stress distribution [54, 58, 59], there are some clinicians who argue that splinting could lead to crestal bone atrophy from "stress shielding" [60]. Rokni et al. [50] in a study found that splinted implants showed more crestal bone loss than non-splinted implants, which could be attributed to disuse atrophy. There have also been several studies that have looked at the outcomes of short implants supporting single posterior crowns. One such study by Lai et al. [19] found a 10-year cumulative survival rate of 98.3%. Villarinho et al. [61] and Rossi et al.[32] had similar results but with less follow up. These findings would suggest that splinting adjacent SDI crowns may not be necessary.

Surgical Preparation of the Osteotomy

There have been several modifications in the osteotomy preparation aimed to increase the initial stability of SDIs, which include making a slightly undersized osteotomy, avoiding countersinking, and slow drilling protocols. The closer the contact between the implant surface and the surrounding bone, the higher the initial stability will be achieved. To achieve high insertion torque levels for SDIs placed in soft bone (type III and type IV), some clinicians have advocated for the use of a slightly undersized osteotomy in order to improve initial implant stability [8, 62]. Vidyasagar et al. [63] reported that countersinking (cervical flaring) should be avoided when placing SDIs in poor-quality bone because it can jeopardize the cortical bone anchorage and compromise initial implant stability. Anitua et al. [64] suggested using a low-speed drilling sequence (50 rpm) to avoid overheating the bone and to allow for retrieval of autogenous graft from the osteotomy. Some clinicians have advocated using disposable surgical burs in order to prevent thermal bone necrosis and to allow for precision drilling. The use of osseodensification burs have also aided in facilitating ridge expansion of compromised sites in order to place larger diameter SDIs [65]. The application of hand osteotomes or reamer burs in the placement of SDIs in the posterior maxilla has been employed by some [66, 67]. Deporter and colleagues [68] reported a technique of using tapered hand osteotomes for indirect sinus elevation and simultaneous placement of rough surface short implants with a mean implant length of 6.9 mm. The study was unique in that they were able to produce a

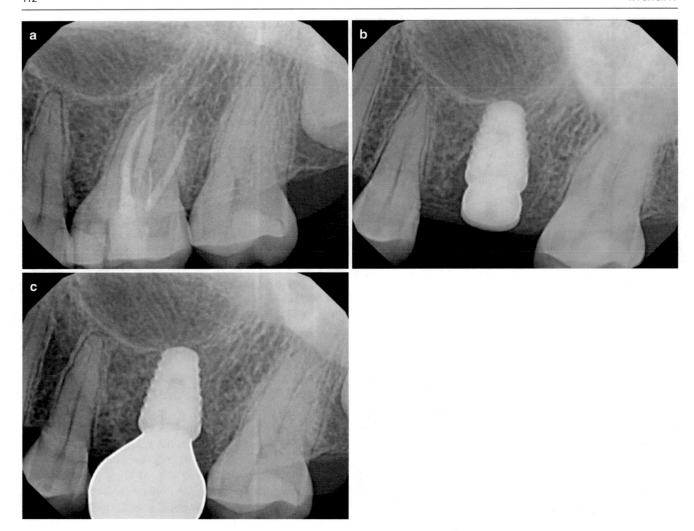

Fig. 15.10 (**a-c**) A 5.8 × 7.5 mm BioHorizons Tapered Internal® implant placed at the left maxillary first molar site. This implant was placed immediately and the final radiograph shows the implant after 2 years of function carrying a single zirconia crown. (Source: Dr. Donald Craig Taylor, Suwanee, GA. Reproduced with permission from Dr. Taylor)

100% success rate in sites with only 3 mm of subantral bone, which is considerably less than the 6 mm originally recommended by Summers. Other clinicians have recommended the application of growth factors to the implant surface in order to enhance osseointegration. Anitua et al. [69] demonstrated a cumulative success rate of 98% for SDIs humidified with platelet rich growth factor (PRGF) placed in posterior sites after 10-year follow-up.

Conclusion

Short (DIL ≤ 8 mm) dental implants have been shown to be a reliable and effective solution to provide implant-supported restorations without the need to vertically augment atrophic edentulous ridges. Finite elemental analysis has changed our understanding of occlusal load distributions on dental

implant surfaces, and it has been reported that implant diameter plays a more substantial role in force dissipation than implant length. Recent literature has shown that short dental implants are an equally efficacious treatment compared with standard length implants, as long as key protocols in implant design and surgical and prosthetic management are followed. Initial stability can be improved by employing short dental implants with smaller thread pitch and greater thread depth into underprepared osteotomies. Crestal bone loss can be mitigated by the use of platform switching, wider diameter implants, and implant neck retentive features. It has been established that high crown to implant (C/I) ratios are not related to increased biologic complications or implant failure. Splinting adjacent short implants is still a topic of debate with no clear consensus within the literature. The key advantage of short dental implants is that they can be utilized to restore the posterior jaws with less morbidity associated with

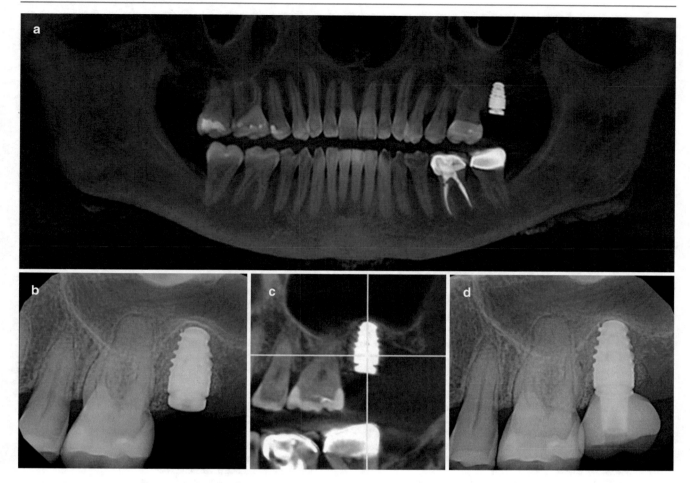

Fig. 15.11 (**a-c**) A 5.0 × 8.0 mm Nobel Active® implant placed at the left maxillary second molar site. This implant was placed immediately utilizing osseodensification burs. (**d**) This radiograph shows the implant after 2 years of function carrying a single Emax crown with a titanium base. (Source: Dr. Ian Mackenzie Farnham, Jacksonville, FL. Reproduced with permission from Dr. Farnham)

grafting procedures, in less time and with less overall treatment costs. The dental implant surgeons wishing to utilize short dental implants need to employ the considerations outlined in this chapter.

References

1. Pagni G, Pellegrini G, Giannobile WV, Rasperini G. Postextraction alveolar ridge preservation: Biological basis and treatments. Int J Dent. 2012;2012:151030.
2. Ashman A. Postextraction ridge preservation using a synthetic alloplast. Implant Dent. 2000;9(2):168–76.
3. das Neves FD, Fones D, Bernardes SR, do Prado CJ, Neto AJ. Short implants—an analysis of longitudinal studies. J Prosthet Dent. 2006;96(4):288.
4. Renouard F, Nisand D. Impact of implant length and diameter on survival rates. Clin Oral Implants Res. 2006;17(SUPPL. 2):35–51.
5. Deporter D. Short implants. In: Minimally invasive dental implant surgery. 1st ed. Hoboken: Wiley Blackwell; 2016. p. 193–207.
6. Lum LB. Biomechanical rationale for the use of short implants. J Oral Implantol. 1991;17(2):126–31.
7. Pierrisnard L, Renouard F, Renault P, Barquins M. Influence of implant length and Bicortical Anchorage on implant stress distribution. Clin Implant Dent Relat Res. 2003;5(4):254–62.
8. Renouard F, Nisand D. Short implants in the severely resorbed maxilla: a 2-year retrospective clinical study. Clin Implant Dent Relat Res. 2005;7(s1):s104–10.
9. Anitua E, Tapia R, Luzuriaga F, Orive G. Influence of implant length, diameter, and geometry on stress distribution: a finite element analysis. Int J Periodontics Restorative Dent. 2010;30(1):89–95.
10. Srinivasan M, Vazquez L, Rieder P, Moraguez O, Bernard JP, Belser UC. Survival rates of short (6 mm) micro-rough surface implants: a review of literature and meta-analysis. Clin Oral Implants Res. 2014;25(5):539–45.
11. Annibali S, Cristalli MP, Dell'Aquila D, Bignozzi I, La Monaca G, Pilloni A. Short dental implants: a systematic review. J Dent Res. 2012;91(1):25–32.
12. Menchero-Cantalejo E, Barona-Dorado C, Cantero-Álvarez M, Fernández-Cáliz F, Martínez-González JM. Meta-analysis on the survival of short implants. Med Oral Patol Oral Cir Bucal. 2011;16(4):e546–51.
13. Ravidà A, Barootchi S, Askar H, Suárez-López del Amo F, Tavelli L, Wang HL. Long-term effectiveness of extra-short (≤ 6 mm) dental implants: A systematic review. Int J Oral Maxillofac Implant. 2019;34(1):68–84a.

14. Kotsovilis S, Fourmousis I, Karoussis IK, Bamia C. A systematic review and Meta-analysis on the effect of implant length on the survival of rough-surface dental implants. J Periodontol. 2009;80(11):1700–18.

15. Nisand D, Renouard F. Short implant in limited bone volume. Periodontol 2000. 2014;66(1):72–96.

16. Wennerberg A, Albrektsson T. Effects of titanium surface topography on bone integration: a systematic review. Clin Oral Implants Res. 2009;20(SUPPL. 4):172–84.

17. Pommer B, Frantal S, Willer J, Posch M, Watzek G, Tepper G. Impact of dental implant length on early failure rates: a meta-analysis of observational studies. J Clin Periodontol. 2011;38(9):856–63.

18. Fugazzotto PA, Beagle JR, Ganeles J, Jaffin R, Vlassis J, Kumar A. Success and failure rates of 9 mm or shorter implants in the replacement of missing maxillary molars when restored with individual crowns: preliminary results 0 to 84 months in function. . A Retrospective Study. J Periodontol. 2004;75(2):327–32.

19. Lai HC, Si MS, Zhuang LF, Shen H, Liu YL, Wismeijer D. Long-term outcomes of short dental implants supporting single crowns in posterior region: a clinical retrospective study of 5-10 years. Clin Oral Implants Res. 2013;24(2):230–7.

20. Malchiodi L, Ghensi P, Cucchi A, Pieroni S, Bertossi D. Peri-implant conditions around sintered porous-surfaced (SPS) implants. A 36-month prospective cohort study. Clin Oral Implants Res. 2015;26(2):212–9.

21. Deporter D, Ogiso B, Sohn D-S, Ruljancich K, Pharoah M. Ultrashort sintered porous-surfaced dental implants used to replace posterior teeth. J Periodontol. 2008;79(7):1280–6.

22. Deporter D, Pharoah M, Yeh S, Todescan R, Atenafu EG. Performance of titanium alloy sintered porous-surfaced (SPS) implants supporting mandibular overdentures during a 20-year prospective study. Clin Oral Implants Res. 2014;25(2):189–95.

23. Deporter D, Watson P, Pharoah M, Todescan R, Tomlinson G. Ten-year results of a prospective study using porous-surfaced dental implants and a mandibular overdenture. Clin Implant Dent Relat Res. 2002;4(4):183–9.

24. Misch CE. Scientific rationale for dental implant design. In: Contemporary implant dentistry. 3rd ed. St. Louis: Elsevier; 2008. p. 200–29.

25. Abuhussein H, Pagni G, Rebaudi A, Wang HL. The effect of thread pattern upon implant osseointegration: review. Clin Oral Implants Res. 2010;21(2):129–36.

26. Manikyamba YJ, Rao B, Raju RA, Sajjan MCS, Nair K. C. Implant thread designs : an overview. Trends Prosthodont Dent Implantol. 2017;8(1 & 2):11–9.

27. Ryu HS, Namgung C, Lee JH, Lim YJ. The influence of thread geometry on implant osseointegration under immediate loading: a literature review. J Adv Prosthodont. 2014;6(6):547–54.

28. Misch CE, Steigenga J, Barboza E, Misch-Dietsh F, Cianciola LJ, Kazor C. Short dental implants in posterior partial Edentulism: a Multicenter retrospective 6-year case series study. J Periodontol. 2006;77(8):1340–7.

29. Iplikçioğlu H, Akça K. Comparative evaluation of the effect of diameter, length and number of implants supporting three-unit fixed partial prostheses on stress distribution in the bone. J Dent. 2002;30(1):41–6.

30. Baggi L, Cappelloni I, Di Girolamo M, Maceri F, Vairo G. The influence of implant diameter and length on stress distribution of osseointegrated implants related to crestal bone geometry: a three-dimensional finite element analysis. J Prosthet Dent. 2008;100(6):422–31.

31. Esposito M, Pellegrino G, Pistilli R, Felice P. Rehabilitation of posterior atrophic edentulous jaws: prostheses supported by 5 mm short implants or by longer implants in augmented bone? One-year results from a pilot randomised clinical trial. Eur J Oral Implantol. 2011;4(1):21–30.

32. Rossi F, Ricci E, Marchetti C, Lang NP, Botticelli D. Early loading of single crowns supported by 6-mm-long implants with a moderately rough surface: a prospective 2-year follow-up cohort study. Clin Oral Implants Res. 2010;21(9):937–43.

33. Urdaneta RA, Daher S, Leary J, Emanuel KM, Chuang S-K. The survival of ultrashort locking-taper implants. Int J Oral Maxillofac Implants. 2014;27(3):644–54.

34. Gargiulo AW, Wntz FMOB. Dimensions and relations of the Dentogingival junction in humans. J Periodontol. 1960;32:261–7.

35. Shin Y, Han C, Heo S. Radiographic evaluation of marginal bone levels around dental implants with different designs after 1 year. Int J Oral Maxillofac Implant. 2006;21(1):789–94.

36. Nevins M, Shapoff CA, Hezaimi K, Kim DM. Engineering biologic width and tissue levels with implant and abutment surface preparation. In: Minimally invasive dental implant surgery. 1st ed; 2017. p. 107–18.

37. Geurs NC, Vassilopoulos PJ, Reddy MS. Histologic evidence of connective tissue integration on laser microgrooved abutments in humans. Clin Adv Periodontics. 2011;1(1):29–33.

38. Nevins M, Kim DM, Jun S-H, Guze K, Schupbach P, Nevins ML. Histologic evidence of a connective tissue attachment to laser microgrooved abutments: a canine study. Int J Periodontics Restorative Dent. 2010;30(3):245–55.

39. Pecora GE, Ceccarelli R, Bonelli M, Alexander H, Ricci JL. Clinical evaluation of laser microtexturing for soft tissue and bone attachment to dental implants. Implant Dent. 2009;18(1):57–66.

40. Alexander H, Ricci JL, Hrico GJ. Mechanical basis for bone retention around dental implants. J Biomed Mater Res – Part B Appl Biomater. 2009;88(2):306–11.

41. Hansson S. The implant neck: smooth or provided with retention elements. Clin Oral Implants Res. 1999;10:394–405.

42. Zuffetti F, Testarelli L, Bertani P, Vassilopoulos S, Testori T, Guarnieri R. A retrospective Multicenter study on short implants with a laser-microgrooved collar (≤7.5 mm) in posterior edentulous areas: radiographic and clinical results up to 3 to 5 years. J Oral Maxillofac Surg. 2020;78(2):217–27.

43. Lazzara RJ, Porter SS. Platform switching: a new concept in implant dentistry for controlling postrestorative crestal bone levels. Int J Periodontics Restorative Dent. 2006;26(1):9–17.

44. Telleman G, Meijer HJA, Vissink A, Raghoebar GM. Short implants with a nanometer-sized CaP surface provided with either a platform-switched or platform-matched abutment connection in the posterior region: a randomized clinical trial. Clin Oral Implants Res. 2013;24(12):1316–24.

45. Telleman G, Raghoebar GM, Vissink A, Meijer HJA. Impact of platform switching on Peri-implant bone Remodeling around short implants in the posterior region, 1-year results from a Split-mouth clinical trial. Clin Implant Dent Relat Res. 2014;16(1):70–80.

46. Aslam AAB. Platform-switching to preserve Peri-implant bone : a meta analysis. J Coll Physicians Surg Pakistan. 2016;26(4):315–9.

47. Stanford CM, Brand RA. Toward an understanding of implant occlusion and strain adaptive bone modeling and remodeling. J Prosthet Dent. 1999;81(5):553–61.

48. Felice P, Pellegrino G, Checchi L, Pistilli R, Esposito M. Vertical augmentation with interpositional blocks of an organic bovine bone vs. 7-mm-long implants in posterior mandibles: 1-year results of a randomized clinical trial. Clin Oral Implants Res. 2010;21(12):1394–403.

49. Cannizzaro G, Leone M, Torchio C, Viola PEM. Immediate versus early loading of 7-mm-long flapless-placed single implants. Eur J Oral Implantol. 2008;1(4):227–92.

50. Rokni S, Todescan R, Watson P, Pharoah M, Adegbembo AO, Deporter D. An assessment of crown-to-root ratios with short sintered porous-surfaced implants supporting prostheses in partially edentulous patients. Int J Oral Maxillofac Implants. 2005;20(1):69–76.

51. Schincaglia G. Pietro, Thoma DS, Haas R, Tutak M, Garcia A, Taylor TD, et al. randomized controlled multicenter study comparing short dental implants (6 mm) versus longer dental implants (11-15 mm) in combination with sinus floor elevation procedures. Part 2: clinical and radiographic outcomes at 1 year of loading. J Clin Periodontol. 2015;42(11):1042–51.

52. Anitua E, Piñas L, Orive G. Retrospective study of short and extra-short implants placed in posterior regions: influence of crown-to-implant ratio on marginal bone loss. Clin Implant Dent Relat Res. 2015;17(1):102–10.

53. Tawil G, Aboujaoude N, Younan R. Influence of prosthetic parameters on the survival and complication rates of short implants. Int J Oral Maxillofac Implants. 2006;21(2):275–82.

54. Hingsammer L, Watzek G, Pommer B. The influence of crown-to-implant ratio on marginal bone levels around splinted short dental implants: a radiological and clinical short term analysis. Clin Implant Dent Relat Res. 2017;19(6):1090–8.

55. Rangert BR, Sullivan RM, Jemt TM. Load factor control for implants in the posterior partially edentulous segment. Int J Oral Maxillofac Implants. 1997;12:360–70.

56. Yilmaz B, Seidt JD, McGlumphy EA, Clelland NL. Comparison of strains for splinted and nonsplinted screw-retained prostheses on short implants. Int J Oral Maxillofac Implants. 2011;26(6):1176–82.

57. Vazouras K, de Souza AB, Gholami H, Papaspyridakos P, Pagni S, Weber HP. Effect of time in function on the predictability of short dental implants (≤6 mm): a meta-analysis. J Oral Rehabil. 2020;47(3):403–15.

58. Kim Y, Oh TJ, Misch CE, Wang HL. Occlusal considerations in implant therapy: clinical guidelines with biomechanical rationale. Clin Oral Implants Res. 2005;16(1):26–35.

59. Guichet D, Yoshinobu DCA. Effect of splinting and interproximal contact tightness on load transfer by implant restorations. Implant Dent. 1998;7(4):377.

60. Korabi R, Shemtov-Yona K, Rittel D. On stress/strain shielding and the material stiffness paradigm for dental implants. Clin Implant Dent Relat Res. 2017;19(5):935–43.

61. Villarinho EA, Triches DF, Alonso FR, Mezzomo LAM, Teixeira ER, Shinkai RSA. Risk factors for single crowns supported by short (6-mm) implants in the posterior region: a prospective clinical and radiographic study. Clin Implant Dent Relat Res. 2017;19(4):671–80.

62. Degidi M, Daprile G, Piattelli A. Influence of underpreparation on primary stability of implants inserted in poor quality bone sites: an in vitro study. J Oral Maxillofac Surg. 2015;73(6):1084–8.

63. Vidyasagar L, Salms G, Apse P, Teibe U. The Influence of Site Preparation (Countersinking) on Initial Dental Implant Stability. An in vitro Study Using Resonance Frequency Analysis. Stomatol Balt Dent Maxillofac J. 2004;6:14–6.

64. Anitua E, Orive G, Aguirre JJ, Andía I. Five-year clinical evaluation of short dental implants placed in posterior areas: a retrospective study. J Periodontol. 2008;79(1):42–8.

65. Padhye NM, Padhye AM, Bhatavadekar NB. Osseodensification — a systematic review and qualitative analysis of published literature. J Oral Biol Craniofacial Res. 2020;10(1):375–80.

66. Nizam N, Gürlek Ö, Kaval M. Extra-short implants with osteotome sinus floor elevation: a prospective clinical study. Int J Oral Maxillofac Implants. 2020;35(2):415–22.

67. Taschieri S, Karanxha L, Francetti L, Weinstein R, Giannì AB, Del Fabbro M. Minimally-invasive osteotome sinus floor elevation combined with short implants and platelet-rich plasma for edentulous atrophic posterior maxilla: a five-year follow-up prospective study. J Biol Regul Homeost Agents. 2018;32(4):1015–20.

68. Deporter D, Todescan R, Caudry S. Simplifying management of the posterior maxilla using short, porous-surfaced dental implants and simultaneous indirect sinus elevation. Int J Periodontics Restorative Dent. 2000;20(5):476–85.

69. Anitua E, Piñas L, Begoña L, Orive G. Long-term retrospective evaluation of short implants in the posterior areas: clinical results after 10-12 years. J Clin Periodontol. 2014;41(4):404–11.

Vertical Ridge Augmentation Technique

Reza Tabrizi and Mohammad Jafarian

The shape and volume of the alveolar process depend on tooth form, the direction of tooth eruption, and the presence or absence of teeth [1]. The alveolar process undergoes atrophy following tooth removal. The horizontal and vertical changes in dimensions of jaws occur in the tooth extracted sites [2]. It was reported that vertical change in the alveolar process was 11–22% at 6 months [1]. A rapid reduction in the alveolar process happens in the first 3–6 months, followed by a gradual decrease in dimension.

Sufficient alveolar bone volume is crucial to gain ideal functional and aesthetic outcomes following implant therapy [3]. In the mandible posterior, the atrophic ridge and other vital structures such as the inferior alveolar nerve prevent to place a dental implant with optimum length.

There are several techniques for restoration of the edentulous area with insufficient vertical height: guided bone regeneration (GBR), alveolar distraction osteogenesis, interpositional block grafts, onlay bone grafting, and the use of short implants [4]. Every technique has advantages and disadvantages, which are discussed in this chapter.

Radiographic Evaluation of the Alveolar Ridge

Radiological evaluation of the maxilla and mandible is a crucial stage of the presurgical dental implant treatment planning. In the initial diagnostic phase, radiographic evaluation combined with the clinical examination provides valuable information about the recipient sites' anatomical and architectural features. Panoramic radiographs, conventional periapical, and cone beam computed tomography (CBCT) are radiography modalities in dental implant surgeries. CBCTs provide precise information about the anatomy of the surgical sites. CBCTs can assess the width and height of the alveolar ridge. Three-dimensional anatomical topography of jaws can be evaluated in the CBCT modality [5] (Fig. 16.1). Moreover, CBCT can be used to assess voxel gray values and bone density through Hounsfield units [6]. Generally, CBCTs are taken with 2 mm interval slices. Edentulous cases may have a skeletal deformity (Fig. 16.2). The lateral cephalometric view helps assess any anterior-posterior discrepancy. In this situation, correction of the skeletal deformity should be managed in combination with bone augmentation.

Tent Pole Grafting (TPG) Technique

TPG technique is suggested for vertical augmentation when 2 to 5 mm bone gaining is considered. TPG is used for augmentation of the limited area (1 to 3 teeth). In this technique, titanium screws (1.5–2 mm) are placed in the alveolar ridge so that approximately 3 to 6 mm of screw threads are exposed. For the primary stability of screws, 3 to 4 mm should be embedded in the recipient's bone. Particulate bone substitutes are placed to cover the screws. Generally, polytetrafluoroethylene (PTFE) reinforced with titanium mesh membrane is applied to cover the augmented area. PTFE membrane has enough rigidity to maintain space for bone substitutes. The disadvantage of using the PTFE membrane is the risk of exposure [7]. Soft tissue dehiscence is the main drawback of vertical bone augmentation. Enough releasing of the soft tissue to passive closure of the augmented area is crucial for preventing exposure and dehiscence [8]. Sometimes, fixtures can be used as screws. In this technique, fixtures are placed in the recipient site with good primary stability. Three to five mm of fixtures are exposed and act like screws. The bone

R. Tabrizi (✉)
Department of Oral and Maxillofacial Surgery, Dental School, Shahid Beheshti University of Medical Sciences, Tehran, Iran
e-mail: rtabrizi@sbmu.ac.ir

M. Jafarian
Department of Oral and Maxillofacial Surgery, School of Dentistry, Shahid Beheshti University of Medical Sciences, Tehran, Iran
e-mail: Mjafarian@sbmu.ac.ir

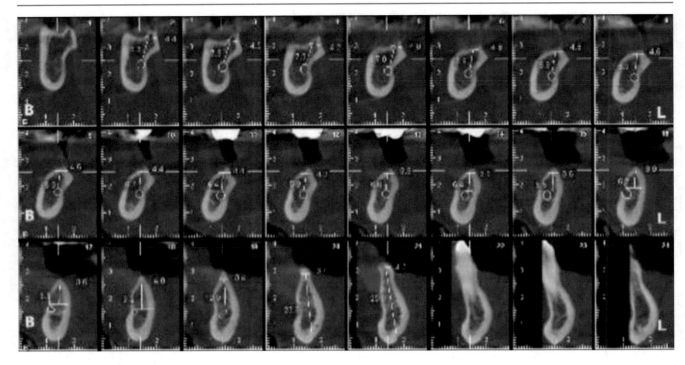

Fig. 16.1 Insufficient bone height with a concavity in the posterior of the mandible

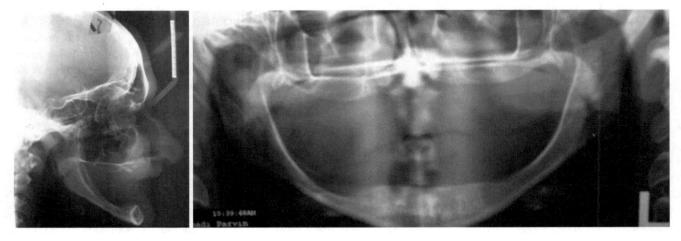

Fig. 16.2 Severe maxillomandibular resorption following teeth loss results in a class III deformity

substitutes are placed around the fixtures, and a membrane covers the augmented site (Fig. 16.3a–d).

Onlay Bone Grafting

The use of onlay bone grafting is a well-known approach to the vertical restoration of the alveolar ridge. Generally, autogenous corticocancellous bone is used. Autogenous grafts are a gold standard for ridge augmentation. However, autogenous grafting needs a second surgery for harvesting bone and has the potential of donor site complications.

Allograft block can be used for vertical augmentation of the deficient ridges [9]. It was showed that freeze-dried cancellous allogeneic bone blocks had a similar resorption rate as autogenous bone blocks [10].

Various donor sites are available intraorally and extraorally for vertical augmentation. In a limited area (1 to 3 cm), the lateral ramus is a suitable donor site. Piezosurgery increases surgery accuracy and reduces the possible complication (bad fracture and neurosensory disturbance) (Fig. 16.4a–d).

The use of extraoral donor sites is recommended for augmentation of an extensive area. For example, iliac bone grafting is a good idea for onlay grafting of the total mandible.

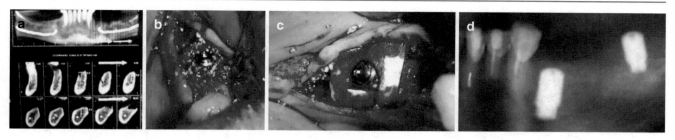

Fig. 16.3 (**a**) A vertically deficient area on the left side of the mandible posterior. (**b**) The xenograft bone substitute was placed around the fixture to cover 4 mm of it. (**c**) A membrane was used to cover the grafted area. (**d**) The post-implantation radiographic view after 6 months

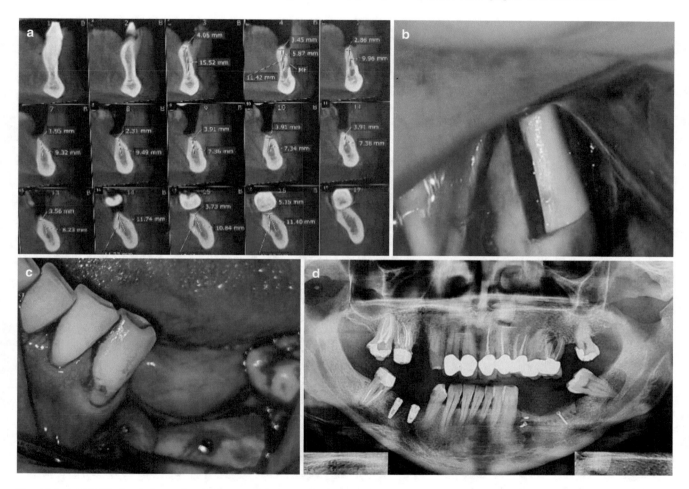

Fig. 16.4 (**a**) CBCT view indicates insufficient vertical bone on the left side of the mandible posterior. (**b**) The lateral ramus bone was harvested. (**c**) Only bone was placed and fixed with mini-screws. (**d**) The post-augmentation view in OPG

Calvaria is another option for the donor site (Fig. 16.5a–c). It is believed that calvaria graft is associated with a lower resorption rate than other extraoral donor sites [11].

It was shown that a significant bone loss happened during the first 12 months, after which the resorption declined, and grafted bone eventually stabilized. The total vertical bone loss was estimated at approximately 27.51% in 10 years after onlay grafting [12]. The average bone gain was reported up to 4 mm with autogenous bone grafting.

The survival rate of allogenic block bone graft was 79.3%, with a mean of 37 months follow-up time [9]. A significant challenge to the augmentation of large vertical bone defects in the soft tissue dehiscence is the excessive tension during flap closure. Proper flap design with sufficient releasing decreases the risk of bone exposure after the vertical augmentation. Periosteal transposition flap has been suggested for coverage of the augmented area [13]. Flap elevation through making a tunnel reduces dehiscence risk [14].

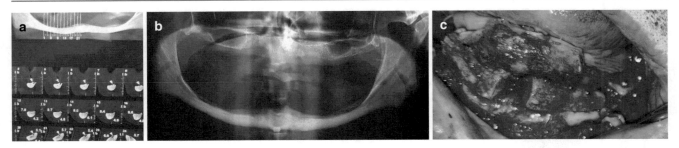

Fig. 16.5 (**a**) An atrophic mandible with the risk of fracture. (**b**) OPG view. (**c**) The bone graft was harvested from the iliac crest and placed as an onlay bone graft

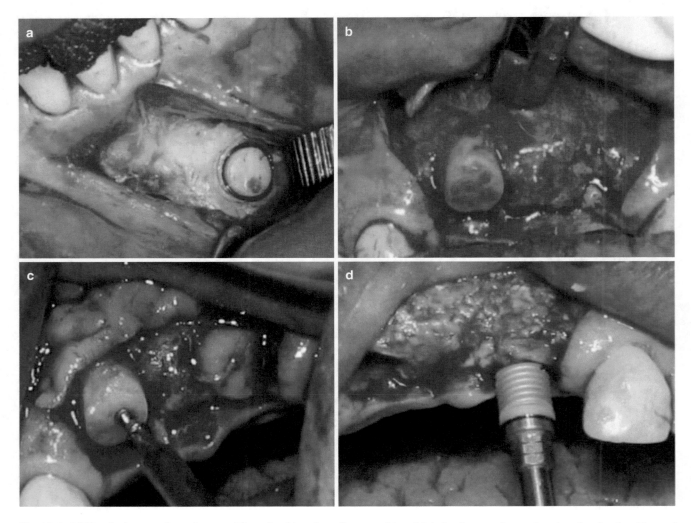

Fig. 16.6 (**a**) The ringbone graft was harvested from the chin using a 7 mm trephine. (**b**) A ring bone graft was placed on the alveolar ridge and fixed with a mini-screw. (**c**) Fixation ring bone graft using a screw. (**d**) Four months later, a fixture was placed

Surgeons should smooth the sharp edges of bone blocks to decrease bone exposure.

Bone ring graft is a technique for vertical augmentation in a limited area of fresh sockets. Generally, the chin is used as a donor site. A circular osteotomy is outlined and drilled. The bone discs outline is placed 3–4 mm away from the mandibular anterior teeth' apices. The trephine is slightly torqued to loosen the bone discs without fracture [15]. A bone ring is placed in a shallow tooth socket and fixed with a screw. Implants can be placed 4 months after grafting (Fig. 16.6).

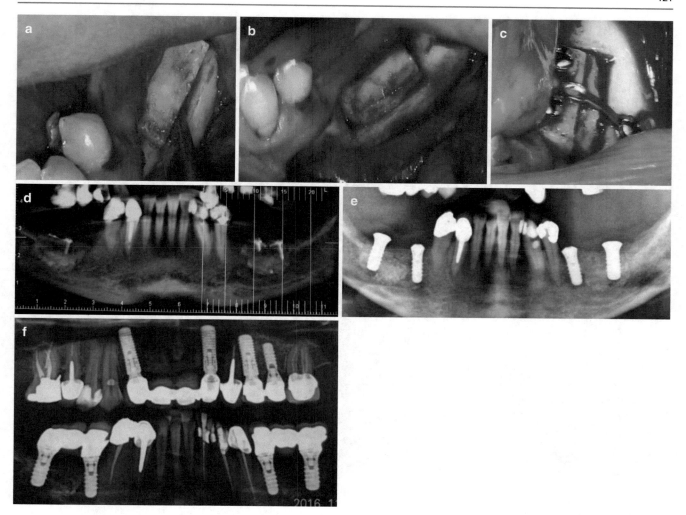

Fig. 16.7 (**a**) The sandwich technique was performed in the posterior of the mandible. (**b**) An autogenous bone graft (from the lateral ramus) was placed between the two segments. (**c**) The bone segments were fixed with a mini-plate. (**d**) Radiographic view after augmentation. (**e**) Two implants were placed after 4 months of radiographic view after loading. (**f**) Radiographic view 6 months after loading

Interposition Sandwich Technique

Onlay bone grafting is associated with unpredictable resorption. Vascularity is the main factor in determining the stability of the grafted bone. The interposition sandwich techniques (IST) basis relates the theory of rapid and complete healing of bone substitutes with graft incorporation and a lower percentage of resorption when biomaterials are placed between two segments of pedicled bone with internal cancellous [16]. The interposition sandwich osteotomy provides adequate blood supply to maintain new bone growth. The correction of the vertical dimension can be achieved through the sandwich technique. The IST in the posterior mandible needs a great surgical precision to prevent injury to the inferior alveolar nerve. Various bone materials such as xenograft, allograft, and cancellous bone can be used in this technique. In IST, vertical bone gaining was reported as 7.5 mm [17]. It seems the bone gaining and stability of augmented bone in IST is associated with a better clinical outcome than simple onlay grafting (Fig. 16.7a–f).

Alveolar Distraction Osteogenesis

Alveolar distraction osteogenesis (ADO) is a well-known and reliable technique for augmentation of the alveolar ridge in the vertical or horizontal directions. ADO has several advantages: no need for a donor site, reducing the risk of dehiscence because of simultaneous soft tissue formation, a low risk of postsurgical infection, and reduced treatment time. ADO is a sensitive technique and is associated with complications, for example, the inferior alveolar nerve injury, basal bone or transport segment fracture, breakage of ADO devices, incorrect distraction vector, and occlusal

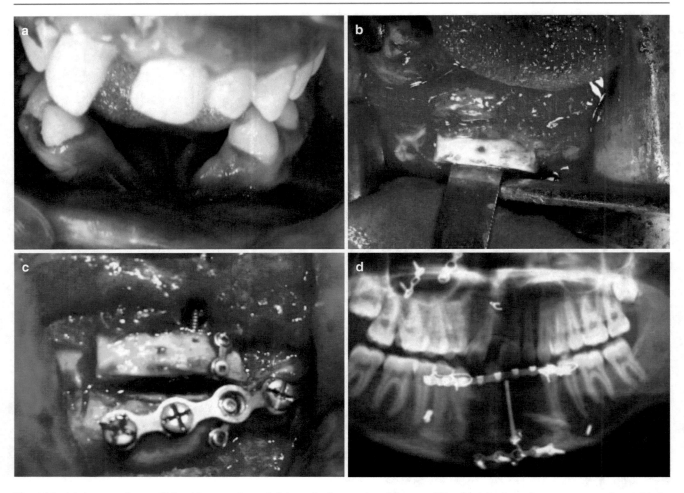

Fig. 16.8 (**a**) A traumatic mandible with severe bone deficiency in the anterior of the mandible. (**b**) A horizontal osteotomy was done with the preservation of the lingual soft tissue. (**c**) An ADO device was placed to distract the osteotomy site vertically. (**d**) The distracted bone after 3 months

interference [18]. In mild alveolar bone height deficiency, up to 7 mm, onlay bone grafting or IST can provide an adequate bone height in a single-stage operation, although in moderate to severe vertical deficiency (more than 7 mm), ADO is a better treatment option [19]. ADO aims to maintain the vascularity of the transported bone segment. Subsequently, the transported bone has a low resorption rate, and new bone forms between the two segments. The other drawbacks of ADO include patient cooperation and the possibility of a second surgery to remove the distraction device (Fig. 16.8a–d).

Alternative Techniques for the Vertical Ridge Augmentation

Three alternative techniques have been introduced for the vertical ridge augmentation: short implants, nerve lateralization, and buccally or lingually tilted implants. Generally, the mentioned techniques are used to restore the posterior of the mandible.

Short implants are a reliable treatment option. Dias et al., in a systematic review, compared short implants and standard-length implants with vertical bone augmentation. They reported that short implants' survival rate was more than traditional-length implants after 1 year (97% versus 92.6%, respectively). The probability of the proportion of patients with complications in short implants was lower than standard-length implants with bone augmentation [20].

Dental implant survivals in the nerve lateralization and transposition are associated with a higher survival rate than vertical bone augmentation in 5 years. However, the complication rate of nerve lateralization or transposition is more than vertical bone augmentation [21]. The main complications in nerve lateralization are a neurosensory disturbance and the risk of fracture in atrophic mandibles [22].

Buccally or lingually tilted implants are a sensitive technique used to place dental implants in the atrophic mandible [23]. This technique depends on the bone thickness between the inferior alveolar canal and the buccal bone plate. In CBCT, the inferior alveolar canal's position should be pre-

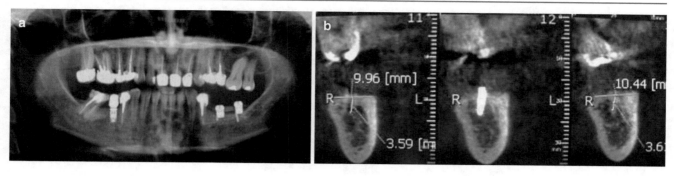

Fig. 16.9 (**a**) An allograft was used to augment the mandible posterior and fixed with two micro-screws—the patient complaint paresthesia following augmentation. (**b**) CBCT showed that a micro-screw involved the inferior alveolar canal

cisely evaluated for consideration of the tilted implants. Tilted implants' disadvantages are nerve injury, inappropriate implant position, and high dependence on operator experience.

The Prognosis and Outcomes of Various Vertical Augmentation Techniques

In 4 mm vertical bone augmentation, the TPG or guided bone regeneration (GBR) using titanium-reinforced membrane is recommended. If more than 4 mm vertical bone gain is desired, ADO, onlay bone grafting, and IST are suggested. The least complication rate was reported for the GBR technique [24]. ADO was associated with the highest bone gain than other vertical bone augmentation techniques (19). The complication rate between ADO and onlay bone grafting is not different [25].

The main complications in vertical bone augmentation techniques are soft tissue dehiscence, bone resorption (common in onlay bone grafting), neurosensory disturbance (common in IST), and infection (Fig. 16.9).

References

1. Tan WL, Wong TL, Wong MC, Lang NP. A systematic review of post-extractional alveolar hard and soft tissue dimensional changes in humans. J Coir. 2012;23:1–21.
2. Van der Weijden F, Dell'Acqua F. Alveolar bone dimensional changes of post-extraction sockets in humans: a systematic review. Slot DEJJocp. 2009;36(12):1048–58.
3. Schropp L, Wenzel A, Kostopoulos L, Karring TJIJoP, Dentistry R. Bone healing and soft tissue contour changes following single-tooth extraction: a clinical and radiographic 12-month prospective study. 2003;23(4).
4. Camps-Font O, Burgueño-Barris G, Figueiredo R, Jung RE, Gay-Escoda C, Valmaseda-Castellón E. Interventions for dental implant placement in atrophic edentulous mandibles: vertical bone augmentation and alternative treatments. A meta-analysis of randomized clinical trials. JJop. 2016;87(12):1444–57.
5. Omami G, Al YF. Should cone beam computed tomography be routinely obtained in implant planning? Dent Clin N Am. 2019;63(3):363–79.
6. Parsa A, Ibrahim N, Hassan B, Motroni A, der Stelt PV, Wismeijer D, et al. Reliability of voxel gray values in cone beam computed tomography for preoperative implant planning assessment. JIJoO. 2012;27(6):1438.
7. Le B, Rohrer MD, Prassad HS. Screw "tent-pole" grafting technique for reconstruction of large vertical alveolar ridge defects using human mineralized allograft for implant site preparation. JJoo Surg M. 2010;68(2):428–35.
8. Deeb GR, Tran D, Carrico CK, Block E, Laskin DM, Deeb JGJJoO, et al. How effective is the tent screw pole technique compared to other forms of horizontal ridge augmentation? 2017;75(10):2093–8.
9. Nissan J, Ghelfan O, Mardinger O, Calderon S, Chaushu G. Efficacy of cancellous block allograft augmentation prior to implant placement in the posterior atrophic mandible. JCID ResR. 2011;13(4):279–85.
10. Kloss FR, Offermanns V, Kloss-Brandstätter A. Comparison of allogeneic and autogenous bone grafts for augmentation of alveolar ridge defects—A 12-month retrospective radiographic evaluation. JCoir. 2018;29(11):1163–75.
11. Mertens C, Decker C, Seeberger R, Hoffmann J, Sander A, Freier K. Early bone resorption after vertical bone augmentation–a comparison of calvarial and iliac grafts. JCoir. 2013;24(7):820–5.
12. Schmitt C, Karasholi T, Lutz R, Wiltfang J, Neukam FW, Schlegel KA. Long-term changes in graft height after maxillary sinus augmentation, onlay bone grafting, and combination of both techniques: a long-term retrospective cohort study. JCoir. 2014;25(2):e38–46.
13. Kermani H, Tabrizi R. Periosteal transposition flap for graft coverage and ridge preservation in the aesthetic zone. JJoCS. 2015;26(6):1967–8.
14. Restoy-Lozano A, Dominguez-Mompell J, Infante-Cossio P, Lara-Chao J, Espin-Galvez F, Lopez-Pizarro V, et al. Reconstruction of mandibular vertical defects for dental implants with autogenous bone block grafts using a tunnel approach: clinical study of 50 cases. JIJoO. 2015;44(11):1416–22.
15. Omara M, Abdelwahed N, Ahmed M, Hindy M. Simultaneous implant placement with ridge augmentation using an autogenous bone ring transplant. Int J Oral Maxillofac Surg. 2016;45(4):535–44.
16. Laino L, Iezzi G, Piattelli A, Lo Muzio L, Cicciù M. Vertical ridge augmentation of the atrophic posterior mandible with sandwich technique: bone block from the chin area versus corticocancellous bone block allograft—clinical and histological prospective randomized controlled study. JBri. 2014;2014.
17. Rachmiel A, Emodi O, Rachmiel D, Israel Y, Shilo D. Sandwich osteotomy for the reconstruction of deficient alveolar bone. JIjoo Surg M. 2018;47(10):1350–7.

18. Yun KI, Choi H, Wright RF, Ahn HS, Chang BM, Kim HJ. Efficacy of alveolar vertical distraction osteogenesis and autogenous bone grafting for dental implants: systematic review and meta-analysis. Int J Oral Maxillofac Implants. 2016;31(1):26–36.

19. Rachmiel A, Shilo D, Aizenbud D, Emodi O. Vertical alveolar distraction osteogenesis of the atrophic posterior mandible before dental implant insertion. JJoO Surg M. 2017;75(6):1164–75.

20. Dias FN, Pecorari V, Martins C, Del Fabbro M, Casati M. Short implants versus bone augmentation in combination with standard-length implants in posterior atrophic partially edentulous mandibles: systematic review and meta-analysis with the Bayesian approach. JIjoo Surg M. 2019;48(1):90–6.

21. Khojasteh A, Hassani A, Motamedian SR, Saadat S, Alikhasi M. Cortical bone augmentation versus nerve lateralization for treatment of atrophic posterior mandible: a retrospective study and review of literature. Clin Implant Dent Relat Res. 2016;18(2):342–59.

22. Palacio García-Ochoa A, Pérez-González F, Negrillo Moreno A, Sánchez-Labrador L, Cortés-Bretón Brinkmann J, Martínez-González JM, et al. Complications associated with inferior alveolar nerve reposition technique for simultaneous implant-based rehabilitation of atrophic mandibles. A systematic literature review. J Stomatol Oral Maxillofac Surg. 2020;121(4):390–6.

23. Özkan BT, Eskitascioglu G, Cigerim L, Kaplan VJB. Equipment B. Insertion of Buccally tilted and placed implants in edentulous atrophic posterior mandibular sites. 2012;26(4):3163–6.

24. Elnayef B, Monje A, Gargallo-Albiol J, Galindo-Moreno P, Wang H-L, Hernandez-Alfaro F, et al. Vertical ridge augmentation in the atrophic mandible: a systematic review and meta-analysis. JIJoO. 2017;32(2).

25. Hameed MH, Gul M, Ghafoor R, Khan FR. Vertical ridge gain with various bone augmentation techniques: a systematic review and meta-analysis. JJoP. 2019;28(4):421–7.

Mandibular Bone Block Graft Techniques in Alveolar Ridge Preservation

17

Andrew C. Jenzer ⓘD

Mandibular block grafts represent a tried and true method of block graft harvesting. The benefit of using an autogenous source from the mandible is multifold. First, by choosing an intra-oral source, the surgeon mitigates the need for a secondary, often extra-oral, site harvest, for example, the iliac crest. This reduces the surgery's morbidity and obviates the need for a second surgical site, which can bring along its own host of complications and problems. Especially in an office-based practice, mandibular bone block harvest and application can be a much easier procedure to attempt than a more invasive harvest from another site, which often have financial and time implications. This can be accomplished easily under intravenous sedation or under local anesthesia [1].

One must balance this technique against the evolving nature of grafting. The evolution of biologic agents like rhBMP-2, the common use of bone marrow aspirate concentrate, and the widespread availability of cadaveric bone all support moving away from autogenous harvest, simply because one can reduce patient morbidity but not creating a harvest site [2]. These techniques in combination with titanium mesh, newer and continually improving membranes, and other techniques outside of block grafting are increasing the size of a practitioner's "tool box" and allowing a myriad of options to restore lost hard tissue volume [3]. Of course, cost remains a chief constraint with all of these products and that can be an excellent reason to use an autogenous mandibular block graft as it will generally incur less cost than these other aforementioned options [4].

The workhorse of this technique is the mandibular ramus graft. In a broad sense, this is simply removing a cortical square shape of bone from the lateral ramus, posterior to the dentition. Patients often have ample bone in this area, especially those with a pronounced oblique ridge. The other option for mandibular bone block harvest is to obtain your block graft from the anterior mandible in the area of the symphysis. There are drawbacks to this technique when compared to the ramus graft harvest. Overall, harvesting from the anterior mandible is associated with higher morbidity and a greater rate of permanent post-operative paresthesia and pain [5]. The bone itself in this area tends to be more unpredictable and can be softer or thicker than a ramus graft, which reliably gives a cortical block that is neither too thin nor thick and of consistent cortical bone quality. Limitations of harvesting block grafts from the mandible are chiefly the size; one to three teeth can be reconstructed with a single block graft, and so for cases requiring a large size of hard tissue augmentation, other sources should be considered [6].

Technique: Ramus Graft

1. Pre-operative planning: Pre-operatively, the surgeon should plan several things. First, one must determine which side to harvest. This decision is made based on the site of surgery and radiographic information about the inferior alveolar nerve's position, ideally selecting the site where the inferior alevolar nerve is as far away from the harvest site as possible. I strongly recommends three-dimensional imaging, typically a cone beam CT scan, for this purpose, speaking as someone who has dealt with the complications of not having it.

   Determining which side to harvest is somewhat arbitrary and surgeon's preference. Let us consider this in a clinical context to illustrate the thought process and considerations better; a patient is edentulous at site #19 with a ridge defect that will be restored with a ramus graft. Harvesting the graft from the same side will mean that the surgeon only needs to make one incision, anteriorly releasing the papilla to expose the defect and a third molar style incision posteriorly with a disto-lateral release. The site can be opened and the ramus graft easily harvested posterior to the site of surgery. An argument to harvest

A. C. Jenzer (✉)
Department of Oral and Maxillofacial Surgery, Eisenhower Army Medical Center, Augusta, GA, USA
e-mail: andrew.c.jenzer.mi@mail.mil

from the contra-lateral side would be whether the patient has paresthesia after the procedure. Was it due to the ramus graft harvest or possible damage from the fixation (typically screws) placed into the graft? With a contra-lateral harvest, a surgeon would know earlier if the screws were impinging on the nerve.

Next, the defect should be measured radiographically and clinically so that an anticipated size of harvest can be known. Then, this measurement can be placed at the harvest site and examined to ensure adequate bone. This step will confirm intra-operatively, but it helps to have an idea prior to surgery.

Finally, it is worthwhile to examine the course of the inferior alveolar nerve around the anticipated harvest area. If the nerve is medial and/or inferior, there is very little risk of damage. However, if the nerve runs lateral and/or superior, right underneath the cortex you plan to access, then the chance of damage to the nerve becomes much higher. My preference is to approach it on a case-by-case basis and make that determination considering the factors above.

2. Incision design: Prior to making an incision to access the graft area, one should open and expose the defect that is planned for grafting. Sometimes, mitigating circumstances that warrant stopping the procedure, for example, a severe infection or osteomyelitis, and given those would be rare and not apparent clinically; however, the worst thing you can do is harvest a graft and then discover that you are unable to use it. For the ramus graft harvest, a standard third molar style incision extended posteriorly is generally adequate to access this area. However, a smaller bilateral sagittal split osteotomy style incision works just

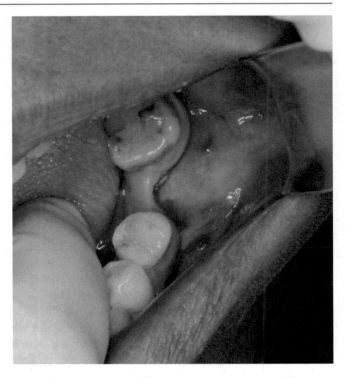

Fig. 17.2 Acquired partial edentulism site #19 demonstrating horizontal bone loss

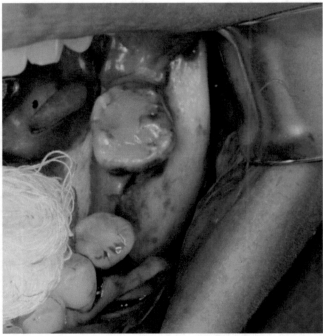

Fig. 17.3 A standard third molar style incision completed with disto-lateral release and anterior papilla release to expose the defect and site of ramus graft harvest

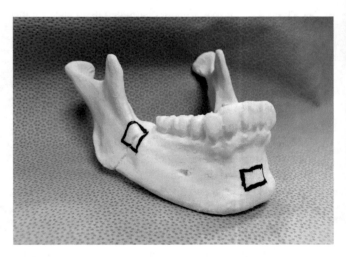

Fig. 17.1 Outlines of harvest sites for mandibular block grafts, demonstrating ramus and symphysis harvest sites

as well (Figs. 17.1, 17.2, and 17.3). This incision is variable and based on surgeon's preference. A key point – not only for this procedure but also for surgery – is one needs vision and access and must design the incision accordingly. This procedure becomes much more difficult if one is fighting the tissues.

3. Harvest: Once the exposure is achieved for both the graft and defect, the next step is measuring. There are several ways to do this. I typically uses an Iwanson or Boley gauge to measure the defect and then mark it on the graft site, either by lightly scoring the bone or by using an electrocautery device. An important principle to remember is your graft will always be smaller than you think! This is because as you use cutting devices to harvest it, you will naturally lose some of the edges. I always over-estimates the size of the graft by at least 2 mm. The graft will need to be trimmed slightly and shaped, but that is much better than not having enough graft. One should consider both anterior-posterior measurements, as well as vertical.

One can employ adjunctive tools to help this measurement. I have used sterile wrappers from sutures to trim to the defect and act as a template, and bone wax to mold into the defect to create a representation of the defect for reference. These techniques are helpful, especially during the learning phase with these techniques.

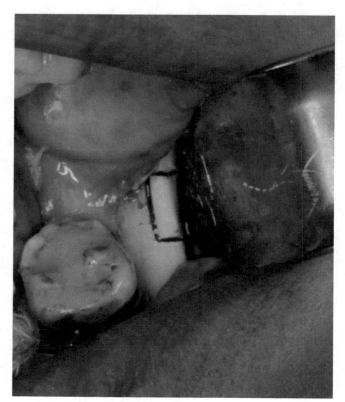

Fig. 17.4 After measuring, the four osteotomies are completed

Once the graft is sized and marked and ready for harvest, four cuts are made (Fig. 17.4). Essentially, one is cutting a square or rectangle into the bone and removing it. The vertical cuts and the superior cut on the ridge itself can be made with a 701 bur, a reciprocating saw, or a piezo-electric type handpiece. These cuts should be connected. An important principle is to go through the outer cortex, and no deeper simply. There is a feeling when the cutting tool drops through the hard outer cortex of the bone and into the softer medullary space. Cutting deeper serves no purpose and only increases the risk of damage to the inferior alveolar nerve. The last cut to consider is the inferior one. This is logistically the hardest to do because access is hard or impossible, given the angulation restrictions. Some piezo-electric units have special burrs with curves that can reach this easily. I generally uses an 8 round burr and simply scores this cut to weaken the bone and allow it to out-fracture.

The next step involves refining these osteotomies with osteotomes. Straight-sharp osteotomes are used to refine the vertical cuts. They must be placed in such a way as not to be too deep; again one can potentially sever the inferior alveoral nerve (IAN) if too deep, and generally placing them half in and half out of the osteotomies is a good way to accomplish this safely. Next, gently curved osteotomes are used along the superior cut in the ridge to out-fracture the graft. The graft should flex and weaken along with the inferior cut until popping off. This harvest's side effect is that the graft will naturally be thicker near the superior aspect and thinner near the inferior. This should be considered against the defect and can be used to bulk up an area that needs it.

With the block graft free, it is taken and placed into a cup or bowl with saline on the back table and the harvest site examined for the IAN and any problems or untoward fracture patterns. As a large area of medullary bone is being exposed, it tends to bleed. A second aspect of the harvest can now be accomplished, that is using a bony safe scraper or other augmenting harvesting devices. Multiple companies manufacture this product, but by scraping the graft edges to smooth them and the cortex around the harvest site, one obtains some autogenous particulate bone to use as an adjunct to the block graft. Next, the sharp edges of bone are smoothed. The wound is irrigated with copious amounts of saline, and this surgeon prefers to place a hemostatic agent at the site, either gel-foam or micro-fibular collagen (Avitene™). The wound is closed with 3-0 chromic gut.

4. Shaping and Application: The graft is then addressed by the surgical team. The first step should be trying it into the defect. It will then need to be shaped and adapted to fit into the defect. Foremost in the surgeon's mind should be the final treatment plan. Generally, where is the implant going to be placed once this heals? This should dictate the

placement of the graft. Common mistakes are trying to achieve too much bone that is unnecessary to the surgical plan. The bigger the graft, the more, the softer tissue envelope becomes stretched, and the higher the likelihood of exposure and failure. It is common knowledge that when thinking about restoring bony alveolar ridge defects, it is much easier to increase horizontal width than vertical. Tissues tend to be much more resistant to vertical stretch and grafting. Using a block graft to obtain a small amount of vertical augmentation can be done; however, one should consider not going more than 1–2 mm.

The shaping process is a series of fine adjustments to the block with a large round or pineapple-shaped bur. My preference for doing this is in a way that minimizes the chances of dropping the graft. With a second surgeon or assistant's help, the graft is grasped between two large hemostats over a large bowl, usually placed or held over the patient's chest, away from the surgical field, and small adjustments are made. One should proceed carefully as one can always remove more graft but never put it back. The small nature of this graft and the brittle nature of the bone make it to jump away from the rotary instrument used to trim it, so solid control of the graft is imperative. Trimming it within a large bowl gives coverage that if the graft falls, it is into saline and not a non-sterile environment.

Once the graft is shaped to the defect, the next step is securing it. I use screws to do that, but plates are another method, though not commonly used for this purpose. Using only one screw is not usually adequate fixation; this will allow the graft to rotate around a single point and micro-motion during heal with cause graft failure. Generally, two screws are used to secure a block graft. Conceptually, the two screws will be lagged into the graft and engage the alveolar bone. This means that the screws will not engage the block graft itself, just the screw heads, and the screw heads will pull the graft to the alveolar ridge and hold it there. Where should the screws go? One must consider the local factors, where tooth roots are, where nerves or other important anatomy is, and try to place the screws in an optimal position. The goal is to maximize the distance between the screws while not placing them too close to the edges. If the screw is near the very edge of the graft, that force can cause a fracture and the graft becomes lost or much more difficult to manipulate during application (Figs. 17.5 and 17.6).

To do this, I consider the local factors, then offsets the screws, so one is high on one side and low on the other. A 702 bur is excellent for making the holes in the graft, controlled as previously mentioned. One should test the screw into each hole, and each screw should passively fit into it. Next, the graft is placed into position, and an appropriate drill to match the screw is used to drill through

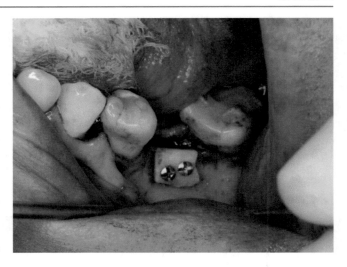

Fig. 17.5 Ramus graft secured using two screws to the site of the defect

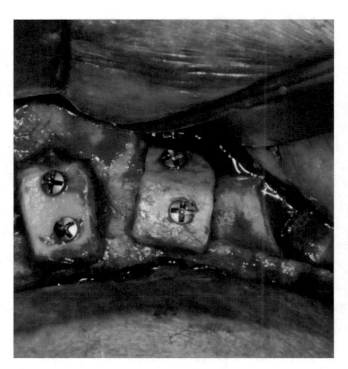

Fig. 17.6 A different case, an example of block graft secured into place using two screws with a slight off-set pattern

the screw hole and into the alveolar ridge under irrigation. In my experience, on average, these screw lengths are 7-9 mm. The goal should be enough screw depth into the ridge to be secure without perforating out the other side. Once drilled, a screw is placed and left slightly loose, and the other drilled and placed and then tightened down in a secure fashion. With the graft now secure in place, any sharp edges can be smoothed and if a safe scraper technique or if any allograft material is being used, material

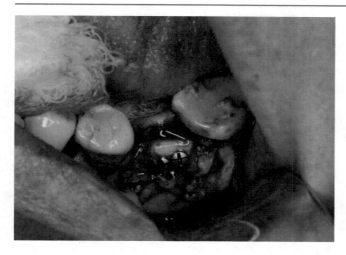

Fig. 17.7 Autogenous bone harvested with a scraper technique mixed with platelet-rich fibrin membranes and placed around the graft

can be packed around the edges, and a resorbable collagen membrane placed over everything to prevent soft tissue in growth into the graft (Fig. 17.7).

A minor variation exists where some surgeons, prior to securing the block graft, like to make a number of small burr holes in the bone of the alveolar ridge or the block graft itself. The concept behind this is the basis of accelerated regional healing; by opening these holes, one can increase blood flow to the area and presumably gain faster healing and better chances of success. Though there is certainly merit to this idea, I do not routinely do this due to a trade-off. By creating lots of small holes, you are potentially jeopardizing your screw placement. If a screw doesn't work or fails, you have much less area to place another screw. That being said, it is certainly reasonable and something to critically think about on each case and weigh the pros and cons.

5. Closure: If the graft becomes exposed, especially in the early phases of healing, there is a much lower chance of success. Thus, maximizing closure is a critical part of the operation. Tension-free flap closure is mandatory and can generally be achieved with periosteal scoring. I prefer longer-lasting sutures to ensure that the wound does not open early, namely 4-0 Vicryl, though any longer-lasting or non-resorbing sutures are acceptable.

6. Follow-up and planning: Maintaining vigilance on the graft allows early intervention if there is a problem. Follow-ups at the one-week and two-week mark should be a minimum, with a four-week follow-up recommended. Planning the time to go back in is equally as important as the initial operation. Too soon, and the graft can just fall off; too late, and the graft can be resorbed. Four to five months is the golden window for going back in to remove the screws and complete the next operation, typically implant placement. Back planning from that time to ensure coordination with

the restoring dentist, surgical implant guides, scheduling a surgical time, etc., should all be planned to hit the optimal window of four to five months [1].

Alternate Technique: Symphysis Block Harvest

Harvesting a block graft from the mandibular symphysis is another option for the harvest site. The site is easily exposed and manipulated through either a vestibular or sulcular incision with releasing incisions. Like the ramus graft, the harvest site is measured, ensuring that tooth roots are safe by staying at least 3 mm inferior to their apices, osteotomies created, and block removed. The site would then be treated just like a ramus graft with any ancillary harvesting completed, smoothing, irrigation, and materials placed as desired. This harvest does convey a higher risk of post-operative paresthesia which should be discussed with patient pre-operatively [7, 8].

Complications

The complications involved in this procedure are several, though often minor. Focusing on the harvest site first, paresthesia is a common post-operative finding given the proximity to the inferior alveolar nerve and should be informed pre-operatively and followed and managed appropriately (outside the scope of this chapter). Graft fracture or being dropped on the floor is a possibility, and I generally consent patients for both sides to mitigate that issue if it should happen and prevent another surgery and anesthetic.

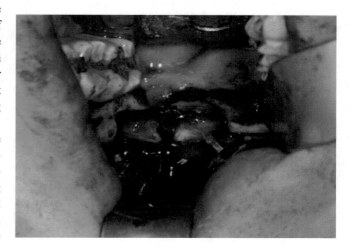

Fig. 17.8 Ramus graft harvest complicated by the transected inferior alveolar nerve. Note additional bone removed to the posterior to fully expose nerve endings

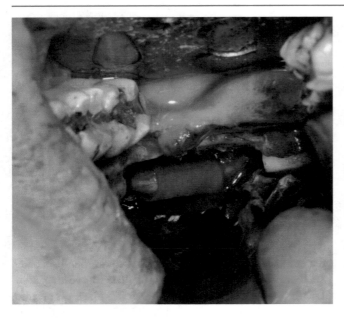

Fig. 17.9 Immediate primary repair accomplished and nerve wrapped with a conduit

One of the most feared complications is damage or transection of the inferior alveolar nerve. Immediate identification of the problem should occur when the graft is removed. If possible, it should be repaired primarily at that time (Figs. 17.8 and 17.9). When the nerve is fully transected, control should be obtained of the ends because the proximal end tends to pull back into the canal in a matter of minutes. Tacking one end with a 7-0 or 8-0 nylon suture will give control of each segment. Sometimes one or both ends cannot be fully identified, or there is not enough area for approximation. Another segment of bone can be removed, almost like another ramus graft, from either side to increase exposure. Suppose this does not occur during the surgery. In that case, consideration should be given to waking the patient up, discussing the complication with the patient and family, and

bringing the patient back to an operating room the next day to repair it. An in-depth discussion of nerve repair is beyond this chapter, but primary repair with a nerve conduit should be considered, and the patient should be informed and followed post-operatively.

Graft exposure is another complication that happens semi-frequently. If infected, it warrants removal. If just exposed, my preference is to get it along to the four- to five-month mark with frequent rinses, of chlorohexidine, give the patient a small syringe and have then irrigate it daily with saline, and have close clinical follow-up. Even if part of the graft is simply dead bone, hopefully, a portion of it does heal and create enough bone to place an implant into, even if some more grafting with a particulate allograft at the time of implant placement is needed. Each case needs to be considered individually based on the clinical conditions.

References

1. Rohrer MD, Prasad HS. Bone Graft Biology and Histology. In: Fonseca, Oral and maxillofacial surgery. 3rd ed. St. Louis: Elsevier; 2018. p. 437–45.
2. Greenwald A, Boden SD, et al. Bone-graft substitutes; facts, fictions, and applications. J Bone Joint Surg. 2001;83(2):98–103.
3. Aghaloo TL, Pi-anfruns J, Jones S, et al. Bone graft techniques and materials. In: Fonseca, editor. Oral and maxillofacial surgery. 3rd ed. St. Louis: Elsevier; 2018. p. 426–36.
4. Tucker MR, Bauer RE, Eans TR, Ochs MW. Implant treatment: advanced concepts and complex cases. In: Hupp JR, editor. Contemporary Oral and maxillofacial surgery. 7th ed. Philadelphia: Elsevier; 2019. p. 281–316.
5. Block MS. Esthetic anterior implant restorations: surgical techniques for optimal results. In: Color atlas of dental implant surgery. 4th ed. St. Louis: Saunders; 2015. p. 362–435e.
6. Misch CM. Maxillary autogenous bone grafting. Oral Maxillofac Surg Clin North Am. 2011;23:229–38.
7. Raghoebar GM, Louwerse C, Kalk WW. Morbidity of chin bone harvesting. Clin Oral Implants Res. 2001;12:503–7.
8. Misch CM. Comparison of intraoral donor sites for onlay grafting prior to implant placement. Int J Oral Maxillofac Implants. 1997;12:767–76.

Alveolar Ridge Preservation

Sindhu Kanikicharla, Thomas J. Balshi,
Muhammad Taimur Khan, and Lovleen Sidhu

The Alveolar Process

The alveolar process constitutes a part of the attachment apparatus known as the periodontium along with the gingiva, connective tissue, periodontal ligament, and cementum. The attachment apparatus helps anchor the tooth in the jaw. Alveolar bone forms by intramembranous ossification and consists of two cortical bone plates separated by an inner cancellous bone layer (see Fig. 18.1). The alveolar bone, along with the attachment apparatus, has an influence on force distribution. The shape and structure of trabeculae in cancellous bone are directly influenced by the forces acting on teeth. Bone is a dynamic tissue that is constantly undergoing formation, resorption, and remodeling due to the functional forces acting on it via the teeth. Alveolar ridge resorption is a progressive and irreversible condition that might result in a plethora of restorative problems that are both aesthetic and functional [1]. The presence and maintenance of alveolar bone depend very much on the presence of teeth [2].

The crest of alveolar bone typically lies 2 mm apical to the cementoenamel junction in health and may migrate apically in the presence of periodontal disease [3].

The loss of a tooth prompts a number of changes in the alveolar process. The healing of a socket is characterized by internal changes, which are mainly histological in nature, and external changes, which consist of structural modifications in alveolar ridge dimensions.

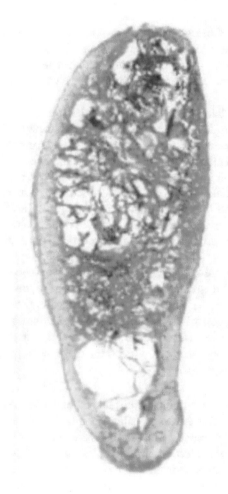

Fig. 18.1 Cross section of an edentulous inter-radicular site a few months after tooth loss. (Reproduced with permission from Tal et al. [2])

Histological Changes As Cardarpoli et al. reported in 2003, varied changes occur throughout the healing process. Immediately after tooth extraction, hemorrhage occurs. On day 1, after extraction, we see a coagulum consisting mainly

S. Kanikicharla (✉)
Division of Prosthodontics, University of Maryland School of Dentistry, Baltimore, MD, USA
e-mail: skanikicharla@umaryland.edu

T. J. Balshi
Prosthodontics Intermedica (Pi Dental Center), Private Implant Mentoring LLC, Fort Washington, PA, USA

M. T. Khan · L. Sidhu
Nova Southeastern University College of Dental Medicine, Ft Lauderdale, FL, USA

© The Author(s), under exclusive license to Springer Nature Switzerland AG 2021
M. R. Stevens et al. (eds.), *Innovative Perspectives in Oral and Maxillofacial Surgery*,
https://doi.org/10.1007/978-3-030-75750-2_18

of erythrocytes and platelets in a fibrin matrix. Within 48–72 hours, granulation tissue begins to infiltrate the clot starting from the socket base. This is followed by changes at days 7 and 14, where there is a greater proliferation of blood vessels. At this time, the primary matrix that is formed transforms into the woven bone. Remodeling of the bone starts around day 30 and continues until days 120 and 180, during which woven bone is replaced by lamellar bone [4]. Healing time may vary depending upon factors such as the socket size, as wider molar sockets take longer to heal compared to the narrower single-rooted teeth sockets. Also, extraction sites where there has been minimal damage to the surrounding bone and soft tissue heal faster.

Structural Changes Literature has shown that loss of teeth leads to remarkable changes in alveolar architecture. Alveolar ridge resorption occurs along with consequent changes in ridge dimensions. Studies have observed certain patterns in these resorptive changes. Recent studies have shown that there is a more significant loss in alveolar ridge width than in height. The reduction in the horizontal ridge width has been reported to reach 50% by Schropp et al. in 2003. Botticelli et al. in 2004 showed that horizontal bone resorption on the buccal aspect could be up to 56%, while on the lingual aspect, they noted up to 30%. Tan et al. in 2012 showed that after 6 months of healing following the extraction, vertical resorption of the alveolar process was 11–22%, while horizontal bone resorption was 29–63% [5]. Iasella et al. (2003), Barone et al. (2008), and Aimetti et al. (2009) all showed that resorption of the buccal plate occurs with a greater magnitude than that of the lingual plate [5]. Various authors have noted that the crest of the residual ridge shifts lingually due to increased buccal resorption when observed from the occlusal aspect. On observing from the lateral aspect, the ridge develops a concavity or flattens [6].

This reduction in ridge width and height due to the resorptive process often leaves the site inadequate for future restoration with implants. Since soft tissue follows the bone, changes in the alveolar process's external profile lead to dimensional changes in the soft tissue as well. Understanding the extent of these bone and mucosal contour changes post-extraction is essential for comprehensive treatment planning as optimal restoration of function and aesthetics during prosthetic rehabilitation might require procedures involving the use of particulate xenografts, allografts, alloplasts, autografts, resorbable or non-resorbable membranes, and growth factors.

Ridge Preservation

Any procedure designed to minimize alveolar ridge resorption and maximize bone formation in the socket at the time of or following an extraction is known as ridge preservation. While most clinical situations allow preservation at the time of extraction, some circumstances like an infection require a delayed procedure. Techniques used to preserve the ridge at the time of extraction include minimally traumatic extraction, immediate implant placement, hard tissue grafting with or without barrier membranes, and use of biologics.

Mechanisms Contributing to Ridge Preservation

Wound Isolation Following an extraction, healing occurs from the apex of the socket and progresses coronally. Soft tissue healing occurs at a faster rate than bone formation. Leaving the extraction site unfilled other than the clot leads to soft tissue invagination into the socket. Inevitable resorption of the buccal plate may also cause soft tissue to collapse into the socket. This might lead to the formation of a defect and reduced bone fill post healing. Using a membrane with or without a graft material that helps stabilize the blood clot and isolate the wound may help concentrate growth factors and other cells necessary for the healing process. The material used for filling the socket also acts as a scaffold and aids in osseoconduction and osteoinduction, helping accelerate bone formation and healing. Due to these properties, a combination of isolation (by the use of a membrane) and an osseoconductive material in the socket helps achieve complete bone fill [1, 7].

Stimulation Multiple authors have proposed that the placement of a graft material in the socket helps stimulate surrounding bone by transmitting forces to the bone in a manner similar to a tooth with a periodontal ligament during normal jaw function. The difference in elastic modulus between the bone and graft material leads to an increase in the density of surrounding bone. Thus forces acting on the graft and being transmitted to the bone when within physiologic limits can aid in preserving surrounding bone [1].

Cellular Activity Bioactive substances placed in sockets can initiate a cellular response from adjacent tissues. Literature shows this response to be different depending upon the material's chemical and surface properties and structure. Particulate graft materials may modify the remodeling process by slowing down the osteoclastic activity or by enhancing the activity of osteoblasts. Biomimetic techniques are also now being used to alter cellular behavior [1].

Ridge Preservation Techniques

Since most alveolar ridge preservation procedures aim to prepare a site for future implant placement, the technique chosen for ridge preservation depends upon the bone defect created due to the extraction and the morphology the ridge presents with. Immediate implant placement combined with a GBR is a preferred approach as it is a one-step treatment. If, however, that is not possible, alveolar ridge preservation can be performed using a combination of a bone graft and membrane or by using them independently.

Atraumatic/Minimally Traumatic Extraction Although the extraction of teeth is a traumatic procedure, appropriate instruments that apply minimal force can minimize the trauma and damage that the surrounding bone and soft tissues experience. Using instruments like luxators and periotomes prior to using forceps helps severe periodontal ligament fibers and loosen the tooth. Procedures like de-coronation and sectioning of multi-rooted teeth also help simplify the extraction procedure. Additionally, timing the extraction as per the planned implant placement is crucial as studies have shown that most of the resorption occurs in the first 3 months post-extraction. Thus, it is useful to plan the extraction so that implant placement if required can be done either immediately or as an early placement [8].

Implant Placement

Studies by Chen et al. in 2004 and Hmmerlee et al. in 2004 proposed that the placement of an implant into a fresh extraction socket will help preserve ridge dimensions and prevent resorption of bone. However, Araujo and Lindhe showed in their canine studies that this does not hold true as they observed a significant reduction of buccal and palatal wall dimensions after 4 months of healing. Grunder, in 2011, showed that despite immediate implant placement combined with a bone graft to seal the buccal gap, significant dimensional changes occurred in the buccal aspect, and he thus concluded that edentulous ridge atrophy could not be prevented by placing an implant into a fresh extraction socket. He also suggested that the use of a soft tissue graft may help in the aesthetic zone [2].

Bone Graft Materials

The four main categories of grafting materials used in dentistry are autografts, allografts, xenografts, and alloplasts. These materials promote bone regeneration by either osteoconduction, osteogenesis, osteoinduction, or a combination of these mechanisms. Osteogenesis occurs when the graft supplies bone-forming osteoblasts even if there are no local undifferentiated mesenchymal stem cells. The graft is osteoinductive if it stimulates the host's undifferentiated stem cells to develop into bone-forming cells (osteoblasts) or the materials that induce osteogenesis, while osteoconduction is the process in which the graft acts as a scaffold to direct the development of bone to conform to the material's surface [9].

Autografts They consist of tissue that is transferred from one site to another within the same individual. The bone can be harvested from intraoral sites such as the chin, mandibular ramus, and maxillary tuberosity or extraoral sites like the iliac crest, ribs, cranium, or tibia. Figure 18.2 shows bone being harvested from the chin and used to graft the same patient's maxillary anterior region. Autografts are most preferred since the graft taken from the same individual has the least chance of graft rejection. Autografts are osteogenic and

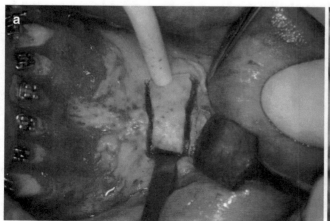
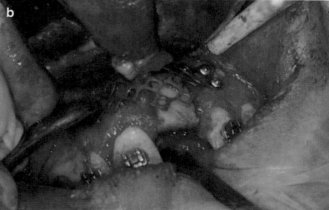

Fig. 18.2 (**a**) Autograft being harvested from the chin. (**b**) Graft used for ridge preservation along with titanium mesh (Photo courtesy Dr. Thomas J Balshi)

also have osteoconductive and osteoinductive potential. Autogenous bone grafts can be cancellous, cortical, or corticocancellous. Generally, cancellous bone is preferred as it has greater osteogenic potential due to the presence of hematopoietic marrow and larger number of undifferentiated stem cells with osteogenic potential. Donor site morbidity, limited availability, and risk of developing postoperative complications such as bleeding and additional pain are the disadvantages associated with the use of these graft materials [10]. These limitations led to the development of alternate graft materials like alloplasts.

Allografts These bone grafts originate from humans but are harvested from a genetically dissimilar individual. They are sourced from cadaver or bone banks. The three types of allografts used are fresh or fresh-frozen bone, freeze-dried bone allograft (FDBA), and demineralized freeze-dried bone allograft (DFDBA). FDBA is mineralized and hence more resistant to resorption than DFDBA. It acts as an osteoconductive scaffold for bone cells to deposit bone at the site of the graft. DFDBA is a demineralized graft material. Removal of the mineral in the allograft exposes the underlying bone proteins and growth factors in the graft and provides it with a greater osteoinductivity than FDBA. The osteoinductivity of an allograft is dependent upon the presence of bone morphogenic proteins. The advantages of using allograft include the unlimited supply of graft material, no secondary donor site, decreased host morbidity, and reduced bleeding and surgical time. As they lack the osteogenic potential that autografts have, bone formation takes longer, but there is also reduced regeneration compared to autografts. Also, there can be concerns of the transmission of infectious diseases from the donor to the host, due to which they undergo very detailed donor screening and processing that reduce this risk of disease transmission [11].

Xenografts These grafts are harvested from species other than humans. Xenografts may be obtained from sources including porcine, bovine, equine, and coralline. Xenografts are biocompatible and integrate with human bone. They are osteoconductive and act as an inert scaffold material for the deposition of bone. Bovine grafts are generally preferred and most commonly used as their mineral content (hydroxyapatite) is very similar to that found in the natural bone in humans. This provides the advantage of rapid revascularization and replacement of the graft by host bone. But these materials present their own set of challenges to the clinician as there is an increased risk of graft rejection due to a host-immune response. Additionally, these materials are resistant to resorption once integrated in bone and have a low turnover that can compromise the grafted site's healing and undermine the mechanical and biological properties of the regenerated bone [11]. In a study by Barone et al., they found that

extraction sites grafted with a combination of xenograft and collagen membrane showed significantly less hard tissue dimensional changes than sockets that were left to heal with no graft material [12]. Kalash et al. found that a mix of PRF and xenograft improves soft tissue healing and also bone regeneration when used in combination with immediate implants placed in fresh extraction sockets, as shown in Fig. 18.3 [13].

Alloplasts These materials are synthetically manufactured bone substitutes. They include inert materials like hydroxyapatite, bioactive ceramics, calcium sulfate, and calcium carbonate. Alloplasts are used as fillers or in combination with the autogenous bone to provide an osteoconductive framework for bone deposition. The synthetic nature of these materials is their most valuable property due to which they are available in unlimited quantities and do not require the presence of a donor site. They do not carry the risk of disease transmission from a donor and have low antigenicity for a host-immune response. Alloplasts are supplied as resorbable and non-resorbable forms and in different particle sizes by the manufacturers.

Hydroxyapatite has a slow resorption rate and can be used for long-term ridge preservation [14]. 100% bone formation has been observed on histological examination after a 3-month healing period with the use of calcium sulfate in extraction sites [15].

Current literature supports autografts as the gold standard for alveolar ridge preservation and augmentation due to their osteogenic, osteoconductive, and osteoinductive properties. Most studies compare other materials to autografts to test the efficacy of the materials in regenerating bone [16]. Although most articles have not concluded on the best graft material for alveolar ridge preservation, in a meta-analysis by Iocca and his group, they found that a combination of freeze-dried bone graft and membrane led to the most effective reduction of bone height remodeling. Autologous bone marrow was best in terms of bone width remodeling. These results serve as guidelines while they need to be interpreted with caution [17].

Barrier Membranes

Barrier membranes have been used extensively for correcting periodontal and other soft tissue defects. Multiple studies have shown that preventing the migration of epithelial cells into the bone defect allows for superior bone regeneration by allowing osteoprogenitor cells and biologic growth factors to repopulate the defect [18]. Dahlin et al. showed in their study that when a membrane isolates an area and maintains contact with the surrounding bone, it only allows cells from the bone

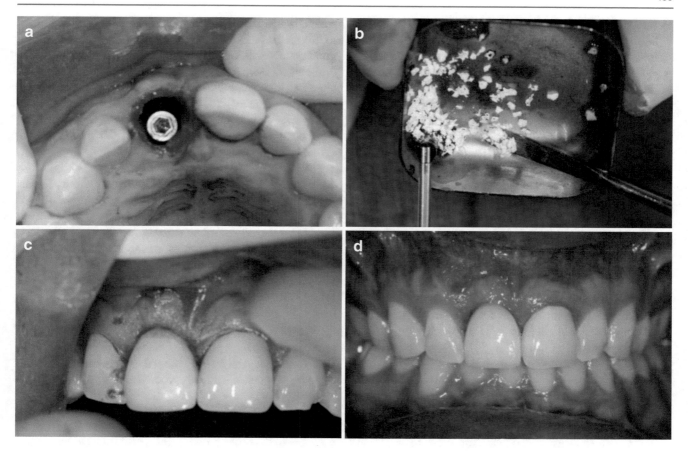

Fig. 18.3 (**a**) Immediate implant placed in the extraction site with the presence of approximately 3 mm buccal gap. (**b**) A mix of PRF and xenograft used for grafting the buccal gap. (**c**) Immediate provisionalization. (**d**) Final restoration. (Photo courtesy Dr. Thomas J Balshi)

and bone marrow around to migrate into the defect and protects the defect from soft tissue ingrowth [11]. Various types of membranes are available based on their ability to resorb and the material that is used to fabricate them. After an extraction, the use of a membrane helps isolate and maintain space, thus preventing tissue ingrowth into the socket/defect and also preventing contamination of the wound. If a membrane is used in conjunction with particulate graft material, it will help prevent graft particles' migration. Membranes should be stable to aid in healing and should be biocompatible. Membranes should be easy to handle and use in order to allow for the efficient surgical procedure

Non-resorbable and resorbable membranes are the two main types of membranes that are currently available. Selection of the specific membrane to be used depends on the expected outcome of the procedure, the length of time the defect needs to be protected and isolated to help with healing, the extent of the bone graft used, etc.

Resorbable Membranes Membranes that are capable of undergoing complete degradation to carbon dioxide and water without requiring a second surgical procedure for their removal are called resorbable membranes. The elimination of the second surgical procedures makes these membranes cost-effective and also helps reduce patient morbidity. These membranes are mainly of two types: collagen membranes and polymeric membranes.

Collagen Membrane These are developed from type I and type III collagen that could be derived from porcine, bovine, or human origin. Collagen membranes can be cross-linked or non-cross-linked. The non-cross-linked membranes have a faster resorption rate. Cross-linked membranes are thus used with graft materials that have a slower rate of substitution. These membranes are easy to use and adapt well to the bone. They are associated with reduced morbidity as they are very mildly immunogenic and they do not require a second surgical procedure for their removal [11]. Studies have shown that the use of a collagen membrane leads to greater bone formation and reduced alveolar dimensional changes in healing extraction sockets compared to sockets where no membrane was used.

Polymeric Membranes (Polylactide and polyglycolide) These membranes are made of synthetic polylactide or polyglycolide polyesters proven to be suitable to the regeneration of bone and soft tissue. One of the advantages of these materials is that they can be manufactured in unlimited quantities. Among the disadvantages of using this membrane are that this can sometimes cause an inflammatory response in the body leading to fibrous encapsulation or sometimes resorbing too soon [11]. Serino et al., in their study, found that the resorption of alveolar bone post tooth extraction can be controlled and reduced by the use of these materials in the tooth socket. They additionally found that the quality of bone found was also suitable for dental implants [19].

Resorbable membranes can also include the acellular dermal matrix (ADM) which is obtained from human skin. Cellular components and epidermis are removed in order to reduce disease transmission risk. Luczyszyn et al. showed in their study that ADM could be used successfully to preserve ridge dimensions after extraction [20].

Non-resorbable Membranes

Titanium mesh, e-PTFE (expanded polytetrafluoroethylene), d-PTFE (high-density polytetrafluoroethylene), and titanium-reinforced PTFE are all different types of non-resorbable membranes.

Titanium Mesh This can be used for alveolar bone regeneration procedures performed at the time of extraction. It helps in treating moderate to severe defects in bone as it tends to be rigid and helps maintain space without collapsing inwards. This allows bone to regenerate without the formation of a defect. Additionally, due to the rigidity of titanium, it can be bent and shaped to suit the defect being regenerated. The presence of a meshwork does not interfere with blood supply and aids healing [11].

e-PTFE Membranes These membranes were developed in 1969 and have been used extensively since the early 1990s. Gore-Tex was the most popular among this class of membranes. This membrane is designed with pores and keeps out any soft tissue cells, thus preventing them from entering the defect. It acts primarily by mechanical isolation of the defect. Multiple studies by Buser, Dahlin, and others have shown that this membrane can predictably allow bone formation in isolated bone defects and can be successfully used for alveolar ridge preservation [11, 21].

d-PTFE Membranes To overcome the weakness of e-PTFE membranes, these membranes were designed with a smaller pore size to reduce microorganisms' migration. Due to this modification, these membranes were able to allow for good bone formation even if they underwent exposure to the oral cavity. The small pore size also kept soft tissue from attaching to the membrane's outer aspect, unlike the e-PTFE membrane, thus making their removal easy. The most commonly used membranes belonging to this class are the cytoplast membranes, and they have been used successfully in alveolar ridge preservation procedures [11].

Titanium-Reinforced PTFE Membranes Both e- and d-PTFE membranes are available in titanium-reinforced forms. This modification helps make the membranes more rigid to be shaped according to the defect. Some studies have shown the titanium-reinforced membranes to have better preserved the original form of the ridge during healing, thus allowing for better preservation and regeneration of alveolar bone [11].

Non-resorbable membranes tend to be more rigid and have better handling properties than resorbable membranes. One of the downsides of using them could be that they require a second surgical procedure for their removal. Another drawback is also that these membranes need primary soft tissue closure. Membrane exposure during healing may increase the risk of infection and adversely affect the outcome of the procedure. It is due to this reason that resorbable membranes are preferred when primary closure is not possible. Studies have shown that particulate graft material in combination with most of the above stated membranes leads to successful bone regeneration and preservation of ridge dimensions compared to non-grafted sockets. Some studies have observed that bone graft material may slow down the process of de novo bone formation compared to non-grafted sockets [11].

Scope of Biologics in ARP

Platelet concentrate products and recombinant growth factors are now being used to accelerate healing of bone and soft tissue.

Platelet-Rich Fibrin (PRF) Choukroun and colleagues developed this platelet concentrate in 2001. PRF is a second-generation concentrate. Venous blood after centrifugation leads to the formation of red blood cells at the bottom, PRF at the intermediate level, and a supernatant consisting of acellular plasma as the top layer (Figs.18.4 and 18.5). PRF contains a fibrin matrix that has a polymerized tetramolecular structure that incorporates platelets, stem cells, cytokines, leucocytes, and growth factors, all of which are released from day 13 through 14 [22]. Due to its fibrin-like consis-

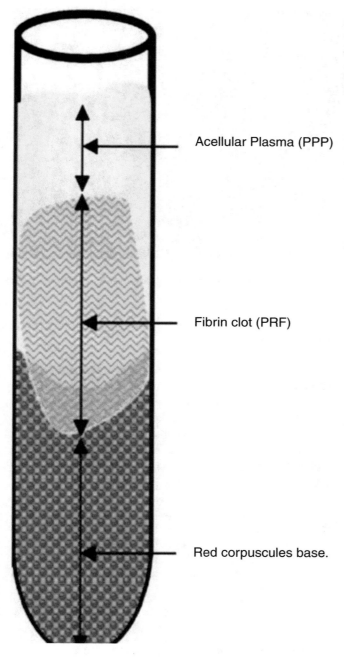

Acellular Plasma (PPP)

Fibrin clot (PRF)

Red corpuscules base.

Fig. 18.4 Blood sample post-centrifugation. Reproduced with permission from Dohan et al. [27]

tency, PRF is slowly destroyed, like that of a natural blood clot [23]. Angiogenesis, harnessing stem cells, and wound protection are crucial properties of PRF that aid in healing [23]. PRF is easy to handle, inexpensive, noninvasive, and is time-efficient. In a study by Dohan et al., they concluded that "PRF membrane sustains a very significant slow release of key growth factors during at least 1 week, which means that the membrane stimulates its environment for a significant time during its remodeling. The properties of this natural

fibrin biomaterial thus offer great potential during wound healing." [23] All of these properties facilitate PRF use in many areas of dentistry, including the treatment of intrabony defects, soft tissue defects, extraction sites, and implant surgery. Despite a number of studies showing that the use of PRF helps with faster soft tissue healing, increased bone fill, increased maturity and density of bone, and reduced bone resorption, some authors have reported no significant benefit with the use of PRF. Articles by Kim et al. where they used platelet-rich plasma on gelatin sponge resulted in good bone formation and ridge preservation [24]. Simon and his colleagues showed minimal dimension changes in extraction sites after platelet-rich growth factor [25].

Growth Factors The use of growth factors can enhance new bone formation and ridge preservation. Growth factors are important for the modulation of cellular development. Among the various growth factors that are important for the regeneration of bone, bone morphogenic proteins (BMPs) and platelet-derived growth factor (PGDF), both play an important role. These molecules are osteoinductive and can be added to various types of bone graft materials to convert them from osteoconductive to osteoinductive. BMP-2 is a recombinant growth factor that is used commonly for alveolar ridge preservation after extraction. A distinct advantage of rhBMP-2 is that it can stimulate new bone formation independently in extraction sites without being combined with other allografts, xenografts, or bone substitutes [25]. In a study conducted by Fiorellini, they found that sockets treated with rhBMP-2 delivered on an absorbable collagen sponge led to a significantly higher amount of bone augmentation compared to sockets treated with absorbable collagen sponge alone [26]. De Freitas et al. stated that rhBMP-2 delivered on an absorbable collagen sponge can be used as an alternative to autogenous bone grafts in ridge augmentation procedures [14]. It should be noted, however, that the rhBMP-2, which is commercially available as INFUSE, (Medtronic, Dublin, Ireland) does produce an inflammatory response in the overlying soft tissue during the initial week of healing.

Although the preliminary results from these materials are very encouraging and these materials may in the future replace the need for bone graft materials, we must keep in mind that the long-term effects of this material in terms of resorption rate of bone, implant success rate in this bone, etc. have not been fully understood yet.

Indications for Ridge Preservation
- Areas where implant placement is being considered more than 6–8 weeks after tooth extraction
- Tooth extraction in the anterior aesthetic zone

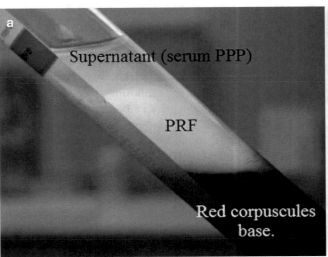 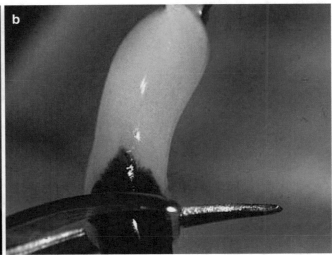

Fig. 18.5 (**a**) Collection of PRF after centrifugation of venous blood. (**b**) resistant autologous fibrin membranes easily obtained by driving out the serum from the clot. (Modified from Dohan et al. [27])

- Presence of a thin buccal plate (<1.5–2 mm)
- Patients with a thin tissue phenotype
- Patients with a high smile line or high aesthetic demands
- Sites where pontic site development might be considered for aesthetic reasons
- Sites where one or more socket walls have been damaged or lost
- Areas in the posterior maxilla or mandible where anatomic structures like the maxillary sinus or the inferior alveolar nerve might complicate future implant placement [8]
- Where immediate implant placement following extraction creates a buccal gap of more than 2.0 mm

Contraindications

- Presence of an acute infection that cannot be completely debrided on the day of the extraction
- Medically compromised patients that cannot undergo multiple procedures
- Areas where maintaining bone and soft tissue volume are not critical for the final restorative result [8]

Limitations

- Longer-term studies are required better to understand the success rates of various materials and techniques.
- No one material or technique can be used in all cases.
- Patient factors, such as health status, smoking, etc., may impact the outcomes of these procedures. [8]

Conclusions

Alveolar ridge preservation has proven to be a successful surgical technique that often allows for optimal implant placement without the need for multiple bone augmentation procedures. Various patient factors have to be considered in order to make the right material choice due to the many options available. Preservation of the ridge in the anterior region is far more critical than other areas and should include both hard and soft tissue grafts.

References

1. Bartee BK. Extraction site reconstruction for alveolar ridge preservation. Part 1: rationale and materials selection. J Oral Implantol. 2001;27(4):187–93.
2. Tal, H., Artzi, Z., Kolerman, R., Beitlitum, I., & Goshen, G. (2012). Augmentation and preservation of the alveolar process and alveolar ridge of bone. Bone Regeneration, InTech Rijeka, 139-184.
3. Gulabivala K, Ng YL. Tooth organogenesis, morphology and physiology. In: Endodontics. St. Louis: Mosby; 2014. p. 2–32.
4. Cardaropoli G, Araujo M, Lindhe J. Dynamics of bone tissue formation in tooth extraction sites: an experimental study in dogs. J Clin Periodontol. 2003;30(9):809–18.
5. Tan WL, Wong TL, Wong MC, Lang NP. A systematic review of post-extractional alveolar hard and soft tissue dimensional changes in humans. Clin Oral Implants Res. 2012;23:1–21.
6. Pietrokovski J. The bony residual ridge in man. J Prosthet Dent. 1975;34(4):456–62.
7. Semeniuk D. Prospective, comparative volumetric assessment of alveolar ridge preservation utilizing different bone grafting materials. 2017.

8. Darby I, Chen S, De Poi R. Ridge preservation: what is it and when should it be considered. Aust Dent J. 2008;53(1):11–21.

9. Albrektsson T, Johansson C. Osteoinduction, osteoconduction and osseointegration. Eur Spine J. 2001;10(2):S96–S101.

10. Kumar P, Vinitha B, Fathima G. Bone grafts in dentistry. J Pharm Bioallied Sci. 2013;5(Suppl 1):S125.

11. Liu J, Kerns DG. Suppl 1: Mechanisms of guided bone regeneration: A review. Open Dent J. 2014;8:56.

12. Barone A, Aldini NN, Fini M, Giardino R, Calvo Guirado JL, Covani U. Xenograft versus extraction alone for ridge preservation after tooth removal: a clinical and histomorphometric study. J Periodontol. 2008;79(8):1370–7.

13. Kalash S, Aboelsaad N, Shokry M, ChouKRouN J. The efficiency of using advanced PRF-xenograft mixture around immediate implants in the esthetic zone: a randomized controlled clinical trial. J Osseointegration. 2017;9(4):317–22.

14. Jamjoom A, Cohen RE. Grafts for ridge preservation. J Funct Biomater. 2015;6(3):833–48.

15. Guarnieri R, Pecora G, Fini M, Aldini NN, Giardino R, Orsini G, Piattelli A. Medical grade calcium sulfate hemihydrate in healing of human extraction sockets: clinical and histological observations at 3 months. J Periodontol. 2004;75(6):902–8.

16. Chavda S, Levin L. Human studies of vertical and horizontal alveolar ridge augmentation comparing different types of bone graft materials: A systematic review. J Oral Implantol. 2018;44(1):74–84.

17. Iocca O, Farcomeni A, Pardiñas Lopez S, Talib HS. Alveolar ridge preservation after tooth extraction: a Bayesian Network meta-analysis of grafting materials efficacy on prevention of bone height and width reduction. J Clin Periodontol. 2017;44(1):104–14.

18. Bartee BK. Extraction site reconstruction for alveolar ridge preservation. Part 2: membrane-assisted surgical technique. J Oral Implantol. 2001;27(4):194–7.

19. Serino G, Biancu S, Iezzi G, Piattelli A. Ridge preservation following tooth extraction using a polylactide and polyglycolide sponge as space filler: a clinical and histological study in humans. Clin Oral Implants Res. 2003;14(5):651–8.

20. Luczyszyn SM, Papalexiou V, Novaes AB Jr, Grisi MF, Souza SL, Taba M Jr. Acellular dermal matrix and hydroxyapatite in prevention of ridge deformities after tooth extraction. Implant Dent. 2005;14(2):176–84.

21. Dahlin C, et al. Healing of bone defects by guided tissue regeneration. Plast Reconstr Surg. 1988;81(5):672–6.

22. Choukroun J, Diss A, Simonpieri A, Girard MO, Schoeffler C, Dohan SL, et al. Platelet-rich fibrin (PRF): a second-generation platelet concentrate. Part IV: clinical effects on tissue healing. Oral Surg Oral Med Oral Pathol Oral Radiol Endod. 2006;101(3):e56–60.

23. Dohan Ehrenfest DM, de Peppo GM, Doglioli P, Sammartino G. Slow release of growth factors and thrombospondin-1 in Choukroun's platelet-rich fibrin (PRF): a gold standard to achieve for all surgical platelet concentrates technologies. Growth Factors. 2009;27(1):63–9.

24. Suttapreyasri S, Leepong N. Influence of platelet-rich fibrin on alveolar ridge preservation. J Craniofac Surg. 2013;24(4):1088–94.

25. Wallace SC, Pikos MA, Prasad H. De novo bone regeneration in human extraction sites using recombinant human bone morphogenetic protein-2/ACS: a clinical, histomorphometric, densitometric, and 3-dimensional cone-beam computerized tomographic scan evaluation. Implant Dent. 2014;23(2):132–7.

26. Fiorellini JP, Howell TH, Cochran D, Malmquist J, Lilly LC, Spagnoli D, et al. Randomized study evaluating recombinant human bone morphogenetic protein-2 for extraction socket augmentation. J Periodontol. 2005;76(4):605–13.

27. Dohan DM, Choukroun J, Diss A, Dohan SL, Dohan AJ, Mouhyi J, Gogly B. Platelet-rich fibrin (PRF): a second-generation platelet concentrate. Part I: technological concepts and evolution. Oral Surg Oral Med Oral Pathol Oral Radiol Endod. 2006;101(3):e37–44.

The Socket Shield Technique

19

Joseph W. Ivory

Introduction

Replacing an anterior maxillary tooth with an implant presents a significant aesthetic challenge to the implant surgeon. The rapid changes in the architecture of the alveolar ridge stemming from bone resorption result in loss of bony width and height with concomitant, dramatic effects on the accompanying soft tissues. The loss of the dental papilla and flattening of the dental arch after a tooth extraction presents a difficult aesthetic challenge. While a successfully integrated anterior implant may restore the function of the arch, the implant will not be considered a "success" if the aesthetics have been compromised, particularly in a patient with a high smile line. The socket shield technique was developed to preserve bony architecture by leaving a thin shelf of dentin in the socket. Understanding how this technique was developed and why it works requires understanding of the anatomy of the alveolar ridge and the biology of ridge remodeling after tooth extraction.

Alveolar Ridge Anatomy and Ridge Resorption

The alveolar process is made up of the inner portion of the socket walls, also known as the lamina dura or "bundle bone," and the remaining hard structure is referred to as alveolar bone [1]. When a tooth is removed from the alveolar process, there are a series of events which have been thoroughly studied in human and animal models [2–4]. As with all bony healing, the healing of an extraction site has an inflammatory phase, a proliferative phase, and bone modeling and remodeling phase.

When a tooth is extracted, the inflammatory phase begins, starting with the formation of a coagulum. This initial coagulum is replaced over 2–3 days by fibrin-rich granulation tissue, as new blood vessels sprout into the wound and bring inflammatory cells and immature fibroblasts to the area. Fibroblasts then replace the granulation tissue with a connective tissue matrix. This matrix is penetrated by new blood vessels and osteoblasts during the proliferative phase, a process referred to as fibroplasia. Osteoblasts then lay down projections of woven bone around these blood vessels to form an osteon. This process occurs over a period of about 2 weeks, and the woven bone remains in place for several weeks. During the bone modeling phase, this woven bone is replaced with lamellar bone and bone marrow, eventually closing the socket. This phase can take several months, during which significant architectural changes can occur.

The majority of changes occur within the first 3 months following extraction. During the first 8 weeks, there is a significant osteoclastic activity which is divided into two phases. During the first 4 weeks (phase 1), there is resorption of the lamina dura of the buccal and lingual aspects of the extraction socket, resulting in loss of buccal width and vertical height. During phase two, there is bone resorption on the socket walls' outer surface [3, 5]. Resorption results in up to 50% loss of buccolingual width in the first 12 months [5]. The loss of buccal bone results in flattening of the dental arch and loss of lip support that is associated with unfavorable changes to facial aesthetics [6]. Additionally, the loss of vertical height results in the loss of the papilla's height, an aesthetic challenge that can be extremely challenging to overcome with subsequent surgical procedures.

There are several predictors of bone loss. A chief factor is the tooth position, with central incisors and canines being much more prone to bone loss than lateral incisors and premolars. Other predictors of bone loss include the presence of an abscess, prior bone loss from trauma, periodontal disease, or extraction [9]. Multiple studies have demonstrated that bone loss is much more significant on the tooth socket's

J. W. Ivory (✉)
Oral and Maxillofacial Surgery, Dwight D. Eisenhower Army Medical Center, Fort Gordon, GA, USA
e-mail: sgtdabney@gmail.com

© The Author(s), under exclusive license to Springer Nature Switzerland AG 2021
M. R. Stevens et al. (eds.), *Innovative Perspectives in Oral and Maxillofacial Surgery*,
https://doi.org/10.1007/978-3-030-75750-2_19

buccal aspect than the lingual [6, 10, 11]. While this increased loss of bone on the buccal aspect may be due to post-extraction trauma to the remaining thin shelf of bone [3], the most significant factor is the loss of the periodontal ligament as the blood supply to the lamina dura [7, 8].

Techniques Developed to Address These Challenges

Dental specialists have developed several techniques over the past several decades to address the challenge of bone loss after tooth extraction. Socket grafting immediately after extraction or "ridge preservation" has enjoyed a great deal of popularity due to its impressive results. This is typically done with an allograft or xenograft bone substitute, barrier membranes [29], or collagen plugs but can be done with connective tissue grafts as well [21]. Socket grafting has been shown to result in a more significant amount of residual bone [13], with a substantial reduction in loss of vertical height [14]. While several different methods have been described in the literature, there is no preponderance of evidence to show that variations in the material or technique make a difference in the outcome [15–17, 19]. Two notable exceptions exist in the literature. Fiorellini showed that the use of rhBMP-2 during socket grafting results in de novo bone formation [20]. In a literature review of 2898 titles, Jambhekar demonstrated that allograft use in socket grafting results in a higher quality of bone than xenografts and allografts after 12 weeks [18].

Following ridge preservation, there is some discussion about when the optimum time is to place the implant into the healed socket. The ideal time to place an implant is dependent on the clinical state of the extraction site, and the treatment plan must be catered to each patient. Jung provided a discussion as to the timing of dental implant rehabilitation after tooth extraction. Based on the literature review, tooth extraction sites with soft tissue defects should have soft tissue preservation techniques completed followed by 6–8 weeks of healing to optimize the soft tissue bed. To optimize the hard and soft tissue bed, the clinician should perform socket grafting with soft tissue preservation, followed by 4–6 months of healing prior to implant placement. For hard tissue defects, such as severe loss of the buccal plate (>50%), hard tissue preservation procedures should be followed by up to 6 months of healing before implant placement [28].

Immediate implant placement after a tooth extraction is another method that has been developed to preserve bone. It has the advantage of a single-stage surgery, which results in increased patient satisfaction (especially with immediate loading), reduced treatment time, and placing the implant into a more physiologic apical position [25–27]. However, it must be noted that immediate implants have a significantly lower survival rate than those placed into healed extraction sites [24]. There is the loss of vertical height and lingual and buccal resorption. However, it has been demonstrated that even in ungrafted sites, there is significant closure of the marginal gap between the socket walls and the bone graft through new bone formation [22]. Grafting around the implant and using a contoured healing abutment reduces the amount of horizontal bone loss [23]. Additionally, the use of bioactive products such as amnion chorion membranes shows promise in promoting soft and hard tissue healing and preserving bone height and width [44].

There have been other methods developed to maintain or restore the original contour of the buccal ridge. Orthodontic extrusion of hopeless teeth before extraction increases bony height in preparation for implant placement [12]. After tooth extraction, it is necessary to try to restore the original contour of the ridge. Block grafting with cortical bone harvested from the ramus, symphysis, calvarium, and iliac crest has long been considered the "gold standard" of bone grafting. Guided bone regeneration using membranes, titanium mesh with membranes, or resorbable mesh are useful methods of restoring the alveolar ridge's contours after extractions. The use of rhBMP-2, stem cells, and blood products has enhanced our ability to reconstruct the atrophic alveolar ridge in preparation for dental implants as well. However, these techniques are limited by the amount of soft tissue available. Post-extraction will be significantly less than before alveolar bone loss has occurred, and the blood supply also becomes reduced with repeated surgeries and scar tissue formation. It is important to note that complete preservation or restoration of the alveolar ridge has not been demonstrated with any of these techniques [30, 31].

Development of the Socket Shield Technique

As noted above, it has been recognized that the majority of bone resorption occurs on the buccal aspect of the alveolar ridge, and the maintenance of this bone is dependent on the blood supply from the periodontal ligament. During tooth extraction, this ligament is disrupted, and the blood supply is lost, resulting in bone resorption and collapse of the buccal, lingual width of the alveolar ridge. This results in loss of soft tissue volume, increasing the likelihood of aesthetic failure in the anterior maxilla. The key to preventing bone resorption, therefore, is the preservation of the periodontal ligament. Several researchers began to develop techniques for preserving tooth structures in order to preserve the PDL and prevent bone loss [39].

In 2001, Filipi demonstrated that by decoronating previously traumatized/ankylosed teeth, the bony height could be preserved and that bone apposition occurred as well [32]. The retention of submerged roots (root submergence technique) to preserve bone was shown to have many applications, including the retention of root canal-treated submerged roots to preserve hard and soft tissue contours underneath a planned implant-supported fixed prostheses (pontic shield technique) [34]. In 2010, Hurzeler demonstrated that retention of a buccal root fragment with immediate implant placement (socket shield technique) not only preserves buccal bone but does not interfere with osseointegration in a dog model [33]. In specimens harvested from the models, he also showed that the dentin shield forms new cementum, filling in the gap between the implant and the shield. In 2013, Kan and Rungcharasseang showed that retention of a mesial and distal root fragment could maintain the height of the papilla in the aesthetic zone (proximal socket shield technique) [35]. Over the next several years, several case reports demonstrated this technique's validity both in the anterior and posterior arches [38, 40–44].

Case series began to be published as the technique gained popularity. In 2014, Glocker published a small case series where the buccal dental shelf was left in place, the socket was grafted and allowed to heal, and implants were successfully placed. Gluckman publishes a ten-patient case series in 2016 showing how the pontic shield technique can be used to develop pontic sites and preserve the ridge [45]. In 2018, Bramanti published a study with 40 patients comparing the socket shield technique to traditional immediate implant placement. He found that the socket shield technique's aesthetic results were superior to traditional immediate implant placement as measured by marginal bone height, implant mobility, signs and symptoms of infection, pain, and the pink aesthetic score [36]. In 2020 Farhan published a 5-year follow-up case series of 14 patients, all of which showed pleasing aesthetics after the socket shield technique on anterior teeth [37].

Case Selection

Gluckman gave the following criteria for case selection of the socket shield technique:

1. A non-restorable tooth or tooth crown indicated for extraction
2. No periapical pathology
3. Intention to preserve the buccolingual alveolar ridge width
4. Immediate implant placement
5. Ridge preservation in conjunction with other partial extraction therapies [39]

Additional considerations would be the mobility of the tooth or a widened PDL [35]. A horizontal root fracture would present an absolute contraindication, and a vertical root fracture represents a relative contraindication if the fracture is through the buccal aspect of the root. Dental decay extending into the buccal aspect of the root, uncontrolled periodontal disease, uncontrolled systemic disease, or poor oral hygiene also constitute contraindications for this technique. Smoking presents a relative contraindication as it theoretically can interfere with the blood supply from the PDL to the bundle bone on the buccal aspect of the alveolar ridge. Severe dental crowding and severe angulations of the tooth to be removed or the adjacent teeth may provide relative contraindications as well. Lastly, the procedure is technique-sensitive, and the operating provider should be a "veteran" at dentoalveolar, implant, and peri-implant surgery.

Surgical Technique

1. Preoperatively, the patient is prescribed Peridex mouth rinse 2 days prior to the appointment BID to reduce bacterial load.
2. Raise a conservative flap, exposing only the tooth root and the top of the crestal bone to prevent disruption of periosteal blood supply.
3. Decoronate the tooth down to 1 mm above the crestal bone (Fig. 19.1).

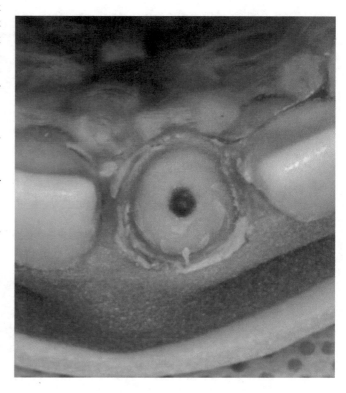

Fig. 19.1 Decoronation of the tooth down to the level of the crestal bone

4. Section the root mesiodistally using a long shank rotary instrument. Ensure the root is sectioned as far apically as possible. In some cases, it is advantageous to section the palatal portion of the root buccolingually to aid in root removal (Fig. 19.2).

5. Using periotomes, root tip elevators, or piezo-type handpiece, remove the palatal portion of the root, taking care not to disrupt the buccal portion of the root (Fig. 19.3).

6. Thin the remaining buccal socket shield using long shank rotary instruments or diamond burs (Figs. 19.3 and 19.4).

7. Use a diamond bur to reduce the crestal portion to bone level and create an internal chamfer. This will help with the emergence profile of the final restoration.

8. Curette the sockets to ensure all debris is removed and irrigate copiously with normal saline.

9. Take radiographs to ensure any root canal treatment material is gone (Fig. 19.5).

10. Verify immobility of the socket shield with an explorer.

11. Prepare the implant site using the palatal portion of the socket to ensure the emergence profile is in line with the lingula of the adjacent teeth and irrigate copiously. Place implant engaging the apical bone against the palatal aspect of the socket. This will typically leave a small

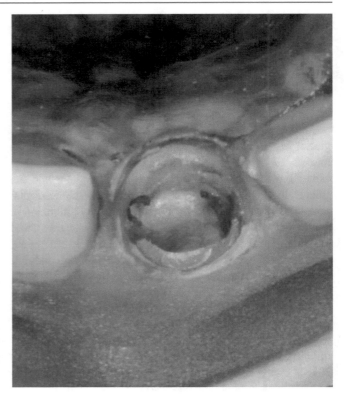

Fig. 19.3 Model demonstrating socket shield after preparation

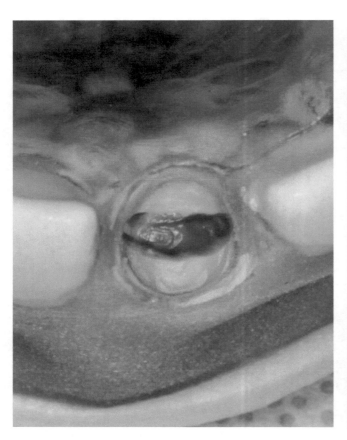

Fig. 19.2 Mesiodistal sectioning of the tooth with fissure bur

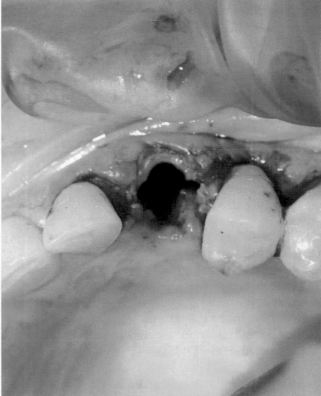

Fig. 19.4 Socket shield after preparation

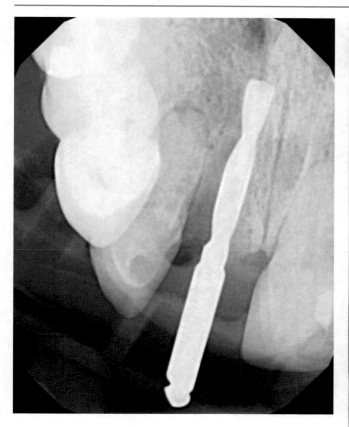

Fig. 19.5 Radiograph taken after preparation to ensure gutta-percha is removed and to check the depth of preparation

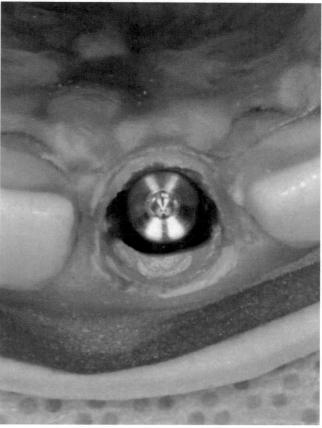

Fig. 19.6 Implant placed with cover screw demonstrating emergence through the lingula and the resultant buccal gap

buccal gap between the dentin and the implant (Figs. 19.6 and 19.7).

12. Graft the buccal gap with bone particulate material, leaving the top of the implant exposed.

13. Seal the socket entrance with membrane, Collaplug, or custom transgingival healing abutment if providing a provisional restoration. The author uses a combination of a Collaplug with an overlying amnion chorion membrane and sews the wound with 4-0 Vicryl sutures if the implant is not immediately loaded (Figs. 19.8 and 19.9).

Management of the implant post-surgery is no different from the management of any immediate implant. The treatment should be tailored to the patient and the surgeon's capabilities. In some of the literature, there are examples of the dentin shelf working through the gingiva on the facial. However, trimming the dentinal shelf down to the level of the crestal bone seems to avoid this complication. The implant is restored in a traditional fashion once osseointegration is confirmed (Figs. 19.10, 19.11, and 19.12).

Conclusion

Extraction of teeth leads to dramatic changes to the alveolar process's architecture, resulting in loss of up to 50% of buccolingual width and loss of vertical height in the first year. This is a particularly vexing problem for the implant surgeon in the aesthetic zone, as even the most advanced tissue engineering techniques cannot fully restore hard and soft tissue volume once it has been lost. The key to maintaining the width and height of the alveolus after extraction is to prevent resorption. While many techniques have been developed to counter the rapid resorption of alveolar bone after tooth extraction, none have been shown to completely prevent absorption. The socket shield technique is an innovative method of preserving hard and soft tissue around extraction sites in the jaws' anterior and posterior aspects. By preserving leaving a "shield" of dentin on the buccal or mesial aspect of the extraction site, the periodontal ligament is left

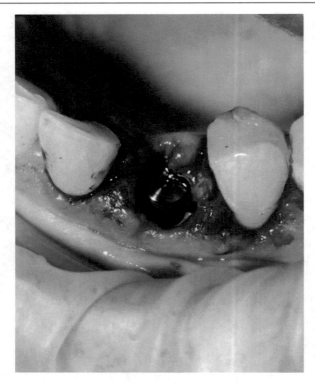

Fig. 19.7 Implant placed in socket shield demonstrating buccal gap to be grafted with particulate

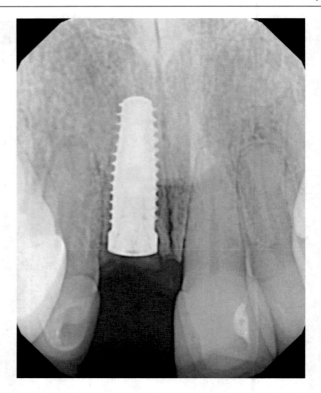

Fig. 19.9 Postoperative radiograph demonstrating socket shield with cover screw in place

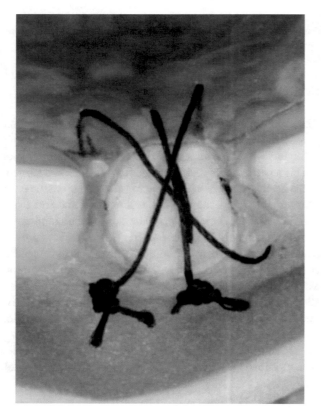

Fig. 19.8 Simulated membrane demonstrating the typical suture pattern utilized by the author to secure the Collaplug and the overlying amnion chorion membrane

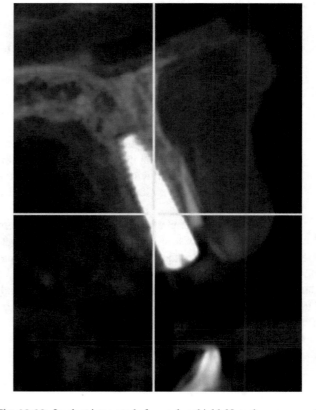

Fig. 19.10 Implant integrated after socket shield. Note the presence of the socket shield and the bony fill in the buccal gap between the implant and the dentin shield

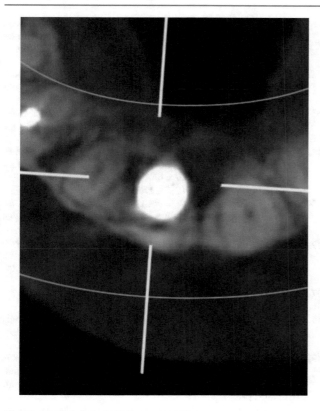

Fig. 19.11 Axial view of the same tooth

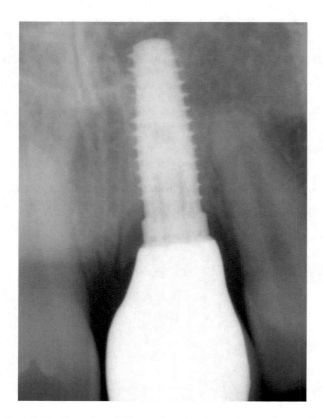

Fig. 19.12 Note the visible socket shield superimposed over the implant and the maintenance of height as compared to the adjacent central incisor

intact, preserving the blood supply to the bundle bone, preventing resorption. Larger prospective studies need to be conducted to document the long-term outcomes of this technique. However, the early literature shows great promise, and the socket shield technique should be in the armamentarium of the modern implant surgeon.

References

1. Araujo MG, Silva CO, Misawa M, Sukekava F. Alveolar socket healing: what can we learn? Periodontology. 2015;68(1):122–34.
2. Amler MH. The time sequence of tissue regeneration in human extraction wounds. Oral Surg Oral Med Oral Pathol. 1969;27:309–18.
3. Araújo MG, Lindhe J. Dimensional ridge alterations following tooth extraction. An experimental study in the dog. J Clin Periodontol. 2005;32(2):212–8.
4. Cardaropoli G, Araújo M, Lindhe J. Dynamics of bone tissue formation in tooth extraction sites. An experimental study in dogs. J Clin Periodontol. 2003;30(9):809–18.
5. Kalsi AS, Kalsi JS, Bassi S. Dental abstracts, 2020-03-01;65(2):111–3.
6. Schropp L, Wenzel A, Kostopoulos L, Karring T. Bone healing and soft tissue contour changes following single-tooth extraction: a clinical and radiographic 12-month prospective study. Int J Periodontics Restorative Dent. 2003;23:313–23.
7. Van der Weijden F, Dell-Acqua F, Slot DE. Alveolar bone dimensional changes of post-extraction sockets in humans: a systemic review. J Clin Periodontol. 2009;36:1048–58.
8. Devlin H, Ferguson MW. Alveolar ridge resorption and mandibular atrophy. A review of the role of local and systemic factors. Br Dent J. 1991;170:101–4.
9. Cosyn J, Cleymaet R, De Bruyn H. Predictors of alveolar process remodeling following ridge preservation in high-risk patients. Clin Implant Dent Relat Res. 2016;18:226.
10. Wennström JL, Lindhe J. Ridge alterations following implant placement in fresh extraction sockets: an experimental study in the dog. J Clin Periodontol. 2005;32:645–52.
11. Fickl S, Zuhr O, Wachtel H, et al. Tissue alterations after tooth extraction with and without surgical trauma: a volumetric study in the beagle dog. J Clin Periodontol. 2008;35:356–63.
12. Salama H, Salama MA. The role of orthodontic extrusive remodeling in the enhancement of soft and hard tissue profiles prior to implant placement: a systematic approach to the management of extraction site defects. In J Periodontics Restorative Dent. 1993;13:312–33.
13. Walker CJ, Prihoda TJ, Mealey BL, et al. Evaluation of healing at molar extraction sites with and without ridge preservation: a randomized controlled clinical trial. J Periodontol. 2016;27:1–14.
14. MacBeth N, Trullenque-Eriksson A, Donos N, Mardas N. Hard and soft tissue changes following alveolar ridge preservation: a systematic review. Clin Oral Implants Res. 2017;28:982–1004.
15. Atieh MA, Alsabeeha NH, Payne AG, et al. Interventions for replacing missing teeth: alveolar ridge preservation techniques for dental implant site development. Cochrane Database Syst Rev. 2015;28:CD010176.
16. Avila-Ortiz G, Rodriguez JC, Rudek I, et al. Effectiveness of three different alveolar ridge preservation techniques: a pilot randomized controlled trial. Int J Periodontics Restorative Dent. 2014;34:509.
17. Barone A, Ricci M, Romanos GE, et al. Buccal bone deficiency in fresh extraction sockets: a prospective single cohort study. Clin Oral Implants Res. 2015;26:823.

18. Jambhekar S, Kernen F, Bidra AS. Clinical and histologic outcomes of socket grafting after flapless tooth extraction: a systematic review of randomized controlled clinical trials. J Prosthet Dent. 2015;113:371.

19. Barone A, Borgia V, Covani U, et al. Flap versus flapless procedure for ridge preservation in alveolar extraction sockets: a histological evaluation in a randomized clinical trial. Clin Oral Implants Res. 2015;26:806.

20. Fiorellini JP, Howell TH, Cochran D, et al. Randomized study evaluating recombinant human bone morphogenetic protein-2 for extraction socket augmentation. J Periodontol. 2005;76:605.

21. Vanhoutte V, Rompen E, Lecloux G, Rues S, Schmitter M, Lambert F. A methodological approach to assessing alveolar ridge preservation procedures in humans: soft tissue profile. Clin Oral Implants Res. 2014;25(3):304–9.

22. Botticelli D, Berglundh T, Lindhe J. Hard tissue alterations following immediate implant placement in extraction sites. J Clin Periodontol. 2004;31:820–8.

23. Tarnow DP, Chu SJ, Salama MA, et al. Flapless postextraction socket implant placement in the esthetic zone: part 1. The effect of bone grafting and/or provisional restoration on facial-palatal ridge dimensional change—a retrospective cohort study. Int J Periodontics Restorative Dent. 2014;34:323.

24. Mello CC, Lemos CAA, Verri FR, dos Santos DM, Goiato MC, Pellizzer EP. Immediate implant placement into fresh extraction sockets versus delayed implants into healed sockets: a systematic review and meta-analysis. Int J Oral Maxillofac Surg. 2017;46(9):1162–77.

25. Lindeboom JA, Tjiook Y, Kroon FH. Immediate placement of implants in periapical infected sites: a prospective randomized study in 50 patients. Oral Surg Oral Med Oral Pathol Oral Radiol Endod. 2006;101:705–10.

26. Agliardi E, Panigatti S, Clerico M, Villa C, Malo P. Immediate rehabilitation of the edentulous jaws with full fixed prostheses supported by four implants: interim results of a single cohort prospective study. Clin Oral Implants Res. 2010;21:459–65.

27. Werbitt MJ, Goldberg PV. The immediate implant: bone preservation and bone regeneration. Int J Periodontics Restorative Dent. 1992;12:206–17.

28. Jung RE, Ioannidis A, Hammerle CHF, Thoma DS. Alveolar ridge preservation in the esthetic zone. Periodontol 2000. 2018;77(10):165–75.

29. Lekovic V, Carmargo P, Klokkevold P, Weinlaender M, Kenney E, Dimitrijevic B, Nedic M. Preservation of alveolar bone in extraction sockets using bioabsorbable membranes. J Periodontol. 1998;69:1044–9.

30. Vignoletti F, Discepoli N, Moller A, de Sanctis M, Muñoz F, Sanz M. Bone modeling at fresh extraction sockets: immediate implant placement versus spontaneous healing. An experimental study in the beagle dog. J Clin Periodontol. 2012;39:91–7.

31. Viglonetti E, Matesanz P, Rodrigo D, Figuero E, Martin C, Sanz M. Surgical protocols for ridge preservation after tooth extraction. A systematic review. Clin Oral Implants Res. 2012;23(Suppl 5):22–38.

32. Filippi A, Pohl Y, von Arx T. Decoronation of an ankylosed tooth for preservation of alveolar bone prior to implant placement. Dent Traumatol. 2001;17:93–5.

33. Hürzeler MB, Zuhr O, Schupbach P, Rebele SF, Emmanouilidis N, Fickl S. The socket shield technique: a proof-of-principle report. J Clin Periodontol. 2010;37:855–62.

34. Wong KM, Christopher Miang CM, Ang CW. Modified root submergence technique for multiple implant-supported maxillary anterior restorations in a patient with thin gingival biotype: a clinical report. J Prosthet Dent. 2012;107:349–52.

35. Kan JYK, Rungcharasseang K. Proximal socket shield for interimplant papilla preservation in the esthetic zone. Int J Periodontics Restorative Dent. 2013;33:e24–31.

36. Bramanti E, Norcia A, Cicciu M, Matacena G, Cervino G, Troiano G, Zhurakivska K, Laino L. Postextraction dental implant in the aesthetic zone, socket shield technique versus conventional protocol. J Craniofac Surg. 2018;29(4):1037–41.

37. Durrani F, Painuly H, et al. Socket shield: an esthetic success? J Indian Soc Periodontol. 2020;24(3):289–94.

38. Glocker M, Attin T, Schmidlin PR. Ridge preservation with modified "socket shield" technique: a methodological case series. Dent J. 2014;2:11–21.

39. Gluckman H, Salama M, Du Toit J. Partial Extraction Therapies (PET) part 1: maintaining alveolar ridge contour at pontic and immediate implant sites. Int J Periodontics Restorative Dent. 2016;36(5):681–7.

40. Holbrook SE. Model-guided flapless immediate implant placement and provisionalization in the esthetic zone utilizing a nanostructured titanium implant: a case report. J Oral Implantol. 2016;42:98–103.

41. Gluckman H, Du Toit J, Salama M. The socket-shield technique to support buccofacial tissues at immediate implant placement: a case report and review of the literature. In Dent Africa Ed. 2015;5:1–7.

42. Mitsias ME, Siormpas KD, Prasad H, Garber D, Kotsiakis GA. A step-by-step description of PDL-mediated ridge preservation for immediate implant rehabilitation in the esthetic region. Int J Periodontics Restorative Dent. 2015;35:835–41.

43. Aslan S. Improved volume and contour stability with thin socket-shield preparation in immediate implant placement and provisionalization in the esthetic zone. Int J Esthetic Dent. 2018;13(2):172–83.

44. Kesting MR, Wolff KD, Nobis CP, Rohleder NH. Amniotic membrane in oral and maxillofacial surgery. Oral Maxillofacial Sur. 2014;18:153–64.

45. Gluckman H, Du Toit J, Salam M. The pontic shield: partial extraction therapy for ridge preservation and pontic site development. Int J Periodontics Restorative Dent. 2016;36:417–23.

Flap Design and Modification to Attain Primary Closure

Alireza Darnahal and Fargol Mashhadi Akbar Boojar

Displaced flaps:

- Apically (APF), coronally (CAF), and laterally (LPF) positioned flaps moved from the original position

None displaced flap:

- The flap is sutured back to its original position.

Modified Widman Flap

In 1974, Ramfjord and Nissle described the "open flap curettage technique" or modified Widman flap technique. Some of the advantages of the modified Widman technique are as follows:

1. Facilitate the adaptation of soft tissue to the root surface.
2. Reduction amount of trauma to the alveolar bone and the exposed soft connective tissues.
3. Less exposure of the root surface, especially in treating the anterior segment of the dentine.
4. Reduce the amount of pocket depths [2].

Three incisions are needed in this flap; first, we should make an initial scalloped incision from the buccal gingival margin or intracervicular incision (if the pockets on the buccal aspects of the teeth are less than 2 mm deep or if aesthetic considerations are important), second intracervicular incision in the teeth about 1 mm (the incision should extend as far as possible in between the teeth, to include maximum amounts of the interdental gingiva in the flap), this incision can facilitate the gentle separation of the collar of pocket epithelium and granulation tissue from the root surfaces (we should continue this incision intrasulcularly until the alveolar bone is connecting with the blade); and third horizontal incision, this technique is a reverse bevel flap procedure.

The initial incision should be placed at least 0.5–1 mm if the buccal or lingual pockets are deeper than 2 mm and the incision should be exaggerated on the palate (1–2 from FGM for flap adaptation). If the pocket is minimal, a sulcular incision is made, and the initial incision should be parallel to the long axis to the teeth in a modified Widman flap.

For the palatal surface, this technique is similar on the buccal aspect; however, placing the knife for the initial incision is at a distance of 1–2 mm from the teeth's mid-palatal surface. A vertical incision is not usually needed on the palatal surface.

This flap is minimally (2–3 mm) reflected to gain access to the tooth surface for scaling and root planing.

For making the initial incision, we use a Bard-Parker #11 or any other appropriate knife that can be directed parallel to the tooth's long axis.

For shallow pockets and when the aesthetic considerations are important, we use intracrevicular incision.

Also, be sure to direct the scalpel slightly palatal to the tooth's long axis aiming for the alveolar process 1–2 mm palatally to the alveolar crest. Otherwise, flap adaptation and flap contour will not be satisfactory [3].

We can achieve postoperative flap adaptation by expelling a minimum of interproximal tissues by eliminating the pocket's epithelial lining; this aim is particularly important for the palatal side because this flap can't be stretched.

This flap design can eliminate the depth of the pockets, but for the lingual surface, pocket elimination surgery is significantly more effective than the modified Widman flap [4]. This flap is the most common flap when we have deep pockets, but this procedure could be unaesthetic in the anterior region. Modified Widman flap could be an appreciated

A. Darnahal (✉)
Tufts University School of Dental Medicine, Boston, MA, USA
e-mail: alireza.darnahal@tufts.edu

F. M. A. Boojar
School of Dentistry, Research committee of Golestan Medical University, Gorgan, Iran

© The Author(s), under exclusive license to Springer Nature Switzerland AG 2021
M. R. Stevens et al. (eds.), *Innovative Perspectives in Oral and Maxillofacial Surgery*,
https://doi.org/10.1007/978-3-030-75750-2_20

choice for treating periodontitis in the anterior maxillary area [2]. Flap elevation is limited and allows only a few millimeters of the alveolar bone crest to become exposed.

Modified Widman flap only can gain interproximal attachment, but subgingival curettage resulted in both lingual and interproximal attachment [4].

The main advantage of the modified Widman flap surgery over any other periodontal surgical procedure is the intimate postoperative adaptation of healthy collagenous tissues to all tooth surfaces. It has been shown experimentally in animals and humans that with a close adaptation of gingival tissues to the tooth surface, a marginal new epithelial attachment forms, which tend to seal off the deeper areas of separation between the tooth and the surrounding tissues [5, 6]. One of the disadvantages of modified Widman flap is unfavorable interproximal architecture promptly taking after the expulsion of the dressing, but with precise oral hygiene, we can heal it [7].

Papilla Preservation Flap

Our objective should be to conserve the interdental papillae to prevent the manifestation of unaesthetic maxillary anterior gingival architecture from making it attractive to the eye. Takei et al. in 1985 established the surgical method to conserve the interdental papillae, who defined the surgery as papilla preservation flap (PPF) technique. PPF emphasized the simplified attachment. It helped in the most favorable interdental coverage and the retention of the bone grafts and averted the graft substance's unfavorable movement [8].

The papilla preservation flap method was founded to apply in coexistence with implants regarding the periodontal osseous flaws [9].

This method involves the construction of a sulcular incision near every tooth without any cuts being done via the interdental papillae. The palatal or lingual flap includes semilunar openings with a minimum measurement of 3 mm apical to the perimeter of the interproximal bony deformity and the papillary incision line minimum of 5 mm from the gingival limit [10].

When making the incisions in the interdental areas, the scalpel blade's tip remains in contact with the root surface. This avoids compromising the blood supply to the interdental papillae and ensures a maximum amount of tissue interdentally. If you cut the papilla, you lose blood supply.

In posterior areas with a narrow interdental space, it may be necessary to trim off the papilla's tip to affect the intact papilla through space. The semilunar incision is made with the scalpel perpendicular to the gingiva's outer surface and extends through the periosteum to the alveolar process. After completing the incisions, the flaps are reflected. A curette and/or interproximal knife is used to carefully free the inter-

dental papilla from the underlying hard tissue. It is important that the interdental tissue, which is a part of the facial or lingual flap, is entirely free and mobile before proceeding to the papilla's reflection. This flap is secured with a cross mattress suture.

We use the papilla preservation flap to achieve a better aesthetic result, so it's better to use this technique in the anterior region [10].

Modified Papilla Preservation Flap (MPPF)

Checchi et al. in 1998 revised the common method. The procedure as per what some declare is that a semilunar cut should be replaced with the horizontal incision in the interproximal area, present in the opposing part of the bone deformity, as it simplifies the maintenance of the regenerated region from the oral surroundings [8]. Cortellini et al. in 1995 introduced the name modified papilla preservation flap [11].

The papilla preservation flap method remodeling has been implemented to accomplish the interproximal tissue's main closure throughout the barrier membranes positioned coronal to the alveolar crest. The conservation of the coronal placement of the interdental tissue, including the main closure, can also be undertaken by this surgical method.

Surgical Technique

In the buccal and interproximal region, the primary incision should continue to the palatal line angle, and a horizontal incision in the buccal surface should perform in the interproximal supracrestal connective tissue, just coronal to the bone crest, to dissect the papilla. Then papilla is elevated toward the palatal aspect. Vertical releasing incision divergent in corono-apical direction extending into the alveolar mucosa can be placed in the interproximal spaces neighboring the defect if coronal advancement of the flap is desired [12].

The restricted interdental areas are observed in the teeth having this flap. Excellent skills are mandatory to execute these flap operations successfully. They heavily rely on efficient dexterity, leading to longer surgical operations, and it is suggested where there is an expectancy of regenerated treatment. The (MPPF and SPPT) improvements and/or vertical internal mattress sutures soothe the tightness in the flap, assist in the passive closure of the interdental tissues, and allow the coronal placement of the flap [13].

Contraindication of MPPF

The coronal reposition of the buccal flap has a poor prognosis. We shouldn't apply this method, e.g., inadequate vestibular depth.

Although the described surgical technique has been specifically designed for use with reinforced barrier membranes, it could be adapted to different regenerative approaches involving the interdental space [12].

Simplified Papilla Preservation Technique (SPPT)

This procedure was designed to provide surgical access to interproximal bony defects while preserving interdental soft tissues, even in narrow interdental spaces and posterior teeth. Actually, we use this technique if the interproximal space is narrow (<2) [14].

Surgical Method

The gingival perimeter is the first step of the main opening at the concerned tooth's buccal line angle. This angled slit is done throughout the papilla from the buccal line angle to the interproximal below the point of union of the adjacent tooth (the blade is to be placed parallel to the longer tooth axis to generate this slanting or angular opening and to prevent the extreme trimming of the rest of the interdental tissue). This angular interdental slit is prolonged intrasulcularly in the buccal aspect of the teeth surrounding the deformity and is then augmented to dissect (slightly) the papillae of the nearby interdental regions. The alveolar bone is made more visible by 2–3 mm with this slit method.

A buccolingual horizontal incision was then performed at the base of the papilla as close as possible to the interproximal bone crest. This incision continues intrasulcularly on the palatal or lingual to neighboring teeth [14].

Advantages of SPPT

1. Allow a simple and safe manipulation of the interdental tissue even in narrow interdental space.
2. Facilitate primary closure of the interdental tissues over bioresorbable membranes without tension.
3. Prevent the collapse of the membranes into the defect because of suture compression [14].
4. This technique requires limited equipment, fast-learning curve, and potentially improved healing.
5. Reduce pain, discomfort, and faster resumption of daily activities.
6. For both patient and provider, these procedures minimize chair time and office visits [15].

Minimally Invasive Surgical Technique (MIST)

The minimally invasive surgical technique (MIST) was initially framed by Harrel and Rees [16].

A complete granulation tissue extraction and root debridement were achieved by applying this procedure with a low flap reflection and the smooth handling of a low flap reflection and the smooth handling of the tissues. To minimize the surgical distress and reform the surgical accuracy, this method was later amended by introducing microsurgical tools and microscopes, thereby resulting in negligible injury and lower flap reflection for and accelerated post-surgical recovery.

Cortellini and Tonetti, in 2007 [17], applied (MIST) to cure the inaccessible intrabony deformities with enamel matrix derivative (EMD). The intrabody deformity in this technique was examined with the preservation flap aid in constricted interdental areas. The cure for deep and shallow intrabony faults is possible with this procedure [14]. (We must evaluate the various layers of the placement level between the interproximal areas of the tooth to detect intrabony deficiency.)

Surgical Technique

1. Intrasulcular incisions are made along with the involved teeth at the interproximal site.
2. Limited extension toward the buccal or palatal/lingual side defects are approached separately.
3. Continuous incisions are avoided.
4. Vertical releasing incisions are avoided.
5. Interproximally, attempts are made to conserve as much interdental tissue as possible.
6. The two intrasulcular incisions are connected with a horizontal incision around 2–3 mm from the papillary crest.
7. In the aesthetic zone, the horizontal incision is placed palatally, whereas in the non-aesthetic zone, it can be placed either buccally or lingually.

Indications for MIST

Isolated interproximal defect, which does not extend beyond the interproximal region.

Multiple, isolated interproximal defects within a quadrant.

Contraindications of MIST

- Generalized horizontal bone defects
- Multiple, interconnected vertical defects

Standard Attributes of MIST

- The affixing of the flap is done by vertical mattress stitches

It's the least invasive method due to its incision outline; extensive reflections are ignored:

Table 20.1 Advantages and disadvantages of MIST

Advantages	Disadvantages
Reduced postoperative healing phase	Technique sensitive due to limited accessibility
Reduced postoperative complications like edema, pain, and root sensitivity	Requires specialized equipment like operating microscope, loupes, and micro-instruments
Enhanced aesthetic results due to minimal reflection and manipulation of the flaps and minimal manipulation of the papillary tissue	This may incur an increased cost to the procedure
Postoperative gingival recession is minimal or non-existent	The operator's skill becomes a dictating factor
Improved papillary soft tissue height and contour	May increase the operating time as the procedure becomes highly technique-sensitive
Increased patient's acceptance	May be difficult to gain access to the palatal defects through the limited buccal window
Limited or no scarring	Cannot be applied universally to all the defects

This table reproduces from: Sultan et al. [18]

- The flap reflection is done with acute dissection.
- The usually inaccessible areas (numerous) can be entered one at a time instead of a single flap system.
- Magnification is the surgical method by utilizing the operating loupes, microscopes, etc.
- The evasion of extracted slits or cuts.
- The graft substance or the membrane is fully concealed whenever applied to ensure the regeneration and the conservation of the interproximal papilla.
- Vertical incisions are avoided and continuous incisions are avoided.
- The flaps are secured using vertical mattress sutures.
- The application of ultrasonic scalers and the miniature scale of tools lead to the success of the complete root surface debridement with a restricted flap lift [18].

The table below listed the advantages and disadvantages of MIST [18] (Table 20.1).

Modified MIST

Cortellini and Tonetti (2009) introduced the MMIST method. The imperfections that were related to the interdental papilla were resolved surgically either with a horizontal slit as per the remodeled papilla conservation method at interdental regions broader than 2 mm or the diagonal opening succeeding the sequence of the facilitated papilla preservation flap when the interdental area was 2 mm wide or constricted. The flap elevation was restricted to the buccal flap. There were no procedures like interdental and/or intrasulcular cuts in MMIST:

The objective of the modified minimally invasive surgical technique (MMIST) is to lessen the surgical invasiveness by applying three significant goals:

1. Minimize patient morbidity
2. Minimize the interdental tissue tendency to collapse
3. Enhance the wound/soft tissue stability [18]

Conclusion

This chapter describes flap design, papilla reconstruction techniques, and soft tissue management toward the enhancement of the attached gingiva. Several intraoral flaps and their modifications have been reported in this chapter. We also mentioned some standard flap techniques (modified Widman flap, papilla preservation flap, modified papilla preservation flap, simplified papilla preservation technique, minimally invasive surgical technique, and modified minimally invasive surgical technique) and their advantages and disadvantages. It is important to understand the patients' needs for applying these flaps. Choosing appropriate flap design would affect the final aesthetic outcome or postoperative morbidity, so it is essential for medicolegal and economic impacts.

References

1. Furness J. Contemporary oral and maxillofacial surgery. Br Dent J. 2013;215(2):99.
2. Shekar CB. Modified widman flap and papilla preservation flap in maxillary anterior region-a comparative study (Doctoral dissertation, RGUHS); 2006–2009.
3. Ramfjord SP, Nissle RR. The modified widman flap. J Periodontol. 1974;45(8):601–7. https://doi.org/10.1902/jop.1974.45.8.2.601. PMID: 4529305.
4. Burgett FG, Knowles JW, Nissle RR, Shick RA, Ramfjord SP. Short term results of three modalities of periodontal treatment. J Periodontol. 1977;48(3):131–5.
5. Caffesse RG, Ramfjord SP, Nasjleti CE. Reverse bevel periodontal flaps in monkeys. J Periodontol. 1968;39(4):219–35.
6. Sullivan H, Dinner D, Carman D. Clinical evaluation of the laterally positioned flap. Int Ass Dent Res. 1971;49:169.
7. Ramfjord SP, Knowles JW, Nissle RR, Shick RA, Burgett FG. Longitudinal study of periodontal therapy. J Periodontol. 1973;44(2):66–77.
8. Checchi L, Schonfeld SE. A technique for esthetic treatment of maxillary anterior infrabony lesions. Quintessence Int. 1988;19(3):209–13. PMID: 3269576.
9. App GR. Periodontal treatment for the removable partial prosthesis patient. Another half-century? Dent Clin N Am. 1973;17(4):601–10.
10. Takei HH, Han TJ, Carranza FA Jr, Kenney EB, Lekovic V. Flap technique for periodontal bone implants: papilla preservation technique. J Periodontol. 1985;56(4):204–10.
11. Checchi L, Montevecchi M, Checchi V, Bonetti GA. A modified papilla preservation technique, 22 years later. Quintessence Int. 2009;40(4):303–11.

12. Cortellini P, Prato GP, Tonetti MS. The modified papilla preservation technique. A new surgical approach for interproximal regenerative procedures. J Periodontol. 1995;66(4):261–6.

13. Dohan DM, Choukroun J, Diss A, Dohan SL, Dohan AJ, Mouhyi J, Gogly B. Platelet-rich fibrin (PRF): a second-generation platelet concentrate. Part I: technological concepts and evolution. Oral Surg Oral Med Oral Pathol Oral Radiol Endod. 2006;101(3):e37–44.

14. Cortellini P, Prato GP, Tonetti MS. The simplified papilla preservation flap. A novel surgical approach for the management of soft tissues in regenerative procedures. Int J Periodontics Restorative Dent. 1999;19(6):589–99.

15. Trombelli L, Simonelli A, Minenna L, Vecchiatini R, Farina R. Simplified procedures to treat periodontal intraosseous defects in esthetic areas. Periodontol 2000. 2018;77(1):93–110.

16. Harrel SK, Rees TD. Granulation tissue removal in routine and minimally invasive procedures. Compend Contin Educ Dent (Jamesburg, NJ: 1995). 1995;16(9):960–2.

17. Cortellini P, Tonetti MS. A minimally invasive surgical technique with an enamel matrix derivative in the regenerative treatment of intra-bony defects: a novel approach to limit morbidity. J Clin Periodontol. 2007;34(1):87–93.

18. Sultan N, Jafri Z, Sawai M, Bhardwaj A. Minimally invasive periodontal therapy. J Oral Biol Craniofac Res. 2020;10:161–5.

Mahmood Dashti and Maneli Ardeshir Zadeh

Introduction

Gingival recession is the subjection of the root surface due to the gingival margin's advancement to the cementoenamel junction (CEJ). It can be generalized or restricted to be linked with a single or multiple tooth regions [1]. Gingival recession is defined to distinguish the marginal gingiva's apical progression from the standard location on the crown of the tooth to different layers on the surface of the root past the cementoenamel junction [2]. Gingival recession can be related to abrasion and/or cervical wear, decay due to the subjection of the root region to the oral surroundings, a rise in the buildup of dental plaque, root caries, and dentin hypersensitivity [3]. Research validates that it's prevalent in a minimum of a single tooth or multiple tooth regions in 23% of the American adults in the age bracket of 30–90 years, making it a reasonably familiar clinical affliction [4]. The mucogingival defects and ailments nearing the teeth and edentulous ridges comprise gingival extreme and unusual coloration, absence of keratinized gingiva, abnormal frenal pull/muscle location, low vestibular depth, and, lastly, gingival/mucosal tissue recession as per the grading framework established by the American Academy of Periodontology [5].

Etiology

The etiology of gingival recession is mostly dependent on numerous factors. Chan et al. list the gingival recession's etiological features as per induced aspects and the precipitating aspects [6].

M. Dashti (✉)
Private practice, Tehran, Iran
e-mail: dashti.mahmood72@gmail.com

M. A. Zadeh
Private practice, Irvine, CA, USA
e-mail: ardeshirzadehmaneli@yahoo.com

Despite the induced aspects being related to anatomical elements like the thickening gingival biotype and underlying bone, this could also indicate inflammation.

Other anatomical influencing elements comprise an absence of sufficient keratinized gingiva [7] and the frenal pull.

Research that differentiated regions with inadequate mucosa that was being affixed identified that a fixed loss or recession did not advance with time [8]. In a modern meta-analysis, after analyzing 1647 regions of the buccal gingival recession, 78.1% of the patients saw a development in the gingival recession on further examination after 2 or more years.

There was a rise in the likelihood of recession formation on a long-term basis (probability ratio 2.43; $p = 0.03$) or the total regions revealing gingival recession (probability ratio 2.16; $p = 0.0005$) according to combined approximations. The Not treating gingival recession can lead to a greater likelihood of its advancement, despite receiving the necessary home supervision as per the writers' deduction [9].

The Etiology List

(a) Calculus: The link between gingival recession to the subgingival and supragingival calculus can be recognized due to the poor availability of prophylactic dental treatment [9].

(b) Brushing of Tooth: Khocht et al. highlighted the utilization of a hard toothbrush being a cause of recession [10].

(c) High Frenal Attachment: This could obstruct plaque extraction due to a pull on the margin of gingiva [11].

(d) The Tooth's Location: Tooth that reveals a discharge near the mucogingival line can reveal concentrated gingival recession due to the absence of or inadequate keratinized tissue [12].

(e) Orthodontic Forces Causing Tooth Displacement: The enlargement of the arch and the extreme proclination of incisors classified as tooth displacements are related to a much higher risk of gingival recession [13].

(f) Poor Design of the Partial Dentures: The preservation or shape of the partial dentures that leads to the accumulation of plaque and the occurrence of gingival distress has the likelihood to give rise to gingival recession [14].

(g) Smoking: The prevalence of gingival recession is higher among smokers than nonsmokers. The regions of the recession were discovered on the mandibular central incisors, premolars, and buccal surfaces of maxillary molars [15].

(h) Restorations: The rise in plaque formation, alveolar bone depletion, and gingival inflammation are due to the subgingival restoration margins [16].

(i) Chemicals: Gingival erosions and ulcerations are due to topical cocaine implementation [17].

Categorization

The two significant categories of marginal gingival recession have been discovered. The first category is more generic, which constitutes interproximal regions, and is usually situated in the populations which is not receiving any treatment and showing bad oral health or care. The second category is mostly about distressing elements and frequently includes a cluster of or fewer teeth. The second category is observed in buccal regions where the abrasions are usually linked with smooth, well-polished hard tissue disproportions and lack of plaque [18, 19].

Miller came up with a handy flaw in the recession that was categorized as per the height of the interdental bone and interproximal papillae close to the faulty region, including the mucogingival association junction [20].

The practicality of this categorization helps in choosing different remedies [18].

Shortcomings of Gingival Recession Categorized By Miller

- *Class I.* Marginal tissue recession that does not advance to the mucogingival junction (MGJ). An absence of a periodontal loss (tender tissue or bone) in the interdental region and a comprehensive root coverage are most anticipated.
- The anticipation of 100% coverage
- *Class II.* The advancement of the marginal tissue recession until or after the MGJ. The absence of periodontal loss (tender tissue or bone) in the interdental region and a comprehensive root coverage are to be expected.
- Prediction of 100% coverage

- *Class III.* The progression of marginal tissue recession until or after the MGJ. A faulty placement of the teeth is evident, and so is the occurrence of the loss of tender tissue or bone in the interdental region, which is an obstacle to strive for 100% root coverage. An incomplete root coverage can be foreseen. Before the operation, the extent of the root coverage can be diagnosed with the help of a periodontal probe. The probe is positioned in a made-up line in a horizontal manner linking the layer of tissue at the center of the face of both the teeth situated on one of the positions of the teeth or tooth showing symptoms of a recession. Root coverage is expected within that layer.
- Prediction of an incomplete coverage
- *Class IV.* The advancement of the marginal tissue recession until or after the MGJ. The soft tissue or bone loss in the interdental region and/or arrangement of the teeth is quite extreme, hence ruling out the hope of root coverage.
- No hope of a coverage

Alternative Categorization

1. Ullivan and Atkins et al. – This categorization, despite being easy, is put through an open examination because of the inconsistencies in the inter-examiner and examiner. Hence, it cannot be replicated [21, 22].
2. Mlinek et al. – The variable assessment can exist at different lengths, and hence this categorization does not define the milestone for the horizontal evaluation [23].
3. Smith in 1990 – In situations of a sizeable vertical portion as suggested by the author, additional horizontal parts can be administered at an intermediate length between the base and the CEJ of the imperfection that does not have a clear description. Additionally, the allocation of distinct assessments can be done for teeth with multiple roots, leading to an increase in complexity. It can result in extreme anticipation of the ailment as the sensitivity adopted here is based on one's personal understanding. The distal and mesial surfaces' central points are also hard to identify when a flawless interdental papilla exists [24].

Mahajan suggested a revision to Miller's categorization in 2010. The complete clinical ailments are absent in this revision, e.g., as there is no reference to the implementation of MGJ in class III [25], a tooth having a gingival recession without advancing up to MGJ but with interdental hard and tender-tissue loss cannot be placed in class I and class III, respectively [25].

After reviewing the above drawbacks, a modern categorization structure is being presented that has the attribute of it being clear and educative, according to Miller's categorization. This current categorization can be carried out for lingual and facial regions of mandibular teeth, and the facial area of maxillary teeth and the grading of interdental papilla recession are also feasible.

The grading structure that is recommended here permits a simple technique to evaluate the advancing degrees of gingival recession by utilizing anatomical milestones as a knowledgeable source that is discerned at will. The degree of gingival recession's explanation is also included.

The implementation of this technique should act as a guideline for interactions between researchers and clinicians in the future [26].

It is grouped into four categories, including subdivisions a and b [26]:

- Class I – Apical movement in the crest of the marginal gingiva, 1–2 mm from CEJ I
    (a) The absence of any interproximal loss of tissue
    (b) Presence of interproximal tissue loss coronal to clinical interproximal CEJ
- Class II – Apical movement in the marginal gingiva crest, greater than 2 mm and less than 3 mm from CEJ
    (a) Absence of any clinical interproximal loss of tissue
    (b) Presence of interproximal loss of tissue coronal to clinical interproximal CEJ
- Class III – Apical movement in the crest of the marginal gingiva >=3 mm from CEJ
    (a) Absence of any clinical interproximal loss of tissue
    (b) Presence of interproximal tissue loss apical to clinical interproximal CEJ
- Class IV – Apical movement in the marginal gingiva crest >3 mm from CEJ with an extremely malposed tooth
    (a) Absence of any clinical interproximal loss of tissue
    (b) Presence of interproximal tissue loss apical to clinical interproximal CEJ

The categories specified above have their shortcomings, comprising:

1. The various systems of prognosis for root coverage are not stated.
2. In a few circumstances, the CEJ is untraceable or misplaced due to lesion, restorations, and abfraction that make it hard to categorize recession, as CEJ is a milestone that is utilized in this recommended categorization.

Prognosis

A prognosis is defined as foreseeing the possible time, course, and result of an ailment according to a common understanding of the ailment's pathogenesis and the occurrence of the dangers associated with the ailment.

Prognostic elements are the circumstances that foresee the results of the existence of the ailment.

On a few occasions, the prognostic aspects and factors of threat are the same, e.g., diabetic patients or those with a history of smoking have a greater chance of suffering from a periodontal ailment. Once they show the symptoms, they usually exhibit a more serious prognosis.

The categorization of prognosis in the past has been outlined according to researches that assess tooth mortality [27–31].

One system allocates the grouping as given below [29–31]:

1. Good prognosis: Sufficient periodontal aid and management of etiological elements confirm that the tooth will be simple to preserve by the clinician and the patient.
2. Fair prognosis: An estimated loss of 25% of the attachment or grade I furcation invasion (depth and placement enable the correct preservation with a sound acceptance of the patient).
3. Poor prognosis: An attachment loss of 50%, grade II furcation invasion (depth and placement make preservation tough but feasible).
4. Questionable prognosis: bad root formation, attachment loss of 50%, bad crown-to-root ratio, grade II furcation invasion (depth and placement make it hard to approach), or grade III furcation invasion; closeness to the root; mobility no 2 or 3.
5. Hopeless prognosis: Insufficient attachment to look after one's daily functions, well-being, and contentment.

One must identify that moderate, sound, and dreadful prognosis can be set up with a rational degree of precision in this grouped structure. But, doubtful and bad prognoses will mostly continue to different classes as they rely on many elements that can associate with numerous methods that are uncertain [32–34].

Kwok and Caton [29] put forward a system that was different from the procedures related to tooth mortality on "the possibility of achieving rationality of the periodontal supporting apparatus." This system relates to the likelihood of advancing the ailment connected to the systemic and regional aspects.

Every aspect is critical and should be taken into deliberation to allocate a prognosis, despite a few of these elements that can influence the advancement of the ailment than others.

This system is explained below [35]:

1. Useless prognosis: Removal of the tooth.

2. Bad prognosis: The systemic or regional aspects affecting the periodontal standing cannot be supervised. A complete periodontal cure and preservation may not stop a periodontal failure in the future.

3. Doubtful prognosis: The systemic or regional aspects affecting the tooth's periodontal standing may or may not be managed. The periodontal standing, if managed, can be stabilized with a complete periodontal surgery. Otherwise, there may be a possible occurrence of periodontal failure in the future.

4. Good prognosis: The loss of periodontal support is unexpected to occur in the future. A complete periodontal surgery and aftercare will stabilize the position of the tooth.

As periodontal steadiness is evaluated daily with the help of clinical methods, it may be more practical to create resolutions for surgery and to foresee prognosis than striving to establish the possibility of the tooth that will be lost [35].

Perils

The risk aspects are the attributes that can put a person under a more significant threat of contracting an ailment. Evaluation of threats is described by multiple elements [27, 30].

The threat of an ailment is a person's likelihood of contracting a distinct condition at a particular time. The prospects of contracting the ailment will differ from person to person [35].

1. Threatening elements
   (a) Microbial deposits in the tooth and pathogenic bacteria
   (b) Smoking tobacco
   (c) Diabetes
2. Determinants of threats/background attributes
   (a) Age
   (b) Gender
   (c) Genetic factors
   (d) Stress
   (e) Socioeconomic standing
3. Danger signs
   (a) Osteoporosis
   (b) Irregular appointments with the dentist
   (c) Acquired immunodeficiency syndrome (AIDS)/ human immunodeficiency virus (HIV)
4. Signs/estimates of threats
   (a) Bleeding on poking
   (b) Medical history of periodontal ailment

Strategies for Cure

1. *Crowns, Veneer, and Restoration*

Crowns could be attached to expand the clinical height than to conceal the subjected root area.

2. *Manufacturing Gingival Mask*

Patients with multiple teeth having symptoms of a recession may exhibit an unattractive look due to black triangles.

3. *Root Conditioning*

The use of citric acid or tetracycline HCl at the root area before the attachment of a tender- tissue graft.

4. *Frenectomy*

Frenectomy is recommended if the recession is due to a frenal pull in those situations.

5. *Root Coverage Surgical Methods*

Recession may be followed by abraded areas or root caries, where patients may lament about flaws in appearance or root hypersensitivity. The regeneration of the missing attachment apparatus of the teeth is one of the objectives of the periodontal cure. Numerous techniques of regeneration have the potential to rectify the flaws of the gingival recession by achieving a complete or an incomplete root coverage and the increase in the height and width of the affixed or keratinized gingiva [32].

Soft-Tissue Crafting

Root coverage is one of the aims of soft-tissue grating. The success rate of the root coverage techniques is usually hard to estimate. It relies on multiple aspects, comprising the method that is adopted, the placement, and the category of the recession [32].

The frequently computed gingival measurements are the distances between the mucogingival line and tender-tissue limit calculated in millimeters and the height.

A favorable result of gingival augmentation is reckoned by a rise in gingival height, separate from the number of millimeters [36].

Lateral Pedicle Graft

The pedicle flap base in the *pedicle graft* has its own blood reserve by simplifying the recreation of the vascular union with the receiving site and continuing the graft. Pedicle grafts may be entirely or slightly thick [37, 38]. The implementation of laterally positioned pedicle graft (LPPG) is not logical until there is a Significant gingiva lateral to where the recession is located. A shallow vestibule can endanger the results too. The utilization of LPPG imparts a perfect match in color, but it's still usually insufficient to cure numerous recessions [32].

The adoption of pedicle grafts to rectify the defectes of mucogingival has been suggested by using an edentulous region as a donor site [39]. If the secured gingiva on the areas of the face of two or three successive teeth is not sufficient, then this method is specifically practical in such situations. That method carries out the advancement of the incomplete thick flaps near the concerned teeth by sliding the complete flap one-half tooth width and then positioning the interdental papillary tissues beyond the tooth's buccal regions that are to be operated [40]. In most cases, the planting involves a mix of a long junctional epithelium (2.0 mm) and the placing of connective tissue (2.1 mm). The histologic examination validated the tissue damage to be the least and the recovery to be fast.

Cohen and Ross [41] has recommended using a double papilla flap that is repositioned to conceal the flaws in situations where there exists an insufficient portion of gingiva in the adjoining region for a lateral sliding flap or the existence of an incomplete part of the gingiva (Fig. 21.1).

The papilla from all portions of the tooth is rotated and reflected beyond the receiving tooth's midfacial element and sutured. The denudation only of interdental bone and the twofold blood reserve is the only unique benefit of this method. The tearing of the gingival papilla and the pulling of the sutures may constitute its shortcomings [41–44].

Coronally Positioned Grafts

It is a dual-phase process. In the primary phase, an autogenous tender-tissue graft that is free is planted apical to a denuded root region. The flap is coronally repositioned following the patient's recovery.

For the success of CPGs, the following are needed:

- An estimated standard interproximal bone height.
- Shallow crevicular depths on proximal areas should exist.
- The height of the tissue is to be inside 1 mm of the cementoenamel junction, or CEJ, on the adjoining teeth.
- Sufficient flap to avoid retraction while recovering.
- The projection of the root is to be lessened in the plane of the adjoining alveolar bone.
- Sufficient recovery of the free graft (if carried out) before the coronal placement.

The utilization of a split-thickness dissection in the next phase of the process is done with mesial and distal vertical releasing cuts only till accomplishing the necessary flap mobility. The flap is sutured in the range of 0.5–1 mm to the CEJ and is concealed with a periodontal dressing [45].

The lateral sliding flaps were collated with coronally placed flaps to cure the isolated gingival recessions [46–47]. In a half-year study, both the methods provided acceptable outcomes, as there were no variations in sulcus depth or a spread of gingiva, and no variations in the tissue coverage were documented (Figs. 21.2 and 21.3).

An average recession coverage of 67% and a 2.7 mm soft tissue on average were achieved.

The outcomes were consistent for 3 years, but the one and only variation between the two methods was an estimated growth of 1 mm in the subjected root at the lateral sliding flap donor region, as no other recession was noticed in the CPF.

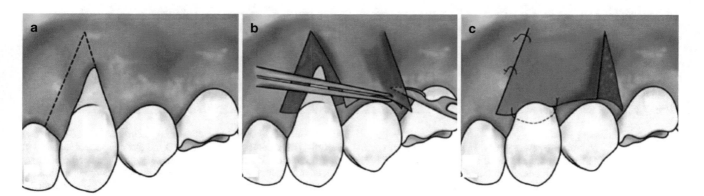

Fig. 21.1 There stages of lateral sliding flap technique. (**a**) Initial incision passes mucogingival junction. (**b**) Releasing the flap at the bucal surface. (**c**) Sliding the partial thickness flap and positioning it on the recession area. (Reproduced with permission from: Wong [50])

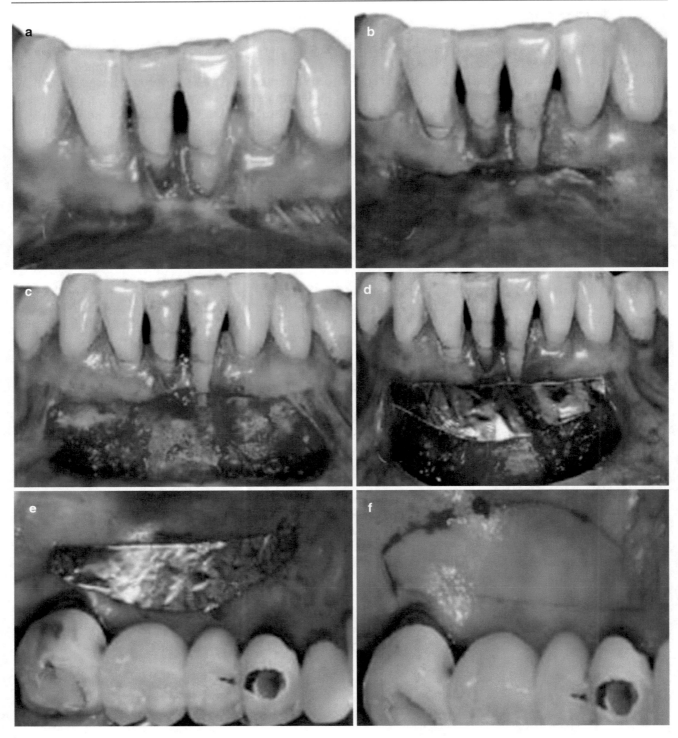

Fig. 21.2 Coronally placed flap

Clinical case of a patient with severe gingival recession defects in mandibular anterior region. The preoperative view shows Miller class IV in central incisors and class III recession in lateral incisor area (**a**). Initial horizontal incision was made (**b**), followed by partial-thickness dissection to remove all loose alveolar mucosa, elastic fibers, and muscle attachments (**c**). A template was trimmed to define the planned dimensions of the free gingival graft (FGG) relative to the recipient bed (**d**) and donor site (**e**). The donor site was outlined (**f**), and a thick FGG (approximately 1.5 mm in thickness) was harvested (**g, h**) and fixated to the recipient bed (**i**). One-week healing results before (**j**) and after suture removal (**k**) showed excellent graft incorporation and donor site healing (**l**). The clinical results after 3 months showed an increase in gingival margin thickness and an increase in attached keratinized gingiva zone (**m**). To harmonize the gingival margins, coronal positioning of the gingival margins was attempted. A trapezoidal flap was made by two distal vertical releasing incisions (**n**) with split-thickness dissection (**o**) and coronal positioning of the flap (**p**). Postoperative results show harmonized gingival margins (**q**). Clinical case, courtesy of Dr. Goncalo Carames. (Reproduced with permission from: Zadeh and Gil [51])

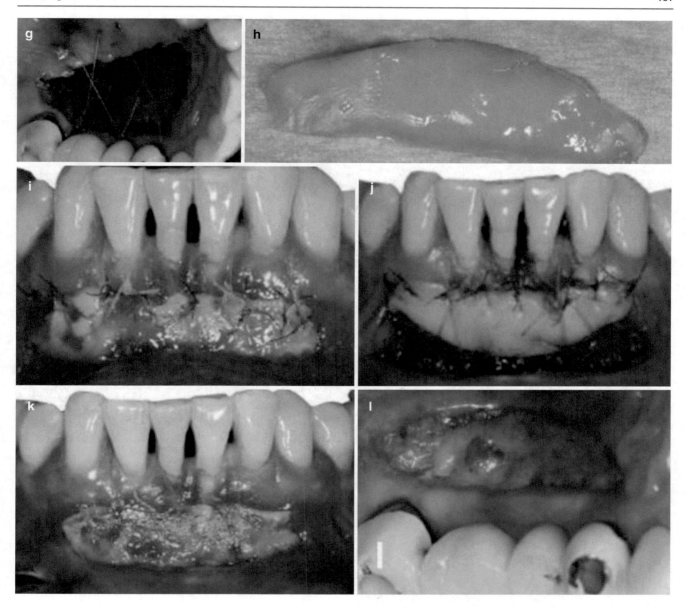

Fig. 21.2 (continued)

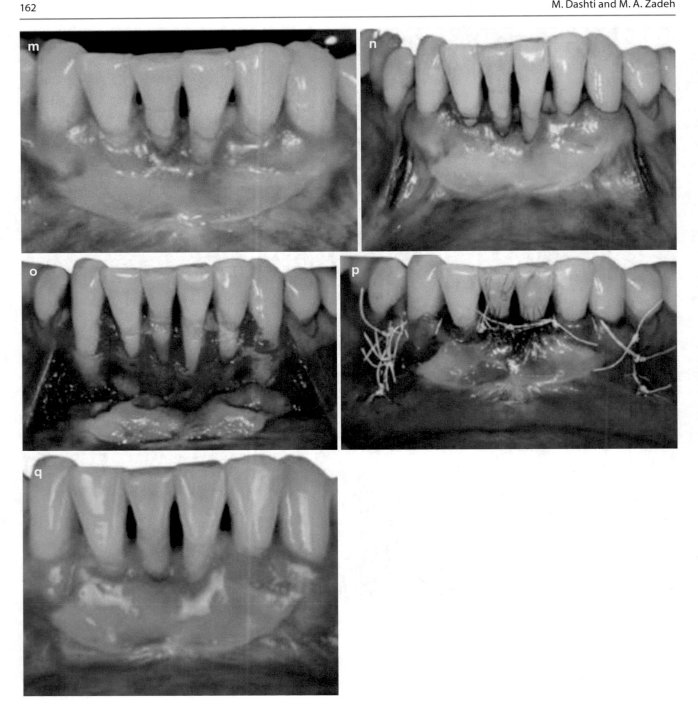

Fig. 21.2 (continued)

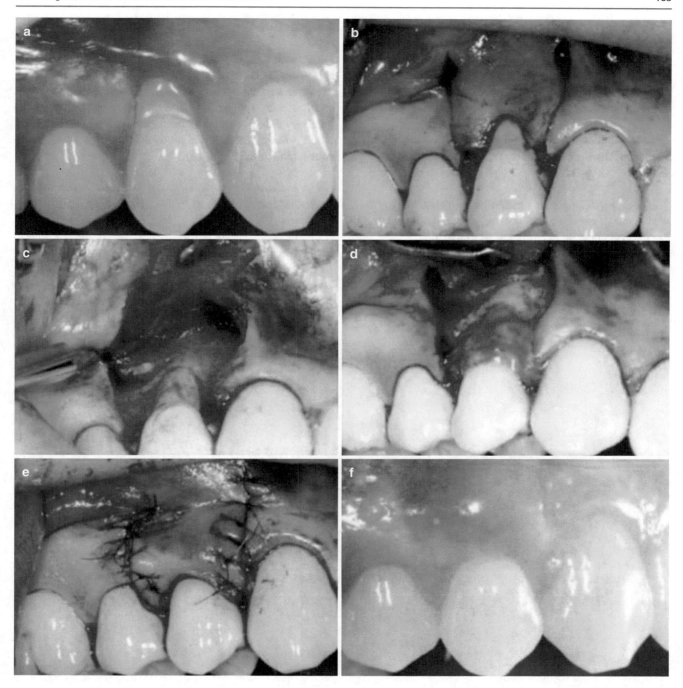

Fig. 21.3 Two coronally advanced flap with a subepithelial connective tissue graft (SCTG), single Miller class I defect. (**a**) Baseline, (**b**) incisions, (**c**) split-full-split preparation, (**d**) SCTG, (**e**) sutures, (**f**) 5-year outcome. (Reproduced with permission from: Windisch and Molnár [52])

Free Autogenous Soft-Tissue Grafts

The dual types of autogenous grafts can be utilized for root coverage; the first graft contains an epithelialized layer. The second graft includes just a tiny epithelialized collar or no collar at all.

Free Epithelialized Autogenous Gingival Grafts

The devising of a receiving site by carrying out subperiosteal dissection to expel the connective and epithelium tissue to the periosteum is an integral part of this method.

A few of the conventional regions for the donor substance comprise palatal gingiva, edentulous ridges, and affixed gingiva [32] (Fig. 21.4).

Connective Tissue Autogenous Grafts

Langer and Langer [48] were the first to document the utilization of CTGs for root coverage. A thick flap (incomplete) with two vertical openings was raised on the receiving site, succeeded by the graft positioning accumulated from the palate by a dual parallel incision method. To avail twice the blood reserve, the flap was placed coronally as an effort to conceal the graft (Fig. 21.5).

Association of Single or Multiple Methods

Numerous clinicians have tried to integrate various methods to improve the success rate of the root coverage. Nelson [43] adopted the CTG, including a twin pedicle graft. Firstly, a free CTG was positioned beyond the root's denuded area, succeeded by a twofold pedicle graft to slightly conceal the CTG.

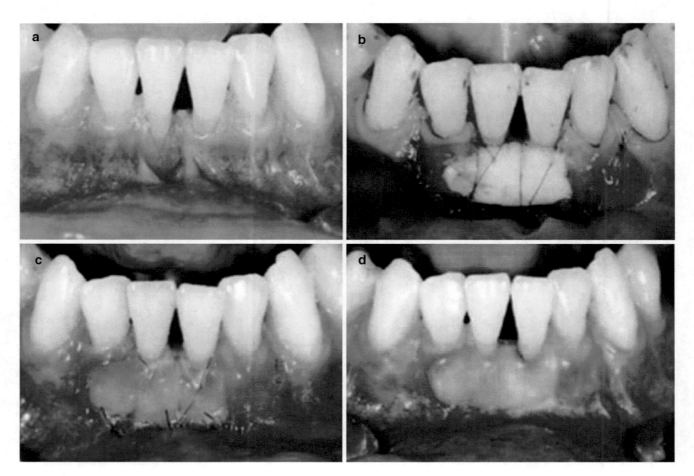

Fig. 21.4 Apically repositioned flap in combination with a free gingival graft for treatment of multiple Miller class IV defects. (**a**) Baseline, (**b**) graft in place, (**c**) 14-day healing, (**d**) 1-year outcome sutures. (Reproduced with permission from: Windisch and Molnár [53])

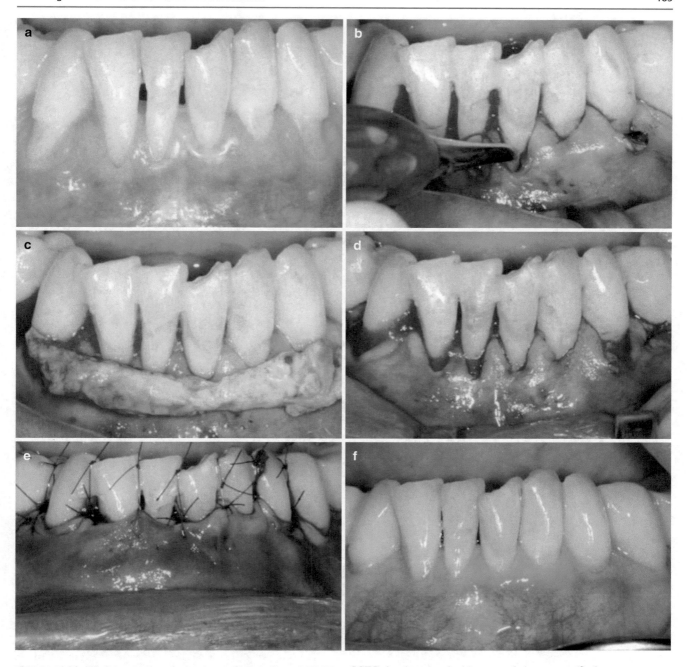

Fig. 21.5 Modified coronally advanced tunnel technique (MCAT) with a subepithelial connective tissue graft (SCTG), multiple Miller class III defects. (**a**) Baseline, (**b**) tunneling, (**c**) SCTG trimmed, (**d**) SCTG in the tunnel, (**e**) suspended sutures, (**f**) 2-year outcome. (Reproduced with permission from Windisch and Molnár [52])

Guided Tissue Regeneration

According to the American Academy of Periodontology, the description of regeneration is "a reconstitution or reproduction of a wounded or missing portion. Hence, it's the biological procedure by which the structure and function of missing tissues are fully repaired" [49]. This suggests the regeneration of the tooth's supporting tissues, the periodontal ligament, the cementum, and the alveolar bone (Fig. 21.6).

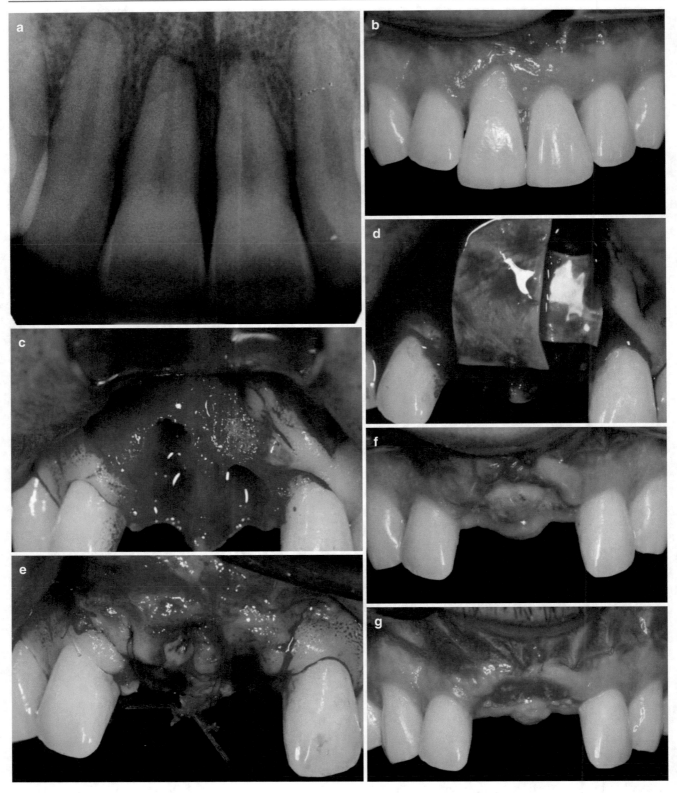

Fig. 21.6 Early wound dehiscence with exposure of mineralized allograft and collagen membrane is better tolerated than with non-resorbable membrane. (**a–e**) Extraction and augmentation of two maxillary central incisor defects with human mineralized allograft and resorbable collagen membrane. (**f**) Early wound dehiscence occurring 1 week after surgery with exposure of collagen membrane and allograft. (**g**) Early granulation of exposed graft. (Reproduced with permission from: Le [54])

Conclusion

The clinician must closely monitor the gingival recession as it can get out of hand (become very serious), and that will eventually result in tooth removal. Clinicians must have the ability to ascertain the prognosis of the tooth related to the category/class of the recession, by which the clinician should be proactive regarding the measures that are needed to be taken to outdo or cure the recession or remove the infected or useless teeth and thereby implement various surgical techniques comprising implants or bridge crowns.

References

1. Kassab MM, Cohen RE. The etiology and prevalence of gingival recession. J Am Dent Assoc. 2003;134(2):220–5.
2. Löe H, Anerud A, Boysen H. The natural history of periodontal disease in man: prevalence, severity, and extent of gingival recession. J Periodontol. 1992;63:489–95. [PubMed: 1625148].
3. Mathur A, Jain M, Jain K, Samar M, Goutham B, Swamy PD, et al. Gingival recession in school kids aged 10–15 years in Udaipur, India. J Indian Soc Periodontol. 2009;13:16–20. [PMCID: PMC2846669] [PubMed: 20376235].
4. Albandar JM, Kingman A. Gingival recession, gingival bleeding, and dental calculus in adults 30 years of age and older in the United States, 1988–1994. J Periodontol. 1999;70:30–43.
5. Armitage GC. Development of a classification system for periodontal diseases and conditions. Ann Periodontol. 1999;4:1–6.
6. Chan HL, Chun YH, MacEachern M, Oates TW. Does gingival recession require surgical treatment? Dent Clin North Am. 2015;59:981–96.
7. Lang NP, Löe H. The relationship between the width of keratinized gingiva and gingival health. J Periodontol. 1972;43:623–7.
8. Kennedy JE, Bird WC, Palcanis KG, Dorfman HS. A longitudinal evaluation of varying widths of attached gingiva. J Clin Periodontol. 1985;12:667–75.
9. Chambrone L, Tatakis DN. Periodontal soft tissue root coverage procedures: a systematic review from the AAP Regeneration Workshop. J Periodontol. 2015;86(Suppl 2):S8–S51.
10. Van Palenstein Helderman WH, Lembariti BS, Van Der Weijden GA, Van't Hof MA. Gingival recession and its association with calculus in subjects deprived of prophylactic dental care. J Clin Periodontol. 1998;25(2):106–11.
11. Khocht A, Simon G, Person P, Denepitiya JL. Gingival recession in relation to history of hard toothbrush use. J Periodontol. 1993;64(9):900–5. [5].
12. Trott JR, Love B. An analysis of localized gingival recession in 766 Winnipeg High School students. Dent Pract Dent Rec. 1966;16(6):209–13.
13. Zachrisson BU. Orthodontics and periodontics. In: Lindhe J, editor. Clinical periodontology and implant dentistry. 3rd ed. Copenhagen: Munksgaard; 1998. p. 741–93.
14. Artun J, Krogstad O. Periodontal status of mandibular incisors following excessive proclination. A study in adults with surgically treated mandibular prognathism. Am J Orthod Dentofacial Orthop. 1987;91(3):225–32.
15. Wright PS, Hellyer PH. Gingival recession related to removable partial dentures in older patients. J Prosthet Dent. 1995;74(6):602–7.
16. Gunsolley JC, Quinn SM, Tew J, Gooss CM, Brooks CN, Schenkein HA. The effect of smoking on individuals with minimal periodontal destruction. J Periodontol. 1998;69(2):165–70.
[10] Parma-Benfenati S, Fugazzato PA, Ruben MP. He effect of restorative margins on post—surgical development and nature of periodontium. Int J Periodontics Restorative Dent. 1985;5:31–51.
17. Quart AM, Butkus Small C, Klein RS. The cocaine connection. Users imperil their gingiva. J Am Dent Assoc. 1991;122(1):85–7.
18. Maynard JG. The value of periodontal plastic surgery-root coverage. Int J Periodont Rest Dent. 2004;24(1):9.
19. Miller PD Jr. Root coverage with the free gingival graft. Factors associated with incomplete coverage. J Periodontol. 1987;58(10):674–81.
20. Miller PD Jr. Root coverage using the free soft tissue autograft following citric acid application. III. A successful and predictable procedure in areas of deep-wide recession. Int J Periodont Rest Dent. 1985;5(2):14–37.
21. Sullivan HC, Atkins JH. Free autogenous gingival grafts. I. Principles of successful grafting. Periodontics. 1968;6:121–9.
22. Camargo PM, Melnick PR, Kenney EB. The use of free gingival grafts for aesthetic purposes. Periodontol 2000. 2001;27:72–96.
23. Mlinek A, Smukler H, Buchner A. The use of free gingival grafts for the coverage of denuded roots. J Periodontol. 1973;44:248–54.
24. Smith RG. Gingival recession. Reappraisal of an enigmatic condition and a new index for monitoring. J Clin Periodontol. 1997;24:201–5.
25. Mahajan A. Mahajan's modification of the Miller's classification for gingival recession. Dent Hypotheses. 2010;1:45–50.
26. Guttiganur N, Aspalli S, Sanikop MV, Desai A, Gaddale R, Devanoorkar A. Classification systems for gingival recession and suggestion of a new classification system. Indian J Dent Res. 2018;29(2):233–7. https://doi.org/10.4103/ijdr.IJDR_207_17.
27. Becker W, Becker B, Berg L. Periodontal treatment without maintenance. A retrospective study in 44 patients. J Periodontol. 1984;55:505.
28. Becker W, Berg L, Becker B. The long-term evaluation of periodontal treatment and maintenance in 95 patients. Int J Periodontics Restorative Dent. 1984;4:54.
29. Kwok V, Caton J. Prognosis revisited: a system for assigning periodontal prognosis. J Periodontol. 2007;78:2063.
30. McGuire MK. Prognosis versus actual outcome: a long-term survey of 100 treated periodontal patients under maintenance care. J Periodontol. 1991;62:51.
31. MK MG, Nunn ME. Prognosis versus actual outcome. II. The effectiveness of clinical parameters in developing an accurate prognosis. J Periodontol. 1996;67:658.
32. Kassab MM, Badawi H, Dentino AR. Treatment of gingival recession. Dent Clin N Am. 2010;54(1):129–40. https://doi.org/10.1016/j.cden.2009.08.009.
33. Chace R Sr, Low SB. Survival characteristics of periodontally involved teeth: a 40-year study. J Periodontol. 1993;64:701.
34. Ghaia S, Bissada NF. Prognosis and actual treatment outcome of periodontally involved teeth. Periodontal Clin Investig. 1996;18:7.
35. Newman M, Takei H, Klokkevold P, Carranza F. Newman and Carranza's clinical periodontology. 13th ed. Philadelphia: Elsevier; 2019.
36. Shapiro N. Retaining periodontally "hopeless" teeth: a case report. J Am Dent Assoc. 1994;125:596.
37. Wennström JL, Zucchelli J. Increased gingival dimensions: a significant factor for successful outcome of root coverage procedures? A 2- year prospective clinical study. J Clin Periodontol. 1996;23:770–7.
38. Pfeifer J, Heller R. Histologic evaluation of full and partial thickness lateral repositioned flaps: a pilot study. J Periodontol. 1971;42:331–3.
39. Sugarman EF. A clinical and histological study of the attachment of grafted tissue to bone and teeth. J Periodontol. 1969;40:381–7.
40. Corn H. Edentulous area pedicle grafts in mucogingival surgery. Periodontics. 1964;2:229–42.

41. Hattler AB. Mucogingival surgery: utilization of interdental gingiva as attached gingiva by surgical displacement. Periodontics. 1967;5:126–31.

42. Cohen DW, Ross SE. The double papillae repositioned flap in periodontal therapy. J Periodontol. 1968;39:65–70.

43. Nelson S. The subpedicle connective tissue graft: a bilaminar reconstructive procedure for the coverage of denuded root surfaces. J Periodontol. 1986;58:95–102.

44. Harris RJ. The connective tissue and partial thickness double pedicle graft: a predictable method of obtaining root coverage. J Periodontol. 1992;63:477–86.

45. Maynard JG. Coronal positioning of a previously placed autogenous gingival graft. J Periodontol. 1977;48:151–5.

46. Guinard EA, Caffesse RG. Treatment of localized gingival recessions, part III: comparison of results obtained with lateral sliding and coronally repositioned flaps. J Periodontol. 1978;49:457–61.

47. Caffesse RG, Guinard EA. Treatment of localized gingival recessions, part IV: results after three years. J Periodontol. 1980;51:167–70.

48. Langer B, Langer L. Subepithelial connective tissue graft technique for root coverage. J Periodontol. 1985;56:715–20.

49. The American Academy of Periodontology. Annals of Periodontology World Workshop in periodontics. Chicago: American Academy of Periodontics; 1996. p. 621.

50. Wong DH. Mucogingival and periodontal plastic surgery: lateral sliding flaps. In: Nares S, editor. Advances in periodontal surgery. Cham: Springer; 2020. https://doi.org/10.1007/978-3-030-12310-9_11.

51. Zadeh HH, Gil A. Coronally positioned flaps and tunneling. In: Nares S, editor. Advances in periodontal surgery. Cham: Springer; 2020. https://doi.org/10.1007/978-3-030-12310-9_9.

52. Windisch P, Molnár B. Recession coverage using autogenous grafts. In: Kasaj A, editor. Gingival recession management. Cham: Springer; 2018. https://doi.org/10.1007/978-3-319-70719-8_8.

53. Windisch P, Molnár B. Surgical management of gingival recession using autogenous soft tissue grafts. Clin Dent Rev. 2019;3. https://doi.org/10.1007/s41894-019-0058-4

54. Le B. Guided bone regeneration for aesthetic implant site development. In: Karateew E, editor. Implant aesthetics. Cham: Springer; 2017. https://doi.org/10.1007/978-3-319-50706-4_13.

Immediate and Early Implantation Versus Delayed Implantation

Shervin Shafiei

Introduction

Conventional dental implant placement is based on achieving complete healing of both the hard and soft tissues before surgery to anticipate favorable osseointegration. Immediate implant placement refers to implant placement in a fresh extraction socket, while early implant placement refers to implant placement after soft tissue coverage of the extraction socket. These techniques offer some advantages over the conventional method and are preferred for some cases.

Different strategies have been introduced over time in implant dentistry to shorten the time lapse between tooth extraction and delivery of final implant prosthesis as much as possible. Pushing forward the loading time of implants, introducing implants with modified surface characteristics to enhance osseointegration, and immediate dental implant placement after tooth extraction are some of these strategies.

There is controversy regarding the exact time of implant placement in the early approach; however, according to the general agreement, implants should be placed within 4–8 weeks after tooth extraction in the early approach and at least 4–6 months after extraction in the delayed approach [1]. The primary rationales for immediate and early approaches include higher patient satisfaction due to fewer surgical procedures, shorter treatment period, considerably shorter edentulism period, hard and soft tissue preservation in the extraction socket, improved esthetics, and even higher implant survival rates. On the other hand, careful patient selection and risk of complications should be taken into account in treatment planning that will be disused in this chapter.

S. Shafiei (✉)
Oral and Maxillofacial Surgery Department, Shahid Beheshti University of Medical Sciences, Tehran, Iran
e-mail: s_shafiei@sbmu.ac.ir

Clinical and Surgical Protocols for Immediate Implant Placement

Clinical evaluation of the soft and hard tissues is imperative before selecting immediate implant placement following tooth extraction. Tooth position relative to the free gingival margin and the adjacent teeth, the form of periodontium and gingival biotype, tooth morphology (especially root configuration), and position and morphology of the alveolar ridge and the alveolar crest are some diagnostic factors that should be considered and carefully evaluated in treatment planning [2].

The surgical techniques in immediate implant placement are mostly similar to those in the conventional method. The primary concerns are bone remodeling following tooth extraction (buccal resorption following tooth extraction and buccal shift of implant) and placing the implant in the dental socket, which would compromise the ideal position and alignment of the implant. Gingival biotype is another important consideration. Patients with a thin gingival biotype are more susceptible to gingival recession after surgical interventions. They also have a thinner buccal bone plate that is more likely to resorb after interruption of its blood supply from the periodontal ligament following tooth extraction [3]. Patients with thick gingival biotype are better candidates for immediate implant placement and have a lower risk of >1 mm gingival recession than those with thin biotype [1, 2].

Different guidelines have been proposed regarding decision-making in immediate implant placement. There is no single recommendation; however, most guidelines mainly rely on the post-extraction socket morphology. Funato et al. [4] introduced a classification guideline to help in decision-making for immediate placement of dental implants. This classification is based on two major concerns regarding socket configurations: gingival biotype and the buccal bone plate.

- Class 1: Intact buccal bone plate and thick gingival biotype
- Class 2: Intact buccal bone plate and thin gingival biotype

M. R. Stevens et al. (eds.), *Innovative Perspectives in Oral and Maxillofacial Surgery*,
https://doi.org/10.1007/978-3-030-75750-2_22

- Class 3: Deficient buccal bone plate in a three-dimensionally favorable alveolar ridge structure
- Class 4: Deficient buccal bone plate deviated from the normal alveolar structure

In this classification, class 1 shows optimal results after the immediate placement of dental implants. Class 2 also yields good results, while implants benefit from careful palatal/lingual positioning and subsequent connective tissue grafting. Class 3 shows acceptable results with simultaneously guided bone regeneration and connective tissue grafting. A delayed approach is recommended for class 4 patients. Needless to say, so many other factors could be part of a favorable outcome in both decision-making and surgical intervention in immediate implant placement; however, the aforementioned classification proposed by Funato et al. [4] could help us determine two simple but important confounding factors before surgery.

Atraumatic tooth extraction is the first determining step in immediate implant placement. Using a surgical blade and periotome would help release the periodontal fibers around the tooth supra- and sub-crestally, respectively. These techniques help to prevent the fracture of alveolar bone. When the tooth becomes adequately mobile, it is removed by forceps with minimal buccolingual movements. Rotational movements are preferred, especially in the anterior maxilla. After tooth extraction, complete debridement and careful examination of the socket should be necessarily performed. Some authors recommend deep curettage or using rotary instruments in the dental socket for maximum intrabony penetration and bleeding before implant placement [1, 5, 6]. The implant's ideal final position is 2–3 mm below the cementoenamel junction of the adjacent teeth apicocoronally (or gingival margin in case of recession). The implant should be placed palatally to avoid contact with the buccal bone plate, and >2 mm distance from the buccal bone would be favorable. In terms of prosthetic considerations, the implant's best position in buccolingual direction is at the lingual cusp or between the incisal edge and cingulum of the future prosthetic crown. The socket free space in the alveolar ridge, the slope of the axial walls, and the extracted tooth's apex position can compromise the implant's ideal buccolingual position, and special care should be taken in the drilling sequence. The implant should ideally have a 1.5–2 mm distance from the adjacent teeth [7, 8].

One challenging decision after immediate implant placement is to determine the need for bone grafting. Bone healing at the implant osteotomy site occurs from the apical toward the coronal; thus, the coronal part is the most challenging and critical site in the healing process. Spontaneous healing of the gap between the implant and bone and favorable results by using interventions such as bone augmentation have been reported in the literature [9–11]. Botticelli et al. [12] reported that gaps larger than 1.25 mm in the midfacial buccal surface and 2.25 mm in mesiodistal locations would benefit from bone grafting to facilitate the healing process of the bone. Quirynen et al. [13] proposed a classification for different types of gaps and bone defects between immediately placed implants and the peripheral bony socket. Type 0 refers to no gap between the implant and the surrounding bone; types 1a and 1b point to circumferential gaps ≤2 mm and >2 mm around the implants, respectively. Types 2a and 2b refer to three-wall mesiodistal and three-wall buccal/lingual defects. Type 3 and type 4 defects only have two walls and zero to one wall, respectively. They concluded that bone augmentation procedures would be necessary for patients with type 1b, 3, and 4 defects around their implants. In a clinical study, Botticelli et al. [12] measured different marginal defects under direct surgical observation before immediate implant placement and at the re-entry surgery 4 months later. Implants were placed in the extraction sockets without using any bone substitute or membrane. After implant insertion, the flaps were returned and sutured around the healing caps of implants. They showed that marginal gaps between the implant and bone were predictably filled with new bone. They even reported a major improvement in marginal bone defects >3 mm after re-entry surgery at 4 months (52 defects >3 mm at baseline compared with 8 defects after 4 months). Even with this optimistic result, they observed considerable resorption of the buccal bone plate (about 56% horizontal resorption of the buccal bone plate with a mean vertical resorption of 3 mm). Moreover, in decision-making regarding bone grafting for immediately placed implants, complications of bone augmentation should be taken into account.

Optimal primary stability is another critical factor to consider in immediate and early implant placement. A minimum of 4–5 mm crestal width and 10 mm height have been proposed to be necessary for immediate implant placement in the literature. Also, 3–5 mm of apical drilling into the native bone beyond the socket or use of larger-diameter implants is highly important to achieve optimal primary stability in immediate and early implant placement [1, 5]. Gaining higher stability should not cause excessive pressure on the alveolar bone plate, especially the buccal plate, because such pressure could cause micro- and/or macro-fractures in the bone plates and prolong the healing period or even cause bone resorption and subsequent failure.

Controversy exists regarding implant placement in infected dental sockets; however, according to recent reports, immediate implant placement in an infected site with a periapical lesion is safe given that the infective tissue is completely debrided and the implant is inserted with optimal primary stability as in non-infected areas [1, 14]. Significant differences have not been reported regarding the overall survival rate of implants placed in infected sockets compared with immediately placed implants in non-infected sites.

Surgical Protocols for Early Implant Placement

Early implant placement is mainly similar to immediate implant placement. In early implant placement protocol, dental implants are inserted in the early stage of the healing process after tooth extraction (at 4–8 weeks, post-extraction). The primary rationales that support the early implant placement protocol include increased risk of infection at the sites with periapical pathosis when the immediate protocol is used, less need for bone augmentation procedures, and adequate amount of soft tissue coverage when it is necessary to submerge the implant or bone grafting is performed [15]. This technique also benefits from the use of socket walls similar to immediate implant placement before their complete resorption or remodeling [16].

Immediate or Early Loading

Immediate and early implant restorations could be functional or non-functional in terms of loading. The results have been different regarding immediate or early loading of immediately/early placed dental implants. Some authors have reported a reduction in the overall implant survival rate in immediate loading of immediately placed implants [13]. However, most studies believe that a good prognosis and success of immediately or early placed implants would not be compromised by their immediate or early loading. On the other hand, obtaining good primary stability is the main factor predicting the safe early loading of implants [11, 17].

The Overall Survival Rate of Immediate and Early Implant Placement

Regardless of the adopted protocol, 5% implant loss can be expected. Most available reports about implant survival in the immediate or early approach compared to the conventional method have a short-term loading follow-up [11]. Recent systematic reviews and meta-analyses indicate that the timing of immediate, early, and delayed implant placement does not significantly affect the overall implant survival rate, and all three protocols can bring about promising outcomes regarding the survival rate [13, 15, 18, 19].

Bassir et al. [19] compared the overall survival rate of dental implants between the immediate and early protocols

in their meta-analysis on recent reports. They reported an overall survival rate of 95.88% and 93.8% for early and immediate implant placement protocols, respectively. They found no significant difference between the two protocols and in comparison with the delayed conventional method.

Preservation of Post-extraction Socket

Following a tooth extraction, the alveolar ridge undergoes remodeling with the highest magnitude within the first year. Morphological changes of the alveolar ridge will compromise optimal final esthetics, especially in the anterior region, and ideal implant position that is necessary for favorable long-term biomechanical loading. These alterations occur in both vertical and buccolingual dimensions and may involve up to 4 mm of the ridge height and 25% of the total volume of the alveolar ridge in the first year after tooth extraction [1]. A previous report demonstrated a higher rate of resorption at 6 months after tooth extraction when no implants were inserted, and no bone augmentation/socket preservation was performed [20]. Immediate implant placement can preserve the extraction socket and the alveolar bone [11].

Despite the conflicting results, it may be concluded that immediate implant placement may preserve the alveolar ridge. However, it should be kept in mind that both immediate and early placements of dental implants, atraumatic tooth extraction, and socket preservation are the most fundamental factors determining the future resorption and morphology of the alveolar ridge.

Changes in Peri-implant Hard and Soft Tissues

Bassie et al. [19], in their systematic review and meta-analysis regarding peri-implant bone and soft tissue resorption after implant placement by immediate, early, and delayed protocols, demonstrated significantly lower marginal bone loss in the early protocol as compared with the immediate protocol (0.14 mm less marginal bone loss). Moreover, there was no significant difference between the early and delayed approaches in terms of marginal bone loss and probing depth. In their study, midbuccal soft tissue recession was also more significant in the immediate protocol; however, it was not significant. Sanz et al. [15] also reported 13.11% and 19.85% reduction of bone resorption in vertical and horizontal directions, respectively, in early implant placement.

The greater marginal bone loss and sometimes soft tissue alterations in immediate implant placement may be related to the hard and soft tissue resorption that begins immediately after tooth extraction; these alterations after immediate implant placement could be part of the natural post-extraction process that occurs in great magnitude early after extractions.

Esthetic Outcomes

Soft tissue recession after implant placement is one of the major concerns, especially in the esthetic regions such as the anterior maxilla. In some cases, even loss of dental papilla and/or midbuccal gingiva smaller than 1 mm could be a failure in terms of esthetic considerations. A provisional crown before the final restoration could manage and shape the gingival contour, especially immediately after tooth extraction. According to the literature, the use of provisional restoration and gingival formers after immediate implant placement without flap elevation could significantly improve the peri-implant gingival form and support the interdental papilla [5].

Although esthetic outcomes seem to be acceptable in both techniques, systematic reviews published by Chen and Buser [21] and Bassir et al. [19] both demonstrated more significant midbuccal soft tissue recession in the immediate group, in comparison with early implant placement protocol.

Potential Disadvantages and Complications of Immediate/Early Implant Placement

Despite the promising overall outcome of immediate/early implant placement and higher patient satisfaction [22], clinical complications should be taken into account.

Difficult control of the final implant position, obtaining favorable primary stability, concerns regarding complete flap closure and possible contamination because of diminished soft tissue coverage (in the immediate approach), and difficulty in the drilling sequence and implant placement are the most common issues encountered in immediate/early implant placement.

Conclusion

Immediate and early dental implant placement protocols have shown promising results in overall survival rate and functional and esthetic outcomes. However, care must be taken in pre-surgical evaluation and surgical considerations to achieve successful treatment outcome.

References

1. Koh RU, Rudek I, Wang H-L. Immediate implant placement: positives and negatives. Implant Dent. 2010;19(2):98–108.
2. Kois JC. Predictable single tooth peri-implant esthetics: five diagnostic keys. Compend Contin Educ Dent (Jamesburg, NJ: 1995). 2001;22(3):199.
3. Kao RT, Fagan MC, Conte GJ. Thick vs. thin gingival biotypes: a key determinant in treatment planning for dental implants. J Calif Dent Assoc. 2008;36(3):193–8.
4. Funato A, Salama MA, Ishikawa T, Garber DA, Salama H. Timing, positioning, and sequential staging in esthetic implant therapy: a four-dimensional perspective. Int J Periodontics Restorative Dent. 2007;27(4):313–23.
5. Bhola M, Neely AL, Kolhatkar S. Immediate implant placement: clinical decisions, advantages, and disadvantages. J Prosthodont Implant Esthet Reconstr Dent. 2008;17(7):576–81.
6. Nemcovsky CE, Artzi Z, Moses O, Gelernter I. Healing of marginal defects at implants placed in fresh extraction sockets or after 4–6 weeks of healing: a comparative study. Clin Oral Implants Res. 2002;13(4):410–9.
7. Tarnow DP, Magner AW, Fletcher P. The effect of the distance from the contact point to the crest of bone on the presence or absence of the interproximal dental papilla. J Periodontol. 1992;63(12):995–6.
8. Gastaldo JF, Cury PR, Sendyk WR. Effect of the vertical and horizontal distances between adjacent implants and between a tooth and an implant on the incidence of interproximal papilla. J Periodontol. 2004;75(9):1242–6.
9. Schropp L, Kostopoulos L, Wenzel A. Bone healing following immediate versus delayed placement of titanium implants into extraction sockets: a prospective clinical study. Int J Oral Maxillofac Implants. 2003;18(2):189–99.
10. Chen ST, Wilson TG Jr, Hammerle C. Immediate or early placement of implants following tooth extraction: review of biologic basis, clinical procedures, and outcomes. Int J Oral Maxillofac Implants. 2004;19(Suppl):12–25.
11. Schropp L, Isidor F. Timing of implant placement relative to tooth extraction. J Oral Rehabil. 2008;35:33–43.
12. Botticelli D, Berglundh T, Lindhe J. Hard-tissue alterations following immediate implant placement in extraction sites. J Clin Periodontol. 2004;31(10):820–8.
13. Quirynen M, Van Assche N, Botticelli D, Berglundh T. How does the timing of implant placement to extraction affect outcome? Database of Abstracts of Reviews of Effects (DARE): quality-assessed Reviews [Internet]. Centre for Reviews and Dissemination (UK); 2007.
14. Lindeboom JA, Tjiook Y, Kroon FH. Immediate placement of implants in periapical infected sites: a prospective randomized study in 50 patients. Oral Surg Oral Med Oral Pathol Oral Radiol Endod. 2006;101(6):705–10.
15. Sanz I, Garcia-Gargallo M, Herrera D, Martin C, Figuero E, Sanz M. Surgical protocols for early implant placement in post-extraction sockets: a systematic review. Clin Oral Implants Res. 2012;23:67–79.
16. Buser D, Halbritter S, Hart C, Bornstein MM, Grütter L, Chappuis V, et al. Early implant placement with simultaneous guided bone regeneration following single-tooth extraction in the esthetic zone: 12-month results of a prospective study with 20 consecutive patients. J Periodontol. 2009;80(1):152–62.

17. Attard NJ, Zarb GA. Immediate and early implant loading protocols: a literature review of clinical studies. J Prosthet Dent. 2005;94(3):242–58.

18. Esposito M, Grusovin MG, Polyzos IP, Felice P, Worthington HV. Interventions for replacing missing teeth: dental implants in fresh extraction sockets (immediate, immediate-delayed and delayed implants). Cochrane Database Syst Rev. 2010;(9).

19. Bassir SH, El Kholy K, Chen CY, Lee KH, Intini G. Outcome of early dental implant placement versus other dental implant placement protocols: a systematic review and meta-analysis. J Periodontol. 2019;90(5):493–506.

20. Schwartz-Arad D, Chaushu G. The ways and wherefores of immediate placement of implants into fresh extraction sites: a literature review. J Periodontol. 1997;68(10):915–23.

21. Chen ST, Buser D. Clinical and esthetic outcomes of implants placed in postextraction sites. Int J Oral Maxillofac Implants. 2009;24 Suppl:186–217.

22. Schropp L, Isidor F, Kostopoulos L, Wenzel A. Patient experience of, and satisfaction with, delayed-immediate vs. delayed single-tooth implant placement. Clin Oral Implants Res. 2004;15(4):498–503.

Biologically Oriented Preparation Technique (BOPT)

Ghida Lawand, Abdullah Ajili, and Yara Ismail

Introduction

One of the most commonly applied procedures for substituting missing teeth is tooth-supported fixed dental prosthesis (FDP) since it offers an excellent clinical constancy. There are various problems with FDP as a treatment choice, with the most common being marginal gingival recession. This recession generally bares the tooth-restoration interface and compromises esthetics, especially in the anterior region, leading to biological and functional problems [1]. Accordingly, maintaining the stability of gingival tissue around fixed prosthetic restorations remains a challenge for most dentists. This type of complication has been linked with chronic inflammation due to inadequate marginal fit; gingival biotype, i.e., quantity and quality of keratinized gingival tissue; trauma such as aggressive tooth brushing; and, above all, iatrogenic consequences of tooth preparation [2].

The invasiveness of tooth preparation for a prosthetic crown remains an issue due to the irreversible tooth structure loss. Several efforts have been made to develop the best approach of tooth preparation and lessen enamel and dentin tooth loss. Many clinical factors, including the pulp's vitality, the patient's age, the number of units (single crown/bridge), the type of material used, and the crown's convexity, play a significant role in guiding the dentist to choose the ideal type of tooth preparation [3, 4].

Tooth preparation prior to placing an FDP is divided into two categories: horizontal and vertical preparation. Horizontal preparation is divided into chamfer (regular, beveled) and shoulder (regular, beveled, rounded, bevel rounded)

G. Lawand (✉) · Y. Ismail
Prosthodontics and Esthetic Dentistry Department, Faculty of Dentistry – Saint Joseph University, Beirut, Lebanon
e-mail: ghida.lawand@net.usj.edu.lb; yara.ismail@net.usj.edu.lb

A. Ajili
Oral Surgery Department, Universitat Internacional de Catalunya, Barcelona, Spain
e-mail: ain143320@uic.es

finish lines. Chamfer-type preparation is a horizontal preparation at a 45-degree angle. It is used when metallic restorations are indicated, including metal cast crowns or ceramo-metallic crowns with full metal on the lingual surface. This type of preparation is also shown in milled Computer-aided design & computer-aided manufacturing (CAD/CAM) crowns and pressed full ceramics. Depending on the rising taper of the preparation, shoulder-less types of vertical tooth preparation can be further classified into chisel, feather, or knife-edge. The limitation of this type of preparation includes a high risk of postoperative sensitivity as a result of hard tissue loss (up to 50%), dentin exposure, and lack of marginal seal due to imperfections in the fabrication that leads to a marginal gap followed by bacterial penetration [5].

Vertical preparations are of two types: shoulder-less and edgeless. Shoulder-less types of vertical tooth preparation can be further classified into chisel, feather, or knife edge. This generally depends on the rising taper of the preparation. Researchers agree that a shoulder-less preparation is the most conservative method and the least susceptible to the marginal gap but has been abandoned due to its countless flaws. Vick Pollard and Rex Ingraham have introduced the other type of vertical preparation, known as the edgeless type, which is also called "gingitage" or "rotary gingival curettage method." Later on, Di Febo, Carnevale, and recently Ignazio Loi have updated its name to the "biologically oriented preparation technique" (BOPT) [5].

BOPT, being the current trend, is a prosthodontic procedure based on tooth preparation receiving a fixed prosthesis without a finish line [6]. Unlike other types of preparation, BOPT creates an axial vertical plane between the root and crown areas, eliminating the emergence of an anatomic crown above the cemento-enamel junction (CEJ), creating a new prosthetic junction situated according to the desired location of the gingival margin [6, 7]. This type of preparation produces a convergent-shaped tooth where the crown can slide telescopically onto the tooth cervically before its

© The Author(s), under exclusive license to Springer Nature Switzerland AG 2021
M. R. Stevens et al. (eds.), *Innovative Perspectives in Oral and Maxillofacial Surgery*,
https://doi.org/10.1007/978-3-030-75750-2_23

cementation [7]. As a result, the marginal space between the restoration and the tooth usually formed with horizontal preparations is eliminated [7–9]. Also, BOPT is a restorative technique that consists of an intentional modification of the tooth-restoration union, generating changes at the gingival level, thus guiding its healing. This is why this technique integrates the soft tissue's response to dental preparations, unlike conventional prosthetic preparations where the prosthesis does not highly influence the shape of soft tissue placed [9].

Several prospective and retrospective studies of crowned teeth with BOPT preparations have shown reliable results instead of traditional techniques. However, many researchers have criticized this technique for it being the reason behind "over-contours" and "inflammation." This posed an ambiguity to many prosthodontists who traditionally performed horizontal preparations. This chapter demonstrates the step-by-step BOPT, analogically and digitally, highlighting the clinical differences among conventional techniques. It also tackles this technique's advantages and disadvantages in terms of biological, mechanical, and histological behavior and discusses whether it can be an alternative to horizontal preparations. Finally, it explains how this revolutionary practice has been recently applied not only in teeth-supported crowns but also in implants.

BOPT in Teeth-Supported Crowns

Being a very delicate technique, the clinician should follow the steps cautiously in order to obtain successful results. These steps are summarized in Table 23.1.

Bone Sounding and Probing

Before beginning the procedure, a precise intra-sulcular mapping is carried out using a graduated periodontal probe to evaluate the health of the tooth and the level of the epithelial attachment. "Double probing" is first done to measure the depth of the gingival sulcus "sulcus probing" and then to measure the bone level "bone sounding," allowing the clini-

Table 23.1 Summary of the step-by-step procedure of biologically oriented preparation technique on teeth-supported restorations

Steps of BOPT in teeth-supported crowns
1. Bone sounding and probing
2. BOPT tooth and tissue preparation
3. BOPT temporization
4. BOPT impression
5. BOPT laboratory procedures
6. BOPT restoration
7. BOPT cementation

cian to locate the CEJ. In the soft tissue de-epithelialization stage, sulcus probing is essential to assess soft tissue preparation's vertical extent. This is important because "gingitage" must always be performed while considering the epithelial insertion, and the de-epithelialization is performed while taking into account epithelial insertion. Bone sounding controls the boundary of preparation of the dental abutment. Bone level should also be determined to avoid contact during tooth preparation [6, 7].

BOPT Tooth and Tissue Preparation

BOPT preparation is divided into two main steps: tooth preparation and soft tissue preparation. The preparation aims to create space for tissue stabilization and conform to normal dental anatomy. This generates an angle at the emergence of the restoration between the crown and the tooth that supports the soft tissue [6] .

In the first stage, the tooth's extra-gingival part is prepared with a diamond flame-shaped bur. The preparation is done in the following order: mesial and distal, occlusal/incisal, buccal aspect at a 45-degree inclined plane, and ending with a supra-gingival circumferential axial reduction (Fig. 23.1a–d). The second stage is the soft tissue preparation, which is done by creating a "rotational abrasion-induced bleeding," "gingiabrasion," or "gingitage." The bur, obliquely tilted in the sulcus, works simultaneously with the gingival sulcus's internal wall and the epithelial component of the gingival junction that produces bleeding. The bur simultaneously contacts the tooth, creating an even vertical surface also termed as the "finishing area" (Fig. 23.1e). Bleeding will produce a blood clot supported by the provisional crown. The even vertical plane will remove the existing CEJ or any finish line in a previously prepared tooth. Four to 6 weeks later, scarring occurs with an increase in volume at the soft tissue's horizontal level in the marginal area. This is a result of the maturation of the clot produced and stabilized in the preparation phase [6, 11].

BOPT Temporization

The dental preparation is followed by BOPT temporization. The fabrication and adaptation of the provisional restoration are key to the success of the technique. Its objective and function lie in protecting the abutment, providing function and esthetics, and stabilizing the gingival preparation clot. It also helps protect the soft tissue during the maturation period and plays a role in subsequent modeling, achieving a new gingival architecture [6].

In BOPT temporization, a lab-fabricated indirect provisional restoration based on the diagnostic wax-up must be

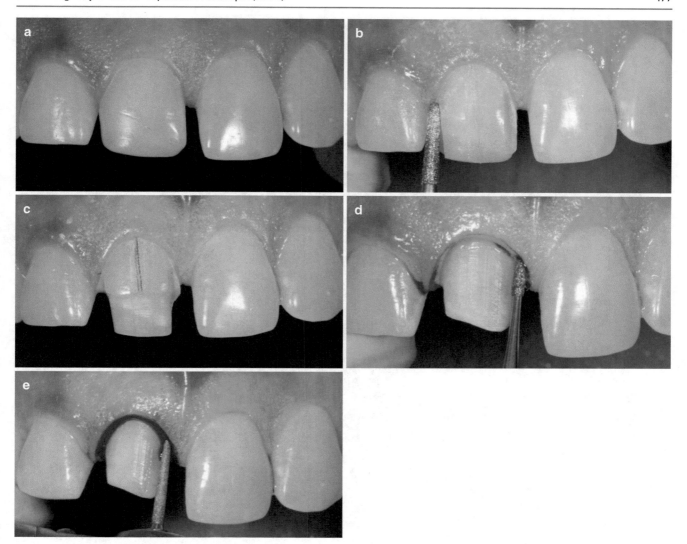

Fig. 23.1 (**a**) Preoperative picture. (**b, c**) Preparation of the mesial and distal sides. (**d**) Supra-gingival circumferential reduction of the tooth. (**e**) Soft tissue preparation by inserting the bur in the sulcus until bleeding results. (With permission from Dr. Ruben Planco)

used. The wax-up must maintain the initial gingival architecture of the patient, even if it is asymmetric. Using a silicone key to duplicate the wax-up, the laboratory should fabricate an acrylic eggshell temporarily (Fig. 23.2a–c). Besides, since these temporary restorations are going to be in the mouth for a long period of time and will need to be relined, acrylic resin is the material of choice. The type of acrylic resin should have optimum dimensional stability and the least possible shrinkage because excessive resin shrinkage in this type of preparation would make the process difficult. The next step is relining (Fig. 23.2d, e). The purpose of relining is to adjust the provisional in a way that stabilizes the blood clot and supports the soft tissue during the period of healing. After relining, the temporary crown is adjusted and trimmed (Fig. 23.2f). Eliminating the vestibular excess should preferably be avoided as it aids in recording the provisional gingival margin. The temporary crown should have

two different margins: a thin internal margin, which registers the intra-sulcular part of the prepared tooth, and an external thick margin that marks the external part of the gingival margin. The space between both margins must reinforce the provisional restoration and give it a correct emergence profile. In the case of single-unit restorations, filling the space can be performed with flowable composite, whereas in multiple restorations or restorations to be placed intraorally for a long time, acrylic resin is the material of choice [6, 11].

Before filling in the space, the provisional's internal margin is marked with a pencil to delimit the contour of the abutment and avoid invading it during relining. Upon connecting both margins, the provisional emergence profile is connected with the gingival margin by trimming the excess. Once the provisional has been placed in the mouth, the gingival margin is drawn around its contour to evaluate how much is trimmed (Fig. 23.3e–g). The provisional is then removed,

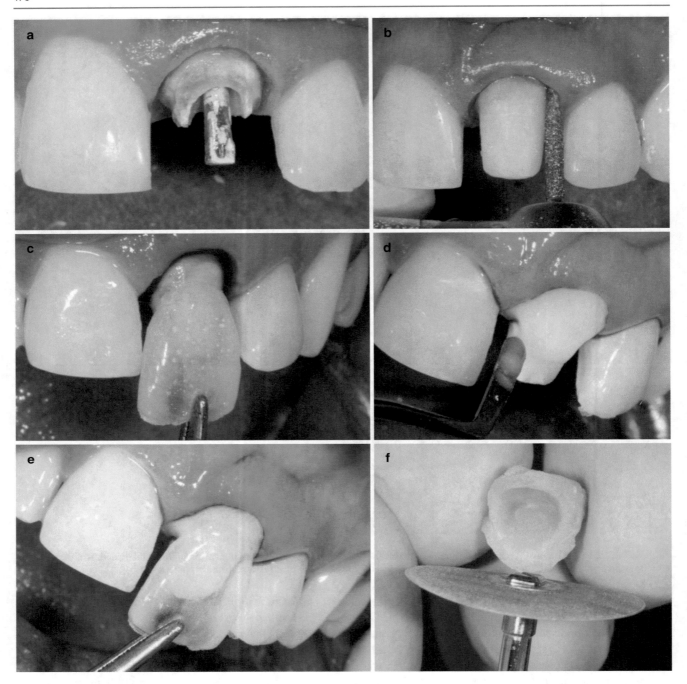

Fig. 23.2 (**a**) Preoperative picture showing an old post that was replaced with a fiber post followed by a composite buildup. (**b**) Tooth and soft tissue preparation following the BOPT. (**c**) Lab-fabricated eggshell temporary based on previous wax-up made. (**d**, **e**) Relining of the eggshell by placing acrylic resin on the tooth and on the inner surface of the shell. (**f**) Trimming of the provisional respecting the space created for the blood clot to occur. (**g**, **h**) Healing of the gingival margin after 4 weeks of placing the provisional. (**i**) Impression of the tooth preparation with polyvinyl siloxane material. (**j**) Lab dye delineating the red line that represents the location of the finish line and the blue line that represents the depth of the sulcus. (**k**) Provisional before cementing the definitive restoration. (**l**) Final BOPT restoration after cementation. Notice the healthiness and thickness of the gingival margin. (With permission from Dr. Ruben Planco)

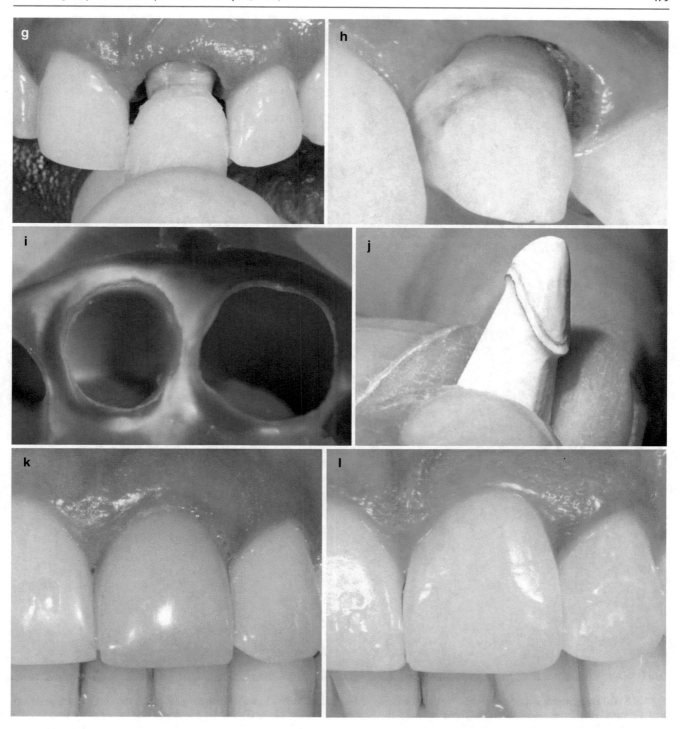

Fig. 23.2 (continued)

followed by the reduction of the internal margin to create a new CEJ line extending not deeper than 0.5–1 mm. This removal is done to respect the clot's space and respect the biological width during healing, thus controllably invading the gingival sulcus. The provisional must also respect the interproximal gingival scallop. For that reason, spaces should be left for the mesial and distal sides of the papillae, both vertically and horizontally. Finally, the provisional must be accurately finished and polished to achieve the objectives listed previously [6, 11].

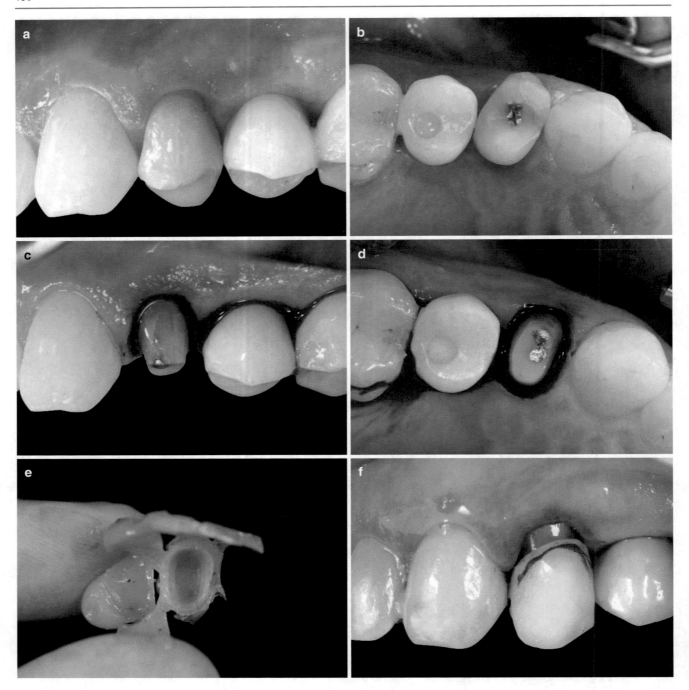

Fig. 23.3 (a) Preoperative frontal photo showing the dark shade of the first premolar. (b) Preoperative occlusal photo showing the wrong angulation of the first premolar. (c) Frontal photo after tooth and tissue preparation. (d) Occlusal photo after tooth and tissue preparation. (e) Provisional restoration made of acrylic resin. (f) Provisional partially placed intraorally where the accurate position of the gingival margin is marked with a pencil. (g) Provisional at the day of temporary cementa-tion. (h) Provisional after healing (4 weeks) showing an increase in gingival thickness. (i) and (j) Frontal photo showing the shape of the gingiva that is exactly a replica of the provisional. (k) Occlusal photo showing complete healing of the tissue with the appropriate emergence profile. (l) Final impression with polyvinyl siloxane material. (m) Definitive restoration on the cast. (n) Final restoration cemented. (With permission from Dr. Lucas Pedrosa)

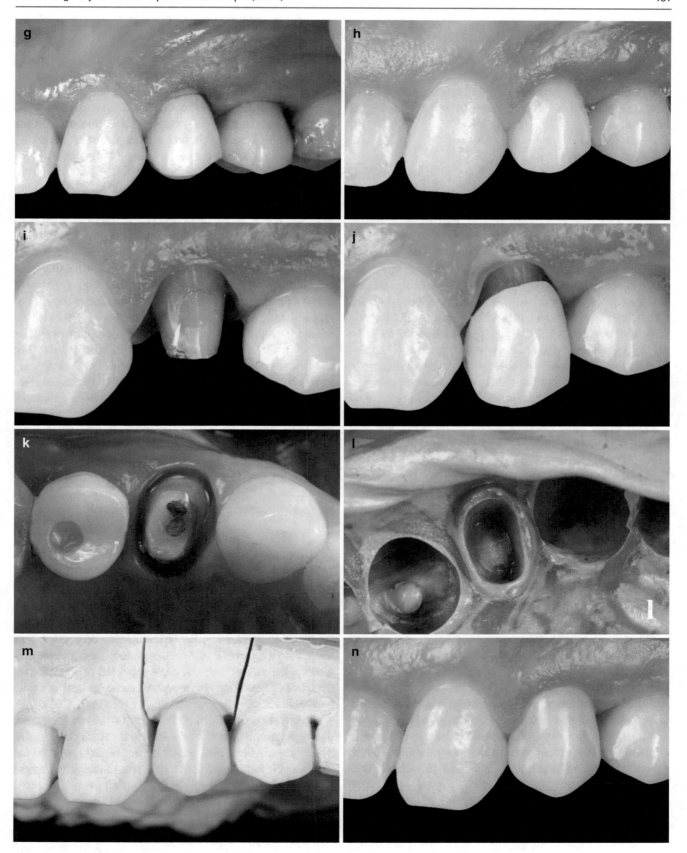

Fig. 23.3 (continued)

BOPT Impression

In around 4 weeks, after the temporization has stabilized the tissues (Fig. 23.2g, h), an impression is taken for the fabrication of the definitive restoration. Two impression techniques are available: the analogical impression and the digital impression.

Analogical Impression

In a horizontal preparation, the impression's accuracy is determined by the clarity of the finish line. However, in vertical preparations, the impression's accuracy is determined by the sulcus's visibility in the impression. Regarding the necessity of placing retraction cords, the double cord technique is applied in BOPT impressions. The double cord technique allows the practitioner to have a good reading of the sulcus, helps the technician during laboratory procedures, and prevents some elastomeric material from going deep into the sulcus, keeping it from tearing when removing the impression from deeply recorded areas [6]. The first thread to be placed is generally the three zeros thread, preferably the aluminum chloride impregnated thread to correctly register at that level. The second thread that varies between zero and one (depending on the thickness of the fabric) must not be completely submerged. The thread should be placed first in the area where the greatest tissue thickness exists, which is usually the interproximal area. After 5 minutes of waiting to achieve the desired effect of the astringent and the retraction thread, the preparation is washed and dried before removing the second thread, and the injection material is injected. If washing and drying are done after removing the second thread, the first thread could be moved. Polyvinyl siloxane (PVS) is the material of choice due to its mechanical and physical properties (Figs. 23.2i and 23.3l). Unlike other more rigid materials that could tear after the first casting, PVS allows obtaining more than one casting without losing information. The impression technique performed is the one-step technique with two consistencies, heavy and light, to facilitate the material's injection throughout the subgingival perimeter [11].

Digital Impression

An error in registering the intra-sulcular area is often frequent in conventional techniques because there's a high possibility for the gingiva to collapse in an inward direction after removing the provisional restoration. This generally presents a serious problem when using this analogical workflow knowing that the gingiva and the sulcus' reproduction is one of the crucial steps in the BOPT. Moreover, alteration of the original gingival margin and sulcus can result from the retraction cords' aggressive placement. Thus, it is essential to stick to an impression procedure that will replicate the gingiva's actual level when the temporary restoration is placed on the abutment tooth and does not rely on the operator's clinical skills. Augustin et al. used a digital technique for reproducing the subgingival region of a tooth prepared according to the BOPT and its adjacent gingival sulcus without having the gingiva collapse. This technique is keen to produce a "virtual gingiva" with a matching emergence morphology as if the temporary restoration is cemented on the tooth [10]. To achieve this, an intraoral scanner is needed to create a standard tessellation language (STL) file. The primary STL file is attained by scanning the temporary prosthesis placed firmly on the tooth as adjacent teeth in the arch are scanned as well. The second scan accounts for the provisional's inner surface since reproducing the intra-sulcular emergence of the cervical area of the crown is of prime importance as this will delineate the invasion of the sulcus by the prosthesis, both horizontally and vertically, given a healthy periodontium. These two scans, when aligned properly, will create a three-dimensional virtual reproduction of the temporary crown. The third scan records teeth prepared with no finish line, registering the gingival region that collapses after removing the temporary crown and all tooth walls. The fourth scan captures the teeth and the gingiva of the opposing arch. The fifth and sixth scans register occlusion on the right and left when in maximum intercuspation. A digital model of the gingiva is then created by exporting the generated digital files to the design software. This process of "virtual gingiva" starts by overlaying all the STL files that will allow a proper digital alignment development. After the "virtual gingiva" is created, it's transferred to the CAD software that will help the technician design a definitive crown following the gingival anatomy generated by the temporary crown [10].

BOPT Laboratory Procedures

Contrary to what other authors have suggested for restorations with feather-edge preparations, the BOPT relies on the observation in which the gingival profile automatically adapts in a specular manner to the coronal emergence profile – not vice versa. Based on this concept, the profiles created on the master cast eliminate the need of the gingival component, resulting in morpho-functional and esthetic ideal contour.

At least two models of plaster type IV are obtained from the impression. The first model is the die-cut which is used to make the structure. The second master model keeps all the soft tissue information intact and serves to check and adjust the gingival parabola finally. After pouring the master casts, a series of lines are drawn on the model to serve as a reference for the fabrication of the definitive restoration. The first line (marked in black) is drawn perpendicular to the longitudinal axis of the tooth in 360 degrees, resting on the cervical margin. It is usually traced with a 0.5 mm pencil over the gingival contour projecting it on the abutment's wall. Then, ditching is performed to remove the soft tissue from the model to the groove's depth and reveal the subgingival area of the prosthetic preparation produced on the model. The second line (marked in blue) is the apical part of the model that is now exposed. The third line (marked in red) is the line that falls into what is known as the "finishing area," which is generally located between the first and the second line. This line, referred to as the "finishing line," is marked by the technician onto which coronal margin lies. Whether more apically or coronally, the position of this line is determined by the depth of the sulcus and on the esthetic needs, but the crown margin will never invade the epithelial attachment (Fig. 23.2j) [6].

The prosthetic restoration is then transferred to the model with the gingiva to evaluate the contours tridimensionally. To fit the crown on the model, the technician uses a sharp scalpel to eliminate any small interferences with the marginal gingiva, hence simulating the interaction between the prosthetic contours and the gingiva that exists in vivo within the oral tissues [6].

BOPT Restoration

Analogical Technique

In the restorative phase, it's important to duplicate the contour achieved with the provisional (Fig. 23.2k, l). Therefore, an impression of the provisional should be transferred to the lab technician to guide the fabrication of the definitive prosthesis. Despite having to copy the contours of the provisional, the technician can slightly modify the gingiva in the plaster or the digital model. The new tissue thickness is directly influenced by the amount of over-contouring of the prosthesis and plaster modification depth (Fig. 23.3m, n). Therefore, the more over-contoured the prosthesis is and the deeper the cut, the greater the thickness of tissue achieved, meanwhile maintaining the limits of the patient's biological width. The main objective is to maintain a thick biotype if already present and thicken those of the thin biotype while modifying the heights of the gingival margins.

The finish line's depth is esthetically important but mainly critical because it allows the clinician to support the modified gingival tissues during the temporization phase. The technician, especially interproximally, can modify the finish line and prosthetic emergence profile to improve gingival scalloping. During the try-in stage, the clinician must pay special attention to the interproximal areas because technicians tend to overextend these areas' limits. Therefore, when there is an overextension, it must be modified during this test [11].

Metal ceramic was initially the material of choice for BOPT restorations. However, zirconia and lithium disilicate are now being used due to the generally high survival rates of all-ceramic restorations on teeth prepared with BOPT as revealed by recent studies. Studies have proved the predictability of this technique's results with scarce reports of mechanical and biological failures [12].

Digital Technique

A CAD-CAM software intended for fabricating dental restorations is used to design and mill all-ceramic crowns using full digital workflows upholding the exact morphology of the temporary crown that was used to create the "virtual gingiva." This ideal morphology will ensure the future crown's sustainable periodontal health and its full adaptation buccally and palatally.

Whenever this full-ceramic crown design protocol is used, it is desirable to mill a transparent resin block that will act as a sample test to check the fit of the crown and assess its size, contact points, morphology, as well as occlusion. Sometimes this sample crown may require some modifications in its anatomy or adaptation. In this case, composite resin may be added for adjustments, and anything in excess can be removed with a bur. Subsequently, using the intraoral scanner, the revised crown is scanned to produce an STL file that is then sent to the laboratory for milling. This protocol ensures that the definitive crown anatomy is not manipulated nor altered when placed on the tooth. In addition, when applying BOPT, the clinician must avoid ischemia in the gingival sulcus from both facial and occlusal views, which could be caused by the prosthetic emergence [10].

BOPT Cementation

Cementation of BOPT restorations is a highly debatable topic given that rubber dam isolation is not an option due to the absence of a clear finish line that guides the level at which the rubber dam clamp is placed. However, several studies investigating the adhesive failures associated with the BOPT cementation phase have revealed high success rates even with lithium disilicate where cementation was performed without rubber dam [13].

Advantages and Disadvantages of BOPT

Several advantages are associated with BOPT. First, the vertical preparation allows maximum preservation of sound tooth structure making it a less aggressive substitute to horizontal preparation. The teeth prepared include periodontally and endodontically treated teeth, vital teeth in young patients requiring modifications in shape and color, or teeth that are affected by pathologies like erosion and abrasion; and carious teeth, mainly at the cervical third of the clinical crown [14]. Furthermore, due to its minimally invasive characteristic, this approach limits irritation of the pulp in vital teeth as it preserves the pulp preparation distance cervically, thus sparing the area most sensitive for the pulp [15].

Second, this type of preparation allows clinicians to correct the position of the anatomic cemento-enamel junction in non-prepared teeth (Fig. 23.3a–d) and eliminate previously prepared finish lines. Meanwhile, new "prosthetic cemento-enamel junction (PCEJ)" is created with the chance of relocating the prosthetic finish line at altered levels of the gingival sulcus, at a depth less than 0.5–1 mm, depending on the existing biological width. Accordingly, the clinician invades the sulcus but in a controlled manner [6].

BOPT also allows the clinician to level the emergence profile and adapt it to the new PCEJ. As a result of the reorganized CEJ, the gingival thickness is increased, and the soft tissue is further stabilized, in the medium and long term (Fig. 23.3h–k) [7]. On a physiological level, after this type of preparation, the gingival tissue proliferates in the same manner that occurs in the process of wound healing [16]. In this phase, new blood vessels are formed, and the fibroblasts and myofibroblasts of the degranulation tissue cultivate and seal the gap caused by the "gingitage." During this stage, the soft tissues relocate coronally due to the surrounding myofibroblasts' contraction caused by the conical dental preparation. The phenomenon upon which tissue growth is established is called the transduction mechanism. In this phenomenon, the fibroblasts located in the connective tissue mechanically trigger the extracellular matrix, i.e., chewing or pressure of the lip during speaking. These mechanical triggers are transformed into chemical ones that excite cell growth and multiplication [16]. Due to the telescopic design of the prosthesis, this technique also improves prosthetic retention, simplifies the impression procedure as compared with dental preparation with finish lines, and allows ideal adaptation between the tooth and restoration (optimal restoration-tooth margin) [6]. Complete marginal openings with the feather-edge finish line are considerably less than those of the chamfer, shoulder, and mini-chamfer finish line types [17]. More recent evidence highlights that vertical preparations without a finish line do not seem to jeopardize the final restorations' longevity. This allows the clinicians to use definitive prosthesis made of metallo-ceramics and lithium disilicate and zirconia [8]. Many studies have concluded that these ceramic materials, in the vertical type of preparation, resist fracture even in the absence of horizontal support on dental abutments in the anterior region. Hence, it only can be concluded that ceramic materials do not result in mechanical complications [18].

Despite the several advantages mentioned, one of the main issues with vertical preparations is the difficulty in accurately locating the prosthetic margin as there is no visible finish line. This makes the technique more complex and time-consuming, resulting in a longer learning curve and chairside time. This technique also makes it hard for the cli-

nician to assess the crown's final fitting and remove all the excess cement. Therefore, the dentist and the lab technician must be highly experienced to prevent uncontrollable invasion and damage in the sulcus [6]. Moreover, although this technique allows optimal gingival stability and thickness, it requires a 4-week healing period in the temporization phase, which many patients may oppose [9].

Histological Alterations After BOPT Preparation

Histological sections of teeth obtained with intact periodontal tissues after a BOPT restoration showed that when this technique partially removes acellular cementum, the root dentin's dentinal structure does not change. When moving apically, the structure of the intact cementum and the compact bone of the alveolar crest is found to be normal. No signs of inflammation were detected in the periodontal ligaments embedded in the cementum and periodontal bone where it displays normal quantity and spatial organization of collagen bundles, cell density, and vascularization. Signs of inflammation were also absent in the attached gingiva covered by a keratinized stratified squamous epithelium lining normal connective tissue. Nevertheless, normal histological structure is found in the regenerated sulcular epithelium, free gingiva, and gingival margin after BOPT preparation is performed. The connective tissue underneath demonstrated a slightly augmented number of defensive cells but no evident inflammation signs. The organization and spatial distribution of the collagen bundles corresponding to the dento-gingival and dento-periosteal fascicles are normal. Finally, the newly formed junctional epithelium attached to the new dentin-cementum area created after BOPT, has been found to extend from the bottom of the gingival sulcus to a variable height. The length generally depends on the slice that is histologically examined. Specific sections showed tiny and wide junctional epithelium far from the alveolar crest, unlike other sections that showed longer epithelial attachment lining the tooth near the alveolar crest. Number of layers was found to decrease apically, ending with only one row of cells firmly attached to the intact acellular cementum [19].

BOPT in Implants

The success of implants in the esthetic region is achieved on both hard and soft tissue levels, i.e., by osseointegration and the presence of healthy and stable peri-implant mucosal soft tissues, respectively (Fig. 23.4a–h). The stability of soft tissues results in a natural outcome and prevents bone resorption, which ensures the implant's long-term success [20]. Marginal bone loss around implants is related to dif-

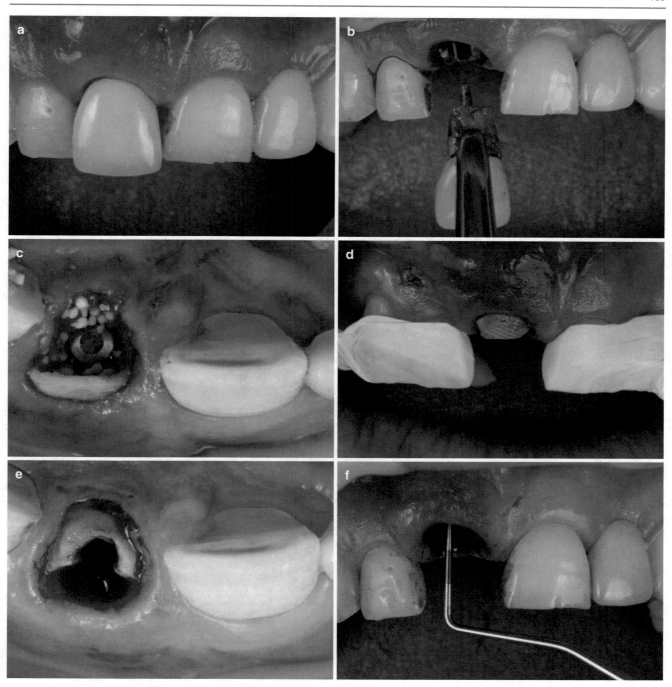

Fig. 23.4 (**a**) Preoperative photo. (**b**) Deep vertical root fracture of the central. (**c**) Occlusal photo demonstrating the vertical fracture. (**d**) Deep bone sounding where there's lack of buccal bone. (**e**) Placing **OSSIX®** Plus resorbable collagen membrane to determine its size. (**f**) **OSSIX®** Plus in place for guided bone regeneration with the ice cream cone technique. (**g**) Occlusal photo showing the **KeraOs®** ß-tricalcium phosphate bone graft, the Prama implant, and the membrane. (**h**) Placing Teflon on adjacent teeth. (**i**) Non-rotational titanium interface used as a provisional abutment. (**j**) VOCO® Structur 3 self-curing composite used to pick up the titanium abutment. (**k**) Provisional placed on the titanium abutment. Notice the convergent collar design of the provi-sional. (**l**) Periapical X-ray showing the Prama implant (3.8 × 13 mm) just after its surgical placement. (**m**) Provisional restoration screwed intraorally over the implant. (**n**) Frontal photo of the provisional after 6 months of healing. (**o**) Occlusal photo of the provisional after 6 months of healing. (**p**) Occlusal photo showing the healing of the gingiva and its architecture and emergence profile. (**q**) Side view photo of the gingiva after healing. (**r**) Titanium-anodized abutment used for the BOPT. (**s**) Final restoration made of bilayered zirconia screwed intraorally. (**t**) Periapical X-ray of the Prama implant with the final restoration. (**u**) Final restoration under cross-polarization. (With permission from Dr. Lucas Pedrosa)

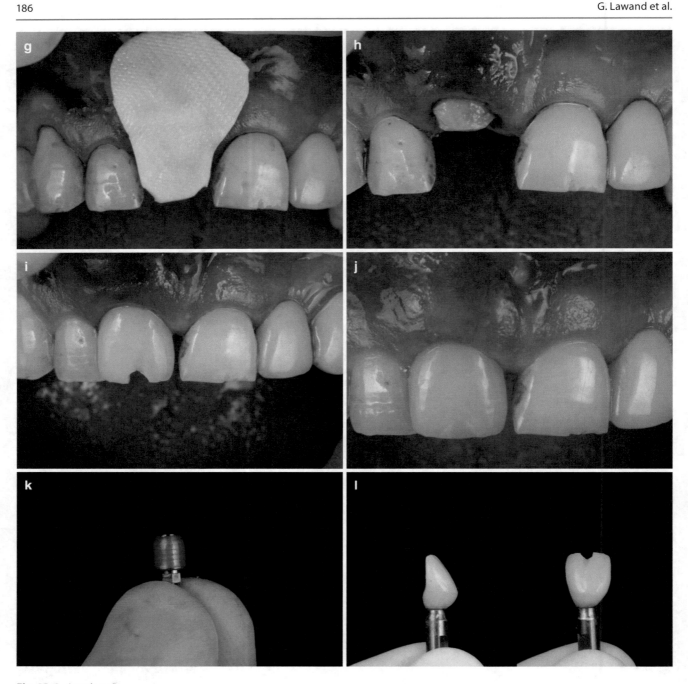

Fig. 23.4 (continued)

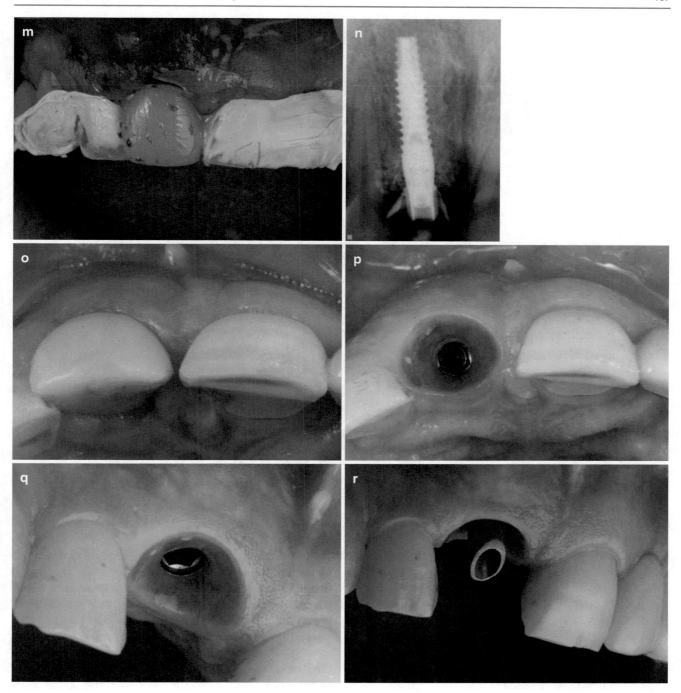

Fig. 23.4 (continued)

Fig. 23.4 (continued)

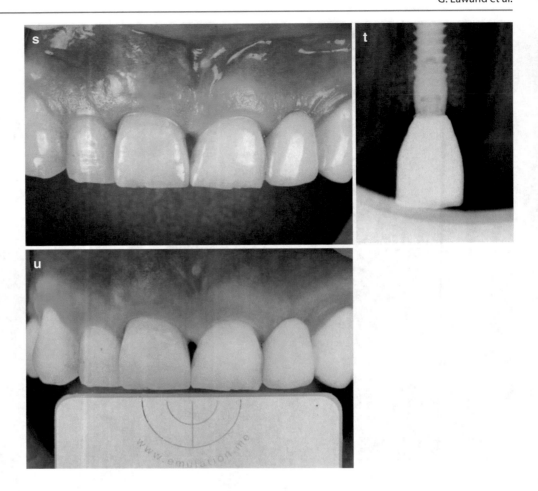

ferent parameters including peri-implant mucosa thickness [21], inter-implant distance [22], macro- and microscopic characteristics of the implant [23], inevitable bacterial contamination of the implant-abutment connection irrespective of the assembly of implant used [24], and most importantly the design of the implant-abutment interface [25]. Hence, the quality of the peri-implant mucosa is determined by the prosthetic accessory materials in contact with the mucosa and the topography of the implant [20, 23]. The development of new dental implants, prosthetic abutments, and crowns offers novel surfaces and designs capable of improving soft tissue insertion while attempting to avoid microbial contamination of vital bone and hence its resorption [26, 27]. Tissue-level implants have been suggested as a reliable method to hinder marginal bone loss [28]. The crestal module's design plays a critical role in the overall success of the implant and prosthesis, particularly in the esthetic area. The crestal module is a portion of a two-piece metal dental implant designed to hold the prosthetic components in place and create a transition zone to the load-bearing implant body, including the implant-abutment connection, the collar, and the more coronal portion of the abutment. Two collar designs are present, the divergent and the convergent. Most tissue-level implants' divergent collar design has been proven to generate excessive compression on the soft tissues, resulting in recession [29]. The second design introduced is the transmucosal implant with a convergent peculiar collar design of a conical shape and parabolic profile to increase peri-implant tissue space. The connection between the implant and the corresponding tapered abutment resembles that of a feather-edge tooth preparation with a crown, following the principles of BOPT. The crown's margin is seated within the peri-implant sulcus, and its emergence profile supports and shapes the gingival margin [26].

Advantages of BOPT in Implants

BOPT in implantology is considerably attracting clinicians today. This is because it allows the practitioner to level the margin of the soft tissues surrounding the implant by using interim crowns (Fig. 23.4i–n). Through the interim crowns, the clinician can controllably invade the sulcus and alter the emergence profile of the definitive prosthesis [6, 30]. To that end, a convergent collar lacking a definite finish line allows the clinician to place the prosthesis limit on the implant rather than on the abutment. The dentist can cement the definitive crown immediately on the neck of the implant, which consequently seals the interface between the implant and the abutment and provides optimal marginal fit due to the lack of a line supporting the restoration on the abutment [29].

Moreover, collagen fiber distribution in this technique appears to increase mucosal fixation. The convergent abutment collar has micro-grooves that create micro-roughness, which directs the fibroblasts and stabilizes adhesion to titanium [31]. This type of abutment helps in the formation of connective tissue fibers with a functional perpendicular orientation called circular fibers. From a clinical perspective, the collar's micro-grooved surface promotes a perpendicular, functional physical connective tissue attachment, which helps stabilize the peri-implant soft tissue over the long term. This, in turn, plays a role in resisting the early inflammation in the peri-implant region, thus reducing peri-implant crestal bone loss [24].

Furthermore, BOPT represents a viable alternative to divergent collars because it improves peri-implant health and esthetics (Fig. 23.4o–u), without the prerequisite of more aggressive and expensive hard or soft tissue regeneration methods [33]. Concerning peri-implant health, the supracrestal position of the junction between the implant and the abutment, with the absence of an implant-abutment interface at the bone level (Fig. 23.4t), prevents bacterial penetration into the critical area of the bone and connective tissue, thus reducing the inflammatory reaction that may form due to this penetration [34]. In terms of esthetics, the biological width around dental implants is established according to the principles of healing of soft tissue by secondary intention, represented by myofibroblasts' contraction. Therefore, the contraction of connective tissue around a coronally convergent conical abutment may produce an attachment located more coronally along with the thickening of soft tissues [29].

Moreover, attempts at reducing marginal bone loss around implants have introduced the concept of switching platform. In this method, the abutment is one size smaller than the implant platform, and this decreases bone loss by retaining the implant-abutment border away from the crestal bone and allowing the soft tissue to grow on top of the implant, resulting in a defensive seal [35]. When Agustín-Panadero et al. compared three types of implant-supported prosthesis (con-

ventionally cemented crowns, screw-retained, and cemented crowns with BOPT) all having a switching platform design, greater keratinized mucosal width, less pocket depth, lower incidence of bleeding on probing, and less bone loss of cemented prosthesis with BOPT were observed in comparison to conventionally cemented and screw-retained prosthesis. Therefore, according to the principle of BOPT, the interface between the abutment and the crown is located further from the bone in two planes, horizontally and vertically, presenting what is called "double switching platform" [36].

Analogical and Digital Workflow of BOPT in Implants

As mentioned earlier, the peri-implant mucosal sealing capacity depends largely on the prosthesis design and specifically on its emergence profile. Thus, both the dentist and the lab technician play an indispensable role in determining the best emergence profile design of the implant-supported prosthesis to achieve optimum esthetics and preservation of peri-implant soft tissue, all of which eventually lead to the survival of the peri-implant hard tissues as well. Two workflow options are suggested for BOPT prosthesis over implants: (1) the analogical and (2) the digital workflow. Both options involve modifications to the existing peri-implant gingiva in order to create an emergence profile optimized to the BOPT prosthesis.

Analogical Workflow

Following the final silicone impression with either an open or a closed tray and prior to pouring of the impression, an O-ring silicone of 1 mm thickness is inserted surrounding each analog's head to form a minimal area exempt of plaster (Fig. 23.5). Adding this O-ring will clear the way to prepare the correct emergence profile by selectively reducing the plaster model without interfering with the edges of the analog, which is usually located slightly beneath the gingiva level (Fig. 23.6a, b) [37].

At first, the crown's cervical contour of the proper emergence profile is traced on the cast based on the objective clinical criteria: gingival thickness and radiographic bone profile. The plaster is then manually trimmed using either a laboratory scalpel or a diamond bur to obtain the best ovoid profile of the future BOPT crown (Fig. 23.6). To maintain sufficient papilla thickness, proper festooning in the interproximal surface is indicated. Regarding the cervical crown

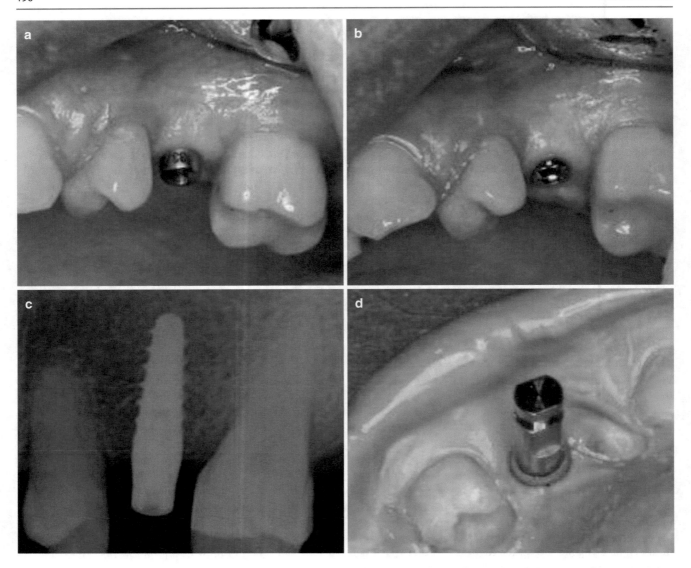

Fig. 23.5 (**a**) Prama implant with the healing abutment. (**b**) Prama implant without the healing cap. (**c**) Periapical photo showing the osseointegration of the implant having the transmucosal convergent collar. (**d**) Final impression of the BOPT implant with the insertion of the O-ring silicone. (With permission from Dr. Guillermo Cabanes Gumbau)

morphology, over-contouring in a buccolingual direction is necessary to generate a prominent emergence profile [37].

Selective gingival compression allows the definitive crowns with proper emergences to create a correct cervical profile where the appropriate gingival morphology created on the cast is transferred to the patient's mouth (Fig. 23.7). Eventually, the thickness and color of the peri-implant mucosal tissues improve with time (Fig. 23.8) [37].

Digital Workflow

Due to the recent advancements in technology, the aforementioned procedure can also be done in a digital setting thanks to an intraoral scanner's presence. In this digital workflow, the practitioner can scan the implant position and design the emergence profile of the crown according to the coronal position indicated for this individualized implant-supported BOPT prosthesis.

Just like a pencil was used in the conventional impression technique, the clinician can use the intraoral scanner's digital software to trace the limits of the cervical contour according

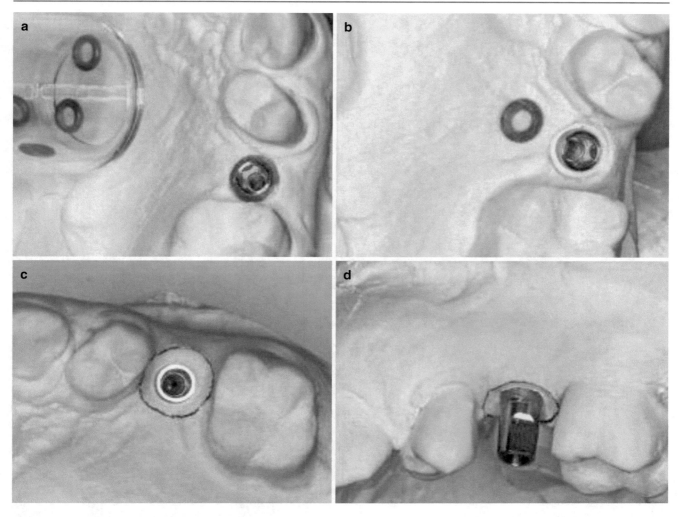

Fig. 23.6 (**a**) O-ring silicone on the plaster model. (**b**) Space created by the O-ring silicone clearing the way for emergence profile preparation. (**c**) Tracing the cervical contour of the desired emergence profile on the plaster model. (**d**) Abutment placed on the implant analog. (With permission from Dr. Guillermo Cabanes Gumbau)

to the desired emergence profile. The clinician should digitally trace the cervical contours and specify the exact starting point of the emergence profile of the crown, either from the head of the implant or from the abutment. The needed distance's depth should be specified interproximally, buccally, and lingually and should ideally be not more than 1–1.5 mm. Accordingly, the lab technician can determine before printing the digital model the required amount and morphology of reduction around the implant to create an accurate unique emergence profile. In this way, the model is printed with modifications that include details about the soft tissue contour. Since this resin model has analogs that can be extracted, the prosthesis is fabricated faster. Clinicians can more easily

check the prosthesis adaptation, the interferences of friction areas, and the contact points [37].

The plaster model can also be conventionally prepared through manual reduction and modeling in the lab and chairside by the clinician who might wish to control this critical phase of the prosthesis more closely. The clinician can manually prepare the model by obtaining the cast and using rotary/manual instruments in the dental clinic. Nonetheless, most dentists will find it more practical to use the digital computer design option prior to obtaining the resin prototype. Besides, the emergence profiles initially printed with the prototype model will often necessitate extra minor manual modifications that can be effortlessly done with burs by either the lab technician or the dentist. Therefore, the digital

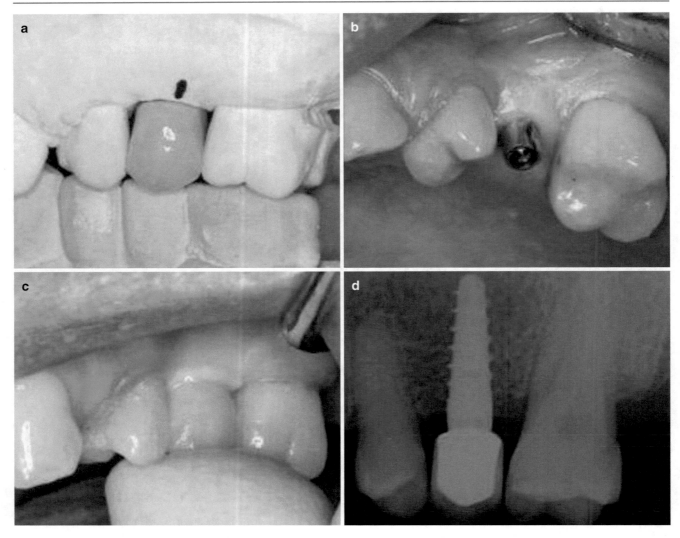

Fig. 23.7 (**a**) Final BOPT implant-supported restoration on the model cast. (**b**) BOPT implant abutment placed intraorally. (**c**) Slight blanching of the gingival margin due to compression created by the BOPT restoration. (**d**) Periapical X-ray of the Prama implant with the BOPT restoration. (With permission from Dr. Guillermo Cabanes Gumbau)

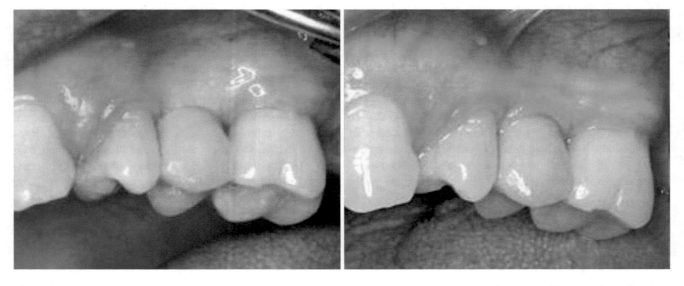

Fig. 23.8 Final BOPT implant-supported restoration after gingival color improvement. (With permission from Dr. Guillermo Cabanes Gumbau)

technique allows the dentist to better control these primary yet significant parameters in preparing the BOPT crowns in a simpler and more applicable manner [37].

However, this digital workflow has several drawbacks. First, since these analogs are extractable, problems in precision may arise compared to the analogical technique. Second, the digital technique's accuracy is also affected by the scanning procedure itself, the type of intraoral scanner used, the software used to design the prosthesis, the type and quality of printer, and the analogs used [38]. Finally, designing the crown on the software is not as real as designing it on a plaster model. This demands a dentist highly experienced in the digital field and who is trained to see virtual three-dimensional objects [39].

Conclusion

The purpose of this chapter is to briefly discuss the BOPT with its analogical and digital clinical steps, benefits, and drawbacks on teeth and implants. Various researches on the concept have advanced the technique from the skeptical to the predictable with commendable success rates. The results have shown the effectiveness of this type of preparation in thickening the gingiva and decreasing marginal gingival recession, to make up for the errors that might prevail in conventional horizontal preparations. However, being a very sensitive technique both at a clinical and laboratory level, it requires additional training by the clinician and lab technician before starting its implication. In addition, studies concerning digital workflows in BOPT on teeth and implants are scarce. This underpins the need for additional research on how to best establish completely digitalized workflows with vertical preparations knowing that they suffer certain limitations and require changes in working protocols. Finally, BOPT seems to provide promising results as long as it is used correctly and its limitations are understood.

References

1. Merijohn GK. Management and prevention of gingival recession. Periodontology. 2016;2000(71):228–42.
2. Podhorsky A, Rehmann P, Wöstmann B. Tooth preparation for full-coverage restorations—a literature review. Clin Oral Investig. 2015;19:959–68.
3. Aboushelib MN. Fatigue and fracture resistance of zirconia crowns prepared with different finish line designs. J Prosthodont. 2011;21:22–7.
4. Schmitz JH, Cortellini D, Granata S, Valenti M. Monolithic lithium disilicate complete single crowns with feather-edge preparation design in the posterior region: a multicentric retrospective study up to 12 years. Quintessence Int. 2017;48:601–8.
5. Łabno P, Drobnik K. Comparison of horizontal and vertical methods of tooth preparation for a prosthetic crown. J Pre-Clin Clin Res. 2020;14:25–8.
6. Loi I. Biologically oriented preparation technique (BOPT): a new approach for prosthetic restoration of periodontically healthy teeth. Eur J Esthet Dent. 2013;8:10–23.
7. Agustín-Panadero R, Solá-Ruíz MF. Vertical preparation for fixed prosthesis rehabilitation in the anterior sector. J Prosthet Dent. 2015;114:474–8.
8. Agustín-Panadero R, Solá-Ruíz MF, Chust C, Ferreiroa A. Fixed dental prostheses with vertical tooth preparations without finish lines: a report of two patients. J Prosthet Dent. 2016;115:520–6.
9. Agustín-Panadero R, Serra-Pastor B, Fons-Font A, Solá-Ruíz M. Prospective clinical study of zirconia full-coverage restorations on teeth prepared with biologically oriented preparation technique on gingival health: results after two-year follow-up. Oper Dent. 2018;43:482–7.
10. Agustín-Panadero R, Loi I, Fernández-Estevan L, Chust C, Rech-Ortega C, Pérez-Barquero JA. Digital protocol for creating a virtual gingiva adjacent to teeth with subgingival dental preparations. J Prosthodont Res. 2020;64:506–14.
11. Ruiz R. Técnica B.O.P.T.: líneas generales y guía práctica. Editorial Quintessence, S.L., Barcelona, España; 2018.
12. Serra-Pastor B, Loi I, Fons-Font A, Solá-Ruíz MF, Agustín-Panadero R. Periodontal and prosthetic outcomes on teeth prepared with biologically oriented preparation technique: a 4-year follow-up prospective clinical study. J Prosthodont Res. 2019;63:415–20.
13. Imburgia M, Cortellini D, Valenti M. Minimally invasive vertical preparation design for ceramic veneers: a multicenter retrospective follow-up clinical study of 265 lithium disilicate veneers. Int J Esthet Dent. 2019;14:3.
14. Schmitt J, Wichmann M, Holst S, Reich S. Restoring severely compromised anterior teeth with zirconia crowns and feather-edged margin preparations: a 3-year follow-up of a prospective clinical trial. Int J Prosthodont. 2010;23:107–9.
15. Wisithphrom K, Murray P, About I, Windsor LJ. Interactions between cavity preparation and restoration events and their effects on pulp vitality. Int J Periodontics Restorative Dent. 2006;26:596–605.
16. Rodríguez X, Vela X. Cutting-edge implant rehabilitation design and management: a tapered abutment approach. Compend Contin Educ Dent. 2017;38:482–91.
17. Comlekoglu M, Dundar M, Özcan M, Gungor M, Gokce B, Artunc C. Influence of cervical finish line type on the marginal adaptation of zirconia ceramic crowns. Oper Dent. 2009;34:586–92.
18. Agustin-Panadero R, Roman-Rodriguez J, Ferreiroa A, Sola-Ruiz M, Fons-Font A. Zirconia in fixed prosthesis. A literature review. J Clin Exp Dent. 2014. https://doi.org/10.4317/jced.51304.
19. Agustín-Panadero R, Martín-de Llano J-J, Fons-Font A, Carda C. Histological study of human periodontal tissue following biologically oriented preparation technique (BOPT). J Clin Exp Dent. 2020. https://doi.org/10.4317/jced.56290.
20. Rompen E, Raepsaet N, Domken O, Touati B, Dooren EV. Soft tissue stability at the facial aspect of gingivally converging abutments in the esthetic zone: a pilot clinical study. J Prosthet Dent. 2007. https://doi.org/10.1016/s0022-3913(07)60015-8.
21. Linkevicius T, Apse P, Grybauskas S, Puisys A. Influence of thin mucosal tissues on crestal bone stability around implants with platform switching: a 1-year pilot study. J Oral Maxillofac Surg. 2010;68:2272–7.
22. Rodríguez-Ciurana X, Vela-Nebot X, Segalà-Torres M, Calvo-Guirado JL. The effect of interimplant distance on the height of the interimplant bone crest when using platform-switched implants. Int J Periodontics Restorative Dent. 2009;29:141–51.
23. Heinemann F, Hasan I, Schwahn C, Biffar R, Mundt T. Crestal bone resorption around platform-switched dental implants with fine threaded neck after immediate and delayed loading. Biomedizinische Technik/Biomed Eng. 2010;55:317–21.

24. Tallarico M, Canullo L, Caneva M, Özcan M. Microbial colonization at the implant-abutment interface and its possible influence on periimplantitis: a systematic review and meta-analysis. J Prosthodont Res. 2017;61:233–41.

25. Canullo L, Pellegrini G, Allievi C, Trombelli L, Annibali S, Dellavia C. Soft tissues around long-term platform switching implant restorations: a histological human evaluation. Preliminary results. J Clin Periodontol. 2010;38:86–94.

26. Canullo L, Tallarico M, Pradies G, Marinotti F, Loi I, Cocchetto R. Soft and hard tissue response to an implant with a convergent collar in the esthetic area: preliminary report at 18 months. Int J Esthet Dent. 2017;12:306–23.

27. Seon GM, Seo HJ, Kwon SY, Lee MH, Kwon B-J, Kim MS, Koo M-A, Park BJ, Park J-C. Titanium surface modification by using microwave-induced argon plasma in various conditions to enhance osteoblast biocompatibility. Biomater Res. 2015. https://doi.org/10.1186/s40824-015-0034-2.

28. Belser UC, Grütter L, Vailati F, Bornstein MM, Weber H-P, Buser D. Outcome evaluation of early placed maxillary anterior single-tooth implants using objective esthetic criteria: a cross-sectional, retrospective study in 45 patients with a 2- to 4-year follow-up using pink and white esthetic scores. J Periodontol. 2009;80:140–51.

29. Cocchetto R, Canullo L. The "hybrid abutment": a new design for implant cemented restorations in the esthetic zones. Int J Esthet Dent. 2015;10:186–208.

30. Sola-Ruiz M, Highsmith JDR, Labaig-Rueda C, Agustin-Panadero R. Biologically oriented preparation technique (BOPT) for implant-supported fixed prostheses. J Clin Exp Dent. 2017. https://doi.org/10.4317/jced.53703.

31. Hamilton DW, Chehroudi B, Brunette DM. Comparative response of epithelial cells and osteoblasts to microfabricated tapered pit topographies in vitro and in vivo. Biomaterials. 2007;28:2281–93.

32. Guarnieri R, Grande M, Zuffetti F, Testori T. Incidence of peri-implant diseases on implants with and without laser-microgrooved collar: a 5-year retrospective study carried out in private practice patients. Int J Oral Maxillofac Implants. 2018;33:457–65.

33. Rancitelli D, Poli PP, Cicciù M, Lini F, Roncucci R, Cervino G, Maiorana C. Soft-tissue enhancement combined with biologically oriented preparation technique to correct volumetric bone defects: a clinical case report. J Oral Implantol. 2017;43:307–13.

34. Jung RE, Pjetursson BE, Glauser R, Zembic A, Zwahlen M, Lang NP. A systematic review of the 5-year survival and complication rates of implant-supported single crowns. Clin Oral Implants Res. 2008;19:119–30.

35. Marconcini S, Giammarinaro E, Covani U, Mijiritsky E, Vela X, Rodríguez X. The effect of tapered abutments on marginal bone level: a retrospective cohort study. J Clin Med. 2019. https://doi.org/10.3390/jcm8091305.

36. Agustín-Panadero R, Bustamante-Hernández N, Labaig-Rueda C, Fons-Font A, Fernández-Estevan L, Solá-Ruíz MF. Influence of biologically oriented preparation technique on peri-implant tissues; prospective randomized clinical trial with three-year follow-up. Part II: soft tissues. J Clin Med. 2019;8:2223.

37. Cabanes-Gumbau G, Soto-Peñaloza D, Peñarrocha-Diago M, Peñarrocha-Diago M. Analogical and digital workflow in the design and preparation of the emergence profile of biologically oriented preparation technique (BOPT) crowns over implants in the working model. J Clin Med. 2019;8:1452.

38. Rebong RE, Stewart KT, Utreja A, Ghoneima AA. Accuracy of three-dimensional dental resin models created by fused deposition modeling, stereolithography, and polyjet prototype technologies: a comparative study. Angle Orthod. 2018;88:363–9.

39. Javaid M, Haleem A. Current status and applications of additive manufacturing in dentistry: a literature-based review. J Oral Biol Craniofac Res. 2019;9:179–85.

The All-on-Four Concept

Ghida Lawand, Hani Tohme, Abdullah Ajili,
and Yara Ismail

Introduction

Periodontal disease, poor oral hygiene, and dental caries are some of the many reasons that lead to complete tooth loss, a condition termed as "edentulism," a commonly occurring condition in the elderly that has a series of deleterious consequences on the oral health-related quality of life as well as the general health [1]. Due to the reported increase in life expectancy by the World Health Organization (WHO) [2], edentulism cases are on the increase. And despite enhancements in preventive dentistry, edentulism is still a main public health problem that underpins the huge need for offering solutions to this condition. Complete edentulism is traditionally treated with a conventional maxillary denture and mandibular overdenture with two implants. However, this restorative option may not be satisfactory to the patient in the long term as bone loss continues in the maxilla with possible acceleration in the premaxilla, resulting in further prosthetic complications [5]. A major shift in the fully edentulous treatment began when Prof. Per-Ingvar Brånemark discovered the osseointegration process of implants, which was then approved for clinical use in 1978 [3]. His breaking innova-

tion has disrupted treatment modalities where dental implants became widely used due to their predictable long-term survival rate [4]. Dental implants are usually placed in an upright straight position. Nevertheless, patients with complete edentulism suffer from severe bone resorption and poor bone quality and quantity. This makes implant placement challenging due to anatomical limitations like the inferior alveolar nerve and maxillary sinus in the mandible and maxilla, respectively, which entail bone grafting and sinus lift procedures. To address this problem, the concept of distally tilting the implants was introduced by Krekmanov et al. [6]. Soon after Krekmanov proved this theory, Malo and his colleagues developed the "all-on-four" immediate function concept in 2003 [7]. This concept was based on placing four implants in a fully edentulous mandibular arch: two implants placed vertically in the anterior region and two implants placed in the posterior para-symphysis region with a distal angulation ranging from 30° to 45° [7]. These implants, also referred to as "cornerstones" by Malo, are immediately loaded with a full fixed acrylic prosthesis in a time frame of 2 hours post-surgery. Building on this achievement, Malo applied the same concept in the maxilla in 2005 [8]. Although high success rates using four implants in the upper maxilla were reported in several short clinical studies [9, 10], several studies advocate the use of two more additional implants in the maxilla because better biomechanical behavior of the implants and prosthesis is observed [10, 11].

G. Lawand (✉)
Prosthodontics and Esthetic Dentistry Department, Faculty of Dentistry – Saint Joseph University, Beirut, Lebanon
e-mail: ghida.lawand@net.usj.edu.lb

H. Tohme
Removable Prosthodontics Department, Founder and Head of Digital Dentistry Unit, Faculty of Dentistry – Saint Joseph University, Beirut, Lebanon
e-mail: hani.tohme@usj.edu.lb

A. Ajili
Oral Surgery Department, Universitat Internacional de Catalunya, Barcelona, Spain
e-mail: ain143320@uic.es

Y. Ismail
Prosthodontics and Esthetic Dentistry Department, Faculty of Dentistry – Saint Joseph University, Beirut, Lebanon
e-mail: yara.ismail@net.usj.edu.lb

Advantages and Disadvantages of the "All-on-Four Concept"

The All-on-four concept offers various advantages. The first main benefit of this concept is that it allows a fixed rehabilitation of edentulous patients without bone grafting or advanced augmentation procedures even in severely resorbed ridges that are close to anatomical structures in both the maxilla and the mandible such as the maxillary sinus and inferior alveolar nerve, respectively [7]. This reduces the overall treatment duration, decreases the healing time, significantly reduces the treatment cost, and guarantees lower rates of neurologic and anatomical complications [12]. Furthermore, from a prosthodontic perspective, using fewer implants simplifies prosthetic procedures such as taking impressions, producing a passive prosthetic structure that ensures a good fit [13]. From a surgical perspective, this technique often requires only one surgical procedure as the implants do not have to be uncovered in a second appointment. From a mechanical aspect, tilting distal implants posteriorly on each side of the edentulous arches may reduce the length of the cantilever and consequently better distribute occlusal loads on the prosthesis and implants. The tilted implants may also allow the placement of longer implants, thus improving cortical anchorage and primary stability as it follows a dense, bony structure, i.e., the anterior sinus wall in the maxilla and the anterior wall of the mental loop in the mandible, respectively. Besides, the final rigid full-arch prosthesis reduces the forces on the implants [6]. The rigid prosthesis associated with the all-on-four concept and the enhanced distribution of masticatory load reduces any considerable movement and stress concentrated at the level of marginal bone [6, 12, 14, 15]. Furthermore, the trapezoidal configuration of the prosthesis enables the transfer of masticatory loads into the distal molar area, thus reducing stresses in the implants [12, 16, 17]. Although the distal implants are tilted, the implant/prosthetic outcome resembles that of traditional axial loaded cases due to the increase in the anterior-posterior (A-P) spread, shortening cantilever by increasing the distance between implants, coupled with cross-arch stabilization [18, 19]. Due to the 30- to 45-degree angulated distal implants, the final prosthesis provides adequate function by containing 10 to 12 teeth per arch [13]. Moreover, only four implants allow them to spread out in a position that allows good accessibility for oral hygiene measures by the patient [20]. The major advantage that pertains to patients is the ability to deliver a prosthesis in the day of surgery, i.e., immediately loading the implants, thus providing immediate function and esthetics. In addition, depending on the patient's desires and within the clinical situation, the final restoration can be fixed or removable [21]. Lastly, compared to the traditional technique, which may take years to complete, the all-on-four treatment can be completed in a very short duration of time (in a few weeks) [22].

However, this technique also has many other disadvantages. First, the length of the final prosthesis's cantilever is very limited as it could compromise the durability of the final restoration and implant survival. Second, this technique cannot always be performed freehandedly as implant placement is completely prosthetically driven [21]. Third, in some cases, sound anterior teeth have to be extracted for the sake of carrying out this treatment option. Furthermore, the All-on-four may not satisfy patients' expectations of maximum masticatory efficiency or the prosthesis's overall appearance as it is limited to the first molar distally. Finally, despite the advantages of the all-on-four treatment, regular maintenance on the patient's part is crucial to the treatment's success. For example, patients with a hybrid prosthesis might find it difficult to clean a hybrid prosthesis and so must regularly visit the dentist for this matter [22].

Indications and Limitations of the All-on-Four Concept

The most important criteria to consider when performing this protocol are the width and height of the remaining crest of the bone. In the mandible, a minimum of 4 mm in width should be present as well as 8 mm or more in height in the interforaminal region between the canines, also known as the mandibular symphysis. In the maxilla, the crestal bone ridge should be at least 4 mm in width and 10 mm or more in height between the two maxillary sinuses from canine to canine [13, 23]. This technique is particularly useful when patients present with maxillary sinus pathologies contraindicating sinus grafting procedures. Edentulous or partially edentulous patients with very limited bone height above the mandibular canals in the posterior mandible and sub-antral bone height in the posterior maxilla are also candidates of this treatment [22]. Furthermore, the all-on-four prosthesis provides future benefits in cases of complete overdentures that present with severe ridge resorption. The prosthesis with the tilted posterior implants increases support to the denture and prevents soft tissue abrasion and further bone loss in the posterior region. Even in patients with partial dentures and few intact natural teeth in the anterior region, the all-on-four technique is an alternative permanent solution [22]. Patients presenting with worn-out dentitions and periodontally compromised mobile teeth requiring extraction and replacement of all teeth can benefit from the all-on-four treatment as well. In addition, this protocol is only applied for patients without severe parafunctional habits like bruxism and with a normal mouth opening of 40 mm [24].

Clinical Planning Protocol

Medical History Review

Like any other implant placement procedure, the first step is to evaluate the patient's medical history to see if he/she is a good surgical candidate for implant treatment. Risk factors such as smoking, unmanaged diabetes, and certain medications may interfere with osseointegration, leading to high early failures or increased late failures. The more medically compromised the patient, the higher the chances of implant failure [25].

Patient's Complaints and Expectations

Upon discussing treatment options for partially or edentulous patients, patients must be informed of the continuous bone resorption naturally associated with conventional treatment options that exclude implant placement. However, the most important decision to make for an all-on-four patient is whether the patient wants a fixed or removable prosthesis. Patients will often decline the removable option as it does not satisfy their psychological needs of wanting to have a prosthesis that feels like a part of their body. Some patients, however, are more concerned with restoring function. In this case, a removable prosthesis would serve the purpose. Accordingly, a patient should be informed of the several treatment options of both fixed and removable restorations and the difference in treatment cost. The clinician must also discuss the importance of compliance with oral hygiene maintenance throughout and after the treatment. For example, the treatment plan for a not so compliant patient might be a more easily cleaned removable implant-supported prosthesis. A patient must be aware that compliance is not limited to personal oral hygiene measures and requires regular evaluation by the clinician and maintenance appointments up to four times a year.

Dental History

Any previous dental failures, including those related to periodontal disease and parafunctional habits, must be recognized in the examination session. If a patient presents with parafunctional habits, a removable prosthesis is indicated, as it can be removed at night to reduce the risk of nocturnal parafunction [5]. For the partially edentulous patient, the periodontal status of the remaining teeth and soft tissue must be examined to evaluate their restorability and the benefits of whether to keep or extract the teeth.

Preoperative Photographs

Preoperative photographs must be taken in facial and sagittal views, while the patient is smiling and at rest and in a retracted view, with and without the prosthesis. The photographs will help evaluate the facial and lip support and communicate to the dental technician any details related to tooth or gingival color.

Primary Impressions

Primary impressions and bite registration are taken in the examination session to mount the articulator's study models. If the VDO (vertical dimension of occlusion) is to be increased, a new bite registration is recorded with the occlusal rims tried in. The mounted study casts are necessary to evaluate the available prosthetic space and the inter-maxillary relationship and develop a wax-up for the planned final prosthesis reflecting their position on the arch and their distribution. Accordingly, the impressions must accurately register the edentulous saddles.

Radiographic Examination

Panoramic X-Ray and CBCT
The clinician can use the panoramic X-ray to estimate the amount of bone available in three radiographic zones that serve as guidelines. Evaluation of the three radiographic zones allows the clinician to Pre-operatively evaluate the presence of adequate support for a full-arch fixed prosthesis. However, a panoramic radiograph does not allow the measurement of the width of the residual alveolar bone available [26]. For a more accurate analysis, the use of a Cone-beam computed tomography (CBCT) scan, later discussed in the chapter, can accurately measure the residual ridge's width and guide the clinician in determining the final treatment outcome, including the patient's prosthetic end position.

Maxilla
For a systematic evaluation of the residual ridge available for placing implants, Bedrossian et al. divided the edentulous maxilla into three radiographic zones: (1) zone 1, maxillary anterior teeth; (2) zone 2, premolar region; and (3) zone 3, molar region [26]. This schema enables the restorative and surgical team to construct an initial treatment plan [Fig. 24.1].

- *Variations of the "All-on-Four Concept" in Maxilla*

All-on-four: Zygomatic Implants and Quad Zygoma
In this technique, developed by Branemark, the implant's apex engages to the zygoma's body, transversing the maxillary sinus and emerging from the first molar position at a 45 angle. The end results are two implants placed axially in the anterior position and two zygomatic implants placed posteriorly [27].

All-on-four Shelf: Maxilla
The "All-on-four Shelf: Maxilla," described by Jensen and colleagues, is a variation where the thin crestal bone is reduced to allow the strategic placement of the implant within the premaxilla in an "M" configuration when viewed

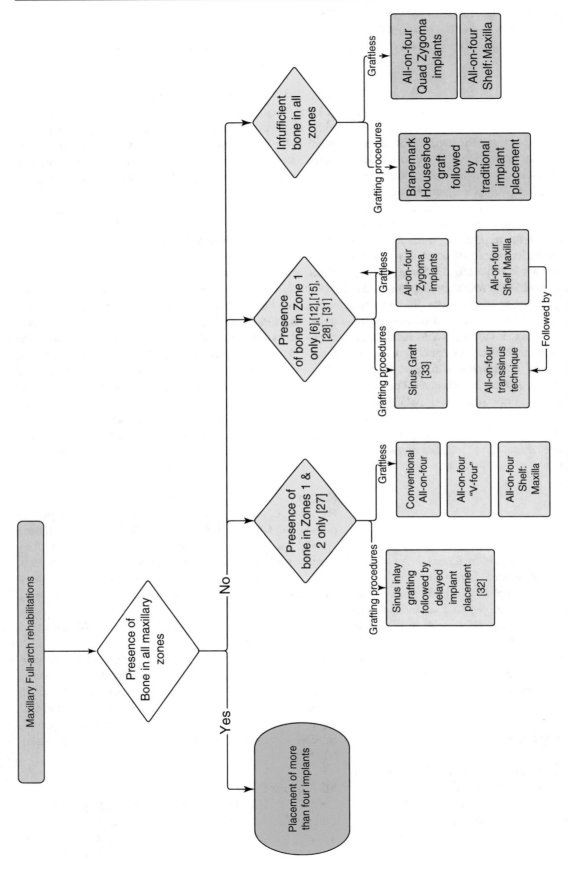

Fig. 24.1 Schematic diagram showing several treatment options for maxillary arch rehabilitations according to the maxillary bone zones

frontally [28]. The alveolectomy reduces alveolar bone until the denser basal bone is reached and increases the inter-arch space required for the definite restoration. The anterior and posterior implants are placed with an apical convergence at a 30-degree angulation. This technique is only indicated in case if an indistinction is present between the maxillary sinus and nasal fossa, in which case it appears as one continuous cavity. In this case, zygomatic implants are indicated [28].

All-on-four Transsinus Technique

An alternative to zygomatic implants is the all-on-four transsinus technique described by Jensen and colleagues. In this procedure, transsinus implants are placed along with a graft of the sinus floor, with the end result of the immediate function. This variant of the all-on-four concept is indicated for patients with extensive sinus pneumatization, atrophic maxillary arches, or post-All-on-four Shelf: Maxilla horizontal bone reduction. The implants are also placed in an "M" configuration [28].

Mandible

Tolstunov divided the mandible into two functional zones: (1) the functional zone 3 (FIZ-3) and (2) the functional zone 4 (FIZ-4). FIZ-3, or the interforaminal zone, is a zone of the alveolar ridge of anterior mandible (symphyseal area), including all anterior teeth and first premolars. The first premolars are included as they are often found anterior to the mental foramen and the inferior alveolar canal bilaterally. FIZ-4, or the ischemic zone, is a bilateral zone of the mandibular alveolar ridge extending posteriorly from the second premolar to the retromolar pad. This zone is limited by the mental foramen anteriorly and the inferior alveolar canal posteriorly [29] [Fig. 24.2].

- *Variations of the "All-on-Four Concept" in Mandible*

All-on-four "V-4"

All-on-four "V-4," described by Jensen and Adams, is indicated for patients with severely atrophic mandibles with residual 5–7 mm of alveolar bone height. The four anterior implants are placed in a "V configuration" at angle 30, when viewed frontally [30].

All-on-four Shelf: Mandible

Following their All-on-four Shelf: Maxilla, Jensen and colleagues performed a similar procedure on the mandible, in which the alveolar ridge was reduced to the basal bone. Although the implant is placed in a manner identical to Malo's "All-on-four" concept, when sufficient bone is present above the inferior alveolar nerve, the distal implant is placed posterior to the mental foramen in a transalveolar direction (buccolingually) to engage the lingual cortex for a better anterior-posterior spread [31].

Clinical Examination

Intraoral Examination

Presence or Absence of a Composite Defect

Two types of defects can be present in edentulous patients: a tooth-only and a composite defect resulting from resorption of alveolar bone and soft tissue and tooth loss. The clinician must differentiate between these two forms of defects as it is a crucial step toward producing an esthetically pleasing final prosthesis; recognizing the form of defect guides the clinician in determining the prosthesis design and material along with the restorative space available or required.

To precisely evaluate the degree of the defect, a transparent duplicate of the try-in denture can be used. The confirmed denture is duplicated by the lab technician using a denture duplicator. The result is a transparent acrylic resin that can be

Fig. 24.2 Schematic diagram showing the variations of All-on-four concept in the mandible

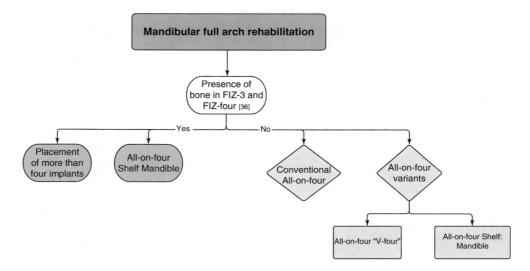

Table 24.1 Guidelines for type of restoration indicated for every restorative space [33]

General guidelines for space requirements	
Space available/obtained (measured from implant head to opposing dentition)	Type of restoration
≥ 10 mm	Monolithic full-contour zirconia fixed restorations
≥ 12 mm	Porcelain fused to metal/zirconia fixed restorations
≥ 15 mm	Acrylic resin bonded to titanium fixed restorations
≥ 16 mm	Implant-supported overdentures *(2–3 mm for heat-cured acrylic resin+ space for acrylic tooth)*

placed intraorally. The defect is then evaluated by comparing the space present between the teeth cervically and the crest of the residual ridge. The transparent denture also helps evaluate the amount of ridge reduction needed to gain the right amount of restorative space, according to the indicated final prosthesis [26]. If no space is present (horizontally or vertically) between the cervical portion of the transparent denture teeth and the residual ridge, a tooth defect is identified. On the other hand, a moderate to a significant amount of space indicates the presence of a composite defect. Nevertheless, the restorative space required for the implant system and final prosthesis will still need to be evaluated.

Restorative Space

Accurately mounted casts are the key to successfully measure the restorative space. When planning an all-on-four prosthesis, the most common error is inadequate restorative space, often realized during the prosthetic space. This error may require either repairing or replacing the veneering material or the entire framework depending on fracture level or choosing another prosthesis design to fit the available space [32]. In cases where space is limited, the clinician must consider one of the three options: altering the vertical dimension, altering the opposing occlusion, and performing an alveolectomy. Accordingly, the clinician must be aware of the restorative space required for the chosen prosthesis design and material (Table 24.1).

A-P Tooth Position

The anterior-posterior spread is the distance between the most anterior and most posterior implants. This distance should be carefully assessed to minimize the cantilever distance of the all-on-four restoration. To determine the A-P tooth position posteriorly in the mandibular prosthesis, Rangert proposed a cantilever of 20 mm for a 10 mm A-P spread, i.e., 2x A-P-spread. On the other hand, English proposed that the A-P tooth position is 1.5x A-P spread, thus allowing a 10–12 mm cantilever posteriorly in the mandible. However, in the maxilla, the cantilever should be limited to 6–8 mm given the low density of the bone [21].

Inter-arch Relation

Before starting the all-on-four implant placement, the clinician must carefully study the inter-arch relation to detect and correct any existing discrepancy [13]. Patients desiring full-arch rehabilitations often present with an unsupported dentition that eventually develops a modified mandibular position during mastication. A clinician should not rely on this habitual inaccurate position during interocclusal record registration; the modified jaw position causes uneven load distribution throughout the prosthesis, resulting in higher rates of fracture of the restoration. Fortunately, this habitual relation can be modified throughout the treatment, during the temporization phase all the way to the definitive prosthesis delivery. In the all-on-four concept, the clinician must record the inter-arch relation in the most predictable position that is in centric relation [34].

Occlusion

The occlusal scheme is an important factor to consider for the long-term prognosis of all-on-four treatments due to occlusal loads' possible effects on implant prosthetic components. Occlusal overloading has been shown to be a primary cause of biomechanical implant complications, including fracture and/or loosening of the implant fixture and/or prosthetic components [35]. Several studies have been conducted to evaluate the effect of various occlusal schemes in full-arch treatments. Turker et al. found that group function occlusion (GFO) is less stressful on screws, abutments, and prostheses as compared to lingualized occlusion (LO) and canine-guided occlusion (CGO) [36]. In cases of opposing natural dentition, Tallarico et al. adopted a mutually protected occlusion with anterior guidance and a balanced occlusion in case of an Fixed dental prosthesis (FDP) and complete removable denture [37]. Another study established a dynamic occlusion with canine/premolar guidance, regardless of the opposite arch's conditions [38]. On the contrary, a study of 109 patients evaluating the treatment outcome and level of patient satisfaction reported no considerable difference among different occlusal schemes in the case of the mandibular implant-supported fixed prosthesis (ISFP) with an opposing maxillary denture [39].

Nevertheless, the occlusal scheme for the fixed full-arch prosthesis is dictated by the opposing dentition; in cases where the opposing dentition is a full denture, the primary aim is to provide a dentition that would not destabilize the opposing denture. However, if natural teeth oppose the prosthesis, the goal is to design an occlusal scheme that would reduce the occlusal overload on the implants placed

[40]. Cantilevers should preferably be infraoccluded (100 μm) [41, 42]. In cases where the implant is placed in the canine region, canine guidance should be avoided as this might lead to occlusal overload followed by mechanical or biological complications of the canine abutment [43]. The case also differs in implant-supported removable overdentures. Some studies have recommended following conventional overdenture occlusal concepts, i.e., bilateral balanced occlusion and lingualized occlusion. In cases where bilateral balanced occlusion seems hard to achieve, the occlusal scheme can take the form of three balanced points in protrusive and lateral movements [44, 45]. However, other clinical studies reported no major difference in terms of patients' satisfaction among the different occlusal schemes [39, 46, 47].

Extraoral Examination

Vertical Dimension

The vertical dimension of occlusion (VDO) can be determined based on the subjective clinical signs related to esthetics and phonetics. The vertical dimension is registered using a base plate and bite with the removable prosthesis in the mouth or before extracting the teeth maintaining the VDO. To measure the VDO, the patient's chin and the tip of the nose are marked. The distance between these two marks is then measured. The distance will serve as a reference point whether the clinician decides to maintain or increase the vertical dimension when placing the immediate full-arch restoration [13].

Facial and Lip Support

Examining the facial and lip support is extremely important when treating an edentulous maxillary arch. Tooth and alveolar ridge loss alter the position of the orbicularis oris muscle and sagittally intrude the upper lip resulting in a typical wrinkled appearance of the edentulous patient. Facial and lip support are assessed with and without the patient's denture in both frontal and lateral profiles [13]. In the case of inadequate facial support, it can be restored mainly by the buccal flange of a removable prosthesis. If a patient with deficient facial support refuses a removable overdenture, a Marius bridge is indicated [26]. However, if a patient with inadequate lip support insists on a fixed prosthesis, the clinician must then evaluate the possibility of this treatment option before proceeding to the next step. A buccal flange cannot be incorporated into a fixed prosthesis due to the impeded access to oral hygiene resulting from the concave intaglio surface. Accordingly, a surgical approach would be required where bone is reduced to a level where the implant is placed higher in order to elevate the restoration's emergence profile [34]. Furthermore,

because the resorption pattern in the maxilla starts labially and inward, a mismatch will exist between the desired teeth position and the residual ridge. In other words, a discrepancy results between the planned implant positions relative to the teeth. This discrepancy cannot be overlooked as it is the key to fabricating a satisfactory prosthesis on both the esthetic and functional levels. If the desired location of teeth and implants is far from the ridge's horizontal limits, a large horizontal discrepancy will result. In such cases, options will include bone reduction followed by deeper implant placement, LeFort I osteotomy, or the use of prosthesis with a flange or fabrication of an implant-supported overdenture [34].

Smile Line and Transition Line of the Prosthesis

For an ultimate esthetic result, the transition between the alveolar ridge's soft tissue and prosthesis should never be visible in both the anterior zone and buccal corridors. This treatment goal sets the rule for the prosthesis design. Upon examination, the patient must be assessed while smiling without the maxillary denture. If the residual ridge's soft tissue is not visible, the transition between the soft tissue of the crest of the ridge and the prosthesis cannot be seen. This implies more flexibility in fabricating a design with harmonious matching colors and contours. However, if the soft tissue can be seen during smiling, then the transition between the prosthesis and the ridge is visible. In this case, the esthetic requirements will depend on whether the patient also has a composite defect. If the ridge has minimally resorbed, conventional metal ceramic- or zirconia-based restorations are indicated, with further enhancement of the present soft tissues to produce an esthetic result. However, suppose a profile prosthesis is used with a visible residual ridge crest. In that case, the junction between the natural soft tissue and artificial gingiva, and the difference in texture and contour, might be detected.

In such situations, an alveolectomy must be considered before placing implants to reduce the ridge's height to a level where it is no longer visible during smiling. At this point, a profile prosthesis may be indicated. If an alveolectomy is not performed, this esthetic challenge can be resolved with a Marius bridge with a flange that hides the junction. The patient can remove the Marius bridge to maintain his/her oral hygiene, along with the stability of a fixed prosthesis offered by this type of restoration [26].

Surgical Phase

After the clinical planning protocol is established, the clinician can start with the surgical phase that is of two types: freehand surgery and guided surgery (Fig. 24.3).

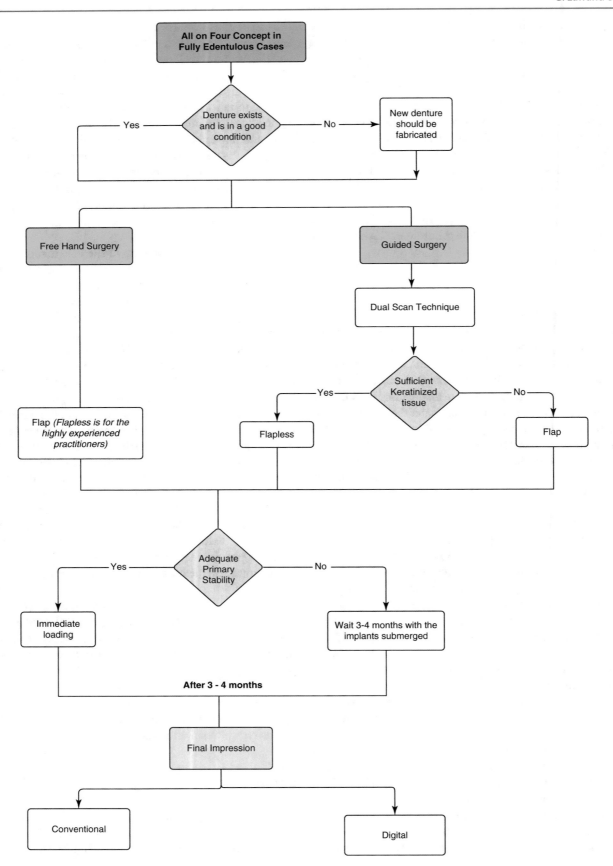

Fig. 24.3 A flowchart showing the different treatment options available for the All-on-four concept in fully edentulous patients

Freehand Surgery (Non-guided Flap Approach)

Freehand surgery in the all-on-four concept involves opening a flap in order to visualize the bone clearly.

All-on-Four in the Mandibular Arch

Knowing the anatomical limits is crucial before performing a freehand surgery [13]. The clinician can easily identify the mental foramen by carefully elevating the flap. The amount of bone available can be determined after checking the loop of the inferior alveolar nerve by inserting a periodontal probe in the foramen, in front of which at least 5 mm is left in order to avoid the loop [48]. After anesthetizing the region, a crestal incision is made, followed by bilateral oblique releasing incisions at the second molar position. A full-thickness mucoperiosteal reflection is created with careful attention to the anatomical landmarks as mentioned previously. In order to start with the drilling process, a marked drill guide specific to the all-on-four concept is used. Each implant system has its own guide that aids in inserting the posterior implants in the appropriate angulation. If the clinician discards this guide's use, there's a chance of angulating the implant more than 45 degrees, which may pose a risk on the implant survival and prosthesis design.

An osteotomy of approximately 8 mm length and 2 mm width is placed in the midline using a 2 mm twist drill to place this guide. After stabilizing the guide in its correct position, the clinician must first place the posterior tilted implants to avoid inter-implant interference by leaving space for the anterior implants. The posterior implants are placed at a 30–45 angle using the precision drill, distally relative to the guide and to the planned depth. The precision drill is then used anteriorly, where it is placed parallel to the vertical lines at 0 next to the midline. An intraoperative radiograph is then taken to verify the angulation and depth of the total four drills. Then, the subsequent drills follow in a sequential manner until the 2.0 mm twist drill is reached. This drill is the most important as it reflects the implant's length and bone density. The implant is then placed depending on the bone density present.

1. If the bone is soft, a 2 mm twist drill is used until the desired implant length is reached, and the subsequent drills are only used on the cortical aspect.
2. In medium-density bone, both 2 mm twist drill and step drill are used until the desired implant's length with the last step drill acting on the cortical aspect only.
3. In dense bone, all the drills are used to the full length of the implant's size. Tapping the osteotomy is necessary if the dense bone is encountered before placing the implant [34].

The surgeon must make sure the drill is kept centered within the bone to avoid perforating the buccal or lingual cortices during drilling. Once the drilling is finalized, the implants are placed, and an insertion torque of 35 Ncm must be achieved in the final seating. In cases of immediate loading, a 35 to 45 Ncm must be obtained to ensure implant stabilization. The insertion torque must not exceed 45 Ncm as it can lead to bone necrosis or implant fracture. When implant insertion is met with resistance, the surgeon should preferably shift to bone tapping. The implants should be finally seated at the level of the bone, with a minimum of 4.3 and 3.5 mm in diameter for the posterior and anterior sites, respectively.

In cases where an alveolectomy procedure is indicated, as mentioned in the clinical planning phase, bone reduction is performed using the rongeur, round bur, or piezoelectric device. The rongeur's advantage is that it allows obtaining autogenous bone that can be used in bone defects if present. The mandibular soft tissue should not be reduced regarding soft tissue considerations but apically positioned due to the limited quantity of keratinized tissue.

All-on-Four in the Maxillary Arch

The procedure followed for the maxillary arch is the same as in the mandible. However, several few steps are added because the anatomical landmarks in the maxillary region differ. The maxilla's anatomical limits are the floor of the nasal cavity in the anterior zone and the anterior wall of the sinus in the lateral zone. Accordingly, a small opening on the maxillary sinus's lateral wall must be drilled to identify the anterior wall of the maxillary sinus. Through that opening, the surgeon explores the wall with a probe. Once identified, the position of the anterior wall is marked with a surgical marker. It's also advisable to start the preparation as posteriorly as possible in order to allow the implant to be at a minimum of 4 mm distance from the sinus. The surgeon then proceeds with all the previous steps already mentioned in the mandibular procedure. Before suturing, the palatal soft tissue of the palatal side must be reduced to avoid covering the abutment or resulting in excess soft tissue, which may interfere during impression making of a multiunit coping with a resultant maladaptation of the prosthesis. However, the buccal soft tissue should not be reduced to maintain adequate keratinized tissue surrounding the abutments [49].

Guided Surgery (Flapless Approach)

The armamentarium of guided surgery in the All-on-Four concept includes [50]:

1. CBCT to apply the dual scan approach
2. Digital planning software
3. 3D printer to print the surgical guide
4. Designing software for the final prosthesis
5. Milling machine

Guided surgery has presented promising results in improving the precision of implant placement in incomplete and partially edentulous patients [51] (Fig. 24.4 (21,22)). One of its main advantages is that it allows the clinician to set the treatment plan on both a prosthetic and anatomic basis. Accordingly, computer-guided implant placement has witnessed an increase in implants' survival rate compared with freehand surgery [52]. There are two types of computer-guided implant surgeries mentioned in the literature: a static one that is mainly based on transferring data from a digital planning software to a surgical guide and a dynamic one that allows the practitioner to continuously visualize the implant placement site through a monitor and accordingly change his planning at any time during the surgery. The static technique, being a simple and cost-effective procedure, is the procedure that is mostly used [53]. Performing a static guided surgery in fully edentulous patients is different from dentate or partially edentulous cases. However, several studies are ongoing on increasing the accuracy and precision of surface scanning completely edentulous jaws using an intraoral scanner, and it is still hard to create reference points necessary for superimposition on a flat mucosa; this is why in the all-on-four concepts, a method known as "dual scan protocol" is used [54].

Before carrying out the "dual scan protocol," a radiographic guide must be obtained. This guide can either duplicate an old complete denture in a good condition, both esthetically and functionally, or a newly fabricated transparent vacuum-formed template (Fig. 24.4(1)). The fabrication of this template is done by preparing a complete denture wax-up following the same steps of complete denture fabrication in terms of establishing denture teeth setup with proper phonetics, vertical dimension of occlusion, and esthetics. A proper radiographic guide is critical because it represents the future prosthetic rehabilitation, and any varia-

tions in its dimensions can cause deviations in the implants' angulations [55]. The guide should have a minimum thickness of 2.5–3 mm to prevent fractures in the future surgical guide. After producing this radiographic guide, the practitioner can proceed with the dual scan protocol. This protocol requires taking two CBCT scans. The first CBCT scan captures the radiographic guide placed on a foam base with six to eight radio-opaque markers. These radio-opaque markers, generally made of gutta-percha, are placed after preparing marker holes of 1.5 mm in diameter using a rose cut bur, making sure not to drill through the guide's full thickness. They are located on the palatal and buccal flanges with fair distribution in order to facilitate future alignment. Caution should be taken on not placing the radio-opaque markers on the occlusal surfaces of teeth because they are important for matching both scans given it's a prosthetically driven procedure.

The second scan is taken with radiographic guide placed intraorally (Fig. 24.4 (2)). According to the patient's centric relation and vertical dimension of occlusion, the guide is stabilized in the mouth by right and left bite indices made of rigid polyvinyl siloxane material. The bite indices stabilize the denture in place, guarantee correct articulation, and permit scanning in an open bite position so that the teeth occlusal surfaces are visible. Two Digital Imaging and Communications in Medicine (DICOM) files are obtained and are imported into a digital planning software. Superimposition of both scans is performed by choosing a minimum of three reference points, creating mutual landmarks that facilitate alignment. Now, the practitioner can vividly examine the amount and density of the bone in relation to teeth position. It's highly important to evaluate the fusion accuracy when using the double scan protocol as all the following steps will rely on it. In addition, to increase the

Fig. 24.4 (1) Previously fabricated complete denture and full edentulous ridge. (2) CBCTs of the two scans according to the dual scan protocol. (3–4) Planning implant placement on the digital planning software called Implant Studio. (5) Designing the surgical guide. (6) Evaluating the angulations of the implants. (7) Digital planning protocol formed by the planning software that will assist the surgeon in the drilling steps. (8) Sending the STL file of the surgical guide to a 3D printing machine. (9) Printed surgical guide with sleeves. (10) Bite indices to stabilize the surgical guide in place. (11) Surgical guide placed intraorally with the aid of the bite index. (12) Occlusal guide of the surgical guide intraorally. (13) Punching the areas of the mucosa to perform a flapless surgery. (14) Fixing the surgical guide with fixation screws and starting the drilling protocol. (15) Implants placed through the surgical guide. (16) Occlusal picture showing the implants' position. (17) Placement of abutments prior to turning the complete denture into a temporary prosthesis. (18) Marking the location of the implants by a pencil. (19) Removing the palate of the old denture and making holes according to the locations of the implants. (20) Placing acrylic to attach it with the abutments. (21) Implant location of the planning software. (22) Panoramic showing the implants' angulations exactly as the planning. (23) Occlusal view showing healing after 3 months of immediate loading. (24) Placing scan bodies over the implants. (25) Pre-preparation scan with the Trios intraoral scanner of the temporary prosthesis, emergence profile scan, and scan with scan bodies. (26) Bite registration. (27) Virtually positioning the implants by adding reference points on the scan bodies. (28) Designing the metallic framework over the implants. (29) STL file showing the design of the framework. (30) Metallic framework fabricated by the selective laser melting additive technique. (31) Lack of passive fit intraorally that necessitated sectioning for soldering again. (32) Adding Duralay to the sectioned part to help the technician reassemble the parts. (33) Soldered metallic framework. (34) Occlusal view of the soldered metallic framework. (35) Try-in of the teeth setup and framework. (36) Acrylic final prosthesis. (37) Frontal view of the final prosthesis. (38) Occlusal view of the acrylic final prosthesis. (With Permission from Dr. Hani Tohme)

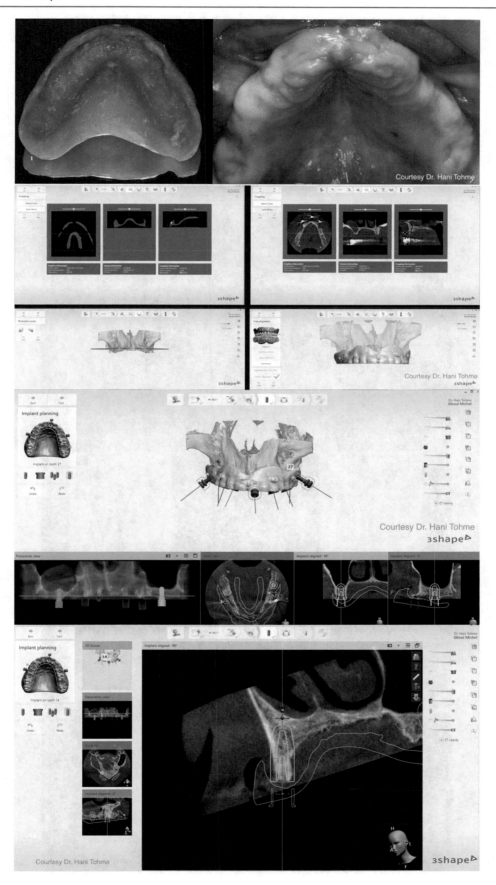

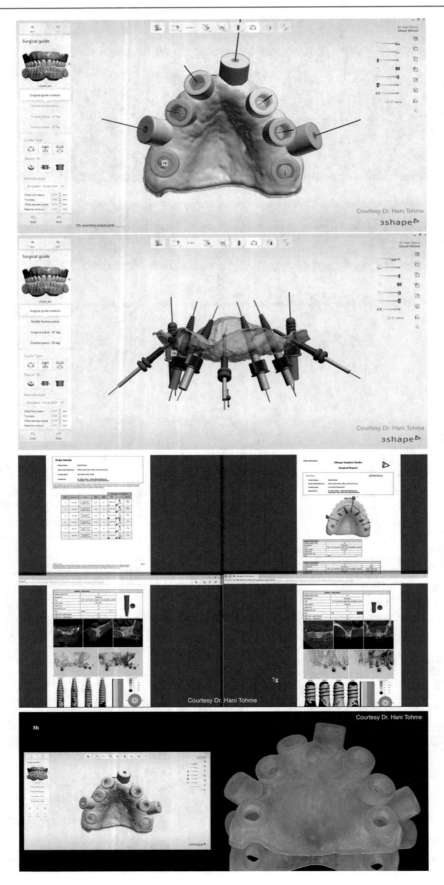

Fig. 24.4 (continued)

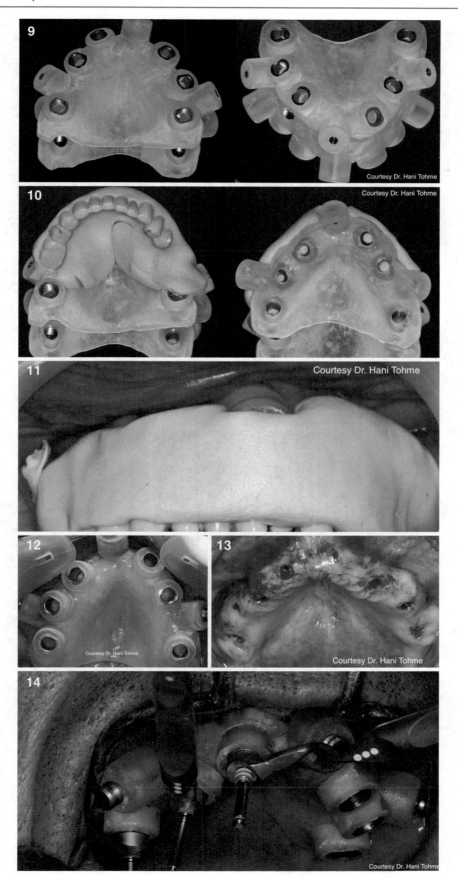

Fig. 24.4 (continued)

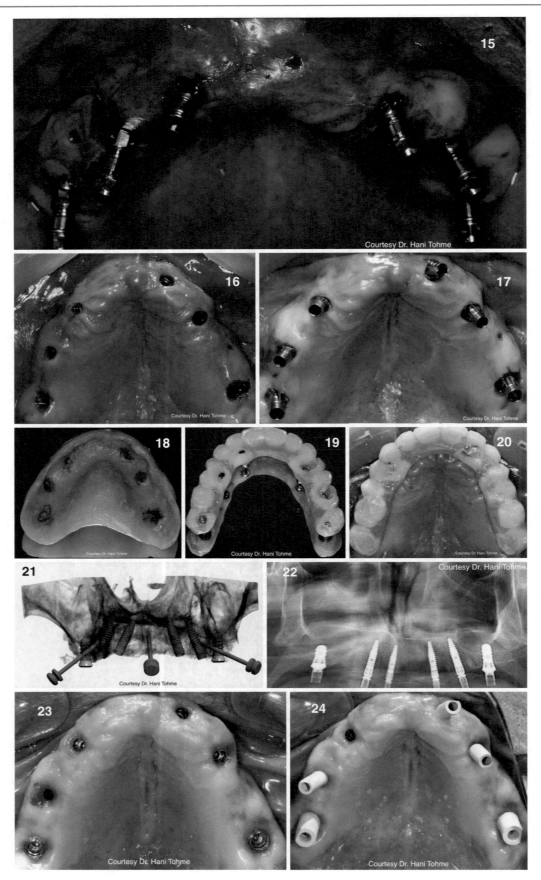

Fig. 24.4 (continued)

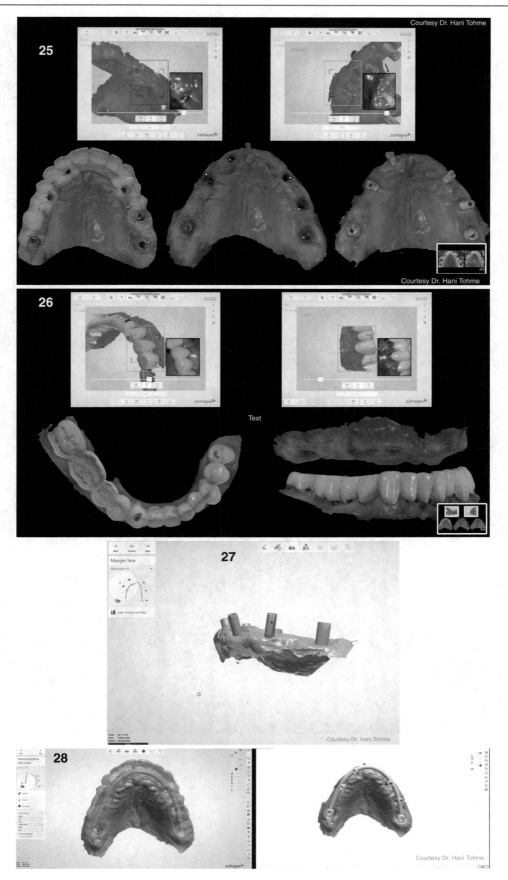

Fig. 24.4 (continued)

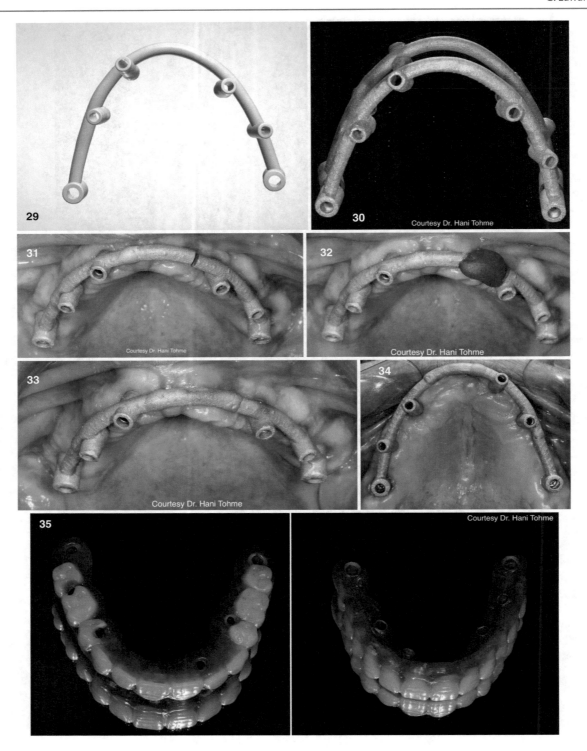

Fig. 24.4 (continued)

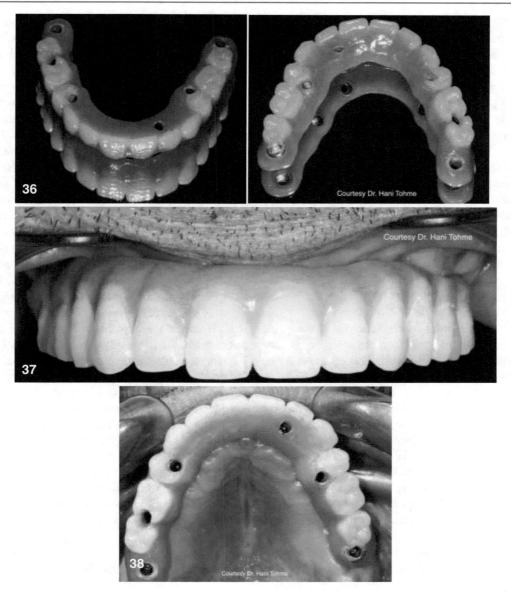

Fig. 24.4 (continued)

accuracy, Oh et al. proposed inserting resin markers on the palate before CBCT scanning to increase the number of reference points and, hence, increase the accuracy of superimposition [56].

After proper alignment is achieved, the practitioner can start planning his surgical guide (Fig. 24.4(3–6)). What's advantageous of this guided protocol is the dentist's flexibility in choosing the type of guide that best suits the clinical condition. The surgical guide can either be tissue-, bone-, or tooth-supported. The tooth-supported guide rests on the teeth occlusal surface, so it is often used in the all-on-four concept when terminal dentition exists. However, it is the least used type because some teeth are present in the area where the implant should be placed, thus limiting its applicability. It

can be contraindicated in some cases because the existing tooth used to support the guide may exist in a place where the implant should be placed. Using bone- or tissue-supported guides is often determined according to whether the surgery is done with or without a flap (flapless) and to whether a terminal dentition exists in the arch or not. Flapless approaches are indicated when a sufficient amount of keratinized tissue exists when the ridge doesn't require preprosthetic surgeries and when the range of jaw movement is not less than 40 mm. In case of limited mouth opening, a mucosa-supported guide is used. Flapless techniques are advantageous because they minimize the possibility of losing peri-implant soft tissue postoperatively and spare the necessity of managing soft tissue during or after surgery

[57]. In addition, the technique is less traumatic with decreased operative time, fewer postoperative complications, and increased patient comfort [58, 59]. However, if an insufficient amount of keratinized tissue is present or bone reduction is required, opening a flap is mandatory, and a bone-supported guide is used. After choosing the type of surgical procedure and surgical guide, planning the four implants' position follows according to the all-on-four concept. While planning the guide, two or three fixation screws must be added to the surgical guide to secure it in place as displacement may occur when drilling. In some cases where osteotomies must be performed, two surgical guides should be planned and printed. The first will guide the practitioner in the bone reduction procedure, and the second one that follows will assist in implant placement after once bone has been reduced. After the surgical guide is designed, the standard tessellation language (STL) file is sent to a 3D additive printing machine ([Fig. 24.4 (8,9)). When printed, sleeves are placed in the surgical guide. The guide is then placed in the patient's mouth in order to check its fit. If the guide doesn't fit perfectly, trimming from the fitting surface is done to reach the ideal fit already planned. Consequently, a bite registration is inserted to ensure the stability (no rocking or rotation) of the surgical guide throughout the surgery (Fig. 24.4 (10, 11)). Following this step, punching is done to remove the keratinized tissue in the area where implants will be placed (Fig. 24.4 (12,13)). The surgical guide is removed to take out the punched tissues and then placed again in the same position using the bite index. Fixation pins are inserted in place to start the surgical phase of the guided surgery. The drilling protocol that the clinician should follow is given by the planning software, ensuring that the implants are placed as planned (Fig. 24.4 (7, 14)).

This case aims at describing all the steps of guided surgery. Although it's an all-on-six case, the protocol followed in the all-on-four concept is typically the same (Fig. 24.4).

Prosthetic Phase

Immediate Loading

Reducing the duration of treatment has become a goal and demand in modern-day implantology. Patients now expect a shorter duration of time between placing implants and installing the definite prosthesis [60]. Furthermore, not all of the elderly find it easy to adapt with their removable prosthesis; thus, the demand for fixed restorations has also been increasing [61]. Accordingly, clinicians must succeed at delivering immediate loading prosthesis, especially in fully edentulous patients who often wish to replace their conventional dentures as soon as possible. Immediately loaded dental implants must achieve adequate primary stability [62] and

should be rigidly splinted around the arch's curvature. In the present day, various diagnostic analyses have been proposed to evaluate primary stability, but the most common are torque and resonance frequency analysis (RFA). In the all-on-four cases, implant torque must be confirmed to be greater than 35 Ncm. The other diagnostic analysis, known as resonance frequency analysis (RFA), utilizes a small transducer tightened to the implant or abutment by a screw. The transducer comprises two elements: vibrated by sinusoidal signals and the other serving as a receptor. Osstell is an RFA device with a measurement unit called implant stability quotient (ISQ), ranging from 0 to 100. A high value indicates more excellent stability. The measurements are objective and can be repeated in a noninvasive, dynamic way to monitor the development of osseointegration. The RFA measures the stiffness of the implant-bone interface throughout the entire body of the implant. In immediate loading, ISQ values greater than 65 have been regarded as most favorable for implant stability, whereas ISQ values below 45 indicate poor primary stability [63]. If one of the implants present did not have optimum primary stability, this might not pose a problem since all implants are splinted with a rigid connection. Upon achieving good primary stability, the immediate loading concept is applied through the temporary prosthesis, in which the existing denture is transferred into a temporary prosthesis (Fig. 24.4 (18,19,20)) . The following steps represent the sequence to achieve temporization (Table 24.2).

In some cases where the opposing dentition is a natural dentition or when the patient has parafunctional habits like bruxism, the acrylic denture is highly susceptible to fracture. This issue is resolved by reinforcing the denture with titanium or metal frameworks to increase its strength [64].

Types and Materials of the Final Prosthesis

The clinical decision-making algorithm on what type of all-on-four final prosthesis to choose depends on the presence or absence of composite defects, as mentioned previously. Figure 24.5. summarizes the options available. If the case is a tooth-only defect, a fixed bridge prosthesis is indicated. However, if a composite defect exists, choosing a fixed hybrid prosthesis or a removable fixed prosthesis depends on the visibility of the residual ridge while assessing the patient's high smile line. Fixed hybrid prosthesis (profile prosthesis) (Fig. 24.6 (9–19)) is appropriate for a nonvisible alveolar ridge, while a fixed-removable prosthesis (Marius bridge) is indicated when the ridge is visible [13]. In fixed hybrid prosthesis, the framework can either be metal-based, zirconia-based, or polyether ether ketone (PEEK)-based. The metal framework can either be casted, milled, or printed by a selective laser melting (SLM) technology. Casted metal can either be cobalt-chromium or noble metals such as silver

Table 24.2 Summary of the steps of changing a complete denture to a temporary prosthesis

Steps for converting the complete denture into a temporary prosthesis

1. Confirm implant torque. A value greater than 35 Ncm must be obtained
2. Take a bite registration
3. Place 30 or 17 and 0 or 17 multiunit abutments on posterior and anterior implants, respectively. The anterior abutments are placed as such so they could emerge toward the occlusal surface of the denture
4. Confirm seating with a radiograph and then torque the abutments to 15 Ncm and 30 Ncm, for the posterior and anterior abutments, respectively
5. Index the denture with polyvinyl siloxane impression material
6. Using an acrylic bur, create adequate space in the denture where index markings are present
7. Remove the protective healing cap, and place temporary coping (multiunit) onto the multiunit abutments
8. Ensure adequate clearance needed for temporary coping (multiunit) and denture
9. Recheck occlusion before placing acrylic
10. Attach the fitting surface of the denture to the temporary coping with acrylic
11. Reduce excess so that the temporary coping is flushed with the denture surface
12. Insert provisional prosthesis with prosthesis screws torqued 15 Ncm
13. Seal access holes with temporary filling

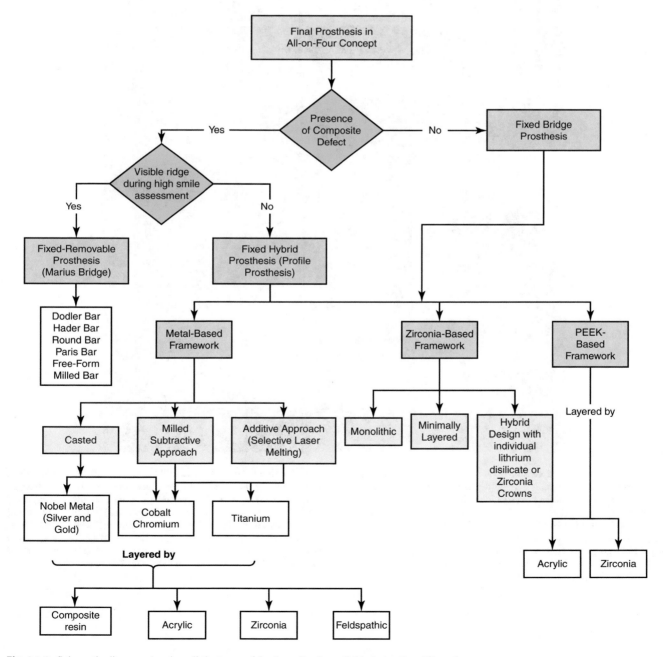

Fig. 24.5 Schematic diagram showing all the types of final prosthesis available to treating All-on-four cases

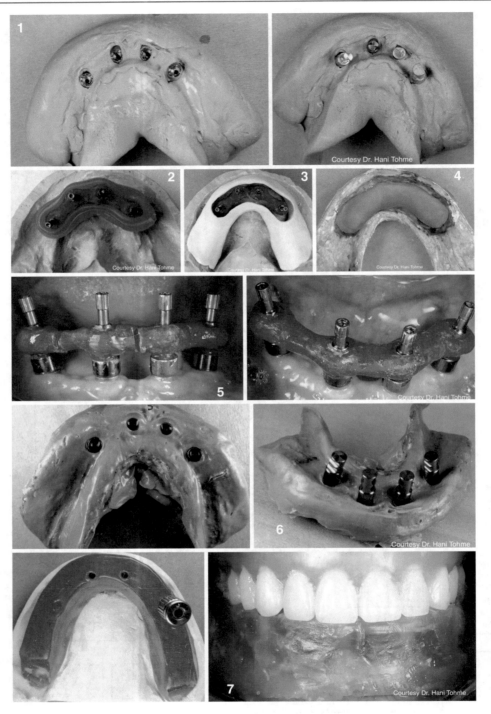

Fig. 24.6 (1) Primary impression of an All-on-Four case using polyvinyl siloxane. (2) Impression coping joined with Duralay. (3) Special tray fabrication. (4) Placing adhesive in the fitting surface and covering the whole with wax. (5) Placing the splinted impression copings intraorally. (6) Final impression with polyether. (7) Record blocks for bite registration. (8) Facebow mounting and teeth setting that aids in the digital design of the framework. (9) Desktop scanning of the cast in order to design the final Toronto bridge All-on-four prosthesis. (10) Superimposing the design of the trial denture in order to design a similar one. (11) Digitally designing the framework. (12) Digitally designing the teeth relative to the framework. (13) Framework trial. (14) Zirconia design of crowns on framework. (15) Zirconia crows and metallic framework. (16) Layering the framework so that it's esthetically appealing. (17) Final Toronto bridge prosthesis ready. (18) Framework screwed in place. (19) Zirconia crowns cemented over the framework. (With permission from Dr. Hani Tohme)

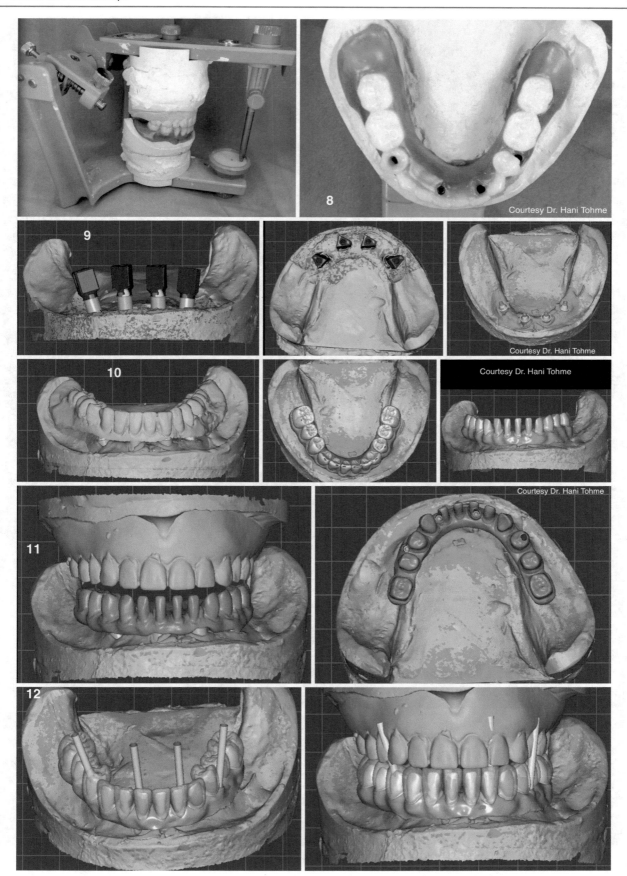

Fig. 24.6 (continued)

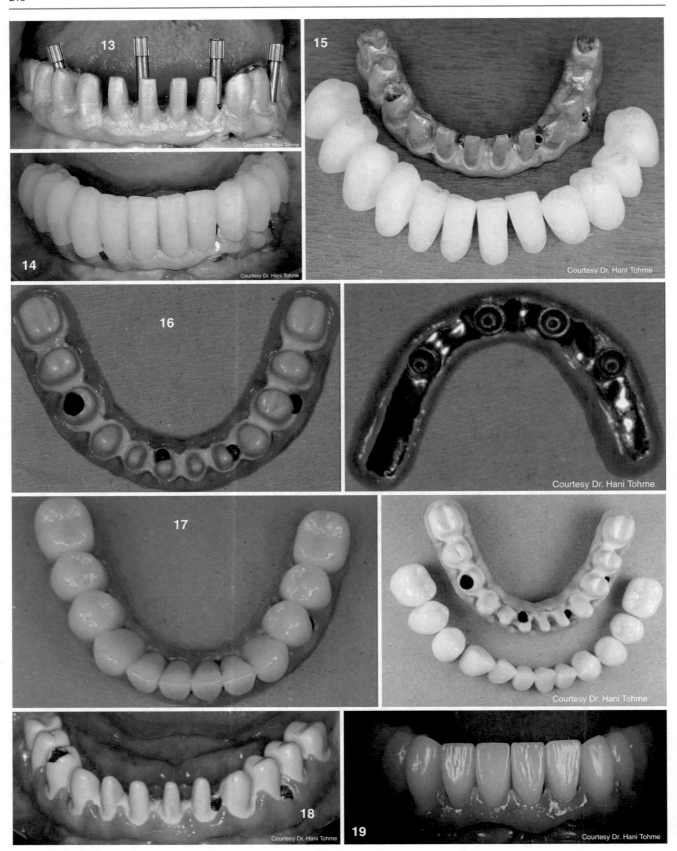

Fig. 24.6 (continued)

and gold. Milled subtractive technique and printed additive technique metals are either titanium or cobalt-chromium. The metal framework can then be either layered with feldspathic ceramic, acrylic (Fig. 24.5. (24–30)), zirconia, or composite resin. Over the last 10 years, zirconia has become increasingly used as the material of choice for full-arch implant prostheses. The main advantage of zirconia is its biocompatibility, low bacterial surface adhesion, high flexural strength, and esthetics [65, 66, 67]. The tooth-like color of zirconia and the excellent wear resistance indicate its use in both the anterior and posterior regions. Zirconia frameworks were previously milled and veneered by porcelain to combine the advantages of maximum strength and esthetics of both materials [68]. However, some clinical studies have reported the complication of chipping associated with the unsupported veneering ceramic [69]. To overcome these drawbacks, it has been recommended that the framework is designed where the occlusal contacts lie in the monolithic zirconia with minimal labial veneering with porcelain, under the condition it is adequately supported. Thus, when designing zirconia-based implant frameworks, the clinician should focus on maximizing the connector dimensions buccolingually and occlusogingivally and decreasing the length of cantilevers. Another alternative to overcome the complication of chipping is using monolithic zirconia. However, further evidence is required to assess the long-term survival of monolithic full-contour frameworks. Nevertheless, some short-term clinical studies have shown that monolithic zirconia CAD/CAM-milled framework restorations for full-arch implant-supported cases are more accurate with no veneer chipping, minimal occlusal adjustment requirements, and high success rates in terms of function, esthetics, and patient's satisfaction [70].

The third type in the zirconia classification is the hybrid design with individual ceramic crowns that can be either zirconia or lithium disilicate. This type of zirconia provides maximal esthetics, especially in the interproximal region, and allows equal distribution of stresses. It also allows easier resolutions of complications associated with single crown fractures as they can be individually replaced in this type of prosthesis.

Polyether ether ketone (PEEK) is a new material recently used in implant fixed prosthesis. This material is claimed to have shock-absorbing properties that may reduce the stresses transferred to the bone-implant interface [71]. As compared to titanium, the modulus of elasticity of PEEK is far lower, but the material remains stiff enough to maintain its rigidity. PEEK's other advantages also include its strength and long-term survival due to its ability to withstand cyclic loads [72]. Fabricating PEEK prosthesis using the CAD/CAM technology has made it much more user-friendly. Despite the several advantages of this material, current studies on the material have been limited to case studies, although the first formal clinical studies are emerging. Malo et al. performed a short-term clinical study to evaluate PEEK layered by acrylic resin in all-on-four fixed prosthesis. The study revealed promising results rendering PEEK a treatment option in all-on-four cases [73]. The last all-on-four restorative option is fixed-removable prosthesis. An overdenture made of acrylic was supported on one of the following types of bars: Dolder, Hader, Round, Paris, and/or free-form milled bar. There are different types of attachments available depending on the clinical case. The attachments can be locators, bars, or clips.

Fabrication of an All-on-Four implant-supported prosthesis must be accurately done in order to ensure its long-term survival. An essential key to such implant treatments' success is the accurate fit of the implant-supported prosthesis, i.e., passive fit, which has been described by Branemark to be ideally in the 10 μm range [3]. A clinically acceptable fit is described as one in which occlusal stresses are well tolerated and within the physiological limits that would enable proper bone remodeling in response to occlusal loads once the prosthesis has been connected. An inaccurate fit between the various parts of the screw-retained denture produces uncontrolled stresses in the prosthetic components and peri-implant tissues, which results in complications including bone loss, screw loosening, component fractures, and possibly eventual loss of the implants, the prosthesis, or both [74, 75, 76]. Highly precise clinical and laboratory procedures are the key to fabricating a well-fit multiple implant prosthetic framework. Heckmann et al. proved that half of the misfits and strains are caused by the impression procedures, while the other half are due to inaccuracies during laboratory procedures such as casting and fabrication of the prosthesis [77]. This is why the impression step is of great importance in determining the prosthesis's passivity and in determining misfit incidences. Today, either conventional or computer-aided approaches can be utilized in order to obtain the needed impression.

Conventional Approach

The conventional impression has several approaches. First, it can be an implant-level or an abutment-level impression. In the abutment-level approach, a multiunit abutment is torqued on the implant, followed by all prosthetic steps done over the abutments. In the implant-level approach, the prosthetic impression components are directly connected to the implant platform. The abutment-level approach allows the easy management of all prosthetic aspects such as impressions, jaw relations, and trials. The choice of impression approach may be determined by the restorative space required. In case of limited restorative space, the implant-level approach may be more suitable as it allows a space gain of 2–3 mm. Regardless of the approach used, the procedural steps will not differ; the only difference is in each component. Second, the impression can be made in an open-tray or closed-tray technique. Both techniques are usually used when taking implant impressions in partially edentulous situations (either single or multiple implants). However, with the all-on four-technique, the closed-tray or indirect transfer technique is not very suitable as it requires implants to be placed parallel to each other. Thus, an open-tray impression is utilized in the all-on four concept, decreasing the distortion's risk associated with the indirect approach [78].

When evaluating several impression protocols with all-on-four cases, Ozan et al. found that in cases of 20-degree or greater angulations between impression copings, open-tray impression techniques proved to be more accurate than the closed-tray. Among highly discrepant implants (30 degrees), cast accuracy is improved by using the sectioned re-splinted open-tray technique [79]. In addition, in fully edentulous implant cases, rigid custom trays have proven to be more accurate in open-tray implant impressions than the polycarbonate stock trays. Rigid custom trays are fabricated either from auto-polymerizing or light-curing acrylic resin or metal [80, 81].

There are three types of impression material preferred for all-on-four cases: (1) polyether, (2) polyvinyl siloxane, and (3) impression plaster as it is a highly accurate and dimensionally stable material. Among the three options, impression plaster is the material of choice when it comes to accuracy. Due to this material's high accuracy, the copings do not have to be splinted; the impression is taken with the copings directly picked up by the impression plaster once it has set in the custom tray. However, impression plasters can only be used with an abutment-level and not impression plaster. If used with implant-level impressions, the plaster might break in the posterior region where angulations are present. Polyether has high rigidity and dimensional stability and can produce accurate impressions in fully edentulous and multiple implant cases. However, the tray is more easily removed using an impression material with higher elastic recovery, such as polyvinyl siloxane. This choice of material will reduce the permanent deformation caused by the stress between impression copings, especially in the case of non-parallel and internal connection implants [82, 83, 84].

When using polyether and polyvinyl siloxane, splinting the coping is recommended to provide more rigid fixation of the impression material's copings. Although numerous studies have examined the effect of splinting vs. non-splinting the impression copings [85–90], the results remain inconsistent with no reports of one technique's superiority over the other [80], [91–93]. Nevertheless, the standard deviation in the splinted techniques is much smaller, and this is why authors advocate its use [93]. Impression copings can be splinted in several ways. These techniques include using auto-polymerizing resin, dual-cured resins, plaster, splinting with prefabricated resin bars, and splinting of copings with auto-polymerizing resin splints, which are sectioned and reconnected after setting [90, 94, 95]. Among these techniques, the majority of literature exists on auto-polym-

erizing acrylic resin (Fig. 24.6 (1–6)). The major disadvantage of resin is its polymerization shrinkage which reduces its accuracy in impression-taking. This drawback is compensated for by sectioning and re-splinting of the acrylic resin [93, 96]. The resin's shrinkage value was found to be at its lowest after 24 h of polymerization [97]. The impression copings should be splinted extraorally on the primary cast with dental floss. Then the resin is applied and sectioned after 24 h. A custom tray is then fabricated on top to be used for the impression procedure. Using a fast-setting resin, the resin jig is then reconnected in the patient's mouth to achieve a passive fit of all the copings. Upon connecting the copings, radiographs of the copings must be taken to verify that all components are properly seated. A pickup impression is then made using a custom tray. Although this technique requires an additional step, it is less messy and saves much chairside time. A study done by Assif et al. on the efficacy of impression plaster as splinting material revealed that it has several advantages including its rapid set, high accuracy and rigidity, resistance to bending or distortion, ease of manipulation, reduced cost and time consumption, and a negligible exothermic reaction [95]. Nissan et al. and Eid also described using impression plaster with implant impressions and reported the material's accuracy, ease in manipulation, and decreased working time [98, 99].

A new method of performing an impression in the all-on-four concept is using a prosthetic guide. The prosthetic guide is a transparent duplicate of the complete denture. This technique is superior to the aforementioned techniques because it combines multiple steps into one single step. First, the clinician can take an accurate final impression with a technique that provides a passive fit for the final prosthesis. Second, a bite registration can be taken at the same time as the impression with the prosthetic guide. Third, the prosthetic guide gives the lab a reference for the prosthetic corridors and teeth setup all at the same time. To perform this technique, it is necessary to follow the steps listed in the table (Table 24.3).

Interocclusal Records (Fig. 24.6 (7,8))

Using tissue-supported bases to register interocclusal records, such as the ones fabricated for complete dentures, is not recommended to compress soft tissue while recording the jaw relation, leading to errors [100, 101]. Instead, interocclusal records should more ideally be obtained on a rigid base that is screw-retained to the implants or abutments. However, using such rims can be very time-consuming as they have to be unscrewed for every adjustment. To overcome this inconvenience, a two-piece rim has been proposed. The rigid primary component is screw-retained to the abutments or implants and has retentive grooves to receive the secondary component, which snaps directly onto the primary part. This technique may require using denture adhesive. This approach is highly advantageous as it allows the clini-

Table 24.3 Steps of taking a final impression using the prosthetic guide

Steps for taking an impression using the prosthetic guide
(a). Take a primary impression with alginate (there's no need to remove the healing caps) in order to prepare primary models (Fig. 24.7 (1–5))
(b). Prepare record blocks
(c). Adjust the record blocks in the patient's mouth along with the occlusal plane, and then take a bite registration according to the centric relation (Fig. 24.7 (6))
(d). Mount the casts on an articulator (Fig. 24.7 (7))
(e). Set the teeth according to the appropriate height and distance (Fig. 24.7 (8,9))
(f). Try the teeth in the patient's mouth making sure that phonetics, function, and occlusion are satisfied
(g). Send it back to the lab technician, so a prosthetic guide made of transparent resin is fabricated (Fig. 24.7 (10–14)])
(h). After receiving the prosthetic guide, check the fitting intraorally. Make sure that there's no interference between the intaglio of the prosthetic guide and the healing cap. If there's any interference, the intaglio is trimmed to remove all the excess resin and achieve a perfect fit (Fig. 24.7 (15))
(i). Remove the healing caps
(j). Place the temporary abutments. Temporary abutments are placed instead of impression copings because the impression coping is long in height, so it may interfere when taking a bite registration. The temporary abutments must be tried to check for further need of adjustments according to the prosthetic height. In case the prosthetic height was 20–25 mm due to severe resorption, an impression coping can be used but remains a risky procedure (Fig. 24.7 (16–18))
(k). Perforate the prosthetic guide in the area of the temporary abutment so that it can be removed and inserted without interference (Fig. 24.7 (19–21))
(l). Take a surface impression. This is done with polyether. In this stage, the temporary abutments should not be connected with the guide since taking the impression with polyether won't be highly accurate because it's a resilient material unlike the rigid plaster (Fig. 24.7 (22))
(m). After the polyether sets, remove the impression where the abutments are still screwed in
(n). Remove the polyether surrounding the abutments
(o). Create a gap between the temporary abutment and the transparent resin
(p). Place the guide with the polyether back in place, and connect the temporary abutments with the guide using pattern resin (Fig. 24.7 (23))
(q). Upon setting of the resin, unscrew the temporary abutments, and remove the impression. The impression now contains polyether that is a replica on the surface and the temporary abutments that reflect the position of the implants. Make sure of the bite by taking a silicone bite registration (Fig. 24.7 (24))
(r). Connect the analogs and pour the impression. Continue fabricating the final prosthesis (Fig. 24.7. (25–30))

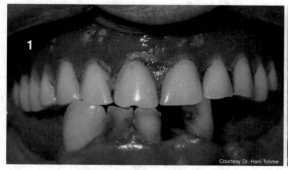
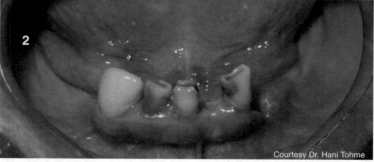

Fig. 24.7 (1) Upper old denture and lower terminal dentition. (2) Teeth of the lower arch. (3) Occlusal view of the lower arch. (4) Panoramic X-ray showing the preoperative condition. (5) Final impression of the upper arch. (6) Record blocks of the lower and upper arch with bite registration. (7) Bite registration shown on the cast. (8) Setting of teeth of the upper arch. (9) Setting of teeth in the lower arch. (10) An index of the lower natural and acrylic teeth. (11) Removal of the teeth on the cast. (12) Fabrication of the prosthetic guide according to the planned final prosthesis. (13) Prosthetic guide with the bite index on the right side. (14) Prosthetic guide and the bite index on the left side. (15) Prosthetic guide placed in the mouth. (16–18) All-on-four implant placement. (19) Perforations of the prosthetic guide at the site of implant. (20) Perforated prosthetic guide placed in the mouth. (21) Placing adhesive coating on the fitting surface of the perforated prosthetic guide. (22) Surface impression with polyether. (23) Connecting the temporary abutment with the prosthetic guide using Duralay. (24) Bite registration. (25) Lower final prosthesis. (26) Upper and lower final prosthesis. (27) Healing after 2 months. (28) Lower final prosthesis screwed over the implants. (29) Panoramic X-ray showing the all-on-four prosthesis where specifically in this case implants were not tilted. (30) Upper final complete denture and lower all-on-four prosthesis

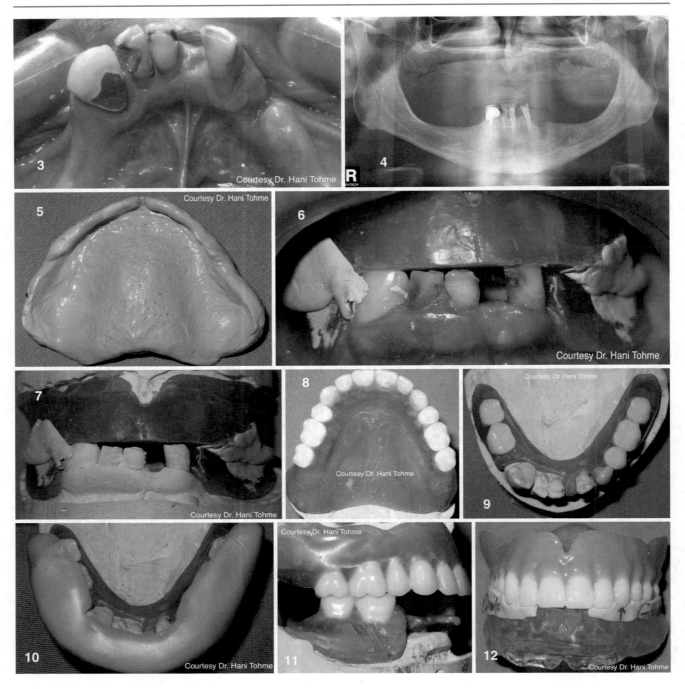

Fig. 24.7 (continued)

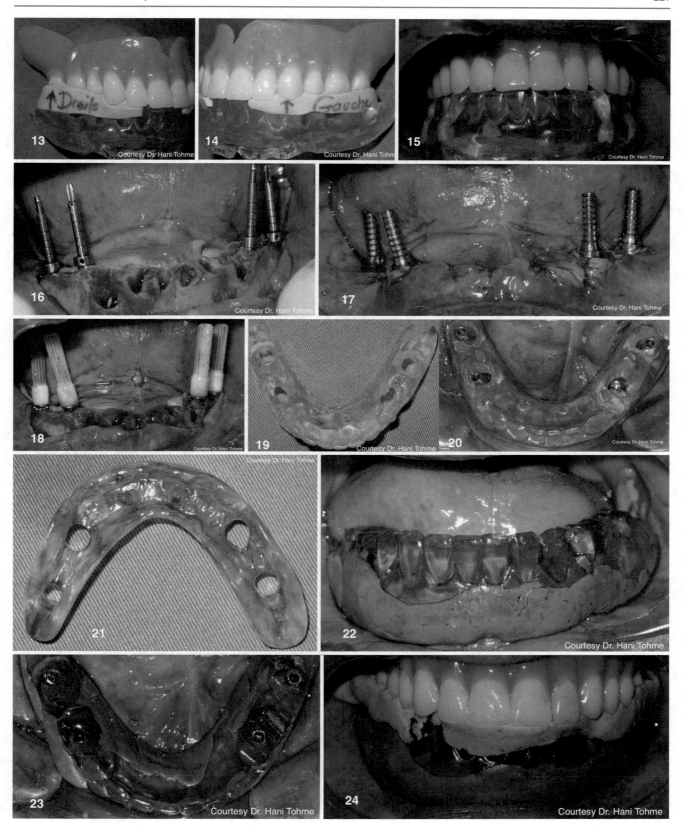

Fig. 24.7 (continued)

Fig. 24.7 (continued)

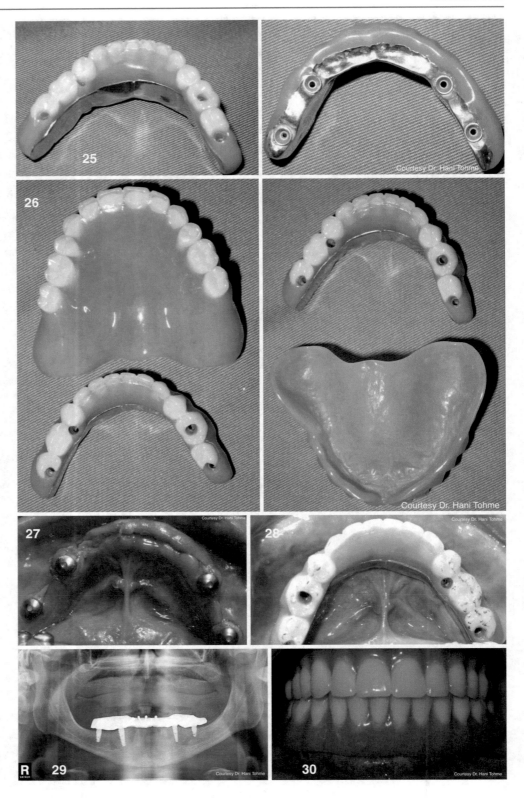

cian to adjust the rim without having to unscrew it constantly. Once the upper rim is retained, a facebow record is registered for accurate orientation of the maxillary cast on the articulator.

Impression Verification

After pouring the master cast, the master cast must be verified prior to milling. This step is invaluable and should not be overlooked by the clinician as it will spare the clinician the possibility of re-making the framework, thus significantly reducing treatment duration and costs. To confirm the accuracy of the master cast, a verification jig connecting all the implants is fabricated on it [102]. This jig must be fabricated of a rigid and non-expanding material [103]. Although acrylic resin jig has been commonly used, it still produces a false-positive result due to its flexibility. Instead, the use of a verification jig made of impression plaster has been recommended. This plaster jig must be secured with one screw. Because plaster is brittle, it will break in the misfit case, indicating the presence of a problem that should be resolved prior to moving to the framework fabrication step.

Framework Fabrication

The types of frameworks were discussed previously in the "Types and Materials of the Final Prosthesis."

Framework Trial

A pickup impression is made with the approved provisional restorations before trying in the framework to transfer information of the soft tissue to the laboratory technician. A full-contour wax-up with controlled cutback should be performed. In complex full-arch cases, the framework is preferably tried to ensure its passive fit [104]. The framework's fitting surface is inspected for any surface irregularities before trying it intra-orally. The clinician must also evaluate the cutback using a putty matrix as a reference to ensure a controlled cutback with even thickness. Once the framework is inspected, the healing abutments or provisionals are removed. The framework is then placed intraorally to verify its passive fit (Table 24.4).

The screw furthest distally is first tightened completely, and a radiograph of the contralateral side is taken to verify the fit of the framework and its flush with the implant/abutment on that side. If a misfit is detected either through the radiograph or screw test (Sheffield test) [104], then the impression must have been inaccurately made. If the misfit occurs with a cast framework, the framework must be sectioned and verified through a radiograph. It is then reconnected intraorally using the pattern resin and resent to the laboratory to be soldered (Fig. 24.4 (31–34)). However, this option may not be possible with milled frameworks such as titanium and zirconia frameworks. At this point, a new impression must be made to re-mill the entire framework.

Table 24.4 Clinical methods available to evaluate passive fit [104]

Clinical methods to evaluate passive fit
"Alternate finger pressure," to evaluate the instability of the prosthetic superstructure and observe the misfit gap for any bubbling around
Direct visualization and tactile sensation by using the explorer tip to confirm the marginal fit, which is restricted by the explorer tip dimension (a pristine explorer tip is approximately 60 mm)
Radiographs: overlap or superimposition is a possible disadvantage; depends on different angulations
"The Sheffield test" ("the one-screw test"): tightening one screw at the end of one side of the framework, and then discrepancies are detected at the other end screw
"Screw resistance test," where one starts with the midline nearest implant; the screws are then tightened one after the other until the initial resistance is met at one of the screws. If the screw needs more than an extra half a turn to reach the optimal screw seating, the framework is considered misfitting
Disclosing media, like "fit checker" (GC), "pressure-indicating paste," or disclosing wax

Second Interocclusal Record

When trying the framework, the jaw relation is preferably verified by registering a second interocclusal record. This clinical step is challenging as the vertical dimension may be altered when registering a new bite and, accordingly, limiting the space available for the veneering ceramic. To avoid this possible complication, the interocclusal record is best registered using an anterior jig. This jig is fabricated on an articulator at the planned vertical dimension and includes a rigid posterior recording material. A second method would be obtaining the framework with three metal occlusal stops fabricated by the laboratory technician. This bite record can then be taken with a bite registration material. The occlusal contacts can then be adjusted by remounting the casts at the desired vertical dimension.

Try-In Stage (Fig. 24.4 (35–38))

All the clinical steps that have been performed during the framework trial stage have to be repeated in the try-in stage. The prosthesis must now be evaluated esthetically to confirm the teeth position relative to the dynamics of the lip and the patient's smile line. In addition, the occlusal scheme must provide maximum intercuspation in centric relation. Bilateral uniform contacts must be confirmed along with anterior guidance that allows disclusion of the posterior teeth during function [105–107]. The anterior guidance must exist within the envelope of function to avoid any interferences [108]. The tissue surface of the prosthesis must maintain positive contact with edentulous areas between the implants. If no such contact exists in the anterior maxilla area, speech sounds would be impeded due to the air escape during the speech. The prosthesis must also have a modified ridge lap or an ovate pontic in both anterior and posterior regions for normal speech and food entrapment avoidance, respectively. A small degree of soft tissue blanching is desired upon screwing the prosthesis over the implants. This blanching should only last for a few seconds or else tissue necrosis will occur if the blanching persists [109]. In case of prolonged excessive blanching, the emergence contour of the prosthesis surrounding the implant must be reduced. After performing the adjustments, the tissue surface of the prosthesis must be highly polished. Lastly, the interocclusal contacts intraorally should match those on the mounted casts. The laboratory technician might have to add ceramic in areas of deficient contacts. However, in case of major discrepancies in occlusion, a new interocclusal record must be resent to the laboratory.

Digital Approach

To make computer-aided implant impressions and transfer three-dimensional implant positions into the digital system, the clinician needs an intraoral scanner and scanning abutments, called scan bodies [110]. These scanning elements have different geometrical properties, such as notches and emersions, which provide information about the implant position in three aspects: rotation, angle, and depth. The scan bodies are either metal-based or manufactured from polyether ether ketone (PEEK). These scan bodies offer the advantages of reducing chair time and simplifying the technique of implant impression-making. From a theoretical aspect, the scan bodies also prevent repeated traumatization of the peri-implant mucosal tissue as the healing abutment is only removed when the final prosthesis is to be delivered. The accuracy of digital impression in All-on-four cases is still questionable. Many studies are ongoing on how to increase the accuracy of digital impressions in the complete implant-supported prosthesis. There are no reference points with the absence of teeth that will help the scanner accurately distinguish the implant positions. Advancements in the intraoral scanners incorporating artificial intelligence present promising results and better scanning strategies.

Protocol for Digitally Scanning All-on-Four Cases
(Fig. 24.4 (23–26)):

1. Pre-preparation scan of the temporary prosthesis and the bite of the patient if all is satisfactory in order to replicate the same design and bite in the final prosthesis.
2. Remove the temporary bridge.
3. Emergence profile scan.
4. Screw the scan bodies over the implants. Two types of scan bodies are available – implant level and abutment level – and scan the arch. Make sure that the flag of the scan body is on the buccal side in order to obtain accurate scanning.
5. Scan the antagonist.
6. Take a bite registration. The bite can be taken either digitally or conventionally. There are two digital scanning

options. The first is to scan the temporary bridge as mentioned previously. The lab will then conduct superimposition. This is why it's indispensable to take a scan of the whole palate if it's an upper arch case in order to superimpose the scan of the temporaries with that of the scan bodies. The second digital bite registration option is done by modifying the temporary bridge. The bridge is cut in half and screwed on one side, and the bite registration is taken on the other side and vice versa. Then the lab conducts superimposition. The third approach is the conventional one, where record blocks are to be made, and the centric relation record is registered conventionally.

7. Send the STL files to the lab. The lab will place reference points to superimpose all the STL files together (Fig. 24.4. (27)). He then will be able to locate the implant position and direction. This allows him to place virtual abutments that are either of abutment level or implant level. He will then design the prosthesis on top of the virtual abutment. The design will differ depending on the choice of prosthesis design and material. The design could be a full monolithic zirconia bridge that doesn't require a framework to be fabricated beforehand, where a full anatomy design is achieved or porcelain fused to metal or fixed hybrid prosthesis. In these two latter cases, a framework should be fabricated (Fig. 24.4 (28,29,30)) where first a full anatomical design is achieved followed by automatic reduction from the software to form the framework design. The STL file is then sent into a milling machine. The framework can then be wax milled and casted or milled immediately into metal (subtractive technique). A different approach can also be applied which is the additive printing approach , also known as selective laser melting or selective laser sintering.
8. After verification layering is performed according to the type of prosthesis, passive fit is checked according to the criteria mentioned previously. In case of a full monolithic zirconia bridge, a verification jig should be made since the framework cannot be sectioned and reassembled like cobalt-chromium in case of lack of a passive fit.

Biological and Prosthetic Complications

In 2018, Malo and colleagues reported cumulative implant survival and success rates of 93% and 91.7%, respectively, after 18 years of follow-up in all-on-four treatment of completely edentulous mandible [111]. These rates were similar to another 15-year follow-up study done in the edentulous maxilla [112]. This means that this concept is viable in long-term studies. However, several complications are still accompanied by this procedure. These complications can be of two types: (1) biological and (2) technical/prosthetic. Biological complications are further divided into intrasurgical and postsurgical.

Biological Complications: Intrasurgical

Intrasurgical complications are various and include [113]:

1. Arterial disruptions during mucogingival flap reflection.
2. Supra-crestal exposure of the mental foramen or inferior alveolar nerve.
3. Pneumatized maxillary sinus extending beyond the anticipated horizontal plane of bone reduction required for All-on-four-style treatment.
4. Hemorrhage from osseous nutrient canals during the reduction of alveolar or basal bone.
5. Accessory mental foramina requiring more mesial placement of dental implants, thus limiting the anterior-posterior spread of the All-on-four-style prosthesis.
6. Damage to the sublingual artery in the anterior mandible leading to life-threatening bleeding complications.
7. Inadequate bone density compromising primary stability.
8. Removal of previously placed dental implants that may lead to bone loss. This may eliminate the possibility of placing a new implant and thus compromise immediate loading of a provisional prosthesis.
9. Perforation through the inferior or anterior wall of the sinus [22].

Biological Complications: Postsurgical

Biological complications related to full-arch implant prosthesis include soft tissue dehiscence, peri-implant bone loss exceeding 2 mm, peri-implant mucositis, tissue inflammation under the fixed prosthesis, and hypertrophy/hyperplasia of soft tissue [76]. Peri-implant mucositis and peri-implantitis have been reported in the literature as the two most frequent causes of late implant failure, resulting from bone loss following the inflammation of soft and hard tissue surrounding the implants [114].

Furthermore, several studies have found that the most frequent biological implant-related complication was excessive peri-implant crestal bone loss exceeding 2 mm [115, 116, 117, 118]. The second most common implant-related biological complication was peri-implant mucositis. According to one study, such biological complications may be reduced by having patients maintain good oral hygiene, which would adequately control plaque [20].

Technical/Prosthetic Complications

Technical complications encountered in all-on-four treatments include fracture of provisional restorations, screw loosening/fracture, veneering material chipping or fracture, need for replacement of resin tooth, framework fracture, loss of screw access filling material, and fracture of the opposing restoration [76, 113]. According to Salvi and Bragger, tech-

nical complications are related to a high crown/implant ratio and the presence of cantilevers [119]. Other studies have reported the fracture of provisional restorations as the most common complication in the all-on-four prosthesis, with rates ranging from 4.17% to 41% [113, 120, 121]. Fractures of the provisional prosthesis during the healing phase are concerning as they eliminate cross-arch stabilizations and disrupt stress distribution patterns. This complication is also worrying to the patients as it results in impaired masticatory function and the restoration's esthetic role. Provisional restorations commonly fracture due to insufficient thickness of the material itself, often caused by under-reduced bone, processing errors, or improper occlusal adjustments [122]. However, in some cases, fractures may occur because of the inherent weakness of the acrylic and polymethyl methacrylate materials, which cannot serve for extended periods of heavy occlusal loads.

Prosthetic complications can also be related to improper or inadequate surgical interventions. These include [34]:

1. Inadequate reduction of the alveolar ridges resulting in an inadequate restorative space for prosthetic material and failure to disguise the transition zone.
2. Placing implants outside the prosthesis's confines resulting in the extension of the prosthesis beyond the limits of the neutral zone. This will result in patient discomfort.
3. Inadequate osseous recontouring of the alveolar ridge which compromises the optimal tissue bed for the intaglio surface of the prosthesis. An appropriate reduction of bone volume ensures a flat or even slightly concave osseous topography that results in a prosthesis's convex intaglio surface. This makes it more favorable for cleansing leading to improved tissue response.

Fracture of the definitive prosthesis at the cantilever area can also occur with all-on-four prostheses. To prevent fracture of the cantilever section, the prosthesis must maintain a minimum bulk of restorative material, immediately distal to the most posterior implant and around channels of the screw access. The prosthetic material's cross-sectional area must be thick enough to acquire strength and rigidity to withstand occlusal loads. This is particularly important for screw channels in the palatal and lingual cross sections of the material. Regarding cantilevers, specifically, the connector size is a significant aspect when dealing with traditional noble metal alloys, titanium, and zirconia frameworks. Frameworks of traditional noble metals are especially indicated in situations where the restorative space is limited.

Nevertheless, when sufficient space exists for the prosthesis and hence connector, the chance of cantilever fracture is reduced, as the connectors can be fabricated with adequate cross-sectional areas [34].

Conclusion

The purpose of this chapter is to provide an overview of the all-on-four concept and the step-by-step procedures of various prosthetic options, along with various material considerations. Providing satisfactory results for completely edentulous patients, on both functional and esthetic levels, is a definite challenge, especially with the increased demand for "same-day delivery." Based on the immediate loading concept, the all-on-four treatment has met the challenge, with numerous studies revealing its long-term success in treating completely edentulous and atrophic arches without the further need of lengthy augmentation procedures. Nevertheless, the clinical success of this technique cannot be achieved without good patient communication, meticulous examination and treatment planning, and knowledge of material options available. Studies on the all-on-four concept are still required in order to resolve or limit inaccuracies in specific clinical procedures, such as the accuracy of soft tissue impressions in the digital workflow. Furthermore, enhancement of the materials' properties can significantly improve this procedure's prosthetic success without compromising implants' survival.

References

1. Van De Rijt LJM, Stoop CC, RAF W, Vries RD, Feast AR, Sampson EL, Lobbezoo F. The influence of oral health factors on the quality of life in older people: a systematic review. Gerontologist. 2019. https://doi.org/10.1093/geront/gnz105.
2. (2018) Life expectancy. In: World Health Organization. https://www.who.int/gho/mortality_burden_disease/life_tables/situation_trends_text/en/. Accessed 25 Sep 2020
3. Branemark P-I. Osseointegration and its experimental background. J Prosthet Dent. 1983;50:399–410.
4. Buser D, Janner SFM, Wittneben J-G, Brägger U, Ramseier CA, Salvi GE. 10-Year Survival and Success Rates of 511 Titanium Implants with a Sandblasted and Acid-Etched Surface: A Retrospective Study in 303 Partially Edentulous Patients. Clin Implant Dent Relat Res. 2012;14:839–51.
5. Misch CE. Dental implant prosthetics. St. Louis: Elsevier Mosby; 2015.
6. Krekmanov L, Kahn M, Rangert B, Lindstorm H (2000) Tilting of posterior mandibular and maxillary implants for improved prosthesis support. Int J. Oral Maxillofac Implants. 15 p. 405–414
7. Maló P, Rangert B, Nobre M. "All-on-Four" immediate-function concept with brånemark system® implants for completely edentulous mandibles: a retrospective clinical study. Clin Implant Dent Relat Res. 2003;5:2–9.
8. Malo P, Rangert B, Nobre M. All-on-four immediate-function concept with branemark systemr implants for completely edentulous maxillae: A 1-year retrospective clinical study. Clin Implant Dent Relat Res. 2005;7(Suppl 1):S88–94. https://doi.org/10.1111/j.1708-8208.2005.tb00080.x.
9. Malo P, Nobre MDA, Lopes A. The use of computer-guided flapless implant surgery and four implants placed in immediate function to support a fixed denture: Preliminary results after a mean follow-up period of thirteen months. J Prosthet Dent. 2007;97(6 Suppl):S26–34. https://doi.org/10.1016/s0022-3913(07)60005-5.
10. Bhering CLB, Mesquita MF, Kemmoku DT, Noritomi PY, Consani RLX, Barão VAR. Comparison between all-on-four and all-on-six treatment concepts and framework material on stress distribution in atrophic maxilla: A prototyping guided 3D-FEA study. Korean J Couns Psychother. 2016;69:715–25.
11. Almeida EO, Rocha EP, Júnior ACF, Anchieta RB, Poveda R, Gupta N, Coelho PG. Tilted and short implants supporting fixed prosthesis in an atrophic maxilla: A 3D-FEA biomechanical evaluation. Clin Implant Dent Relat Res. 2013;17(Suppl 1):e332–42. https://doi.org/10.1111/cid.12129.
12. Aparicio C, Perales P, Rangert B. Tilted implants as an alternative to maxillary sinus grafting: a clinical, radiologic, and periotest study. Clin Implan Dent Relat Res. 2001;3:39–49.
13. Babbush CA. Dental implants: the art and science. Maryland Heights: Saunders Elsevier; 2011.
14. Testori T, Del Fabbro M, Capelli M, Zuffetti F, Francetti L, Weinstein RL. Immediate occlusal loading and tilted implants for the rehabilitation of the atrophic edentulous maxilla: 1-year interim results of a multicenter prospective study. Clin Oral Implants Res. 2008;19:227–32.
15. Calandriello R, Tomatis M. Simplified Treatment of the Atrophic Posterior Maxilla via Immediate/Early Function and Tilted Implants: A Prospective 1-Year Clinical Study. Clin Implant Dent Relat Res. 2005;7:s1–s12.
16. Butura CC, Galindo DF, Jensen OT. Mandibular all-on-four therapy using angled implants: a three-year clinical study of 857 implants in 219 Jaws. Oral Maxillofac Surg Clin North Am. 2011;23:289–300.
17. Bevilacqua M, Tealdo T, Menini M, Pera F, Mossolov A, Drago C, Pera P. The influence of cantilever length and implant inclination on stress distribution in maxillary implant-supported fixed dentures. J Prosthet Dent. 2011;105:5–13.
18. Tada S, Stegaroiu R, Kitamura E, Miyakawa O, Kusakari H. Influence of implant design and bone quality on stress/strain distribution in bone around implants: a 3-dimensional finite element analysis. Int J Oral Maxillofac Implants. 2003;18:357–68.
19. Rangert B, Sullivan RM, Jemt T. Load factor control for implants in the posterior partially edentulous segment. Int J Oral Maxillofac Implants. 1987;12:360–70.
20. Corbella S, Del Fabbro M, Taschieri S, De Siena F, Francetti L. Clinical evaluation of an implant maintenance protocol for the prevention of peri-implant diseases in patients treated with immediately loaded full-arch rehabilitations. Int J Dent Hyg. 2011;9:216–22.
21. Taruna M, Chittaranjan B, Sudheer N, Tella S, Abusaad M. Prosthodontic perspective to all- on-4 ® concept for dental implants. J Clin Diagn Res. 2014;8(10):ZE16–9. https://doi.org/10.7860/jcdr/2014/9648.5020.
22. Singh AV, Singh S. Chapter 22: Full-arch fixed prosthesis: 'All-on-4TM'/'All-on-6' approach. In: Clinical implantology - E-Book. Elsevier Health Sciences; 2013. p. 575–611.
23. Maló P, de Araújo NM, Lopes A, Francischone C, Rigolizzo M. "All-on-4" immediate-function concept for completely edentulous maxillae: a clinical report on the medium (3 years) and long-term (5 years) outcomes. Clin Implant Dent Relat Res. 2012;14:e139–50.
24. Chan MH, Holmes C. Contemporary "All-on-4" concept. Dent Clin N Am. 2015;59(2):421–70. https://doi.org/10.1016/j.cden.2014.12.001.
25. Curtis D, Lin G-H, Fishman A, Sadowsky S, Daubert D, Kapila Y, Sharma A, Conte G, Yonemura C, Marinello C. Patient-Centered Risk Assessment in Implant Treatment Planning. Int J Oral Maxillofac Implants. 2019;34:506–20.

26. Bedrossian E, Sullivan RM, Fortin Y, Malo P, Indresano T. Fixed-prosthetic implant restoration of the edentulous maxilla: a systematic pretreatment evaluation method. J Oral Maxillofac Surg. 2008;66:112–22.

27. Parel S. Chapter 23: The evolution of the angled implants. In: Dental implants: the art and science. 2nd ed. Maryland Heights: Saunders an imprint of Elsevier; 2011. p. 370–88.

28. Jensen OT, Adams MW, Cottam JR, Parel SM, Phillips WR 3rd. The All-on-4 shelf: Maxilla. J Oral Maxillofac Surg. 2010;68:2520–7.

29. Tolstunov L. Implant zones of the jaws: implant location and related success rate. J Oral Implantol. 2007;33:211–20.

30. Jensen OT, Adams MW. All-on-4 treatment of highly atrophic mandible with mandibular V-4: report of 2 cases. J Oral Maxillofac Surg. 2009;67:1503–9.

31. Jensen OT, Adams M, Cottam JR, Parel SM, Phillips WR 3rd. The All on 4 shelf: mandible. J Oral Maxillofac Surg. 2011;69:175–81.

32. Jivraj S, Chee W, Corrado P. Treatment planning of the edentulous maxilla. Br Dent J. 2006;201:261–79.

33. Wicks RA. A systematic approach to definitive planning for osseo-integrated implant prostheses. J Prosthodont. 1994;3:237–42.

34. Jivraj S. Graftless solutions for the edentulous patient. Cham: Springer; 2018.

35. Fu JH, Hsu YT, Wang HL. Identifying occlusal overload and how to deal with it to avoid marginal bone loss around implants. Eur J Oral Implantol. 2012;5(Suppl):S91–103.

36. Türker N, Alkış HT, Sadowsky SJ, Büyükkaplan UŞ. Effects of occlusal scheme on all-on-four abutments, screws and prostheses: A three-dimensional finite element study. J Oral Implantol. 2020;47(1):18–24. https://doi.org/10.1563/aaid-joi-d-19-00334.

37. Tallarico M, Canullo L, Pisano M, Penarrocha-Oltra D, Penarrocha-Oltra M, Meloni SM. An up to 7-year retrospective analysis of biologic and technical complication with the All-on-4 concept. J Oral Implantol. 2016;42:265–71.

38. Niedermaier R, Stelzle F, Riemann M, Bolz W, Schuh P, Wachtel H. Implant-supported immediately loaded fixed full-arch dentures: evaluation of implant survival rates in a case cohort of up to 7 years. Clin Implant Dent Relat Res. 2017;19:4–19.

39. Wennerberg A, Carlsson GE, Jemt T. Influence of occlusal factors on treatment outcome: a study of 109 consecutive patients with mandibular implant-supported fixed prostheses opposing maxillary complete dentures. Int J Prosthodont. 2001;14(6):550–5.

40. Kim Y, Oh T-J, Misch CE, Wang H-L. Occlusal considerations in implant therapy: clinical guidelines with biomechanical rationale. Clin Oral Implants Res. 2004;16:26–35.

41. Shackleton J, Carr L, Slabbert J, Becker P. Survival of fixed implant-supported prostheses related to cantilever lengths. J Prosthet Dent. 1994;71:23–6.

42. Falk H, et al. Occlusal interferences and cantilever joint stress in implant-supported prostheses occluding with complete dentures. Int J Oral Maxillofac Implants. 1989;5:70–7.

43. Wie H. Registration of localization, occlusion and occluding materials for failing screw joints in the Brånemark implant system. Clin Oral Implants Res. 1995;6:47–53.

44. Gross M. Occlusion in implant dentistry. A review of the literature of prosthetic determinants and current concepts. Aust Dent J. 2008;53:S60–8.

45. Wismeijer D, et al. Factors to consider in selecting an occlusal concept for patients with implants in the edentulous mandible. J Prosthet Dent. 1995;74:380–4.

46. Kimoto S, et al. Prospective clinical trial comparing lingualized occlusion to bilateral balanced occlusion in complete dentures: a pilot study. Int J Prosthodont. 2006;19:103–9.

47. Peroz I, et al. Comparison between balanced occlusion and canine guidance in complete denture wearers--a clinical, randomized trial. Quintessence Int. 2003;34:607–12.

48. Jensen OT, Cottam J, Ringeman J, Adams M. Trans-sinus dental implants, bone morphogenetic protein 2, and immediate function for all-on-4 treatment of severe maxillary atrophy. J Oral Maxillofac Surg. 2012;70:141–8.

49. All-on-4® treatment concept Procedures manual. https://www.oldsdenturecentre.com/wp-content/uploads/2019/01/Nobel-Biocare-All-on-4-treatment-concept.pdf. Accessed 11 Oct 2020

50. Whitley D, Eidson RS, Rudek I, Bencharit S. In-office fabrication of dental implant surgical guides using desktop stereolithographic printing and implant treatment planning software: A clinical report. J Prosthet Dent. 2017;118:256–63.

51. Choi W, Nguyen BC, Doan A, Girod S, Gaudilliere B, Gaudilliere D. Freehand versus guided surgery: factors influencing accuracy of dental implant placement. Implant Dent. 2017;26(4):500–9. https://doi.org/10.1097/ID.0000000000000620.

52. Ravidà A, Barootchi S, Tattan M, Saleh MHA, Gargallo-Albiol J, Wang HL. Clinical outcomes and cost effectiveness of computer-guided versus conventional implant-retained hybrid prostheses: A long-term retrospective analysis of treatment protocols. J Periodontol. 2018;89:1015–24.

53. Schneider D, Marquardt P, Zwahlen M, Jung RE. A systematic review on the accuracy and the clinical outcome of computer-guided template-based implant dentistry. Clin Oral Implants Res. 2009;20:73–86.

54. Verstreken K, Cleynenbreugel JV, Martens K, Marchal G, Steenberghe DV, Suetens P. An image-guided planning system for endosseous oral implants. IEEE Trans Med Imaging. 1998;17:842–52.

55. Olin P. Effects of varied dimensions of surgical guides on implant angulations. Yearb Dent. 2006;2006:136.

56. Oh J-H, An X, Jeong S-M, Choi B-H. Digital Workflow for Computer-Guided Implant Surgery in Edentulous Patients: A Case Report. J Oral Maxillofac Surg. 2017;75:2541–9.

57. Rocci A, Martignoni M, Gottlow J. Immediate Loading in the Maxilla Using Flapless Surgery, Implants Placed in Predetermined Positions, and Prefabricated Provisional Restorations: A Retrospective 3-Year Clinical Study. Clin Implant Dent Relat Res. 2003;5:29–36.

58. Arısan V, Karabuda CZ, Özdemir T. Implant surgery using bone- and mucosa-supported stereolithographic guides in totally edentulous jaws: surgical and post-operative outcomes of computer-aided vs. standard techniques. Clin Oral Implants Res. 2010 https://doi.org/10.1111/j.1600-0501.2010.01957.x.

59. Sunitha RV, Sapthagiri E. Flapless implant surgery: a 2-year follow-up study of 40 implants. Oral Surg Oral Med Oral Pathol Oral Radiol Endod. 2013; https://doi.org/10.1016/j.oooo.2011.12.027.

60. Lenzi C. Immediate loading in edentulous jaws: long-term clinical evaluation of 337 immediately loaded implants. Clin Oral Implants Res. 2017;28:361.

61. Elsyad MA, Elgamal M, Askar OM, Al-Tonbary GY. Patient satisfaction and oral health-related quality of life (OHRQoL) of conventional denture, fixed prosthesis and milled bar overdenture for All-on-4 implant rehabilitation. A crossover study. Clin Oral Implants Res. 2019;30:1107–17.

62. Szmukler-Moncler S, Piattelli A, Favero GA, Dubruille J-H. Considerations preliminary to the application of early and immediate loading protocols in dental implantology. Clin Oral Implants Res. 2000;11:12–25.

63. Tettamanti L, Andrisani C, Bassi MA, Vinci R, Silvestre-Rangil J, Tagliabue A. Immediate loading implants: review of the critical aspects. Oral Implantol. 2017;10:129.

64. Soto-Penaloza D, Zaragozi-Alonso R, Penarrocha-Diago M, Penarrocha-Diago M. The all-on-four treatment concept: systematic review. J Clin Exp Dent. 2017; https://doi.org/10.4317/jced.53613.

65. Larsson C, Steyern PVV. Implant-supported full-arch zirconia-based mandibular fixed dental prostheses. Eight-year results from a clinical pilot study. Acta Odontol Scand. 2012;71:1118–22.

66. Abdulmajeed AA, Lim KG, Närhi TO, Cooper LF. Complete-arch implant-supported monolithic zirconia fixed dental prostheses: A systematic review. J Prosthet Dent. 2016; https://doi.org/10.1016/j.prosdent.2015.08.025.

67. Papaspyridakos P, Lal K. Computer-assisted design/computer-assisted manufacturing zirconia implant fixed complete prostheses: clinical results and technical complications up to 4 years of function. Clin Oral Implants Res. 2012;24:659–65.

68. Cheng C-W, Chien C-H, Chen C-J, Papaspyridakos P. Complete-mouth implant rehabilitation with modified monolithic zirconia implant-supported fixed dental prostheses and an immediate-loading protocol: A clinical report. J Prosthet Dent. 2013;109:347–52.

69. Guess PC, Bonfante EA, Silva NR, Coelho PG, Thompson VP. Effect of core design and veneering technique on damage and reliability of Y-TZP-supported crowns. Dent Mater. 2013;29:307–16.

70. Carames J, Suinaga LT, Yu YCP, Pérez A, Kang M. Clinical Advantages and Limitations of Monolithic Zirconia Restorations Full Arch Implant Supported Reconstruction: Case Series. Int J Dent. 2015;2015:1–7.

71. Najeeb S, Zafar MS, Khurshid Z, Siddiqui F. Applications of polyetheretherketone (PEEK) in oral implantology and prosthodontics. J Prosthodont Res. 2016;60:12–9.

72. Sereno N, Rosentritt M, Jarman-smith M, Lang R, Kolbeck C. In-vitro performance evaluation of polyetheretherketone (PEEK) implant prosthetics with a cantilever design. Clin Oral Implants Res. 2015;26(S12):296.

73. Maló P, Nobre MDA, Guedes CM, Almeida R, Silva A, Sereno N, Legatheaux J. Short-term report of an ongoing prospective cohort study evaluating the outcome of full-arch implant-supported fixed hybrid polyetheretherketone-acrylic resin prostheses and the All-on-Four concept. Clin Implant Dent Relat Res. 2018;20:692–702.

74. Toia M, Stocchero M, Jinno Y, Wennerberg A, Becktor J, Jimbo R, Halldin A. Effect of Misfit at Implant-Level Framework and Supporting Bone on Internal Connection Implants: Mechanical and Finite Element Analysis. Int J Oral Maxillofac Implants. 2019;34:320–8.

75. Katsoulis J, Takeichi T, Sol Gaviria A, Peter L, Katsoulis K. Misfit of implant prostheses and its impact on clinical outcomes. Definition, assessment and a systematic review of the literature. Eur J Oral Implantol. 2017;10(Suppl 1):121–38. PMID: 28944373.

76. Papaspyridakos P, Chen CJ, Chuang SK, Weber HP, Gallucci GO. A systematic review of biologic and technical complications with fixed implant rehabilitations for edentulous patients. Int J Oral Maxillofac Implants. 2012;27(1):102–10. PMID: 22299086.

77. Heckmann SM, Karl M, Wichmann MG, Winter W, Graef F, Taylor TD. Cement fixation and screw retention: parameters of passive fit. An in vitro study of three-unit implant-supported fixed partial dentures. Clin Oral Implants Res. 2004;15:466–73.

78. Gallucci GO, Papaspyridakos P, Ashy LM, Kim GE, Brady NJ, Weber HP. Clinical accuracy outcomes of closed-tray and open-tray implant impression techniques for partially edentulous patients. Int J Prosthodont. 2011;24(5):469–72. PMID: 21909490.

79. Ozan O, Hamis O. Accuracy of different definitive impression techniques with the all-on-4 protocol. J Prosthet Dent. 2019;121:941–8.

80. Baig M. Accuracy of Impressions of Multiple Implants in the Edentulous Arch: A Systematic Review. Int J Oral Maxillofac Implants. 2014;29:869–80.

81. Burns J, Palmer R, Howe L, Wilson R. Accuracy of open tray implant impressions: An in vitro comparison of stock versus custom trays. J Prosthet Dent. 2003;89:250–5.

82. Kurtulmus-Yilmaz S, Ozan O, Ozcelik TB, Yagiz A. Digital evaluation of the accuracy of impression techniques and materials in angulated implants. J Dent. 2014;42:1551–9.

83. Vigolo P, Fonzi F, Majzoub Z, Cordioli G. An evaluation of impression techniques for multiple internal connection implant prostheses. J Prosthet Dent. 2004;92:470–6.

84. Sorrentino R, Gherlone EF, Calesini G, Zarone F. Effect of Implant Angulation, Connection Length, and Impression Material on the Dimensional Accuracy of Implant Impressions: An In Vitro Comparative Study. Clin Implant Dent Relat Res. 2010;12:63–76.

85. Hariharan R, Shanker C, Rajan M, Baig MR, Azhagarasan NS. Evaluation of accuracy of multiple dental implant impressions using various splinting materials. Int J Oral Maxillofac Implants. 2010;25:38–44.

86. Vigolo P, Mutinelli S, Fonzi F, Stellini E. An in vitro evaluation of impression techniques for multiple internal-and external-connection implant prostheses. Int J Oral Maxillofac Implants. 2014;29(4):808–18.

87. Öngül D, Gökçen-Röhlig B, Şermet B, Keskin H. A comparative analysis of the accuracy of different direct impression techniques for multiple implants. Aust Dent J. 2012;57(2):184–9.

88. Assuncao WG, Gennari Filho H, Zaniquelli O. Evaluation of Transfer Impressions for Osseointegrated Implants at Various Angulations. Implant Dent. 2004;13(4):358–66.

89. Naconecy MM, Teixeira ER, Shinkai RS, Frasca LCF, Cervieri A. Evaluation of the accuracy of 3 transfer techniques for implant-supported prostheses with multiple abutments. Int J Oral Maxillofac Implants. 2004;19(2):192–8.

90. Filho HG, Mazaro JVQ, Vedovatto E, Assunção WG, dos Santos PH. Accuracy of impression techniques for Implants. Part 2—comparison of splinting techniques. J Prosthodont. 2009;18(2):172–6.

91. Kim J-H, Kim KR, Kim S. Critical appraisal of implant impression accuracies: A systematic review. J Prosthet Dent. 2015;114(2):185–92. https://doi.org/10.1016/j.prosdent.2015.02.005.

92. Baig MR. Multi-unit implant impression accuracy: a review of the literature. Quintessence Int. 2014;45(1):39–51.

93. Moreira AHJ, Rodrigues NF, Pinho ACM, Fonseca JC, Vilaça JL. Accuracy comparison of implant impression techniques: a systematic review. Clin Implant Dent Relat Res. 2015;17(Suppl 2):e751–64. https://doi.org/10.1111/cid.12310.

94. Cabral LM, Guedes CG. Comparative analysis of 4 impression techniques for implants. Implant Dent. 2007;16(2):187–94.

95. Assif D, Nissan J, Varsano I, Singer A. Accuracy of implant impression splinted techniques: effect of splinting material. Int J Oral Maxillofac Implants. 1999;14:885–8.

96. Lee S-J, Cho S-B. Accuracy of five implant impression technique: effect of splinting materials and methods. J Adv Prosthodont. 2011;3:177–85.

97. Lopes-Júnior I, Lucas BDL, Gomide HA, Gomes VL. Impression techniques for multiple implants: a photoelastic analysis. Part I: comparison of three direct methods. J Oral Implantol. 2013;39:539–44.

98. Nissan J, Barnea E, Krauze E, Assif D. Impression technique for partially edentulous patients. J Prosthet Dent. 2002;88:103–4.

99. Eid N. An implant impression technique using a plaster splinting index combined with a silicone impression. J Prosthet Dent. 2004;92:575–7.

100. Hobo S, Ichida E, Garcia LT. Osseointegration and occlusal rehabilitation, vol. 159-162. Chicago: Quintessence; 1989. p. 171–3.

101. Rungcharassaeng K, Kan JY. Fabricating a stable record base for completely edentulous patients treated with osseointegrated implants using healing abutments. J Prosthet Dent. 1999;81:224–7.

102. Ercoli C, Geminiani A, Feng C, Lee H. The influence of verification jig on framework fit for nonsegmented fixed implant-supported complete denture. Clin Implant Dent Relat Res. 2011. https://doi.org/10.1111/j.1708-8208.2011.00425.x

103. Alhashim A, Flinton RJ. Dental gypsum verification jig to verify implant positions: A clinical report. J Oral Implantol. 2012;40(4):495–9.

104. Kan JY, Rungcharassaeng K, Bohsali K, Goodacre CJ, Lang BR, Kan JY, Rungcharassaeng K, Bohsali K, Goodacre CJ, Lang BR. Clinical methods for evaluating implant framework fit. J Prosthet Dent. 1999;81:7–13.

105. Sadowsky SJ. The role of complete denture principles in implant prosthodontics. J Calif Dent Assoc. 2003;31(12):905–9. PMID: 14736042.

106. Quirynen M, Naert I, van Steenberghe D. Fixture design and overload influence marginal bone loss and fixture success in the Brånemark system. Clin Oral Implants Res. 1992;3(3):104–11. https://doi.org/10.1034/j.1600-0501.1992.030302.x.

107. Lundgren D, Laurell L. Biomechanical aspects of fixed bridgework supported by natural teeth and endosseous implants. Periodontology 2000. 1994;4:23–40. https://doi.org/10.1111/j.1600-0757.1994.tb00003.x.

108. Bakeman EM, Kois JC. The myth of anterior guidance: 10 steps in designing proper clearance for functional pathways. J Cosmet Dent. 2012;28(3):56–62.

109. Wittneben JG, Buser D, Belser UC, Brägger U. Peri-implant soft tissue conditioning with provisional restorations in the esthetic zone: the dynamic compression technique. In J Periodontics Restorative Dent. 2013;33(4):447–55.

110. Andriessen FS, Rijkens DR, van der Meer WJ, Wismeijer DW. Applicability and accuracy of an intraoral scanner for scanning multiple implants in edentulous mandibles: a pilot study. J Prosthet Dent. 2014;111(3):186–94.

111. Maló P, de Araújo NM, Lopes A, Ferro A, Botto J. The All-on-4 treatment concept for the rehabilitation of the completely edentulous mandible: A longitudinal study with 10 to 18 years of follow-up. Clin Implant Dent Relat Res. 2019;21(4):565–77. https://doi.org/10.1111/cid.12769.

112. Maló P, de Araújo NM, Lopes A, Ferro A, Nunes M. The All-on-4 concept for full-arch rehabilitation of the edentulous maxillae: A longitudinal study with 5-13 years of follow-up. Clin Implant Dent Relat Res. 2019;21(4):538–49. https://doi.org/10.1111/cid.12771.

113. Holtzclaw D. All-on-4® Implant Treatment: Common Pitfalls and Methods to Overcome Them. Compend Contin Educ Dent. 2016;37(7):458–65;quiz466. PMID: 27548398

114. Lindhe J, Meyle J. Peri-implant diseases: consensus report of the Sixth European Workshop on Periodontology. J Clin Periodontol. 2008;35:282–5.

115. Fischer K, Stenberg T, Hedin M, Sennerby L. Five-year results from a randomized, controlled trial on early and delayed loading of implants supporting full-arch prosthesis in the edentulous maxilla. Clin Oral Implants Res. 2008;19:433–41.

116. Gallucci GO, Doughtie CB, Hwang JW, Fiorellini JP, Weber HP. Five year results of fixed implant-supported rehabilitations with distal cantilevers for the edentulous mandible. Clin Oral Implants Res. 2009;20:601–7.

117. Jemt T, Bergendal B, Arvidson K, et al. Implant-supported welded titanium frameworks in the edentulous maxilla: A 5-year prospective multicenter study. Int J Prosthodont. 2002;16:415–21.

118. Örtorp A, Jemt T. CNC-Milled Titanium Frameworks Supported by Implants in the Edentulous Jaw: A 10-Year Comparative Clinical Study. Clin Implant Dent Relat Res. 2009;14:88–99.

119. Salvi GE, Bragger U. Mechanical and technical risks in implant therapy. Int J Oral Maxillofac Implants. 2009;24(Suppl):69–85.

120. Francetti L, Agliardi E, Testori T, et al. Immediate rehabilitation of the mandible with fixed full prosthesis supported by axial and tilted implants: interim results of a single cohort prospective study. Clin Implant Dent Relat Res. 2008;10(4):255–63. 48.

121. Pomares C. A retrospective study of edentulous patients rehabilitated according to the 'all-on-four' or the 'all-on-six' immediate function concept using flapless computer-guided implant surgery. Eur J Oral Implantol. 2010;3(2):155–63.

122. Holtzclaw D. The effects of reinforcement on the fracture rates of provisional All-on-4 restorations: a retrospective report of 257 cases involving 1182 dental implants. J Implant Adv Clin Dent. 2016;8(3):31–7.

Farhad Zeynalzadeh and Alvaro de la Iglesia Beyme

Introduction

Autologous tooth transplantation refers to relocating an autologous tooth to another extraction site or a surgically formed recipient site. This procedure is for teeth with congenital defects or teeth with ectopic rash, severe caries, periodontal disease, trauma, or endodontics when appropriate donor teeth are available [1–3]. Autologous grafts use the patient's teeth to improve resistance to occlusal loads, maintain periodontal ligaments (PDL) and surrounding bone, and have better aesthetic potential [4, 5].

The most common donor teeth are the third molar (affected or completely erupted), anterior molar, and supernumerary tooth. This surgical procedure offers time and cost advantages when compared to dental implants. This line of treatment for implant surgery's main benefits is proprioception, alveolar bone preservation, and papilla preservation. It is also better than traditional fixed bridges [2, 4, 5]. It is strongly indicated that cases of teeth that cannot be repaired due to the presence of deep cavities, fractures, or periodontal disease must be replaced with healthy donor sites at the recipient site. After the first reported clinical application [6] in 1950, dental autotransplantation's success rate gradually increased thanks to advances in diagnostic and surgical techniques such as computer-assisted rapid prototyping (CARP) models. Since the 1990s, many studies investigating periodontal tissue and periodontal membrane healing and root resorption have aroused new clinical interest [7–9].

F. Zeynalzadeh (✉)
Department of Oral and Maxillofacial Surgery, Faculty of Dentistry- Medical Sciences University, Mashhad, Iran
e-mail: Zeynalzadehf961@mums.ac.ir

A. de la Iglesia Beyme
Department of Oral and Maxillofacial Surgery, Faculty of Dentistry – Universitat Internacional de Cataluyna, Barcelona, Spain
e-mail: Alvarodelaiglesia@uic.es

Indications

Indications for dental autotransplantation include affected or ectopic teeth, premature or traumatic tooth loss, tooth loss due to tumors, or teeth for congenital paroxysmal reasons. It has lost missing teeth in one arch combined with clinical signs of arch length mismatch or tooth congestion in the opposite angle, poor prognosis, and tooth replacement with development.

Autotransplantation guarantees alveolar bone mass maintenance in dental abnormalities, the periodontal ligaments in open apex tooth by physiological stimulation. In closed apex tooth, root canal therapy needs to be done without any demand for maintenance of periodontal [2, 4–12, 48, 49], unlike prosthetic restorations, provide proprioception during function and have an excellent prognosis in growing patients [14]. However, clinical trials in adult patients have good results.

Finally, the total cost of treatment is usually lower than other treatment plans such as dental implants, prosthetic restorations, and closure of orthodontic space [19, 21]. However, in some cases, the patient may be burdened with additional costs for the donor site's rehabilitation.

Prognosis of Autotransplantation

The prognosis of autologous teeth is influenced by the preoperative and postoperative conditions recognized as prognostic factors [2]. The presence of appropriate alveolar bone supports all dimensions of the patient's gender, age, stage of development, recipient site, and donor tooth root anatomy [3, 4, 6, 10].

Use of non-traumatic surgical techniques and proper storage conditions for the donor's teeth are the best ways to obtain and maitain appropraite autogenous teeth. Atraumatic extraction is performed without touching the cementoenamel junction. It is mandatory not to embrace the forceps or elevator below the cementoenamel junction because this could harm the periodontal ligament cells and cause resorption. Also during remodeling the socket, the best solution for

M. R. Stevens et al. (eds.), *Innovative Perspectives in Oral and Maxillofacial Surgery*,
https://doi.org/10.1007/978-3-030-75750-2_25

storing the tooth is saline or Hanks. The degree of adaptation of donor's teeth to recipient alveoli, duration and method of tooth stabilization immediately after transplantation, and their surgery post-care are all characterized by different authors as prognostic factors [19, 24, 25, 47].

In addition, surgeon experience [4–6], candidate patient health and oral hygiene, lack of acute infection and chronic inflammation at the recipient site [16], presence or absence of occlusal contact during healing [2, 9, 10, 14], and autologous teeth [2, 4, 8, 15, 20] also affect the prognosis of autotransplantation.

Endodontic treatment is the basis of dental autotransplantation. To avoid any complications specially in closed apex teeth, it is better to perform root canal therapy which are proved by clinical symptoms and radiographic data [2–13, 48, 49].

The following variables may affect the prognosis of autotransplanted teeth:

1. *Tooth type*
    (i) Eruption status: uninterrupted, partially exploded, or completely exploded
    (ii) Root and apex developmental stages: divergent, parallel, converges on open and closed vertices
2. *Acceptance site and surgery*
    (i) Recipient site location
    (ii) Alveolar bone condition at the recipient site: appropriate or inadequate bone level
    (iii) Surgical difficulty and ease of autologous graft placement
3. *How to stabilize teeth after transplantation*
4. *Endodontic treatment: treatment start time and technique quality of root canal filling (based on radiographic appearance)*
5. *Causes of tooth loss requiring automatic transplantation, for example, trauma, periodontal disease, lacerations, and caries [2–9]*

Complications

In addition to the benefits of this particular procedure, like any other surgery, there are some complications that you may face. The main issues that you may encounter are:

1. Resorption of inflammatory roots
2. Ankylosis
3. Donor tooth loss
4. Fracture of a donor's tooth during extraction
5. Loss of attachment

Inadequate nutrition on the root surface can increase the complication rate of root resorption. Besides, this factor can lead to donor tooth loss [8, 13–25].

Predictability and Prognosis

The prognosis of the procedure is influenced by several factors, including the shapes and conditions of the donor's teeth, the recipient's location, the duration of retention the teeth outside the mouth, the postoperative division method, the start of endodontic treatment and marginal bone loss. The primary and most important factor affecting the prognosis of autologous tooth grafts is the healing of periodontal ligament cells [37]. These cells can be seen attached to the surface of the roots. To achieve recovery, these cells should remain alive. Therefore, non-traumatic extraction is essential for maintaining these cells [3, 9, 19].

The success of treatment depends upon inflammation, stabilization, trauma, root formation, intraoperative storage, medication, and bone quality and quantity. The most critical factors in achieving a success rate are the maintenance of healthy periodontal tissue and the healing process of PDL [37–39]. Maintaining good oral hygiene and proper alveolar bone is very important. 3D replication reduces extraoral exposure time and increases the ease of surgery [8, 13, 15].

Healing Assessment

In the case of PDL healing, non-traumatic extraction is an essential factor in the preservation of root cells and PDL cells, which play an indispensable role [41]. Damage to these cells leads to inadequate healing. After extraction, the extraoral condition is affected by pH, osmotic pressure, dehydration, etc. and thus affects the healing process. If a non-traumatic extract is obtained in a short extraoral time, these cells will heal in a new socket in 2 weeks.

In terms of bone healing, genetically, PDL cells showed bone induction during the healing process from fibroblasts, cementoblasts, and osteoblasts. The latter are the type involved in the appearance of hard thin layers and bone formation through rapid regeneration. Therefore, there is no need to transplant material to fill the space between the bone wall and the root [37].

For root development, the amount of evolution cannot be predicted. In immature roots, continuous development can also be expected when Hertwig's epithelial root sheath conservation is achieved around the apex.

Surgical Considerations and Treatment Plans

Autologous tooth transplantation sequences include clinical and radiological examinations, diagnosis, orthodontic treatment, endodontics, treatment planning, surgical procedures, therapeutic treatment, and follow-up.

To achieve high success and predictable procedures

1. *Thorough clinical and X-ray examination* (Fig. 25.1a).
2. *Appropriate diagnosis and examination of the case*

Cases are examined and diagnosed primarily with clinical and radiological information about whether a transplant is needed. Important information includes the anatomical shape of the donor's teeth and how they fit into the recipient site, the stage of root development, the ease of preparation of the recipient socket, and damage to the donor's teeth during removal.

Correct diagnosis of the case is essential to the success of the procedure. The right test can provide the best option for the patient. The proper diagnosis of a case depends primarily on laboratory and radiological examinations (Fig. 25.1b).

Radiological evaluation requires a focus on many aspects during the examination. It includes morphological and anatomical considerations of the donor's teeth, root development, and potential risk factors for damaging the donor's teeth.

In addition to periapical and panoramic radiography, cone beam computed tomography scan (CBCT scan) plays a vital role in completing the diagnosis to understand the shape, size, location, and difficulty of the case (Fig. 25.1c).

3. *Creating an ideal treatment plan*

Cases are examined and diagnosed primarily with clinical and radiological information about whether a transplant is needed. Important information includes the anatomical shape of the donor's teeth and how they fit into the recipient site, the stage of root development, the ease of preparation of the recipient socket, and damage to the donor's teeth during removal.

4. *Surgical procedure*

A Series of Surgical Procedures

The sequence of surgical procedures is as follows:

1. *Preoperative administration of antibiotics*: It is recommended to administer antibiotics hours before surgery.
2. *Disinfection and anesthesia of the surgical site.*

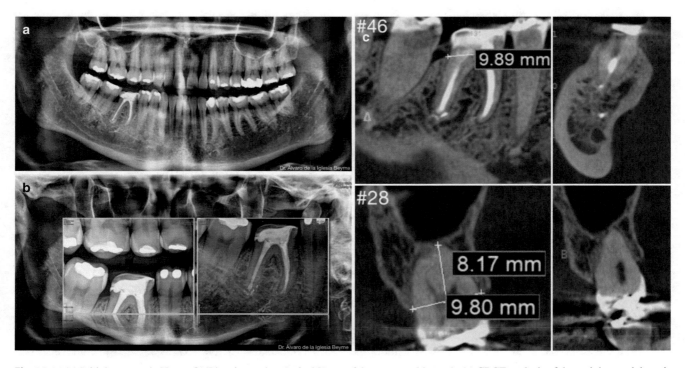

Fig. 25.1 (**a**) Initial panoramic X-ray. (**b**) Bitewing and periapical X-ray of the unrestorable tooth. (**c**) CBCT analysis of the recipient and donor's tooth

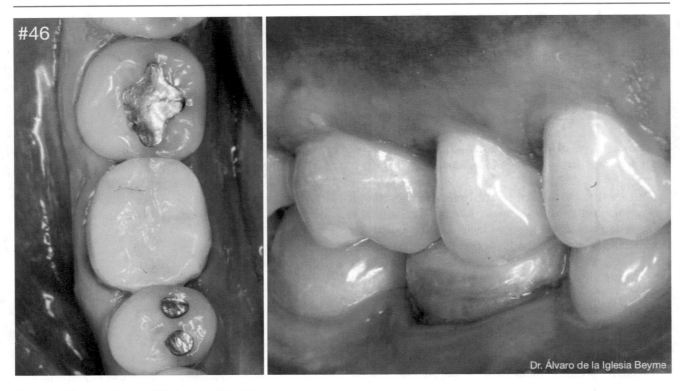

Fig. 25.2 Unrestorable tooth #32 due to a vertical fracture

3. *Extraction of teeth at the recipient site*: For immediate transplantation, the tooth extracted at the recipient site should be removed before the donor's tooth (Fig. 25.2).

4. *Extraction of donor's teeth*: Before preparing the recipient socket, the donor's teeth should be removed to examine the anatomy, size, and condition of the PDL (Fig. 25.1a). To avoid PDL, care must be taken. To preserve as much PDL as possible in the roots, intrasulcular incision is made before dislocation, and the donor tooth is slowly extracted in the most atraumatic way imaginable. Donor teeth must be removed and waited to be inserted into the donor socket before repositioning in the original socket. If extraoral time is planned, the tooth should be stored in a storage medium such as Hanks Balanced salt solution, which maintains periodontal ligament cells' viability. Water is hypotonic and damages periodontal cells and should not be used for this purpose.

5. *Donor tooth measurement*: Measure the mesiodistal width of the root and crown and the donor root's length.

6. *Recipient site preparation* (Fig. 25.5): Recipient sockets are prepared somewhat larger than donors by using a low-speed surgical round bar and cooling with saline. The tooth at the recipient site was removed without the need to raise the mucosal periosteal flap. The teeth were dissected with a tungsten carbide bar to reduce bone trauma and then passively dislocated with forceps (Fig. 25.6). After extraction, the recipient socket was prepared somewhat more massive than the donor using a slow, round surgical bar and was thoroughly washed with saline. After confirming the 3D tooth replica's suitability at the recipient site and the correct placement of the 3D printed guide template, the donor's tooth was extracted.

To minimize trauma during extraction, an intracervical incision was made before dislocation to preserve as much PDL as possible in the roots. The donor's teeth were then passively implanted and dislocated with the beak of forceps placed over the cementoenamel junction. Elevator use is minimized to prevent damage to concrete and PDL. The same dislocation protocol was used after flap elevation and osteotomy around the donor's teeth when the donor's teeth were impacted and surgically removed. Optimal placement of donor's teeth at the recipient site was established using a 3D printed guide template (Fig. 25.4).

7. *Trial and Adjustment:* The correspondence between the recipient and the donor is checked regularly by attempting to place the teeth in the socket with light pressure (Fig. 25.6)

Obstacles on the exit wall will be removed upon encounter. The donor's optimal placement concerning the recipient is to establish a biological width similar to the naturally crashed tooth's width. If possible, avoid deep placement below the occlusal level of adjacent teeth. That way, you don't have to do an orthodontic treatment at a later stage.

8. *Flap cutting and stitching*: The most crucial procedure in surgery is the airtight chain of the gingival flap around the donor's teeth. A tighter fit between the gap and the donor's teeth is achieved by suturing before the donor's placement. This technique is fundamental to the graft when the affected donor is transplanted to an adjacent second mole recipient site. If the donor is sprinted using sutures, one cord from each suture should be left long enough for this purpose.

9. *Donor tooth placement and splinting* (Fig. 25.7): The donor's tooth is lightly inserted into the recipient's alveoli through the opening of the sutured gingival flap. Ideally, a snug fit between the teeth and gingiva should be desired, so the gingival space should be slightly smaller than the donor's diameter. Then perform a sprint using sutures. If the implant is unstable after the suture sprint or a more occlusal adjustment is required, replace the sprint with a wire and adhesive resin sprint. If the implant is dangerous but does not require occlusal adjustment, the wire and resin sprint can be delayed 2–3 days after the suture sprint (Fig. 25.8). Surgical procedures make optimal results difficult.

10. *Occlusal adjustment*: The occlusal should be checked to make sure there is no occlusal interference. When using sutures for stabilization, ideally, occlusal contact should be reduced extraorally before placing the donor, taking care not to damage the PDL (Fig. 25.3). It can also be done in the oral cavity before donor extraction. If you use sprints with wires, you can make occlusal adjustments after placing the sprints. Occlusal adjustment should be conservative. After healing, a complex restoration is needed to adjust the occlusion and aesthetic appearance of the crown.

11. *Radiological evaluation*: X-rays are taken before surgery and before and after the splinting to assess the donor's teeth position in the new socket.

12. *Surgical dressing (periodontal packing)* is applied to protect the graft from infection during the first 3 days of wound healing. This dressing is removed after 3–4 days of surgery.

13. *The suture* is removed after 4–5 days of surgery.

Endodontic Treatment

Pulp healing can be expected with a developing tooth transplant. If so, X-rays are taken monthly for 3 months after surgery to monitor inflammatory absorption or apical periodontitis due to medullary infection. If signs of pulp infection are observed (e.g., inflammatory absorption is observed), root canal treatment should be started as soon as possible (Fig. 25.9) [2–16]. If no signs of pulp infection are

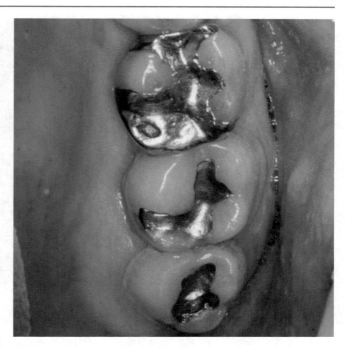

Fig. 25.3 Occlusal picture of the donor tooth #28

observed, X-rays are taken 6 months after surgery to assess continued root development and pulp canal closure. Successful regeneration should inevitably result in pulp tube obstruction and should be considered a positive sign of pulp health. The susceptibility test should be positive in this 6-month booster (root canal) [25, 28, 30].

Treatment should be planned at the right time. If you have access to the donor's teeth, you can complete the endodontic treatment before surgery. Two weeks of endodontic therapy is critical. Endodontic treatment immediately after surgery can cause further damage to the PDL, and if delayed by more than 2 weeks, the infection can cause inflammatory absorption [31, 32, 34, 38]. On the first day of endodontic treatment, the canal is opened, cleaned, and summoned with a creamy mixture of $Ca(OH)_2$ rotated into the canal with a lentulo spiral instrument. Two weeks later, the canal was instrumented and molded, and the canal was filled with gutta-percha and sealant. At this point (4 weeks after surgery), the sprint remains intact [25–32, 43].

Restorative Treatment

Ideally, if the third molar's development is transplanted to another part of the arch, no repair treatment is needed once the flesh has healed. In less ideal situations, crown repair is required, such as filling the cavity for root canal treatment, creating better adjacent interdental contact, or remodeling the crown for occlusion and aesthetic purposes. Composite resins are the first material of choice given their cost advantages and maintaining the enamel's aesthetics. Whitening can be done before repairing the transplanted anterior teeth

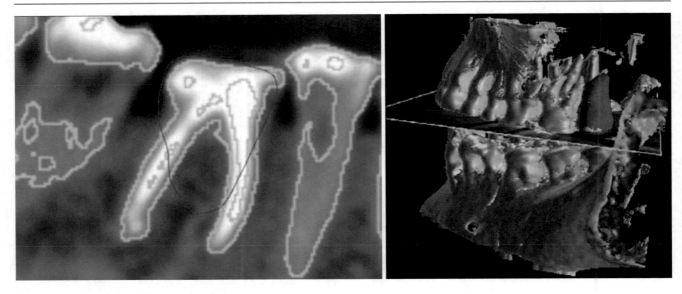

Fig. 25.4 3D donor tooth replica plantation

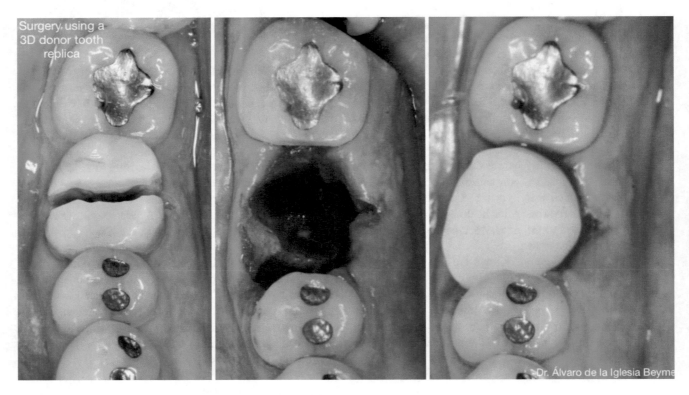

Fig. 25.5 Extraction of the unrestorable tooth and verification of the position of the 3D replica

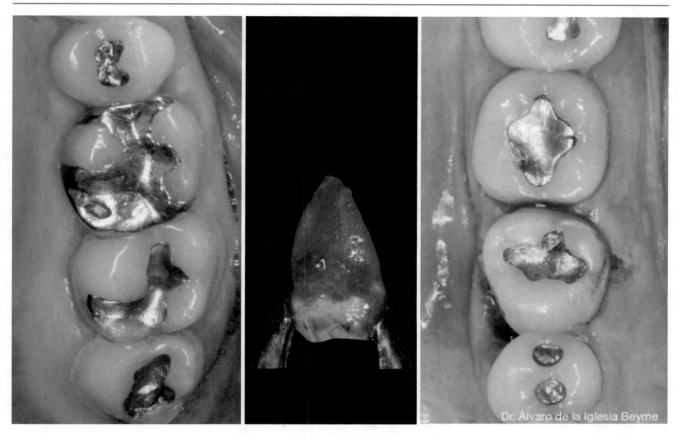

Fig. 25.6 Atraumatic extraction of the donor tooth and adjusting it in the new position

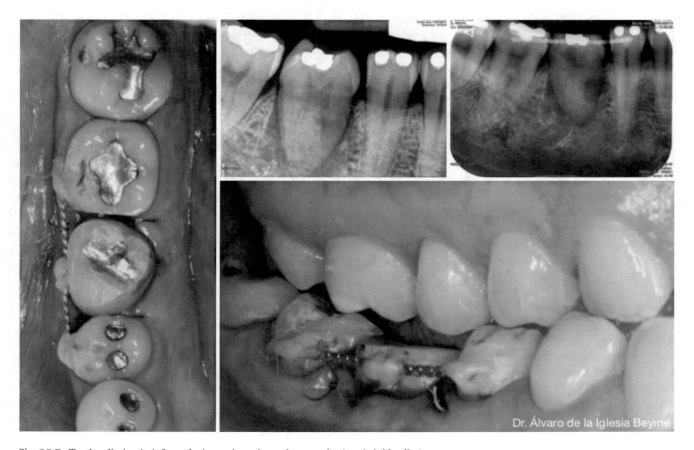

Fig. 25.7 Tooth splinting in infraocclusion, using wire and composite (semi-rigid splint)

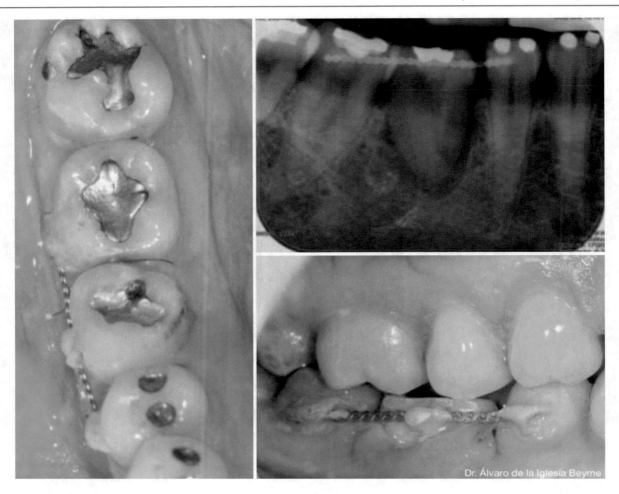

Fig. 25.8 One-week follow-up and suture removal

treated with a root canal. Exposure to dentin causes bacterial invasion and can cause apical periodontitis. If dentin exposure is unavoidable, immediate recovery is required (Fig. 25.11) [8, 12, 19, 42].

Follow-up
A naturally healed transplant tooth will heal and carry the same risks as other natural teeth in caries and periodontal disease. Therefore, regular follow-up should be done as often as the other teeth in the mouth (Fig. 25.10) with compliance. Maintenance is essential to ensure long-term positive results (Figs. 25.12 and 25.13) [42–44].

Postoperative Support

After surgery, a prescription of antibiotics (amoxicillin 500 mg) is mandatory for 1 week and is instructed to rinse with 0.2% chlorhexidine three times a day for 3 weeks. Patients need to be evaluated clinically and radiologically.

Prosthodontic treatment should be given 1 to 3 or 12 months after surgery and 3 to 8 months after transplantation.

Key Factors to Enhance the Success Rate

Several factors are involved in the success and selection of autologous transplant cases. Two basic factors are patient's age and exposure time, should control and limit retainting the donor's teeth outside the mouth not to exceed 15 minutes. Clinicians should be care to maintain and preserve the periodontal ligament cells around the donor's teeth, reduce the timing of endodontic treatment of the donor's teeth to prevent possible pain, occlusal adjustment, and the tooth infrared from the occlusal force is very similar to the method of sprinting on the next tooth. Finally, maintaining patient oral hygiene is a significant factor in achieving successful processes and procedures [33, 44, 48].

It has increased the success rate of transplantation of nonfunctioning immature and mature teeth. Root canals are rec-

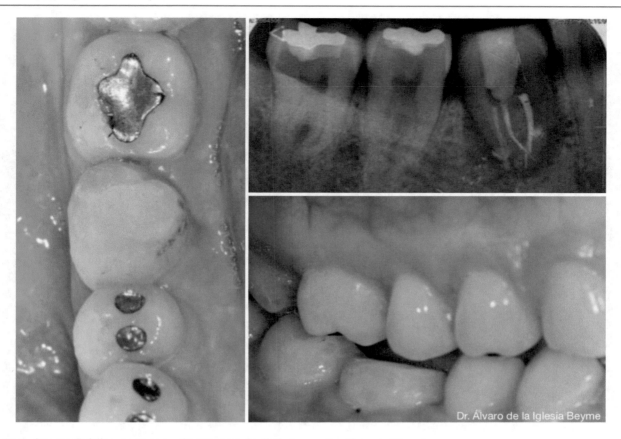

Fig. 25.9 One-month follow-up. Root canal treatment and splinting removal performed at 2 weeks

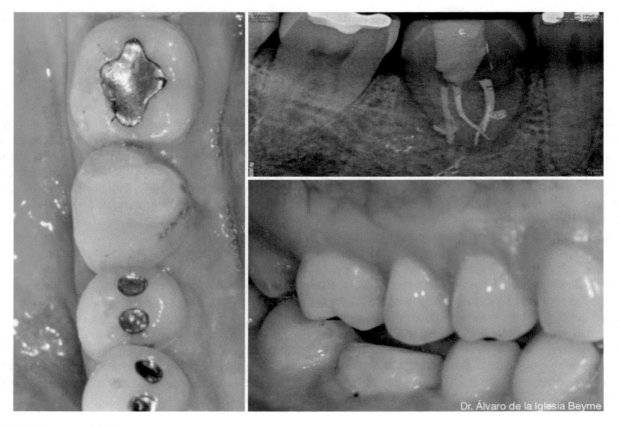

Fig. 25.10 Three-month follow-up

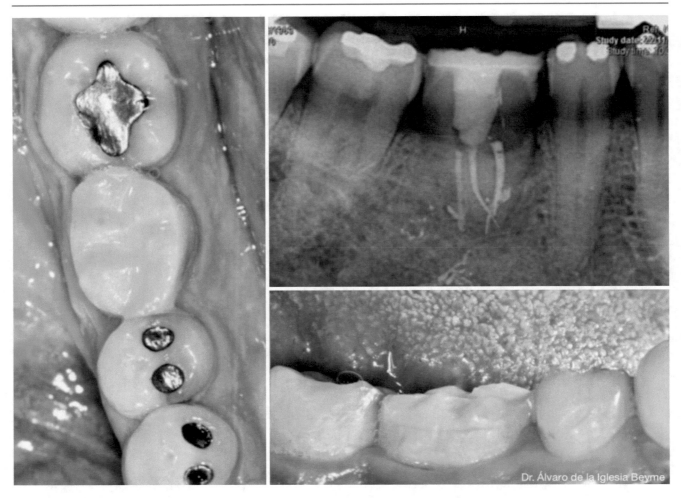

Fig. 25.11 Six-month follow-up with the definitive restoration

ommended before surgery or 2 weeks after transplantation, as no revascularization of the closed apical tooth could be expected. Early endodontic treatment 2 weeks ago can cause further damage to the PDL, and delays of more than 2 weeks can cause the development of inflammatory absorption in the root canal system. In a recent systematic review, Chung et al. concluded that the estimated survival rate was 1–5 years [49, 50]. In cases with clinical and radiological symptoms, it is best to schedule root canal treatment to prevent additional complications. The advantage of performing root canal treatment is that it stops the process of absorption and painlessness. In addition, clinicians should manage toxins and degradation products that may pass through the apical foramen, accessory or dental canal and prevent them to surround tissues. According to the recent systematic review and meta-analysis studies, survival and success rate of open autotransplanted teeth with an open apex was reported greater than teeth with a closed apex. The average of success rate and survival rate was found

between 89 to 96.6% and 98%, respectively. Prognostic factors like the stage of root formation of the donor tooth, type of donor tooth, and receptor site were announced. Moorees et al. [61] and Denys et al. [62] declared that fewer failures were found in stages 3 and 4. The absence of progressive root resorption, ankylosis, mobility, inflammation, and increased probing depth are the highest success variables that were described in studies. Most complications that were reported related to an open apex autotransplantation are ankylosis, root resorption, and pulp necrosis [25, 33, 40, 63, 64].

Recently, using a 3D model to induce donor replication and allow sockets to be prepared before the donor's teeth are removed has improved survival and autotransplantation success rates [49–51]. We study interventions through 3D models and digital schemes by examining the availability and compatibility of donor and recipient sites, the donor tooth root morphology, and the likelihood of extracting the most donor teeth (non-traumatic) [52–54]. The duplicate tooth model is digi-

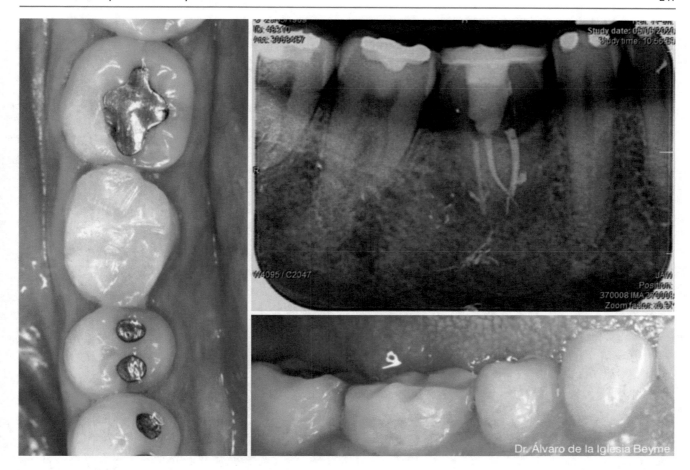

Fig. 25.12 One-year follow-up

tally designed based on the morphology of the donor's tooth. It is designed to prepare the recipient site and verify the socket's availability, and this method follows this evaluation with minimal extraoral tooth time and planned intervention. You get the benefit of gaining accuracy [8, 32, 55].

Evaluation of Healing

In the case of PDL healing, non-traumatic extraction is an essential factor in the preservation of root cells and PDL cells, which play an important role. Damage to these cells leads to inadequate healing. After extraction, the extraoral condition is affected by pH, osmotic pressure, dehydration, etc. and thus affects the healing process. If a non-traumatic extract is obtained in a short extraoral time, these cells will heal in a new socket in 2 weeks [54–58].

In terms of bone healing, genetically, PDL cells showed bone induction during the healing process from fibroblasts, cementoblasts, and osteoblasts. The latter are the type involved in the appearance of hard thin layers and bone for-

mation through rapid regeneration. Therefore, there is no need to transplant material to fill the space between the bone wall and the root.

For root development, the amount of development cannot be predicted. In immature roots, continuous development can also be expected when Hertwig's epithelial root sheath conservation is achieved around the apex [57, 58].

Dental Implant and Autotransplantation

Autotransplantation is a common procedure, particularly in children and adolescents. Although, it is a viable alternative treatment to conventional prosthetic and implant rehabilitation, the long-term outcome is not predictable, and it is a sound treatment option for replacement of a lost or hopeless tooth, usually providing satisfactory clinical, aesthetic, and functional benefit and preserving more amount of quality in alveolar bone [59, 60]. It is inevitable to compare transplants with implants because the two techniques have similar objectives. So, the criteria for choosing each must be discussed.

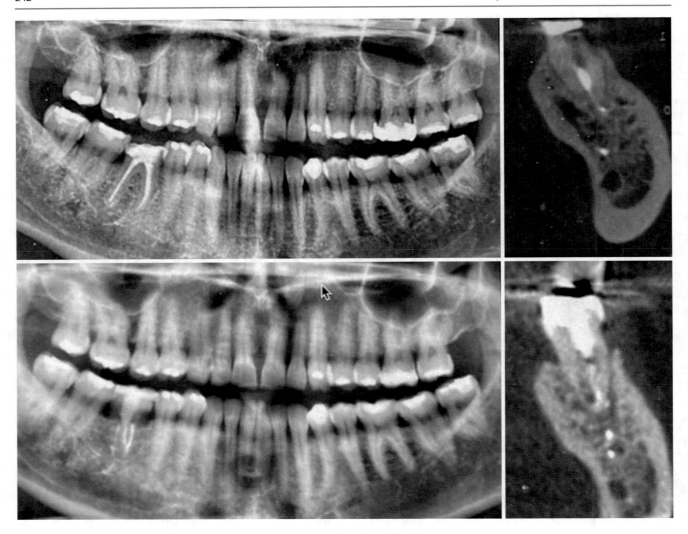

Fig. 25.13 Before and after 1-year follow-up in panoramic view and CBCT analysis

Implants are indicated to all patients (who can afford the cost), while transplants are limited to those who have appropriate donor teeth [34]. The techniques for transplants and implants are similar in difficulty and so is the high prognosis. However, the post-surgical restorative options are generally much simpler for transplanted teeth [5, 8, 32, 34, 61, 62].

Conclusion

Dental transplants performed in children and adolescents have shown high success and survival rates at the fundamental stages of development that affect the healing of the transplanted teeth pulp and PDL. Autologous tooth transplantation is considered a conservative and predictable surgery. Successful autotransplantation procedures include the absence of endodontic damage, root or bone resorption, and subsequent complete root formation. It is essential to have the right treatment plan and

accurate diagnosis of the case and follow the key indications and surgical stages to achieve time and success.

References

1. Czochrowska EM, Stenvik A, Bjercke B, Zachrisson BU. Outcome of tooth transplantation: survival and success rates 17–41 years posttreatment. Am J Orthod Dentofacial Orthop. 2002;121:110–9; quiz193.
2. Zachrisson BU, Stenvik A, Haanaes HR. Management of missing maxillary anterior teeth with emphasis on autotransplantation. Am J Orthod Dentofac Orthop. 2004;126:284–8.
3. Sugai T, Yoshizawa M, Kobayashi T, Ono K, Takagi R, KitamuraN OT, Saito C. Clinical study on prognostic factors for autotransplantation of teeth with complete root formation. Int J Oral Maxillofac Surg. 2010;39:1193–203. https://doi.org/10.1016/j.ijom.2010.06.018.
4. Cohen AS, Shen TC, Pogrel MA. Transplanting teeth successfully: autografts and allografts that work. J Am Dent Assoc. 1995;126:481–5. quiz 500

5. Vriens JP, Freihofer HP. Autogenous transplantation of third molars in irradiated jaws—a preliminary report. J Craniomaxillofac Surg. 1994;22:297–300.

6. Tsukiboshi M. Autotransplantation of teeth: requirements for predictable success. Dent Traumatol. 2002;18:157–80.

7. Miller HM. Transplantation: a case report. J Am Dent Assoc. 1950;40:327.

8. Lundberg T, Isaksson S. A clinical follow-up study of 278 autotransplanted teeth. Br J Oral Maxillofac Surg. 1996;34:181–5.

9. Hillerup S, Dahl E, Schwartz O, Hjørting-Hansen E. Tooth transplantation to bone graft in cleft alveolus. Cleft Palate J. 1987;24:137–41.

10. Czochrowska EM, Stenvik A, Album B, Zachrisson BU. Autotransplantation of premolars to replace maxillary incisors: a comparison with natural incisors. Am J Orthod Dentofac Orthop. 2000;118:592–600.

11. Kristerson L. Autotransplantation of human premolars. A clinical and radiographic study of 100 teeth. Int J Oral Surg. 1985;14:200–13.

12. Paulsen HU, Andreasen JO, Schwartz O. Pulp and periodontal healing, root development and root resorption subsequent to transplantation and orthodontic rotation: a long-term study of autotransplanted premolars. Am J Orthod Dentofac Orthop. 1995;108:630–40.

13. Pogrel MA. Evaluation of over 400 autogenous tooth transplants. J Oral Maxillofac Surg. 1987;45:205–11.

14. Andreasen JO, Hjorting-Hansen E, Jolst O. A clinical and radiographic study of 76 autotransplanted third molars. Scand J Dent Res. 1970;78:512–23.

15. Schatz JP, Joho JP. Long-term clinical and radiologic evaluation of autotransplanted teeth. Int J Oral Maxillofac Surg. 1992;21:271–5.

16. Schwartz O, Bergmann P, Klausen B. Autotransplantation of human teeth. Int J Oral Surg. 1985;14:245–58.

17. Nordenram A. Autotransplantation of teeth. A clinical and experimental investigation. Acta Odontol Scand. 1963;21(Suppl 33):7–76.

18. Slagsvold O, Bjercke B. Indications for autotransplantation in cases of missing premolars. Am J Orthod. 1978;74:241–57.

19. Dixon DA. Autogenous transplantation of tooth germs into the upper incisor region. Br Dent J. 1971;131:260–5.

20. Kahnberg K. Autotransplantation of teeth. (I). Indications for transplantation with a follow-up of 51 cases. Int J Oral Maxillofac Surg. 1987;16:577–85.

21. Marques-Ferreira M, Rabaça-Botelho M-F, Carvalho L, Oliveiros B, Palmeirão-Carrilho EV. Autogenous tooth transplantation: evaluation of pulp tissue regeneration. Med Oral Patol Oral Cir Bucal. 2011;16:e984–9.

22. Mendes RA, Rocha G. Mandibular third molar autotransplantation—literature review with clinical cases. J Can Dent Assoc. 2004;70:761–6.

23. Kristerson L, Johansson LA, Kisch J, Stadler LE. Autotransplantation of third molars as treatment in advanced periodontal disease. J Clin Periodontol. 1991;18:521–8.

24. Bauss O, Schilke R, Fenske C, Engelke W, Kiliaridis S. Autotransplantation of immature third molars: influence of different splinting methods and fixation periods. Dent Traumatol. 2002;18:322–8.

25. Northway WM, Konigsberg S. Autogenic tooth transplantation. The state of the art. Am J Orthod. 1980;77:146–62.

26. Josefsson E, Brattström V, Tegsjö U, Valerius-Olsson H. Treatment of lower second premolar agenesis by autotransplantation: four-year evaluation of eighty patients. Acta Odontol Scand. 1999;57:111–5.

27. Marcusson KA, Lilja-Karlander EK. Autotransplantation of premolars and molars in patients with tooth. 1996.

28. Oswald RJ, Harrington GW, Van Hassel HJ. A postreplantation evaluation of air-dried and saliva-stored avulsed teeth. J Endod. 1980;6:546.51.

29. Andreasen JO, Hjorting-Hansen E. Replantation of teeth. I. Radiographic and clinical study of 110 human teeth replanted after accidental loss. Acta Odontol Scand. 1966;24:263.86.

30. Andreasen JO, Hjorting-Hansen E. Replantation of teeth. Histological study of 22 replanted anterior teeth in humans. Acta Odontol Scand. 1966;24:287.306.

31. Andreasen JO. Relationship between surface and inflammatory ;resorption and changes in the pulp after replantation of permanent incisors in monkeys. J Endod. 1981;7:294.301.

32. Andreasen JO. The effect of pulp extirpation or root canal treatment on periodontal healing after replantation of permanent incisors in monkeys. J Endod. 1981;7:245.52.

33. Melcher AH. On the repair potential of periodontal tissues. J Periodontol. 1976;47:256.60.

34. Ten Cate AR. Oral histology, development, structure and function. 2nd ed. St Louis: Mosby; 1985.

35. Lindhe J. Textbook of clinical periodontology. Copenhagen: Munksgaard; 1984.

36. Melcher AH. Periodontal ligament. In: Bhaskar SN, editor. Orban's oral histology and embryology. St Louis: Mosby; 1986. p. 198.231.

37. Yamamura T, Shimono M, et al. Differentiation and induction of un differentiated mesenchymal cells in tooth and periodontal tissue during wound healing and regeneration. Bull Tokyo Dent Coll. 1980;21:181.222.

38. Inoue T, Shimono M, Yamamura T. Osteogenetic activity of periodontal ligament of rat incisor in vivo and in vitro. J Dent Res. 1988;67:401.

39. Inoue T, Chen SH, Shimono M. Induction of cartilage and bone formation by cells from explants of various oral tissues. In vitro. J Dent Res. 1989;68:416.

40. Hamamoto Y, Kawasaki N, Jarnbring F, Hammarstrom L. Effects and distribution of the enamel matrix derivative Emdogain in the periodontal tissues of rat molars transplanted to the abdominal wall. Dent Traumatol. 2002;18:12–23.

41. Andreasen JO. Interrelation between alveolar bone and periodontal ligament repair after replantation of mature permanent incisors in monkeys. J Periodontal Res. 1981;16:228.35.

42. Andreasen AW, Sharav Y, Massler M. Reparative dentine formation and pulp morphology. Oral Surg Oral Med Oral Pathol. 1968;26:837.47.

43. Skoglund A, Hasselgren G, Tronstad L. Oxidoreductase activity in the pulp of replanted and autotransplanted teeth in young dogs. Oral Surg. 1981;52:205.9.

44. Kvinnsland I, Heyeraas KJ. Cell renewal and ground substance formation in replanted cat teeth. Acta Odontol Scand. 1990;48:203.15.

45. Skoglund A, Tronstad L, Wallenius K. A microangiographic study of vascular changes in replanted and autotransplanted teeth of young dogs. Oral Surg. 1978;45:17.27.

46. Slagsvold O, Bjercke B. Applicability of autotransplantation in cases of missing upper anterior teeth. Am J Orthod. 1978;74:410–21.

47. Andreasen JO, Paulsen HU, Yu Z, Bayer T. A long-term study of 370 autotransplanted premolars. Part A Root development subsequent to transplantation. Eur J Orthod. 1990;12:38.50.

48. Kristerson L, Andreasen JO. Influence of root development on periodontal and pulpal healing after replantation of incisors in monkeys. Int J Oral Surg. 1984;13:313.23.

49. Chung WC, Tu YK, Lin YH, Lu HK. Outcomes of autotransplanted teeth with complete root formation: a systematic review and meta-analysis. J Clin Periodontol. 2014;41:412–23.

50. Almpani K, Papageorgiou SN, Papadopoulos MA. Autotransplantation of teeth in humans: a systematic review and meta-analysis. Clin Oral Investig. 2015;19(6):1157–79.

51. Strbac GD, Schnappauf A, Giannis K, et al. Guided autotransplantation of teeth: a novel method using virtually planned 3-dimensional templates. J Endod. 2016;42:1844–50.

52. Anssari Moin D, Verweij JP, Waars H, et al. Accuracy of computer-assisted template guided autotransplantation of teeth with custom three-dimensional designed/printed surgical tooling: a cadaveric study. J Oral Maxillofac Surg. 2017;75:925.e1–7.

53. Lee SJ, Jung IY, Lee CY, et al. Clinical application of computer-aided rapid prototyping for tooth transplantation. Dent Traumatol. 2001;17:114–9.

54. Bae JH, Choi YH, Cho BH, et al. Autotransplantation of teeth with complete root formation: a case series. J Endod. 2010;36:1422–6.

55. Sange S, Thilander B. Transalveolar transplantation of maxillary canines. A follow up study. Eur J Orthod. 1990;12:140–7.

56. Berthold C, Thaler A, Petschelt A. Rigidity of commonly used dental trauma splints. Dent Traumatol. 2009;25:248–55.

57. Kwan SC, Johnson JD, Cohenca N. The effect of splint material and thickness on tooth mobility after extraction and replantation using a human cadaveric model. Dent Traumatol. 2012;28:277–81.

58. Yu HJ, Jia P, Lv Z, Qiu LX. Autotransplantation of third molars with completely formed roots into surgically created sockets and fresh extraction sockets: a 10- year comparative study. Int J Oral Maxillofac Surg. 2017;46:531–8.

59. Cardona JL, Caldera MM, Vera J. Autotransplantation of a premolar: a long-term follow-up report of a clinical case. J Endod. 2012;38:1149–52.

60. Jang Y, Choi YJ, Lee SJ, et al. Prognostic factors for clinical outcomes in autotransplantation of teeth with complete root formation: survival analysis for up to 12 years. J Endod. 2016;42:198–205.

61. Moorees C, Fanning E, Hunt E. Age variation of formation stages for ten permanent teeth. J Dent Res. 1963;42:1490.

62. Denys D, Shahbazian M, Jacobs R, et al. Importance of root development in autotransplantations: a retrospective study of 137 teeth with a follow-up period varying from 1 week to 14 years. Eur J Orthod. 2013;35:680.

63. Atala-Acevedo C, Abarca J, Martínez-Zapata MJ, Díaz J, Olate S, Zaror C. Success rate of autotransplantation of teeth with an open apex: systematic review and meta-analysis. J Oral Maxillofac Surg. 2017;75(1):35–50.

64. Rohof ECM, Kerdijk W, Jansma J, Livas C, Ren Y. Autotransplantation of teeth with incomplete root formation: a systematic review and meta-analysis. Clin Oral Investig. 2018;22(4):1613–24.

Zygomatic Implants in Implant Dentistry

26

Justin Bonner

Historical Perspective

The first use of implants placed into the zygoma for oral rehabilitation was by Branemark and colleagues in the late 1980s, and by 1998, a clinical protocol was developed and published [1]. During this time and beyond, zygomatic implants have allowed for the reconstruction and rehabilitation of patients with severe maxillary atrophy or the absence of the maxilla due to trauma, pathology, or post-surgical defects [2]. This is done without extensive grafting procedures and can allow for immediate loading of a prosthesis. Today, multiple dental implant companies manufacture zygomatic implants for a variety of clinical scenarios, and implant and prosthesis survival rates are superior to implants placed in grafted bone (Fig. 26.1) [3–6].

Indications and Contraindications

Zygomatic implants are indicated for patients with inadequate posterior maxillary bone and who receive a prosthesis providing cross-arch stability [7]. This lack of bone is most commonly due to pneumatization of the maxillary sinus and resorption of the alveolus, but it may also result from numerous other reasons such as trauma, pathology, or prior surgery.

Zygomatic implants are contraindicated in the setting of maxillary or zygomatic pathology, as well as infection of the adjacent bone and sinuses. Caution should also be used in patients who may have been treated with bisphosphonates and head and neck radiation, are currently smoking, or may not have the ability to maintain a prosthesis.

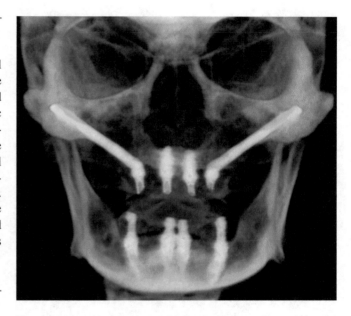

Fig. 26.1 A patient with zygomatic implants and anterior axial implants supporting a fixed provisional prosthesis

Anatomic Overview

The zygomatic bone, or cheek bone, is a paired bone of the midfacial skeleton that forms the prominence of the cheek. Its processes articulate with the frontal bone, sphenoid bone, maxilla, and temporal bone (Fig. 26.2).

The maxillary process of the zygomatic bone articulates with the maxilla to form the inferior orbital rim and the zygomaticomaxillary buttress. The temporal process of the zygomatic bone articulates with the temporal bone to form the zygomatic arch which overlies the temporalis muscle and represents the border between the temporal fossa above and the infratemporal fossa below. The frontozygomatic notch is formed between the frontal and temporal processes of the zygomatic bone and is a key landmark for dissection and retraction during zygomatic implant surgery.

J. Bonner (✉)
Oral and Maxillofacial Surgeon, Private Practice, West, TX, USA
e-mail: DrBonner@BonnerOralSurgery.com

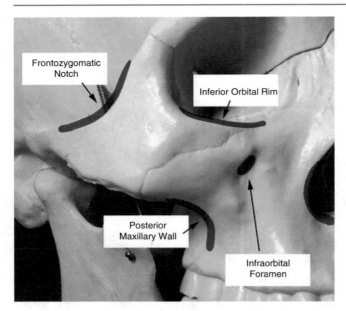

Fig. 26.2 Illustration of zygomatic anatomy

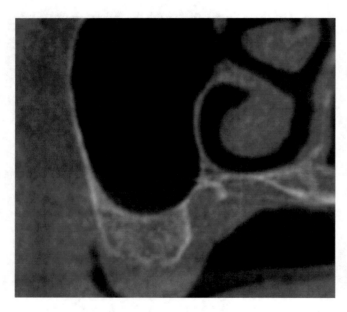

Fig. 26.3 Coronal slice of cone-beam computed tomography (CBCT) demonstrating the patency of the maxillary sinus ostium

The maxilla is a paired bone that is fused to create the majority of the midface. Within the body of the maxilla is the maxillary sinus which typically has thin overlying walls. The maxillary sinus's medial wall is also the lateral wall of the nasal cavity, and the ostium of the maxillary sinus allows for communication between the two structures (Fig. 26.3). The posterior wall of the maxillary sinus is also the anterior wall of the pterygopalatine fossa.

Below the inferior orbital rim on the anterior wall of the maxillary sinus is the infraorbital foramen. The infraorbital

neurovascular bundle exits the infraorbital foramen. The nerve gives sensation to the skin of the lower eyelid, lateral nose, upper lip, and cheek as the facial mucosa of the anterior maxilla.

Case Selection and Pre-surgical Evaluation

Preoperatively the patient is evaluated systematically as described by Bedrossian and colleagues [8].

The first step involves determining whether the patient is only missing teeth or if they have a composite defect, which is present if they are missing hard and soft tissue in addition to their missing teeth. Patients with a history of periodontitis, for example, may be expected to have a composite defect given their loss of alveolar bone from the disease process.

When determining the presence of a tooth-only defect or a composite defect, it is critical to work backward from the ideal position of the maxillary teeth. If it was made with the correct tooth position and vertical dimension of occlusion, a patient's existing denture may be helpful in this assessment.

One technique is to duplicate the existing denture in clear acrylic using a Lang Denture Duplicator Flask. This clear denture can then be worn by the patient to show whether the denture teeth appear to sit on the ridge (indicating a tooth-only defect) or off the ridge (indicating a composite defect) (Fig. 26.4). If the patient's denture is not made with the correct tooth position and vertical dimension, it should be corrected prior to surgery.

If only teeth are missing, then a prosthesis replacing only the crowns of the teeth, such as a porcelain fused to metal bridge, is indicated. If the patient has a composite defect, then a prosthesis such as a hybrid prosthesis is planned.

The next step in the systematic approach is to determine whether or not the patient's gingiva is visible during maximum animation. This is critical because it indicates the transition line's position, which is the transition between a fixed prosthesis and the gingiva (Fig. 26.5).

When reconstructing a composite defect with a fixed prosthesis, the transition line must be hidden by the upper lip during maximum animation, or else the final result will be unaesthetic. The amount of alveoloplasty required to provide restorative space for the prosthesis should also be considered, and if the transition line would still be visible, then additional alveoloplasty should be planned. If this is not possible, then a removable restoration should be planned so that the flange of the prosthesis may hide this transition line.

The third step in the systematic approach is to determine the presence or absence of bone in each of the three zones of bone. Bedrossian et al. have described three zones of the maxilla – zone 1 is the premaxilla, zone 2 is the premolar/bicuspid region, and zone 3 is the molar region (Fig. 26.6). A panoramic radiograph is used to screen these zones quickly,

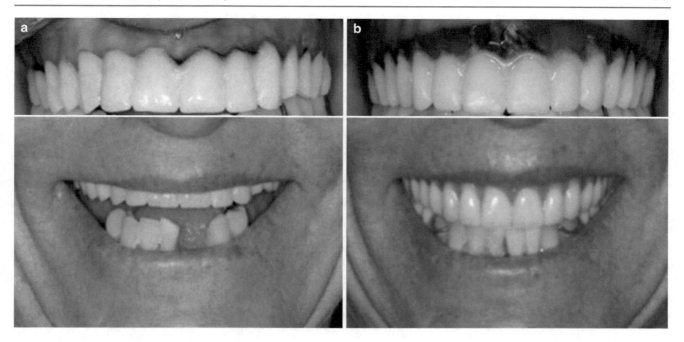

Fig. 26.4 Clear acrylic duplicate dentures with barium-impregnated teeth. (a) shows the patient's existing denture which was made at the incorrect occlusal vertical dimension and incorrectly suggested a tooth-only defect. (b) shows the same patient with a new denture made at the correct occlusal vertical dimension

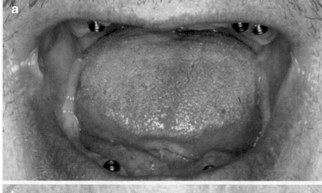

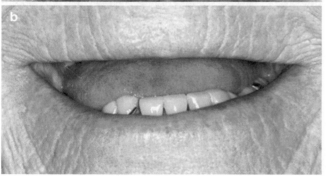

Fig. 26.5 (a) A patient with an overdenture who was referred for evaluation for zygomatic implants and requesting a fixed prosthesis. Gingiva was visible during maximum animation and was concealed by the flange of his removable prosthesis. Transitioning to a fixed prosthesis without addressing this gingival display would be problematic and result in an unaesthetic prosthesis (b)

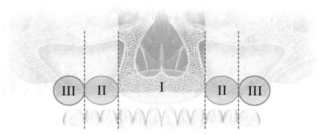

Fig. 26.6 Illustration demonstrating the zones of bone in the maxilla. (Illustration courtesy of Nobel Biocare, Yorba Linda, CA. Used with permission)

and a CT or CBCT can be used to confirm the volume of bone in these zones. A duplicated denture with barium-impregnated teeth when making these radiographs may also be helpful.

The following algorithm provides a graftless approach to the implant reconstruction of the edentulous maxilla (Table 26.1): If bone is present in all three zones, then traditional axial implants are placed. If adequate bone is present in zones 1 and 2 only, then axial implants are placed in zone 1, and titled implants are placed in zone 2 in order to provide posterior support and minimize cantilevers. If adequate bone is only present in zone 1, then axial implants are placed in zone 1, and posterior support is achieved through zygomatic implants. If adequate bone is not present in any of the zones, a quad zygoma treatment plan is indicated (Fig. 26.7) [8].

Table 26.1 Treatment algorithm for graftless, full-arch reconstruction

Zones with adequate bone	Anterior support	Posterior support
1, 2, 3	Axial implants in zone 1	Axial implants in zone 3
1, 2	Axial implants in zone 1	Tilted implants in zone 2
1	Axial implants in zone 1	Zygomatic implants
No zone is adequate	Zygomatic implants	Zygomatic implants

Adapted from Bedrossian et al. [8]

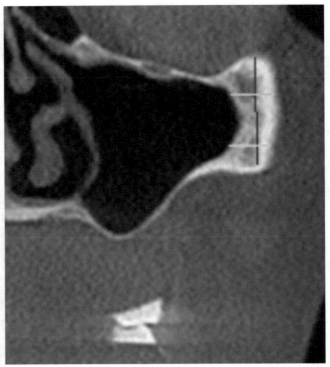

Fig. 26.8 This coronal slice of a CBCT demonstrates the adequacy of bone in the left zygoma, a clear maxillary sinus with a patent ostiomeatal complex, atrophy of the posterior maxilla, and the magnitude of the composite defect as indicated by the barium-impregnated denture teeth

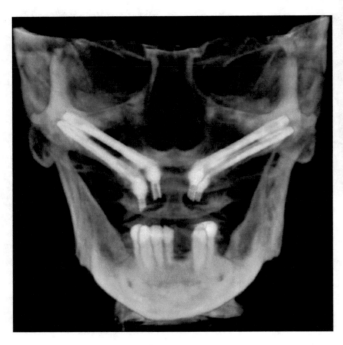

Fig. 26.7 3D image of a patient with four zygomatic implants – "quad zygoma"

In the case of a zygomatic implant treatment plan, a CT or CBCT is often evaluated to confirm the adequacy of bone in the zygomas, as well as to rule out pathology in the maxillary sinuses and demonstrate patency of the ostia (Fig. 26.8).

In preparation for surgery, some clinicians perform model surgery on a 3D printed model of their patient in order to aid in visualization and treatment planning.

Caution is advised with restricted surgical guides as a small deviation from the planned trajectory of the implant can lead to large deviations from the planned implant position. Intraoperative navigation has also been utilized in the placement of zygomatic implants, and all guidance systems should be viewed as an adjunct and not a substitute for the surgeon's ability to perform the procedure without such guides [9].

Surgical Technique

Zygomatic implants may be placed using local anesthesia, IV sedation, or general anesthesia. Local anesthesia should include transcutaneous infiltration of the body of the zygoma and the frontozygomatic notch. The buccal vestibule and palatal gingiva should also be infiltrated, and the superior posterior alveolar and infraorbital nerves should be blocked. Some clinicians have noted improvements when a mandibular block is also given, allowing retraction and manipulation of the mandible with greater comfort.

A crestal incision with bilateral releases over the tuberosity areas is created. A full-thickness mucoperiosteal flap is developed to expose the anterior and lateral maxillary walls. Caution is taken when dissecting superiorly to avoid the infraorbital neurovascular bundle.

The body of the zygoma is exposed, and a retractor is placed in the frontozygomatic notch – this retraction aids in direct visualization of the drills and implants which will follow. The importance of this retraction should not be overlooked. Adequate visualization helps prevent the inadvertent placement of the implant into undesirable locations such as the orbit.

Further aiding the visualization, an approximately 10 mm by 5 mm window is created in the lateral maxillary wall following the posterior maxilla contour. The sinus membrane may be elevated and preserved, though many surgeons make no special efforts to keep this intact [1]. If the maxilla's contour is such that the planned position of the implant will not enter the sinus, this step is omitted.

In most cases, the trajectory begins at the crest of the ridge in the first-second premolar region. It follows the contour of the posterior maxillary wall body of the zygoma. In cases of severe resorption or the absence of maxillary bone due to resection or trauma, the implant's coronal portion may not reside in crestal bone at all. Carlos Aparicio has proposed a classification to describe the zygomatic implant pathway [10].

Sequential osteotomies are created following the manufacturer's drilling protocol, taking care to maintain the instruments' visualization through the maxillary sinus and exiting through the zygoma (Fig. 26.9). A drill guard may protect the soft tissues while drilling, and lateral pressure should not be placed on the drills to prevent breakage.

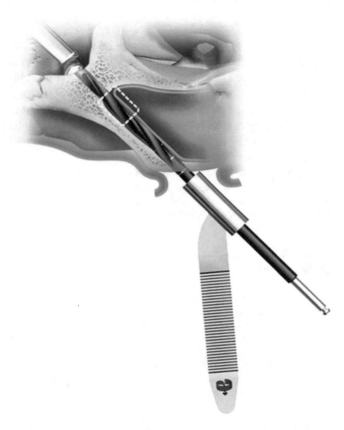

Fig. 26.9 A retractor is placed in the frontozygomatic notch to facilitate direct visualization. The white dotted outline represents the window created in the sinus for visualization. The drill guide is shown to protect the soft tissue. (Illustration courtesy of Nobel Biocare, Yorba Linda, CA. Used with permission)

A measurement is made to determine the implant's appropriate length, and after irrigation of all debris, the implant is placed. The implant is placed using either the surgical drilling unit or manually, taking care not to exceed the manufacturer's recommendations for insertion torque. After the correct placement is verified, the apex is irrigated to ensure no debris remains below the periosteum in the frontozygomatic region, and the retractor is removed.

Implant mounts are disengaged, and a cover screw may be placed. If adequate insertion torque has been achieved, a multiunit abutment may be placed for provisionalization with a prosthesis providing cross-arch stabilization.

Some surgeons choose to drape any extra-maxillary portion of the implant with the buccal fat pad [11, 12] prior to closure. The gingiva is closed with the operator's choice of suture, and the provisional prosthesis is converted.

Complications

As with all surgical procedures, complications can occur in managing patients with zygomatic implants, and the clinician should be familiar with their prevention and management.

Zygomatic implants are considered to be reliable and generally have a high success rate [4, 6, 13] . Aparicio et al. reviewed 20 studies presenting clinical outcomes for zygomatic implant patients and found an overall survival rate of 98.4%, though it was noted that some studies covered the same patient groups and, therefore, the true numbers of unique [13]. Similarly, Block et al. reviewed 21 studies that demonstrated success rates of zygomatic implants ranging from 90% to 100% [14].

One of the most prominent concerns with the placement of zygomatic implants is the effect on the maxillary sinus, and this will be discussed in more detail below.

Another potential complication is the inadvertent placement of the implant into the orbit or the temporal fossa. This should be avoided by thorough knowledge of regional anatomy as well as adequate visualization of the implant's trajectory via a sinus window and retraction at the frontozygomatic notch.

Bleeding can occur intraoperatively and is typically managed with local measures. Postoperative hemorrhage may lead to a facial hematoma, which typically resolves spontaneously over the course of time. Blood may exit the nares for the first few days after treatment as the blood that had accumulated during surgery escapes the sinuses. This generally requires no treatment, but a brisk bleed may require nasal packing.

Paresthesia of the infraorbital nerve distribution may occur, typically from retraction [6]. As long as the nerve is kept intact, this should resolve over a few weeks or months. This should be minimized by gentle retraction near the infraorbital foramen and not traumatizing the nerve with a retractor inadvertently.

A lip laceration may occur during osteotomy creation and can be avoided by adequate retraction and protection of the soft tissues by using a drill guide [15].

Subcutaneous emphysema has also occurred after the placement of zygomatic implants [6], and patients should be cautioned against nose blowing and sneezing.

Similar to traditional endosteal implants, peri-implant mucositis and peri-implantitis can occur with zygomatic implants, and treatment should be focused on prevention. This should at least include (1) careful attention to creating a prosthesis that is cleansable by the patient (i.e., avoiding plaque traps), (2) meticulous home care by the patient, and (3) routine follow-up for removal of the prosthesis and professional cleaning of both the prosthesis and the fixtures. For implants whose crestal component is not encased in maxillary bone, coverage with the buccal fat pad at the time of placement may improve gingival outcomes [11, 12].

Inflammation may occur at the apex of the implant and can manifest overlying skin changes. Copious irrigation of the tissues overlying the apex and the frontozygomatic notch prior to closure may help prevent this. Treatment may require transcutaneous or transoral resection of a portion of the implant's apex, but the remaining parts of the implant are often stable and can be left in place.

An oroantral communication may occur at either an early or late stage and may be amenable to closure by traditional means such as a buccal fat pad flap.

Zygomatic Implants and the Maxillary Sinus

Given the relationship between zygomatic implants and the maxillary sinus, a salient concern involves what effects they might have on the sinuses and the development of sinusitis.

It is important to recognize that the majority of zygomatic implant patients do not experience sinus symptoms [16]. It is also important to understand that sinusitis is common in the general population. In a 2012 survey of adults in the United States, 12% had been told by a doctor or other health professional in the past 12 months that they had sinusitis [17]. Accordingly, it should be expected that some degree of zygomatic implant patients will experience sinus symptoms at some point, just as the rest of the population does, and it has not been shown that zygomatic implant patients experience a higher rate of sinus symptoms than the general population [16].

Investigating the response of the maxillary sinus to a zygomatic implant, Petruson performed sinuscopy in 14 patients who had been functioning with their zygomatic implants for at least 1 year [18]. He found that the implants were either partially or totally covered in the mucosa, and there was no evidence of infection or increased secretions, suggesting that zygomatic implants do not cause a foreign body reaction. This finding is consistent with an animal study that examined the reaction of the sinus to implants placed into the sinuses of dogs [19]. However, radiographic thickening of the sinus mucosa in patients with implants in the sinus has been demonstrated [16, 20].

Regarding the treatment of the zygomatic implant patient who develops sinus symptoms at some point after surgery, Becktor et al. removed three implants due to sinusitis after failing treatment by an otolaryngologist consisting of sinus rinses and antibiotics. However, an attempt at functional endoscopic sinus surgery was not reported in these cases [21]. While removing the implant and draining the infection through the implant osteotomy may resolve the infection, it leaves the patient with a significant disability. In contrast, Branemark et al. reported the surgical management of sinusitis (inferior meatal antrostomy) in four zygomatic implant patients with recurrent sinusitis and found that the infection resolved in all cases without the need for removing the implant [22].

With this in mind, the management of the sinus in the zygomatic implant patient should involve treatment of preexisting sinus disease prior to implant placement and avoiding the creation of an oroantral fistula at the time of surgery. If a sinus infection develops after implant placement and is not resolved by oral antibiotics, functional endoscopic sinus surgery should be preferred over the removal of the implant.

Acknowledgments The author would like to thank Dr. Edmond Bedrossian for his contribution to the author's education as a clinical instructor as well as for the advancement of the profession of oral and maxillofacial surgery and implant dentistry.

References

1. Branemark PI. Surgery and fixture installation. Zygomaticus fixture clinical procedures. Gothenburg: Nobel Biocare AB; 1998.
2. Schmidt BL, Pogrel MA, Young CW, Sharma A. Reconstruction of extensive maxillary defects using zygomaticus implants. J Oral Maxillofac Surg. 2004;62:82–9.
3. Keller EE, Tolman DE, Eckert SE. Maxillary antral-nasal inlay autogenous bone graft reconstruction of compromised maxilla: a 12-year retrospective study. Int J Oral Maxillofac Implants. 1999;14(5):707–21.
4. Alzoubi F, Bedrossian E, Wong A, Farrell D, Park C, Indresano T. Outcomes assessment of treating completely edentulous patients with a fixed implant-supported profile prosthesis utilizing a graftless approach. Part 1: clinically related outcomes. Int J Oral Maxillofac Implants. 2017;32(4):897–903.
5. Bedrossian E. Rehabilitation of the edentulous maxilla with the zygoma concept: a 7-year prospective study. Int J Oral Maxillofac Implants. 2010;25(6):1213–21.

6. Ferna H, Trujillo-Saldarriaga S, Castro-Nu J. Zygomatic implants for the management of the severely atrophied maxilla: a retrospective analysis of 244 implants. 5. J. Craniofacial Surg. 2020. https://doi.org/10.1097/SCS.0000000000006978.

7. Bedrossian E, Stumpel LJ III. Immediate stabilization at stage II of zygomatic implants: rationale and technique. J Prosthet Dent. 2001;86(1):10–4.

8. Bedrossian E, Sullivan RM, Fortin Y, Malo P, Indresano T. Fixed-prosthetic implant restoration of the edentulous maxilla: a systematic pretreatment evaluation method. J Oral Maxillofac Surg. 2008;66(1):112–22.

9. Wang F, Bornstein MM, Hung K, Fan S, Chen X, Huang W, et al. Application of real-time surgical navigation for zygomatic implant insertion in patients with severely atrophic maxilla. J Oral Maxillofac Surg. 2018;76(1):80–7.

10. Aparicio C. A proposed classification for zygomatic implant patient based on the zygoma anatomy guided approach (ZAGA): a cross-sectional survey. Eur J Oral Implantol. 2011;4(3):269–75.

11. de Moraes EJ. The buccal fat pad flap: an option to prevent and treat complications regarding complex zygomatic implant surgery. Preliminary report. Int J Oral Maxillofac Implants. 2012;27(4):905–10.

12. Guennal P, Guiol J. Use of buccal fat pads to prevent vestibular gingival recession of zygomatic implants. J Stomatol Oral Maxillofac Surg. 2018;119(2):161–3.

13. Aparicio C, Ouazzani W, Hatano N. The use of zygomatic implants for prosthetic rehabilitation of the severely resorbed maxilla. Periodontol 2000. 2008;47(1):162–71.

14. Block MS, Haggerty CJ, Fisher GR. Nongrafting implant options for restoration of the edentulous maxilla. J Oral Maxillofac Surg. 2009;67(4):872–81.

15. Aparicio C, Ouazzani W, Garcia R, Arevalo X, Muela R, Fortes V. A prospective clinical study on titanium implants in the zygomatic arch for prosthetic rehabilitation of the atrophic edentulous maxilla with a follow-up of 6 months to 5 years. Clin Implant Dent Relat Res. 2006;8(3):114–22.

16. Davó R, Malevez C, López-Orellana C, Pastor-Beviá F, Rojas J. Sinus reactions to immediately loaded zygoma implants: a clinical and radiological study. Eur J Oral Implantol. 2008;1(1):53–60.

17. Blackwell DL, LJ, Clarke TC. Summary health statistics for U.S. adults: National Health Interview Survey, 2012 [Internet]. Vital Health Stat 10(260).: National Center for Health Statistics; 2014 [cited 2020 Nov 1]. Available from: http://doi.apa.org/get-pe-doi.cfm?doi=10.1037/e403882008-001.

18. Petruson B. Sinuscopy in patients with titanium implants in the nose and sinuses. Scand J Plast Reconstr Surg Hand Surg. 2004;38(2):86–93.

19. Jung J-H, Choi B-H, Zhu S-J, Lee S-H, Huh J-Y, You T-M, et al. The effects of exposing dental implants to the maxillary sinus cavity on sinus complications. Oral Surg Oral Med Oral Pathol Oral Radiol Endod. 2006;102(5):602–5.

20. Jung J-H, Choi B-H, Jeong S-M, Li J, Lee S-H, Lee H-J. A retrospective study of the effects on sinus complications of exposing dental implants to the maxillary sinus cavity. Oral Surg Oral Med Oral Pathol Oral Radiol Endod. 2007;103(5):623–5.

21. Becktor JP, Isaksson S, Abrahamsson P, Sennerby L. Evaluation of 31 zygomatic implants and 74 regular dental implants used in 16 patients for prosthetic reconstruction of the atrophic maxilla with cross-arch fixed bridges. Clin Implant Dent Relat Res. 2005;7(3):159–65.

22. Brånemark P-I, Gröndahl K, Ohrnell L-O, Nilsson P, Petruson B, Svensson B, et al. Zygoma fixture in the management of advanced atrophy of the maxilla: technique and long-term results. Scand J Plast Reconstr Surg Hand Surg. 2004;38(2):70–85.

Role of Lasers in Pre-prosthetic Oral Surgery

27

Mohit Sachdeva

Introduction

Laser is expanded as light amplification by stimulated emission of radiation. It is formulated on Albert Einstein's hypothesis of stimulated emission in 1917. The concept of "laser" was reported in the newspapers by Gordon Gould in 1959. The original laser was defined as "ruby laser" and was worked on by T. H. Maiman in 1960.

The Various Properties of Laser

They are collimated, which makes the rays highly concentrated, contrasting to the light from a bulb. They are rational as all the photons have the same frequency and wavelength, making it a highly structured beam. It is also monochromatic as the light has a distinctive wavelength.

The light has multiple methods of radiation. The laser beam constantly radiates at a specific power level. The laser beam is generated in the "on" and "off" modes (with a variance of a few milliseconds). The laser beam is usually "off" in the long term, preceded by emissions of very small duration. Lasers in dentistry are mostly classified as soft tissue lasers categorized on the magnitude of their penetration and hard tissue lasers [1–3].

The standard lasers utilized in the field of dentistry are argon laser, Nd:YAG laser (neodymium-doped yttrium aluminum garnet), CO2 laser, Er:YAG laser (erbium-doped yttrium aluminum garnet), and diode laser where the 980 nm is suitable for cutting and the 810 nm is better suited for clotting [4].

The Influence of Laser in Dentistry

Transmission is determined by the pace/momentum of power and motion. Reflection is the divergence of the laser for identifying caries. Scattering for the biostimulation, that is accelerated by the movement of heat to the nearby tissues. Absorption is the magnitude of the hydration and tissue pigmentation level that determines the absorption of the laser beam.

Oral surgery uses lasers of multiple wavelengths [2, 4].

Diode Laser

It is commonly known as the soft tissue laser. It is ideal for enhancing the shape and cutting of the oval soft tissue. The diode laser of wavelengths in 810 nm to 980 nm in a pulse or constant mode is implemented in soft tissue operations (Fig. 27.1).

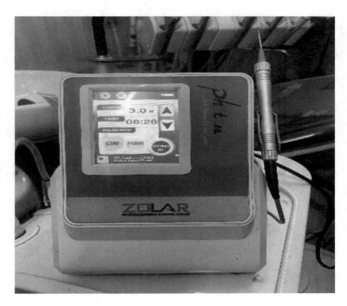

Fig. 27.1 Diode laser

M. Sachdeva (✉)
Rajdhani Dental Care Clinic, Dental and Oral Laser Centre,
New Delhi, India
e-mail: rdcc@live.in

The attributes of tiny size and portability are the primary benefits of using the diode laser.

The diode laser is commonly used for:

Photothermal teeth bleaching at 2 W the 980 nm diode laser is utilized to bleach teeth. The thermal variations at the pulpal position can be avoided at an energy of 2 W [5, 6].

Root canal disinfection it is the introduction of the diode laser optic fiber in the canal that is executed at 3 to 4 mm short of the apex and is slowly removed. It is a highly efficient method in canal sterilization.

Oral Submucous Fibrosis Treatment Lasers are famous for multiple maxillofacial and oral techniques. The inflammation and fibrosis of tissues eventually result in the mouth's restricted opening being an oral submucous fibrosis indicator (Fig. 27.2, laser in oral submucous fibrosis). The blood can make the surgical excisions of the fibrotic bands slightly challenging due to the restricted visibility and accessibility [3–7].

Cutting Fibrotic Bands The energy range of 4–5 W makes the 980 nm diode laser an excellent instrument for cutting fibrotic bands. Hemostasis is instantly accomplished throughout the operation, due to which the diode laser solves the problem of visibility.

Periodontal Therapy To disinfect periodontal pockets, the 980 nm diode is utilized. The tip is introduced at the periodontal to maintain a 1 mm gap from below, which is equidistant to the tooth's long axis to be operated. To effect the expulsion of junctional epithelium and the formation of a clot, quick vertical and horizontal motions are mandatory (Fig. 27.3).

Identifying Caries To locate caries at occlusal fissures/tears, the diode laser fluorescence is regarded as the appropriate procedure.

Aphthous Ulcer Treatment In this procedure, the tip is positioned 5 mm away from the wound, and an aphthous wound is exposed to an energy of 1.5 W (low-level laser beam) that leads to the absorption of the laser beam (photons) by the chromophores, defined as "photobiomodulation." The cure and reduction in pain are accelerated by this methodology (Fig. 27.4) [5, 7, 8].

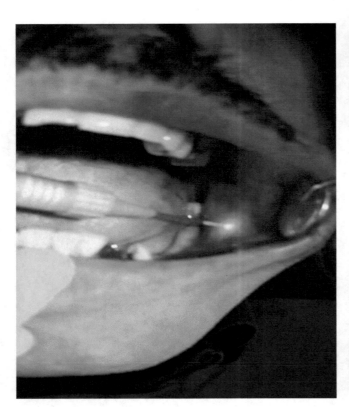

Fig. 27.2 Diode laser

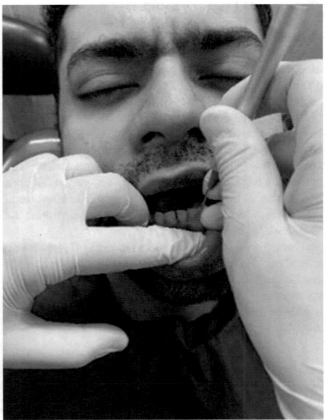

Fig. 27.3 Diode laser for periodontal pocket disinfection

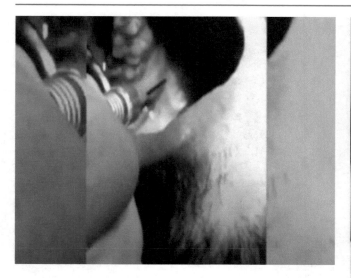

Fig. 27.4 Biomodulation using diode laser

Vestibuloplasty It is defined as the improvement of the mucous and gingiva membrane correlation. The "sulcus deepening surgery" is another common term. The injury can be cured, and the possibility of the occurrence of a mark can be lessened by exposing energy of 1.5 W of the 980 nm diode.

Mucocele Expulsion A usual bruise precedes the irritational fibroma in the oral cavity defined as the "mucocele." It is mostly visible at the lower lip, and a constant emission of 1.5 W (energy) of the diode laser can be utilized to eliminate the mucocele.

Gingivectomy An excessive protrusion of the gingiva mostly occurs due to bad oral hygiene and bacteria or due to drug use. The 980 nm diode laser is implemented, resembling a sequence of a brush from the distal to the mesial pathway. The potency of the laser can be gradually altered in the range of 1–1.5 W. The pain after the surgery is minimal, and sutures are unnecessary (Fig. 27.5).

Using Diode Laser

Frenectomy The diode laser expels the large frenum attachment by the contact method. The recovery is quicker than the standard procedure, and sutures are unnecessary following the operation.

Hypersensitivity The diode laser tip in zero contact mode at an energy of 1.5 W in the altering and liquefying of the

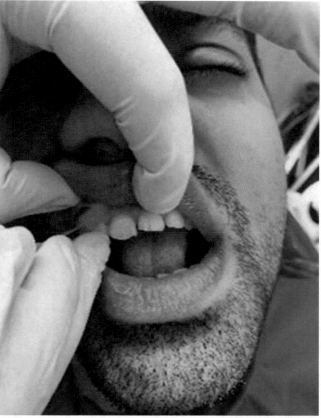

Fig. 27.5 Gingivectomy

dentinal tubules to curb dentinal hypersensitivity [9, 10] (Fig. 27.6).

Crown Extension At an energy of 2 W, the tip of the laser in the contact method can be carried out to raise the height of the abutment crown while the denture operation is partly mended and ongoing.

CO2 Laser It is the surgical CO_2 soft tissue laser in the field of dentistry. A constant gated-pulse technique radiates it. The zero-contact method is implemented for the clotting of tiny blood vessels and tissue ablation *(Lumenis CO2 Laser, 2018)* (Fig. 27.7).

Argon Laser The argon laser is highly absorbed by tissues, melanin, and red pigments with high hemoglobin. The laser delivers great outcomes in clotting and homeostasis. It can be implemented for tissue welding (arterial welding), gingivoplasty, and gingivectomy. At 90–100 °C, the increase in tissue temperature causes the blood vessels to clot.

Lip Reduction Surgery 1:16 is considered the perfect lip ratio. For symmetry, both the lips are narrowed. The opera-

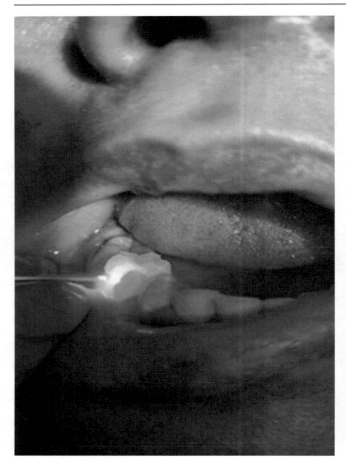

Fig. 27.6 Dentinal hypersensitivity treatment using diode laser

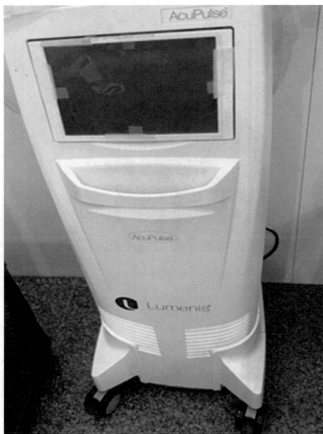

Fig. 27.7 CO2 laser

tion does not involve blood due to the CO2 laser, and the thinning of the lips is implemented by local anesthesia. The stitches are taken off in a week, and the laser diminishes the downtime. It is also utilized for excisional biopsy, frenectomy, and oral fibroma on buccal mucosa (Fig. 27.8). *Lip Reduction using CO2 Laser*

Oral Leukoplakia When utilizing the CO2 laser, precancerous oral bruises can be cured by presenting multiple benefits like minimal post-surgery homeostasis and issues and accurate expulsion. CO2 laser can be implemented to ablate the cut by lessening the post-surgery inflammation and dysfunction. The secondary intention results in recovery (Fig. 27.9) [3, 5, 8].

Benefits of CO2 Laser

The benefits are absence of suture, minimal swelling, minimal marks, and minimal pain due to thickening/clotting of external endings.

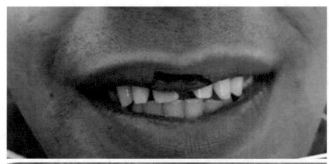
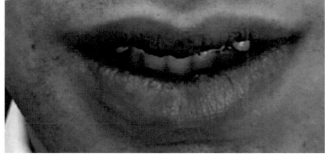

Fig. 27.8 Lip reduction surgery

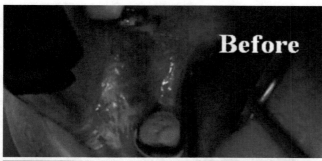

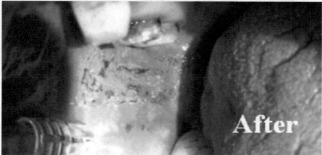

Fig. 27.9 Oral leukoplakia treatment

Er:YAG Laser

This hard tissue laser has a remarkable absorption rate in apatite crystals and water. The Er:YAG laser delivers a small thermal variation at the dentinal level and can be utilized to expel carious and contaminated dentin.

The Er:YAG Laser Is Mainly Utilized In

Enamel hypoplasia, setting up of cavity, elimination of bone in impaction cases, expulsion of caries, osteotomy, and apicoectomy. Mercury vapors are emitted if the Er:YAG laser is carried out to expel amalgam fillings and ceramic fillings. Hence, it is avoided.

Nd:YAG Laser

This laser (soft tissue) has the properties of tissue vaporization and clotting.

It is utilized for frenectomy, thickening of large vascular gashes, gingivectomy, and excision in the tongue's rear portion, which is a sensitive region. There is a higher inflamma-

tion than the CO_2 laser, being the only shortcoming of the Nd:YAG laser [8–10].

Conclusion

	Laser	Conventional operation
Recovery	Fast	Slow
Operation	Slightly complex	More trouble-free
Anesthesia	Mild Or unnecessary	Mandatory
Duration	Minimal duration	Long-lasting
Post-surgery complication	Negligible	High
Suture	Unnecessary	Needed in invasive operations
Bleeding	Absent or negligible	Mandatory

References

1. Strauss RA, Coleman M. Lasers in major oral and maxillofacial surgery. In: Convissar RA, editor. Principles and practice of laser dentistry. New york: Mosby; 2011.
2. Lanzafame RJ, Rogers DW, Naim JO, et al. The effect of CO_2 laser excision on local tumor recurrence. Lasers Surg Med. 1986;6(2):103–5.
3. Lanzafame RJ, Rogers DW, Naim JO, et al. Reduction of local tumor recurrence by excision with the CO_2 laser. Lasers Surg Med. 1986;6(5):439–41.
4. Gatone GA, Alling AC. Laser applications in oral and maxillofacial surgery. Philadelphia: Saunders; 1997.
5. Shafer G, Hine M, Barnet L. Textbook of oral pathology. Elsevier. 6th ed. p. 917.
6. Horch HH, Gerlach KL, Schaefer HE, et al. Erfahrungenmit der LaserbehandlungoberflachlicherMundschleimhauterkrankungen. Dtsch Z Mund-Keifer-Gesichts-Chir. 1983;7:31–5.
7. Sachs SA, Borden GE. The utilization of carbon dioxide laser in the treatment of recurrent papillomatosis: report of a case. J Oral Surg. 1981;39:299.
8. De Souza TO, Martins MA, Bussadori SK, Fernandes KP, Tanji EY, Mesquita-Ferrari RA, Martins MD. Clinical evaluation of low-level laser treatment for recurring aphthous stomatitis. Photomed laser Surg. 2010;28 Suppl 2:S85–8.
9. Bladowski M, Konarska-Choroszucha H, Choroszucha T. Comparison of treatment results of recurrent aphthous stomatitis (RAS) with low-and high-power laser irradiation vs. pharmaceutical method (5-year study). J Oral Laser Appl. 2004;4:191–209. Photomed Laser Surg. 2010;28 Suppl 2:S85–8.
10. Apfelberg DB, Master MR, Lash H, et al. CO_2 laser resection for giant perineal condyloma and verrucous carcinoma. Ann Plast Surg. 1983;11(5):417–22.

Vertical Ridge Augmentation by Titanium Mesh

Farhad Zeynalzadeh and Amir Zahedpasha

Introduction

The presence of sufficient alveolar bone volume is one of the principal prerequisites for implant treatment [2, 5, 6]. Prosthetic-driven implantology requires planning patient rehabilitation in advance, designing the optimal patient's functional and esthetic rehabilitation, and determining where implants will be placed [1, 3, 4]. Early tooth loss, hormonal changes, and increased age are some of the factors contributing to bone resorption, which impairs or even prevents the installation of the osseointegrated dental implant. Several augmentation techniques have been proposed, even in cases with limited bone support and inadequate nourishment. For situations where the ridge height is marginal (i.e., < 10 mm or so), it is often possible to manage osteotomy preparation complications such as bone fenestrations or dehiscence with various graft and barrier materials. In severe cases, however, it becomes necessary to prepare the deficient ridge, and splitting osteotomy [7], distraction osteogenesis [8, 9], guided bone regeneration with resorbable [10] and non-resorbable membranes [11] or Ti mesh [12], and onlay block grafts taken from intraoral or extraoral sites [13] are the most commonly applied methods.

By applying different graft materials in the past, vertical bone augmentation could possibly be done. Some researches have revealed combined risks along with harvesting procedures, potential complications, and intra- or extraoral donor site morbidity [14] despite using autogenous bone as the gold standard augmentation material worldwide [15–17].

The majority of the latest guided bone regeneration surveys emphasized augmentation procedures by applying bone substitution materials of allogenic [18], xenogenic [15, 19, 20], and alloplastic origin [21] due to existing obstacles. Allogeneic bone is widely accessible and has safe application. It relies on impressive donor screening and suitable tissue banking. Theoretically, infinite availability and an optimal alternative scaffold representation have been shown by xenographs since the three-dimensional structure and mineral component composition were taken into consideration. Among mammals, bone tissue does not have a remarkable difference [15]. Recombinant human bone morphogenetic protein-2 (rhBMP-2) and recombinant human platelet-derived growth factor (rhPDGF) are known as growth factor products that are used to enrich tissue regeneration [22–25]. Platelet-rich plasma (PRP) is a combination product that shows progenitor cell employment with highly concentrated bioactive proteins and has led to positive regeneration outcomes [26, 27]. Lack of structural integrity is one of the drawbacks of particulate graft usage. Soft tissue decomposition leads to graft compression or displacement as well as not reaching the desired consequences when there is no containment system [28]. There is a proposed technique to augment bones called guided bone regeneration. A barrier membrane is applied for space creation and maintenance, so we can use titanium-reinforced expanded/nonexpanded polytetrafluoroethylene (ePTFE/PTFE) membrane plus VRA (vertical ridge augmentation). It can be seen that subsequent fraction in a membrane along with its exposure is considered the main obstacle for ePTFE/PTFE material because nothing can penetrate inside [29–32].

Recently, titanium mesh has received growing attention for the reports that document predictable and consistent results in this material. Several benefits of the use of titanium mesh have been suggested. Non-resorbable membranes must be removed if flap dehiscence and exposure occur to prevent infection because exposure in these cases would not heal spontaneously. Conversely, titanium mesh did not appear to affect the final outcome. Titanium mesh provides superior space maintenance, a fundamental prerequisite for any bone regeneration procedure. Furthermore, the titanium mesh

F. Zeynalzadeh (✉)
Department of Oral and Maxillofacial Surgery, Faculty of Dentistry-Medical Sciences University, Mashhad, Iran
e-mail: Zeynalzadehf961@mums.ac.ir

A. Zahedpasha
Department of Oral and Maxillofacial Surgery, Faculty of Dentistry-Medical Sciences University, Babol, Iran

pores are thought to play a critical role in maintaining blood supply to a grafted defect. They provide a thorough tenting effect, thanks to their rigidity, and, being moldable, can be easily given the shape needed to cover the defect under treatment. Moreover, they maintain their shape over time. Yet, they must be removed, not resorbable, and require time-consuming shaping that is ordinarily performed after flap elevation to test the best of the mesh on the defect. This increases both the surgical time and the risk of complications for the patient. Titanium meshes have been used in conjunction with graft materials providing a more efficient scaffold than the blood clot to support cells and vessels.

We use titanium (Ti) mesh vastly in oral and maxillofacial surgery to reconstruct large and small defects. Titanium mesh was first documented successfully by Boyne for the repair of continuity defects in the mandible [33].

For large osseous maxillofacial defect restoration and osseous restoration of deficient edentulous maxillary and mandible ridges, Ti meshes were proposed for the first time [34, 35]. TIME technique was reintroduced by Von Arx et al. for applying Ti meshes. This technique possesses micro-titanium augmentation mesh particularly designed for ridge defect augmentation [36, 37].

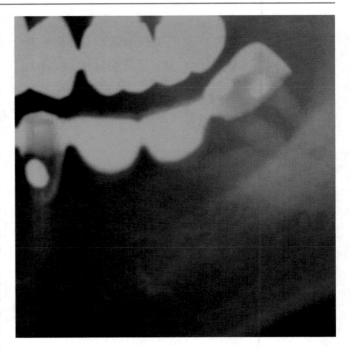

Fig. 28.1 Panoramic view radiography taken before removal of tooth 38 and adjacent crowns

Biochemical Characteristics of Ti Mesh

Ti-based alloys and pure titanium (Ti) are applied in different medical applications as they have excellent biocompatibility, corrosion resistance, and noticeable mechanical performance [38–41]. Topography microstructure and wettability of Ti mesh surface have significant roles in improving in vivo osseointegration: the features of Ti implants surface as the traits of topography and microstructure that persuade the changes of surface wettability which the absorbed proteins degree in blood as well as the growth factor [42]. Stress distribution and peak Von Mises stress of titanium mesh implants declined dramatically at 1 mm thickness. The Ti mesh implant created a relatively lower Von Mises stress on the bone defect spot; it does not have the structure of a triangular bone plus as square one. Two-thirds of space beneath the titanium mesh consists of a bone-like tissue, as histologic tests have shown [43].

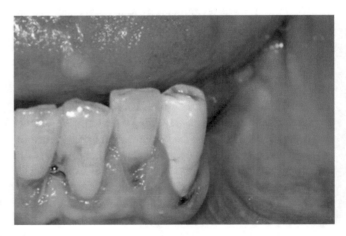

Fig. 28.2 Preoperative photography of mandibular ridge segment in facial view

Surgical Procedure

Radiographic evaluations were performed to assess the precise dimensions of the alveolar process. Nowadays, CT scans and CBCT scans are the best tools for measuring bone dimensions (Figs. 28.1 and 28.2). The surgical procedures are performed in an operating room with strict aseptic conditions, under local anesthesia with/without intravenous seda-

tion, except for severe atrophic ridges. After local infiltration anesthesia, like lidocaine or mepivacaine chlorhydrate, a mid-crestal horizontal incision was made to maximize the keratinized mucosa on each side of the incision, with oblique releasing incisions where needed, in order to mobilize a full-thickness flap (Fig. 28.3). The flap was carefully elevated from the palatal/lingual and buccal aspect of the alveolar ridge, isolating the neurovascular bundle in order to preserve these vessels. All fibrous tissue is removed, and perforations into the marrow space were made using small round surgical burs to improve bleeding and graft incorporation (Fig. 28.4).

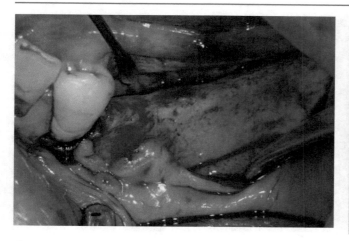

Fig. 28.3 Full-thickness mucoperiosteal flap reflection exposing severe deficiency

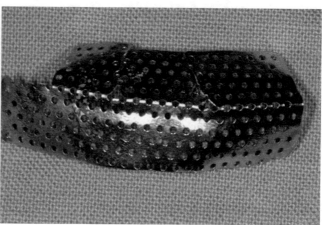

Fig. 28.5 Customized and trimmed titanium mesh to the desired shape of the future alveolar ridge

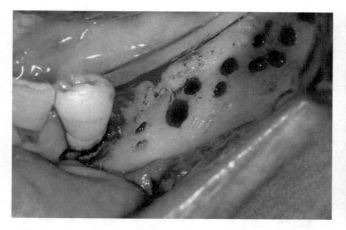

Fig. 28.4 Decortication to perforate cortical plate and expose bone marrow

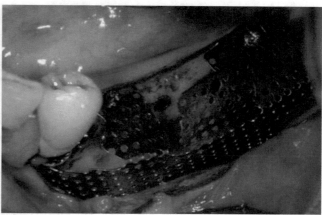

Fig. 28.6 Filling defect and titanium mesh with bone material before mesh placement

The bone graft was particulated using a bone miller. A titanium mesh is then customized to the future alveolar ridge's desired shape and adjusted to maintain and protect the bone graft (Fig. 28.5). Adaptation of the titanium mesh during surgery created a defined space between the mesh and the decorticated area that mimicked the desired ridge's shape. When the stereolithographic model was available, the mesh was shaped and adjusted on it before surgery. The particulate bone graft is positioned at the recipient site and in Ti mesh, and the mesh was fixed in position with two or more titanium microscrews (Figs. 28.6 and 28.7). A collagen membrane is often placed over the mesh to thicken the tissue and prevent the mesh's exposure. With sufficient saline irrigation for a clean surgical field, split-thickness periosteal releasing incisions are also completed, when possible, to aid in primary

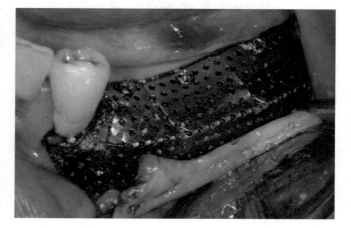

Fig. 28.7 Titanium mesh fixation with miniscrews

tension-free closure. Horizontal mattress sutures were used to obtain tension-free closure.

Postoperatively, the patients were recommended to apply ice packs onto the treated area and keep them in place for at least 4 h. Antibiotics and analgesics are prescribed three times daily for 7 days. The patient is instructed to rinse with chlorhexidine 0.12% twice daily for 2 weeks. Patients were also advised not to brush their tooth and to avoid trauma in the site of surgery for 3 weeks. Sutures are removed 10 days after surgery. After 4–6 months, the site was re-entered with a reflection of the full-thickness flap, and titanium mesh was removed. Newly formed bone is ready for implant insertion (Figs. 28.8, 28.9, and 28.10).

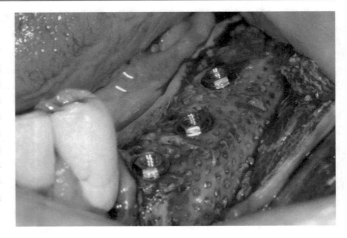

Fig. 28.10 Implant placement into regenerated site at 35, 36, and 37 positions

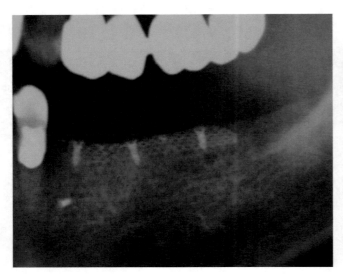

FIG. 28.8 Postoperative panoramic view radiography

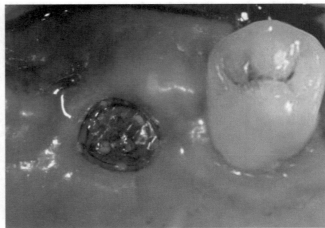

Fig. 28.11 Titanium mesh exposure (circular shape)

In a previous study, by clinical evaluation, the mean of vertical regeneration was 4.91 mm (range 2.26–8.6). The mean is between 20 and 40%, along with the mesh exposure rate (Fig. 28.11). The success rate of mean among implants in augmented ridge is 89.9%. The mean of survival rate is 100% and the failure rate 0%, which can be seen from measuring data [3, 44, 45].

Complications

In previous research, Ti mesh exposure, particularly if early exposure occurs, was reported for the major surgical complication, 20 to 40%. Early titanium mesh exposure does not fail the graft. The amount of keratinized mucosa, flap thick-

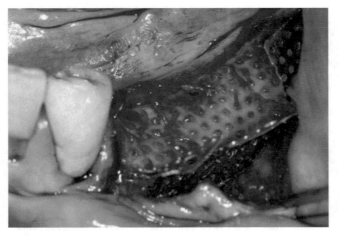

Fig. 28.9 Removing titanium mesh after healing

ness and features, which essentially help to promote primary wound closure are basic factors to have acceptable mucosa. Crestal exposure factors of titanium mesh include incision placement; incision breakdown; lack of blood supply; excessive vertical augmentation; compromised wound bed, especially the soft tissues; distance of angiogenesis; masticatory function abrasion; exposure by sharp edges on the mesh surface of titanium; infection; and loosening titanium device, These are potential reasons.

The incision design incidence of wound breakdown will be declined, consisting of vestibular, crestal, or tunneling approaches. Crestal incision is the most convenient way of performing, but the vestibular incision is located on the thicker part of the tissue where periosteum is not essential to be released for primary closure achievement.

Deep sutures following a mucosal layer can close the wound. Titanium mesh placement technique cannot be done by tunneling approach in spite of having advantages unless this would be used in small defects. It is vital to have wide flap dissection for crestal incision to close the periosteum and mucosa over the crestal wound margin.

By lack of periosteal integrity, the decomposition of mucosa immediately contributes to hardware exposure. Pores make the nutrition and metabolic exchange process easy, so mucosal dehiscence as a risk of complications can disappear compared to titanium-reinforced non-resorbable membranes (ePTFE) [4, 46]. Titanium mesh exposure could be closer to graft resorption with the rate of 15 to 20%; fortunately, it does not interfere with implant placement or any important complicated tasks [31]. Chlorhexidine rinses are the main management of the exposure, using 0.12% chlorhexidine and plaque removal locally in the first stage, and second wound healing will cover the mesh. When there is no obvious infection, the time of mesh removal will be postponed, and the procedures are going according to plan. Total bone resorption with early mesh exposure and infection and partial bone resorption with minor resorption are reported in previous articles at 4.8% and 10%, respectively.

Another postoperative discomfort included swelling, ecchymosis, and pain for the first week and did not require specific additional treatment.

A New Generation of Ti Mesh: Ultraflex Mesh Plate

Ultraflex mesh plate is the next generation of titanium mesh with a Margaret-flower structure (Fig. 28.12). The Margaret-flower structure is flexible with shape and contour, so no cutting or trimming is needed to form the alveolar ridges desirably. This is excellent potential in mesh plate for next generation to prepare the alveolar ridge's desired contour [47].

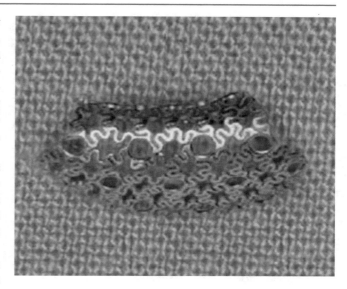

Fig. 28.12 Ultraflex mesh plate

Conclusion

Several augmentation techniques have been proposed, even in cases with limited bone support and inadequate nourishment. Recently, titanium mesh has received growing attention for the reports that document predictable and consistent results in this material. Several benefits of the use of titanium mesh have been suggested. Non-resorbable membranes must be removed if flap dehiscence and exposure occur to prevent infection because exposure in these cases would not heal spontaneously. Conversely, titanium mesh did not appear to affect the outcome. The mean of vertical regeneration was 4.91 mm (range 2.26–8.6). The mean is between 20 and 40%, along with the mesh exposure rate, with a success rate of implant placement and survival rate at 89.9% and 100%, respectively. Titanium mesh provides superior space maintenance, a fundamental prerequisite for any bone regeneration procedure. Furthermore, the titanium mesh pores are thought to play a critical role in maintaining blood supply to a grafted defect. They provide a thorough tenting effect, thanks to their rigidity, and, being moldable, can be easily given the shape needed to cover the defect under treatment.

References

1. Casap N, Rushinek H, Jensen OT. Vertical alveolar augmentation using BMP-2/ACS/allograft with printed titanium shells to establish an early vascular scaffold. Oral Maxillofac Surg Clin North Am. 2019;31(3):473–87.
2. Rocchietta I, Fontana F, Simion M. Clinical outcomes of vertical bone augmentation to enable dental implant placement: a systematic review. J Clin Periodontol. 2008;35(8 Suppl):203–15.

3. Rasia-dal Polo M, Poli PP, Rancitelli D, Beretta M, Maiorana C. Alveolar ridge reconstruction with titanium meshes: a systematic review of the literature. Med Oral Patol Oral Cir Bucal. 2014;19(6):e639–46.

4. Louis PJ, Gutta R, Said-Al-Naief N, Bartolucci AA. Reconstruction of the maxilla and mandible with particulate bone graft and titanium mesh for implant placement. J Oral Maxillofac Surg. 2008;66(2):235–45.

5. Roccuzzo M, Ramieri G, Bunino M, Berrone S. Autogenous bone graft alone or associated with titanium mesh for vertical alveolar ridge augmentation: a controlled clinical trial. Clin Oral Implants Res. 2007;18(3):286–94.

6. Bai L, Ji P, Li X, Gao H, Li L, Wang C. Mechanical characterization of 3D-printed individualized ti-mesh (membrane) for alveolar bone defects. J Healthc Eng. 2019;2019:4231872.

7. Engelke WG, Diederichs CG, Jacobs HG, Deckwer I. Alveolar reconstruction with splitting osteotomy and microfixation of implants. Int J Oral Maxillofac Implants. 1997;12(3):310–8.

8. Jensen OT, Cockrell R, Kuhike L, Reed C. Anterior maxillary alveolar distraction osteogenesis: a prospective 5-year clinical study. Int J Oral Maxillofac Implants. 2002;17(1):52–68.

9. Uckan S, Dolanmaz D, Kalayci A, Cilasun U. Distraction osteogenesis of basal mandibular bone for reconstruction of the alveolar ridge. Br J Oral Maxillofac Surg. 2002;40(5):393–6.

10. Brunel G, Brocard D, Duffort JF, Jacquet E, Justumus P, Simonet T, et al. Bioabsorbable materials for guided bone regeneration prior to implant placement and 7-year follow-up: report of 14 cases. J Periodontol. 2001;72(2):257–64.

11. Simion M, Jovanovic SA, Tinti C, Benfenati SP. Long-term evaluation of osseointegrated implants inserted at the time or after vertical ridge augmentation. A retrospective study on 123 implants with 1-5 year follow-up. Clin Oral Implants Res. 2001;12(1):35–45.

12. Buser D, Dula K, Hirt HP, Schenk RK. Lateral ridge augmentation using autografts and barrier membranes: a clinical study with 40 partially edentulous patients. J Oral Maxillofac Surg. 1996;54(4):420–32. discussion 32-3

13. Schwartz-Arad D, Levin L. Intraoral autogenous block onlay bone grafting for extensive reconstruction of atrophic maxillary alveolar ridges. J Periodontol. 2005;76(4):636–41.

14. Kumar P, Vinitha B, Fathima G. Bone grafts in dentistry. J Pharm Bioallied Sci. 2013;5(Suppl 1):S125–7.

15. Pistilli R, Felice P, Piatelli M, Nisii A, Barausse C, Esposito M. Blocks of autogenous bone versus xenografts for the rehabilitation of atrophic jaws with dental implants: preliminary data from a pilot randomised controlled trial. Eur J Oral Implantol. 2014;7(2):153–71.

16. Sbordone L, Toti P, Menchini-Fabris GB, Sbordone C, Piombino P, Guidetti F. Volume changes of autogenous bone grafts after alveolar ridge augmentation of atrophic maxillae and mandibles. Int J Oral Maxillofac Surg. 2009;38(10):1059–65.

17. Misch CM. Comparison of intraoral donor sites for onlay grafting prior to implant placement. Int J Oral Maxillofac Implants. 1997;12(6):767–76.

18. Spin-Neto R, Stavropoulos A, Coletti FL, Faeda RS, Pereira LA, Marcantonio E Jr. Graft incorporation and implant osseointegration following the use of autologous and fresh-frozen allogeneic block bone grafts for lateral ridge augmentation. Clin Oral Implants Res. 2014;25(2):226–33.

19. Li J, Xuan F, Choi BH, Jeong SM. Minimally invasive ridge augmentation using xenogenous bone blocks in an atrophied posterior mandible: a clinical and histological study. Implant Dent. 2013;22(2):112–6.

20. Barone A, Aldini NN, Fini M, Giardino R, Calvo Guirado JL, Covani U. Xenograft versus extraction alone for ridge preservation after tooth removal: a clinical and histomorphometric study. J Periodontol. 2008;79(8):1370–7.

21. Chiapasco M, Casentini P, Zaniboni M. Bone augmentation procedures in implant dentistry. Int J Oral Maxillofac Implants. 2009;24(Suppl):237–59.

22. Maroo S, Murthy KR. Treatment of periodontal intrabony defects using beta-TCP alone or in combination with rhPDGF-BB: a randomized controlled clinical and radiographic study. Int J Periodontics Restorative Dent. 2014;34(6):841–7.

23. Simion M, Nevins M, Rocchietta I, Fontana F, Maschera E, Schupbach P, et al. Vertical ridge augmentation using an equine block infused with recombinant human platelet-derived growth factor-BB: a histologic study in a canine model. Int J Periodontics Restorative Dent. 2009;29(3):245–55.

24. Froum SJ, Wallace S, Cho SC, Khouly I, Rosenberg E, Corby P, et al. Radiographic comparison of different concentrations of recombinant human bone morphogenetic protein with allogenic bone compared with the use of 100% mineralized cancellous bone allograft in maxillary sinus grafting. Int J Periodontics Restorative Dent. 2014;34(5):611–20.

25. Edmunds RK, Mealey BL, Mills MP, Thoma DS, Schoolfield J, Cochran DL, et al. Maxillary anterior ridge augmentation with recombinant human bone morphogenetic protein 2. Int J Periodontics Restorative Dent. 2014;34(4):551–7.

26. Torres J, Tamimi F, Alkhraisat MH, Manchon A, Linares R, Prados-Frutos JC, et al. Platelet-rich plasma may prevent titanium-mesh exposure in alveolar ridge augmentation with anorganic bovine bone. J Clin Periodontol. 2010;37(10):943–51.

27. Agarwal A, Gupta ND. Platelet-rich plasma combined with decalcified freeze-dried bone allograft for the treatment of non-contained human intrabony periodontal defects: a randomized controlled split-mouth study. Int J Periodontics Restorative Dent. 2014;34(5):705–11.

28. Donos N, Kostopoulos L, Karring T. Alveolar ridge augmentation using a resorbable copolymer membrane and autogenous bone grafts. An experimental study in the rat. Clin Oral Implants Res. 2002;13(2):203–13.

29. Artzi Z, Dayan D, Alpern Y, Nemcovsky CE. Vertical ridge augmentation using xenogenic material supported by a configured titanium mesh: clinicohistopathologic and histochemical study. Int J Oral Maxillofac Implants. 2003;18(3):440–6.

30. Proussaefs P, Lozada J, Kleinman A, Rohrer MD, McMillan PJ. The use of titanium mesh in conjunction with autogenous bone graft and inorganic bovine bone mineral (bio-Oss) for localized alveolar ridge augmentation: a human study. Int J Periodontics Restorative Dent. 2003;23(2):185–95.

31. Roccuzzo M, Ramieri G, Spada MC, Bianchi SD, Berrone S. Vertical alveolar ridge augmentation by means of a titanium mesh and autogenous bone grafts. Clin Oral Implants Res. 2004;15(1):73–81.

32. Miura K, Matsui K, Kawai T, Kato Y, Matsui A, Suzuki O, et al. Octacalcium phosphate collagen composites with titanium mesh facilitate alveolar augmentation in canine mandibular bone defects. Int J Oral Maxillofac Surg. 2012;41(9):1161–9.

33. Haggerty CJ, Vogel CT, Fisher GR. Simple bone augmentation for alveolar ridge defects. Oral Maxillofac Surg Clin North Am. 2015;27(2):203–26.

34. Boyne PJ. Restoration of osseous defects in maxillofacial casualties. J Am Dent Assoc. 1969;78(4):767–76.

35. Boyne PJ, Cole MD, Stringer D, Shafqat JP. A technique for osseous restoration of deficient edentulous maxillary ridges. J Oral Maxillofac Surg. 1985;43(2):87–91.

36. von Arx T, Hardt N, Wallkamm B. The TIME technique: a new method for localized alveolar ridge augmentation prior to placement of dental implants. Int J Oral Maxillofac Implants. 1996;11(3):387–94.

37. von Arx T, Wallkamm B, Hardt N. Localized ridge augmentation using a micro titanium mesh: a report on 27 implants followed

from 1 to 3 years after functional loading. Clin Oral Implants Res. 1998;9(2):123–30.

38. Yu S, Guo D, Han J, Sun L, Zhu H, Yu Z, et al. Enhancing antibacterial performance and biocompatibility of pure titanium by a two-step electrochemical surface coating. ACS Appl Mater Interfaces. 2020;12(40):44433–46.

39. Nakagawa M, Matsuya S, Shiraishi T, Ohta M. Effect of fluoride concentration and pH on corrosion behavior of titanium for dental use. J Dent Res. 1999;78(9):1568–72.

40. Gittens RA, Olivares-Navarrete R, Tannenbaum R, Boyan BD, Schwartz Z. Electrical implications of corrosion for osseointegration of titanium implants. J Dent Res. 2011;90(12):1389–97.

41. Peng P-W, Ou K-L, Chao C-Y, Pan Y-N, Wang C-H. Research of microstructure and mechanical behavior on duplex (α+β) ti–4.8Al–2.5Mo–1.4V alloy. J Alloys Compd. 2010;490(1):661–6.

42. Shih Y-H, Lin C-T, Liu C-M, Chen C-C, Chen C-S, Ou K-L. Effect of nano-titanium hydride on formation of multi-nanoporous TiO2 film on ti. Appl Surf Sci. 2007;253(7):3678–82.

43. Huang MT, Juan PK, Chen SY, Wu CJ, Wen SC, Cho YC, et al. The potential of the three-dimensional printed titanium mesh implant for cranioplasty surgery applications: biomechanical behaviors and surface properties. Mater Sci Eng C Mater Biol Appl. 2019;97:412–9.

44. Deshpande S, Deshmukh J, Deshpande S, Khatri R, Deshpande S. Vertical and horizontal ridge augmentation in anterior maxilla using autograft, xenograft and titanium mesh with simultaneous placement of endosseous implants. J Indian Soc Periodontol. 2014;18(5):661–5.

45. McAllister BS, Haghighat K. Bone augmentation techniques. J Periodontol. 2007;78(3):377–96.

46. Gutta R, Baker RA, Bartolucci AA, Louis PJ. Barrier membranes used for ridge augmentation: is there an optimal pore size? J Oral Maxillofac Surg. 2009;67(6):1218–25.

47. Takahashi T, Yamauchi K. Vertical Augmentation of the Alveolar Ridge with Titanium-Reinforced Devices (Protected Bone Regeneration). 2016. p. 93–109.

Computer-Guided Implant Dentistry

29

Theodoros Tasopoulos, Pindaros-Georgios Foskolos, George Kouveliotis, and Ioannis Karoussis

Introduction

Since its early days, implantology was related to innovative knowledge of biology and technology, and as a result, the need for continuous research and development of clinical techniques placed this field in a knife-edge dental environment. Premature implant surgical and prosthetic protocols were based on primary stability and long-term osseointegration, as described by Branemark. The prosthetic rehabilitation was adapted to the above requirements [1, 2]. However, the establishment of biological principles of implantology led to various clinical options regarding soft tissue plastic surgery and grafting. Major technological developments in three-dimensional diagnostic imaging methods improved the protocol of high-standard implant treatment planning and implant positioning in terms of topography; relation to important anatomical structures such as nerves, vessels, roots, nasal floor, and sinus cavity; as well as clinically relevant pathology [3, 4]. Moreover, the introduction of surface optical scannings such as intraoral scanners and computer-aided design (CAD) and computer-aided manufacturing (CAM) technologies allow a more precise diagnosis, accurate preoperative planning, and a planned treatment outcome.

At that time, researchers realised that besides functionality, emphasis should be put on esthetics, especially on restoring partial edentulism. Treatment planning should be directed by the anticipated restoration rather than the surgery and the definite prostheses and vice versa. Initial articulation, diagnostic wax-up, and construction of radiographic guide, which is converted into a surgical guide, are the typical workflow of conventional implant restorations. The main purpose of such an interdisciplinary approach in implant dentistry is related to the thesis that screw-retained restorations are preferable than cement-retained, regarding retrievability and protection of peri-implant diseases, due to lack of cement excess to peri-implant soft tissue.

The progress of digital technologies made a breakthrough in contemporary implantology. Finest dental imaging and novel software led to laboratory scanners' appearance and then intraoral scanners. These innovations enable clinicians to have a firm and detailed treatment planning concerning precision in implant placement. Subtractive (milling) or additive (3D printing) methods offer a viable alternative to conventional techniques for the fabrication of surgical templates, implant-supported prosthetic components, and custom-made bone grafts.

A fully digital workflow concept is applied to patient in dental implantology as represented in Fig. 29.1. It consists of data file acquisition obtained with optical surface scans (STL files) and CBCT (DICOM files), being merged with the digital design software (CAD design). Within the software, the implant positions are planned virtually, guided by the desired prosthetic design. The next step includes the digital fabrication and the 3D print of the surgical splint to assist implant placement.

T. Tasopoulos (✉)
School of Dentistry, National and Kapodistrian University of Athens, Athens, Greece

Department of Prosthodontics, National and Kapodistrian University of Athens, Athens, Greece
e-mail: tasopoulost@gmail.com

P.-G. Foskolos
Department of Prosthodontics, National and Kapodistrian University of Athens, Athens, Greece
e-mail: pindaros@uic.es

G. Kouveliotis
Department of Prosthodontics, National and Kapodistrian University of Athens, Athens, Greece

Department of Oral and Maxillofacial Surgery, International University of Catalonia, Barcelona, Spain
e-mail: gkouveliotis@gmail.com

I. Karoussis
Department of Prosthodontics, National and Kapodistrian University of Athens, Athens, Greece
e-mail: ikaroussis@dent.uoa.gr

M. R. Stevens et al. (eds.), *Innovative Perspectives in Oral and Maxillofacial Surgery*,
https://doi.org/10.1007/978-3-030-75750-2_29

Fig. 29.1 Digital workflow in dental implantology

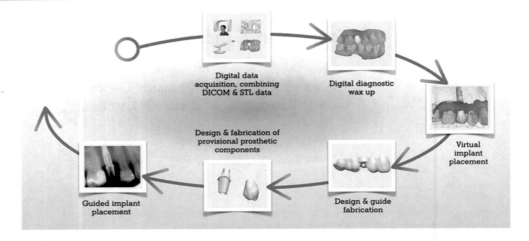

Digital Dental Imaging

CBCT/CT

New acquisition digital imaging devices, such as cone beam computed tomography (CBCT), allow the collection of patient's data and provide critical information about the diagnosis and the treatment decision [5]. Computed tomography (CT) and CBCT create 2D image slices of the patient's jaw, which are then displayed individually or stack rendering 3D radiographic imaging data. CBCT units have a lower radiation dose (92–118 μSv) than CT (860 μSv), are less expensive, and are more compact, allowing in-house use in a dental office [6].

CBCT scans produce volumetric data of the underlying bony structure and teeth, displaying tissue with high density, while soft tissue is displayed unpredictably. In the presence of metal restorations, radiographic images display artifacts. Scatter on a CBCT directly affects the scanned object's trueness and does not display the tooth structure clearly for preoperative planning [7]. Patient moving during scan acquisition may result in motion artifacts [4].

The accuracy of CBCT is critically important in order to achieve a satisfactory and precise treatment planning outcome. According to the Fifth ITI Consensus Conference, a CBCT scan's deviation is at least one voxel (0.3 mm^2). It is unlikely that this deviation would compromise the safety or efficacy of digital implant planning or computer-aided surgery [8].

Optical Non-contact Surface Scans

The digitization of the oral cavity's hard and soft tissues can be achieved via intraoral scanners (IOSs) or extraoral scanners (model scan). Data derived from these two distinct processes are available in the universal stereolithography format as an STL (surface tessellated language) file. This file describes three-dimensional objects' surface geometry, although other information such as color of the teeth and mucosa are not

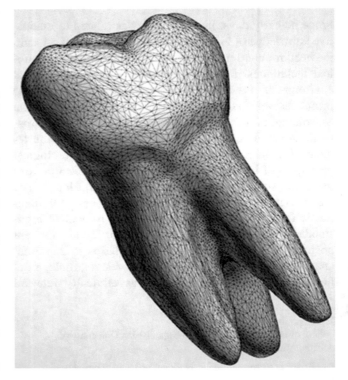

Fig. 29.2 The STL file creation links the continuous geometry of small triangles together to form the intended shape

included (Fig. 29.2). A universal format of intraoral scans containing color information is the OBJ format [9].

Intraoral scans have the advantage of generating a digital replica of the oral cavity and preview of the three-dimensional virtual model directly on the computer screen. The accuracy of the scan is defined by the trueness and precision of measurement [10].

Optical scans may also be obtained from stone casts or dental impressions. Extraoral scans perform high accuracy. Desktop laboratory scanners work with a static light-emitting/light-receiving device and project constantly lines or patterns onto the gypsum stone casts (Fig. 29.3). Two or more cameras detect the reflection and distortion of the projected light for the calculation of the surface geometry [11], [12].

Virtual Implant Planning

After data acquisition, implant planning software allows the merging of DICOM and STL files. Computer-aided implant planning is performed following a set of steps:

1. Visualization of radiographic data (segmentation)
2. Registration of radiographic and optical surface scans (merging)
3. Digital wax-up of future implant-supported restoration
4. Virtual implant positioning
5. Digital design of surgical guide for guided implant placement

Three-dimensional surface models of the bone and teeth in CBCT data are displayed using segmentation (**Step 1**). The superimposition of the radiographic image of DICOM files retrieved by the CBCT and the STL files originated from intraoral and extraoral optical scans produces a virtual 3D model of the patient that constitutes the baseline of the fully digital or partially digital workflow (Fig. 29.4). The latter might include conventional laboratory stages during the process of treatment planification. Moreover, patient's exported data can be directly 3D projected and transferred using com-

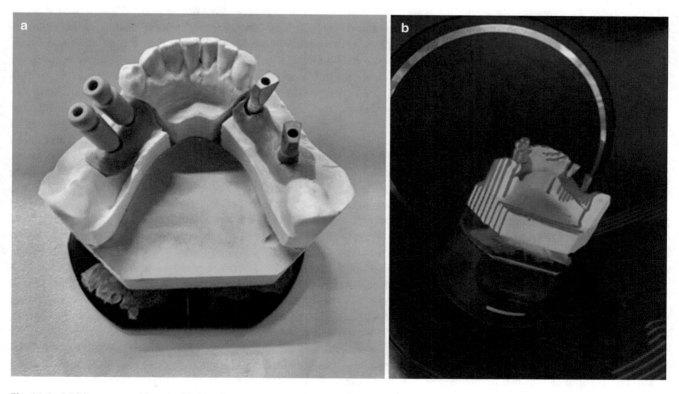

Fig. 29.3 (**a**) Master cast with embedded implant analogs, scan bodies, and gingival mask in place. (**b**) Master cast in a laboratory scanner

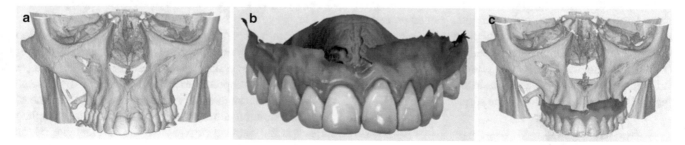

Fig. 29.4 Merging of CBCT and intraoral scan. (**a**) CBCT segmentation. (**b**) Intraoral surface scan. (**c**) Registration

puter-assisted design (CAD) software (**Step 2**). Thus, digital workflows allow team members such as dentists, patients, and dental technicians to significantly improve their communication and share information regarding treatment proposals [13]. The CAD software architecture can be either open or closed. Open software assists the clinician in working in a digital environment without being restrained to a single system. The virtual diagnostic setup can be used for the final restoration of the implant. Various virtual tools are available, including a digital library with standard tooth shapes, shaping tools, and virtual articulators to perform a functional and realistic digital diagnostic tooth wax-up (**Step 3**). When virtually planning the implant, a minimum of 1–1.5 mm of bone is required to surround the implant [14]. A minimum distance of 3 mm is required between two implants. Regarding the depth of the implant, its rough surface should be placed subcrestally. It should be of 3–4 mm depth regarding the planned cementoenamel junction [15] (**Step 4**). The surgical guide ensures accurate implant placement by transferring the planned implant position to the surgical field (**Step 5**).

Types of Surgical Guides

Guided implant surgery systems use a combination of hardware and software to facilitate the planning of implant positions.

There are different concepts proposed for digitally guided implant placement and surgery, such as "static computer-guided surgery" and "dynamic computer-navigated surgery" [16]. In the first method, a surgical template, which is designed according to the virtual 3D data of the patient, is used to transfer the virtually planned implant position on the surgical site by guiding the insertion of the drills and implants. This type of guides was fabricated through CAD/CAM technologies, such as computer numerical control (CNC) subtractive and additive methods [16, 17]. In the second concept, the intra-surgical implant placement is navigated by a computer software, displaying the real-time position of surgical instruments compared to the ideal virtually plannified positioning [18, 19]. However, some studies concerning dynamic implant navigation systems demonstrate equal accuracy with static computer-guided procedure; still it has limited indication and appliance on implant dentistry [20, 21]. Static computer-aided implant surgery (s-CAIS) includes either a guided pilot drilling approach or a fully guided protocol for the entire drilling sequence, including implant placement through the surgical guide [22].

Static Surgical Guides

The classification of surgical guides is based on the anatomical structures that provide support to them [23]:

1. Tooth-supported surgical guide: The template is positioned over teeth.
2. Mucosa-supported surgical guide: The template is positioned over mucosa.
3. Bone-supported surgical guide: The template is positioned over the bone after a mucoperiosteal flap is raised.
4. Special supported, (mini) implant, pin-supported surgical guides: the template is placed over implants that have been inserted on a previous or current surgery.

Bone-supported guides were the first templates used for the treatment of fully edentulous patients [24]. Using this type of guide, it is necessary to open a mucoperiosteal flap and extend the mobilization to access the underlying bone. This surgical process can cause great patient discomfort and possible loss of the alveolar bone crest due to limited blood supply [25]. The accuracy of tooth-supported and implant-supported templates is higher than the mucosa- and bone-supported guides [23, 26, 27]. Mucosa-supported surgical guides are usually based on the double-scan technique. This type of guide presents a statistically significant higher accuracy than the bone one, nevertheless to be executed in a flapless manner. This comes with certain prerequisites: a minimum of 4.5–5 mm of keratinized tissue and minimum bone width of 4–4.5 mm. However, a higher mucosal thickness is associated with more frequent deviation occurrence. Flapless implant placement also includes the risk of thermal damage to the bone, because of the decreased saline irrigation reaching the underlying tissues through the guide. In addition, flapless procedures are 1.75 times more likely to cause failures, and, according to Charchovic et al., this is because of the removal of the surgical guide in the last step of the surgery, which is the implant placement [28]. This is also confirmed by the meta-analysis of Zhou et al., indicating a much higher accuracy of fully guided surgery in angular, entry point, and apex deviation.

Static surgical templates can either guide the pilot drill (partially guided implant placement) or each drill in the drilling sequence (fully guided implant placement) (Fig. 29.5) [28].

Advantages of Guided Implant Dentistry

Guided implant surgery enhances the communication between dental practitioners of different specializations, dental technicians, radiologists, and patients. Therefore, a multidisciplinary approach to treatment is applied by increasing the treatment outcome's overall quality [25, 29]. One of the most common intraoperative complications in implant surgery is the damage proximal to the surgical site of the anatomical structures (inferior alveolar nerve, Schneiderian membrane of the sinus, etc.) [30–32]. Prosthodontically driven implant placement is a crucial factor for implant therapy success, decreasing patient's morbidity and possible

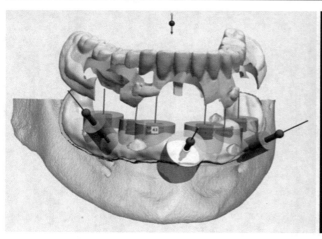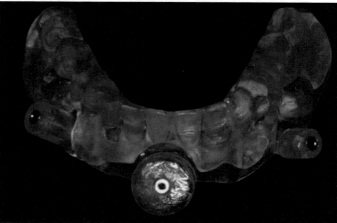

Fig. 29.5 Fully guided, full-arch dual surgical guide

biologic and prosthodontic complications, while it enhances the survival rates of the implant itself [33]. This is a less invasive technique, reducing patient discomfort, postoperative edema, bleeding, pain, and inflammation, eliminating surgical time, and accelerating the healing process [34].

Limitations and Complications of Guided Implant Dentistry

On the other hand, the digital approach presents limitations as well. All the diagnostic and treatment steps such as precision and accuracy of CBCT data, the efficacy of IOSs, surgical guides, accuracy design, and fabrication can cause implant inaccuracy. Moreover, clinicians' continuing education and experience can affect the clinical outcome. The dentist should be familiar with all the relative software/hardware and its evolution, increasing the expenses and his working time [35]. Dental offices should be equipped with new technology devices, software, and hardware that, as a result, raise the treatment cost [36].

According to Schneider et al. (2009), the frequency of early surgical complications in computer-guided implant placement is 9.1%, while prosthetic complications presented an incidence of 18.8% [37]. The most usual complications of guided implant placement protocols are fracture of the surgical template intra-surgically and early implant loss because of a lack of primary anchorage and fracture of the prosthesis [23].

Materials: Method of Production

The fabrication of the surgical guide can be cast-based, CAD/CAM-based, or printed through 3D printing technology [27, 38, 39].

1. **Cast-Based**: The surgical template is formed over a cast model in the laboratory. The most common materials of choice are auto-polymerizing acrylic resin [40–43], heat-polymerizing acrylic resin [44], and vacuum-formed thermoplastic matrix in combination with acrylic resin [45–48].
2. **CAD/CAM-Based:** The surgical template is designed digitally and milled from CAD/CAM machine.
3. **3D printing:** The surgical guide is formed by the additive manufacturing process.
   There are different systems of 3D printers. Some of the ones that use light in order to polymerize the layers of resin are [39, 49]:
   (i) Stereolithography apparatus (SLA)
   (ii) Triple jetting technology (PolyJet)
   (iii) Multijet printing (MJP)
   (iv) Digital light processing (DLP)
   (v) Continuous liquid interface production (CLIP)

The CAD/CAM milled guide seemed to present higher rates of deviation of dimensions between the virtually designed guide and the actual one. Among the 3D printing systems, the CLIP seemed to be the most accurate. However, all the systems have presented dimensional deviations that are clinically acceptable (less than 100 μm) (Fig. 29.6) [50].

Variables Affecting the Positional Accuracy of Static Computer-Aided Implant Surgery Techniques in Both Partially and Fully Edentulous Patients

The accuracy and precision in computer-guided implant placement are higher compared to freehand surgery [51]. The precise transfer of digitally planned implant position, from virtual planning to patient's mouth, involves several factors to

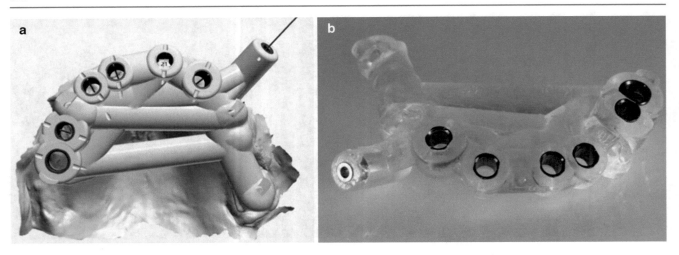

Fig. 29.6 (**a**) Digital design of a full-arch surgical template in CAD software. (**b**) 3D-printed surgical guide (DLP process)

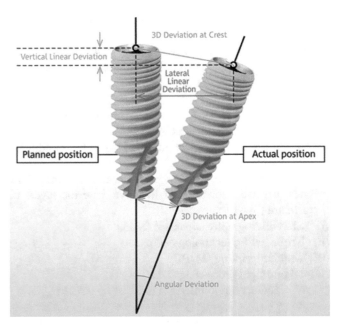

Fig. 29.7 Deviation values measured

reproduce the prosthetically driven result. Errors may occur during CT or CBCT volumetric data acquisition, data transfer, data processing, and treatment planning options. Additionally, optical surface scans via intraoral scanning or model digitalization, surgical guide design and fabrication via CAM technologies or 3D printing workflow, and surgical execution were found to contribute to deviations from the final implant placement and compromise the outcome [52, 53] (Fig. 29.7). Selecting a surgical protocol that includes shorter drilling distance apical to the guided sleeve, lower sleeve height, and longer drill key promotes a more favorable result on the accuracy of static computer-aided implant sur-

gery (sCAIS) procedures [54]. Short surgical templates covering four neighboring teeth produced the equivalent degree of accuracy to that provided by full-arch surgical guides [55]. The macro-design of dental implants affects the accuracy of sCAIS, with tapered designs offering statistically significant positional accuracy compared to parallel-walled macro-designs [56]. Implant abutment connection and tightening for immediate loading may contribute to positional discrepancies due to lack of implant mechanical stability [57].

Even though the latest three consecutive ITI consensus publications demonstrated that there was an overall improvement in accuracy of sCAIS, there was also a great variation in levels of evidence in the digital workflow that can lead to statistically significant inaccuracies [57]. The mean deviations in entry and apex positions were similar as published in previous and novel systematic reviews and meta-analyses, within the clinically acceptable range [28, 56]. A safety "distance" of at least 2 mm should be respected.

Error at entry point: The mean linear deviation for entry point measured at the center of the implant for fully edentulous patients was 1.3 mm and 0.9 mm for partially edentulous cases, treated with guided surgery. Average errors for both fully and partially edentulous cases were 1.2 mm.

Error at the apex: The mean three-dimensional deviation at the apex for fully edentulous cases was 1.5 mm and for partially edentulous cases was 1.2 mm. The average error for all cases treated with sCAIS was 1.4 mm.

Angular deviation: The mean angular deviation for both fully and partially edentulous cases was 3.3°. The average angular deviation for both fully and partially edentulous cases was 3.5° when treated with static computer-assisted guidance systems.

Error in implant height at the apex: The mean vertical linear deviation at the apex was 0.5 mm.

Immediate Loading in Guided Implantology

Contemporary implant therapy includes, as mentioned previously, many different approaches combining the surgical and restorative principles with CAD-CAM technology.

Dental implants were established as a better alternative for restoring partial or fully edentulous patients, even though in modern societies, patients' functional and esthetic needs or demands are not compatible with delay loading implant protocols [58, 59]. Moreover, removable prosthesis as provisional restoration in fully edentulous cases, where osseointegration needs several weeks or months, temporarily worsens function and makes patient feel uncomfortable and insecure. An immediate loading implant protocol must be planned and proposed to achieve acceptable patient satisfaction concerning esthetics and function. In the past few years, immediate loading protocols (loading until 48 hours) or early loading (loading until 14 days) has become popular [60].

All-on-4 protocol, as described by Malo, is a treatment option related to immediate loading in full edentulous cases. Four implants placed in specific distances and angulation can receive a screw-retained superstructure immediately after a minimal invasive surgical approach without grafting [61].

Accuracy of surgical guides, as well as accuracy of CAD-CAM systems, has to be taken into consideration. Those two parameters determine the seating of the prosthesis, interim or definite, which is described as passive fit.

The passive fit of the prosthesis and detailed occlusal adjustments are the key factors for obtaining a predictable immediate loading protocol. Immediate loading refers to definite prosthesis one, and immediate provisionalization refers to interim prosthesis [62, 63]. Clinically, there are two options in guided implant protocol: the one refers to the restoration that can be designed and made before surgery with the abutments attached on it and the other about the prefabricated prosthesis that can be activated postoperatively connecting the prosthesis and the abutment intraorally with resin materials (Fig. 29.8). Then the screw-retained fixed provisional prostheses can be trimmed and contoured in the laboratory and delivered back to the patient at the same appointment. Material selection is important in immediate loading cases due to cytotoxicity that some acrylic-based or resin-based materials have. Concerning small deviation during digital guided implant protocol, the passive fit is obtained accurately with intraoral activation, especially in fully edentulous cases [64, 65].

The prosthesis has to be favorable to the implant osseointegration period. Additionally, cantilevers have to be avoided eliminating both biological and technical complications. The occlusal scheme should be beneficial to the group function,

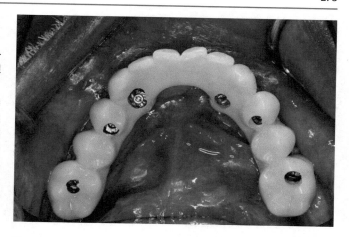

Fig. 29.8 Immediate provisionalization protocol with temporary abutments placed and screwed after implantation. Access holes ensure prosthesis passive fit and create adequate space for resin material to activate the restoration

and the occlusal forces have to be directed to an axis parallel to the implant. Cusps with highly designed cusp walls or deep grooves should also be avoided [66].

Based on clinical trials' findings comparing immediate and early loading with conventional loading protocols, there is a higher risk of implant failure. The number of implants placed, implant surface, number and position of artificial teeth units, type of connection, and bone quality are some of the parameters that affect the decision-making for immediate loading protocol [67, 68].

In conclusion, immediate loading is a beneficial clinical option regarding esthetics and function. Immediate loading protocols show lower implant survival rates than conventional loading, even though there is no difference in marginal bone loss after loading. However, every immediate loading case has to be precisely designed, and a careful patient selection would eliminate possible failures.

Conclusions

Even if guided implant surgery is gaining popularity among dental clinicians, various factors can compromise the treatment outcome.

The thorough training of clinicians plays a key role in the success of the technique. The use of digital technology cannot replace either surgical or prosthetic knowledge or education.

However, if applied following guidelines and indications by clinicians who have the principal knowledge and experience, it can greatly benefit patients.

References

1. Bahat O. Osseointegrated implants in the maxillary tuberosity: report on 45 consecutive patients. Int J Oral Maxillofac Implants. 1992;7(4):459–67.

2. Preston J, Daftary F, Bahat O. Is it a tooth or an implant? J Calif Dent Assoc. 1992;20(5):53–6.

3. Loubele M, Jacobs R, Maes F, Denis K, White S, Coudyzer W, et al. Image quality vs radiation dose of four cone beam computed tomography scanners. Dentomaxillofac Radiol. 2008;37(6):309–19.

4. Bornstein MM, Horner K, Jacobs R. Use of cone beam computed tomography in implant dentistry: current concepts, indications and limitations for clinical practice and research. Periodontol 2000. 2017;73(1):51–72.

5. Pauwels R, Araki K, Siewerdsen JH, Thongvigitmanee SS. Technical aspects of dental CBCT: state of the art. Dentomaxillofac Radiol. 2015;44(1):20140224.

6. Ludlow JB, Ivanovic M. Comparative dosimetry of dental CBCT devices and 64-slice CT for oral and maxillofacial radiology. Oral Surg Oral Med Oral Pathol Oral Radiol Endodontol. 2008;106(1):106–14.

7. Schulze R, Heil U, Groβ D, Bruellmann D, Dranischnikow E, Schwanecke U, et al. Artefacts in CBCT: a review. Dentomaxillofac Radiol. 2011;40(5):265–73.

8. Fokas G, Vaughn VM, Scarfe WC, Bornstein MM. Accuracy of linear measurements on CBCT images related to presurgical implant treatment planning: a systematic review. Clin Oral Implants Res. 2018;29:393–415.

9. Mehl A, Bosch G, Fischer C, Ender A. In vivo tooth-color measurement with a new 3D intraoral scanning system in comparison to conventional digital and visual color determination methods. Int J Comput Dent. 2017;20(4):343–61.

10. Braian M, Wennerberg A. Trueness and precision of 5 intraoral scanners for scanning edentulous and dentate complete-arch mandibular casts: A comparative in vitro study. J Prosthet Dent. 2019;122(2):129–36. e2.

11. Ender A, Zimmermann M, Mehl A. Accuracy of complete-and partial-arch impressions of actual intraoral scanning systems in vitro. Int J Comput Dent. 2019;22(1):11–9.

12. Siqueira R, Chen Z, Galli M, Saleh I, Wang HL, Chan HL. Does a fully digital workflow improve the accuracy of computer-assisted implant surgery in partially edentulous patients? A systematic review of clinical trials. Clin Implant Dent Relat Res. 2020.

13. Joda T, Gallucci GO. The virtual patient in dental medicine. Clin Oral Implants Res. 2015;26(6):725–6.

14. Buser D, Martin W, Belser UC. Optimizing esthetics for implant restorations in the anterior maxilla: anatomic and surgical considerations. Int J Oral Maxillofac Implants. 2004;19(7).

15. Grunder U, Gracis S, Capelli M. Influence of the 3-D bone-to-implant relationship on esthetics. Int J Periodontics Restorative Dent. 2005;25(2):113–9.

16. Jung RE, Schneider D, Ganeles J, Wismeijer D, Zwahlen M, Hämmerle CH, et al. Computer technology applications in surgical implant dentistry: a systematic review. Int J Oral Maxillofac Implants. 2009;24(Suppl):92–109.

17. Vercruyssen M, Jacobs R, Van Assche N, van Steenberghe D. The use of CT scan based planning for oral rehabilitation by means of implants and its transfer to the surgical field: a critical review on accuracy. J Oral Rehabil. 2008;35(6):454–74.

18. Widmann G, Bale RJ. Accuracy in computer-aided implant surgery--a review. Int J Oral Maxillofac Implants. 2006;21(2):305–13.

19. Block MS, Emery RW, Lank K, Ryan J. Implant placement accuracy using dynamic navigation. Int J Oral Maxillofac Implants. 2017;32(1):92–9.

20. Vercruyssen M, Hultin M, Van Assche N, Svensson K, Naert I, Quirynen M. Guided surgery: accuracy and efficacy. Periodontol 2000. 2014;66(1):228–46.

21. Mediavilla Guzmán A, Riad Deglow E, Zubizarreta-Macho Á, Agustín-Panadero R, Hernández Montero S. Accuracy of computer-aided dynamic navigation compared to computer-aided static navigation for dental implant placement: An In Vitro Study J Clin Med. 2019;8(12).

22. Laleman I, Bernard L, Vercruyssen M, Jacobs R, Bornstein MM, Quirynen M. Guided implant surgery in the edentulous maxilla: a systematic review. Int J Oral Maxillofac Implants. 2016;31.

23. D'Haese J, Ackhurst J, Wismeijer D, De Bruyn H, Tahmaseb A. Current state of the art of computer-guided implant surgery. Periodontol 2000. 2017;73(1):121–33.

24. Raico Gallardo YN, da Silva-Olivio IRT, Mukai E, Morimoto S, Sesma N, Cordaro L. Accuracy comparison of guided surgery for dental implants according to the tissue of support: a systematic review and meta-analysis. Clin Oral Implants Res. 2017;28(5):602–12.

25. Rosenfeld AL, Mandelaris GA, Tardieu PB. Prosthetically directed implant placement using computer software to ensure precise placement and predictable prosthetic outcomes. Part 2: rapid-prototype medical modeling and stereolithographic drilling guides requiring bone exposure. Int J Periodontics Restorative Dent. 2006;26(4):347–53.

26. Turbush SK, Turkyilmaz I. Accuracy of three different types of stereolithographic surgical guide in implant placement: an in vitro study. J Prosthet Dent. 2012;108(3):181–8.

27. Ozan O, Turkyilmaz I, Ersoy AE, McGlumphy EA, Rosenstiel SF. Clinical accuracy of 3 different types of computed tomography-derived stereolithographic surgical guides in implant placement. J Oral Maxillofac Surg. 2009;67(2):394–401.

28. Chrcanovic BR, Albrektsson T, Wennerberg A. Flapless versus conventional flapped dental implant surgery: a meta-analysis. PLoS one 2014;9(6):e100624.

29. Rosenfeld AL, Mandelaris GA, Tardieu PB. Prosthetically directed implant placement using computer software to ensure precise placement and predictable prosthetic outcomes. Part 1: diagnostics, imaging, and collaborative accountability. Int J Periodontics Restorative Dent. 2006;26(3):215–21.

30. Greenstein G, Tarnow D. The mental foramen and nerve: clinical and anatomical factors related to dental implant placement: a literature review. J Periodontol. 2006;77(12):1933–43.

31. Greenstein G, Cavallaro J, Tarnow D. Practical application of anatomy for the dental implant surgeon. J Periodontol. 2008;79(10):1833–46.

32. Apostolakis D, Brown JE. The anterior loop of the inferior alveolar nerve: prevalence, measurement of its length and a recommendation for interforaminal implant installation based on cone beam CT imaging. Clin Oral Implants Res. 2012;23(9):1022–30.

33. Papaspyridakos P, Barizan Bordin T, Kim YJ, DeFuria C, Pagni SE, Chochlidakis K, et al. Implant survival rates and biologic complications with implant-supported fixed complete dental prostheses: a retrospective study with up to 12-year follow-up. Clin Oral Implants Res. 2018;29(8):881–93.

34. Tatakis DN, Chien HH, Parashis AO. Guided implant surgery risks and their prevention. Periodontol 2000. 2019;81(1):194–208.

35. Pozzi A, Tallarico M, Marchetti M, Scarfò B, Esposito M. Computer-guided versus free-hand placement of immediately loaded dental implants: 1-year post-loading results of a multicentre randomised controlled trial. Eur J Oral Implantol. 2014;7(3):229–42.

36. Ganz SD. Computer-aided design/computer-aided manufacturing applications using CT and cone beam CT scanning technology. Dent Clin N Am. 2008;52(4):777–808.

37. Schneider D, Marquardt P, Zwahlen M, Jung RE. A systematic review on the accuracy and the clinical outcome of computer-guided template-based implant dentistry. Clin Oral Implants Res. 2009;20(Suppl 4):73–86.

38. D'Souza KM, Aras MA. Types of implant surgical guides in dentistry: a review. J Oral Implantol. 2012;38(5):643–52.

39. Kim T, Lee S, Kim GB, Hong D, Kwon J, Park JW, et al. accuracy of a simplified 3D-printed implant surgical guide. J Prosthet Dent. 2020;124(2):195–201.e2.

40. Engelman MJ, Sorensen JA, Moy P. Optimum placement of osseo-integrated implants. J Prosthet Dent. 1988;59(4):467–73.

41. Adrian ED, Ivanhoe JR, Krantz WA. Trajectory surgical guide stent for implant placement. J Prosthet Dent. 1992;67(5):687–91.

42. Takeshita F, Tokoshima T, Suetsugu T. A stent for presurgical evaluation of implant placement. J Prosthet Dent. 1997;77(1):36–8.

43. Annibali S, La Monaca G, Tantardini M, Cristalli MP. The role of the template in prosthetically guided implantology. J Prosthodont. 2009;18(2):177–83.

44. Espinosa Marino J, Alvarez Arenal A, Pardo Ceballos A, Fernandez Vazquez JP, Ibaseta DG. Fabrication of an implant radiologic-surgical stent for the partially edentulous patient. Quintessence Int. 1995;26(2):111–4.

45. Minoretti R, Merz BR, Triaca A. Predetermined implant positioning by means of a novel guide template technique. Clin Oral Implants Res. 2000;11(3):266–72.

46. Ku YC, Shen YF. Fabrication of a radiographic and surgical stent for implants with a vacuum former. J Prosthet Dent. 2000;83(2):252–3.

47. Becker CM, Kaiser DA. Surgical guide for dental implant placement. J Prosthet Dent. 2000;83(2):248–51.

48. Almog DM, Torrado E, Meitner SW. Fabrication of imaging and surgical guides for dental implants. J Prosthet Dent. 2001;85(5):504–8.

49. Geng W, Liu C, Su Y, Li J, Zhou Y. Accuracy of different types of computer-aided design/computer-aided manufacturing surgical guides for dental implant placement. Int J Clin Exp Med. 2015;8(6):8442–9.

50. Rungrojwittayakul O, Kan JY, Shiozaki K, Swamidass RS, Goodacre BJ, Goodacre CJ, et al. Accuracy of 3D printed models created by two Technologies of Printers with different designs of Model Base. J Prosthodont. 2020;29(2):124–8.

51. Chen Z, Li J, Sinjab K, Mendonca G, Yu H, Wang HL. Accuracy of flapless immediate implant placement in anterior maxilla using computer-assisted versus freehand surgery: a cadaver study. Clin Oral Implants Res. 2018;29(12):1186–94.

52. Cassetta M, Di Mambro A, Giansanti M, Stefanelli L, Cavallini C. The intrinsic error of a stereolithographic surgical template in implant guided surgery. Int J Oral Maxillofac Surg. 2013;42(2):264–75.

53. El Kholy K, Lazarin R, Janner SF, Faerber K, Buser R, Buser D. Influence of surgical guide support and implant site location on accuracy of static computer-assisted implant surgery. Clin Oral Implants Res. 2019;30(11):1067–75.

54. Schneider D, Schober F, Grohmann P, Hammerle CH, Jung RE. In-vitro evaluation of the tolerance of surgical instruments in templates for computer-assisted guided implantology produced by 3-D printing. Clin Oral Implants Res. 2015;26(3):320–5.

55. El Kholy K, Lazarin R, Janner SFM, Faerber K, Buser R, Buser D. Influence of surgical guide support and implant site location on accuracy of static computer-assisted implant surgery. Clin Oral Implants Res. 2019;30(11):1067–75.

56. Tahmaseb A, Wismeijer D, Coucke W, Derksen W. Computer technology applications in surgical implant dentistry: a systematic review. Int J Oral Maxillofac Implants 2014;29.

57. Tahmaseb A, Wu V, Wismeijer D, Coucke W, Evans C. The accuracy of static computer-aided implant surgery: a systematic review and meta-analysis. Clin Oral Implants Res. 2018;29:416–35.

58. Romanos GE, Aydin E, Locher K, Nentwig GH. Immediate vs. delayed loading in the posterior mandible: a split-mouth study with up to 15 years of follow-up. Clin Oral Implants Res. 2016;27:e74–9.

59. Barewal RM, Stanford C, Weesner TC. A randomized controlled clinical trial comparing the effects of three loading protocols on dental implant stability. Int J Oral Maxillofac Implants. 2012;27:945–56.

60. Esposito M, Siormpas K, Mitsias M, Bechara S, Trullenque-Eriksson A, Pistilli R. Immediate, early (6 weeks) and delayed loading (3 months) of single implants: 4-month post-loading from a multicenter pragmatic randomised controlled trial. Eur J Oral Implantol. 2016;9:249–60.

61. Maló P, de Araújo NM, Lopes A, Ferro A, Gravito I. All-on-4[1] treatment concept for the rehabilitation of the completely edentulous mandible: a 7-year clinical and 5-year radiographic retrospective case series with risk assessment for implant failure and marginal bone level. Clin Implant Dent Relat Res. 2015;17(2):531–41.

62. Zembic A, Glauser R, Khraisat A, Hammerle CH. Immediate vs. early loading of dental implants: 3-year results of a randomized controlled clinical trial. Clin Oral Implants Res. 2010;21:481–9.

63. Degidi DM, Nardi D, Piattelli A. Immediate versus one-stage restoration of small-diameter implants for a single missing maxillary lateral incisor: a 3-year randomized clinical trial. J Periodontol. 2009;80:1393–8.

64. Grandi T, Guazzi P, Samarani R, Tohme H, Khoury S, Sbricoli L, et al. Immediate, early (3 weeks) and conventional loading (4 months) of single implants: preliminary data at 1 year after loading from a pragmatic multi- center randomised controlled trial. Eur J Oral Implantol. 2015;8:115–26.

65. Güncü MB, Aslan Y, Tümer C, Güncü GN, Uysal S. In-patient comparison of immediate and conventional loaded implants in mandibular molar sites within 12 months. Clin Oral Implants Res 2008; 19:335–341.

66. Testori T, Bianchi F, Fabbro M, Szmukler-Moncler S, Francetti L, Weinstein R. Immediate non-occlusal loading vs. early loading in partially edentulous patients. Pract Proced Aesthet Dent. 2003;15:787–94.

67. De Bruyn H, Christiaens V, Doornewaard R, Jacobsson M, Cosyn J, Jacquet W, et al. Implant surface roughness and patient factors on long- term peri-implant bone loss. Periodontol 2000 2017;73:218–27.

68. Capelli M, Esposito M, Zuffetti F, Galli F, Fabbro M, Testroi T. A 5-year report from a multicentre randomised clinical trial: immediate non-occlusal versus early loading of dental implants in partially edentulous patients. Eur J Oral Implantol. 2010;3:209–19.

Digital Dentistry in Oral Surgery

Chara Chatzichalepli, Pindaros-Georgios Foskolos,
Federico Hernández-Alfaro, and J. Bertos Quilez

Introduction

Computer-aided dentistry has been effectively introduced to the everyday clinical practice for more than two decades. Among the digital technologies available for dentistry are digital radiography, electronic prescriptions, computerized case presentations, CAD/CAM restorations, digitally based surgical guides, imaging for implant placement, and digital impressions.

Digital dental technology can strengthen the collaboration between the patient, the oral surgeon, the dentist/prosthodontist, and the dental technician by achieving quicker communication for an ideal result. Among the digital technologies available in dentistry science, a variety of categories are already utilized in the field of oral surgery. Those mainly include a combination of the three-dimensional imaging (3D imaging) with the use of CBCT (cone beam computed tomography) and the CAD/CAM (computer-aided design and computer-aided manufacturing) technology, offering a variety of advantages, mainly involving reduction of operational time and precision of surgical actions [20, 21].

C. Chatzichalepli (✉)
Department of Oral and Maxillofacial Surgery, National and Kapodistrian University of Athens, Athens, Greece
e-mail: chatzichalepli.chara@gmail.com

P.-G. Foskolos
Department of Prosthodontics, National and Kapodistrian University of Athens, Athens, Greece
e-mail: pindaros@uic.es

J. B. Quilez
Department of Oral and Maxillofacial Surgery, International University of Catalonia, Barcelona, Spain
e-mail: jorgebertos@uic.es

F. Hernández-Alfaro
Department of Oral and Maxillofacial Surgery, International University of Catalonia, Barcelona, Spain

Teknon Medical Center, Barcelona, Spain
e-mail: h.alfaro@uic.es

Cone Beam Computed Tomography

The cone beam computed tomography imaging is a well-established radiographic tool. CBCT has many advantages since it represents three-dimensional imaging of the oral and maxillofacial region structures in contrast to a two-dimensional orthopantomography (panoramic radiograph) or other types such as periapical radiographs. The detailed, three-dimensional representation of the anatomical geometry can lead to a thorough investigation [2, 19, 20, 36]:

(i) The site and the extension of a pathological lesion located in the bone structures of the maxillofacial region.
(ii) The proximity to vital anatomical landmarks with detailed imaging of their position, such as the inferior alveolar nerve, the incisive canal, and the mental foramen, and critical anatomic boundaries for prevention of neurovascular trauma.
(iii) The neighboring teeth and estimation of their prognosis.
(iv) The accurate dimensions of the alveolar ridge for implant positioning and the assessed bone quality. Cases related to inadequate bone morphology, volume, and quality can be depicted.
(v) Augmentation procedure choices.
(vi) Suspected trauma history of jaws and teeth.
(vii) Presurgical planning and transfer.
(viii) Virtual analogue of the patient.

The virtual analogues of patients occur with computer-aided design and manufacturing technologies combined with radiographic imaging and the superimposition of intraoral scans and occasionally extraoral face scans [22].

A 3D object representing the anatomic site of intervention is created in a layer-by-layer array in a printer. Three-dimensional (3D) printing is a method derived from additive manufacturing technology offering the promising potential for bone reconstruction, rehabilitation, and regeneration and expanding treatment options in many oral surgery fields [28]. Frequently used 3D printing techniques include fused deposition modeling (FDM), stereolithography apparatus (SLA), selective laser sintering (SLS), and 3D spray (3DP). A wide range of materials can be used for 3D printing, including natural and synthesized polymers, metals, and ceramics [17].

3D printing in the field of oral surgery can be applied for:

(i). Rehabilitation of small and large hard and soft tissue defects following tumor excision or trauma in the craniomaxillofacial region in combination with prosthetic analogues

(ii). Reconstruction using devices for fixation and guides for cutting or drilling so as to precise and stabilize the surgical field

(iii). Regeneration by the preservation of existing bone and stimulation of bone remodeling

Bone regeneration represents a promising dentistry approach and is considered an ideal clinical strategy in treating diseases, injuries, and defects of the maxillofacial region. Regeneration by preserving existing bone and stimulation of bone remodeling using 3D printing allows the production of innovative scaffolds with patient-specific dimensions using computer-aided design (CAD). Those scaffold designs are materials acting as a biological platform for repair, restoration, or augmentation of the involved tissues. Currently, tissue engineering's ultimate goal is to create a three-dimensional (3D) biocompatible support that can be inserted into a tissue to repair a lesion or correct a defect by allowing the adhesion and proliferation of a specific cell type. Three-dimensional tissue regeneration using computer guidance has been recently applied in many aspects of oral surgery [5, 17].

Three-dimensional bioprinting technology allows for the fabrication of artificial grafts that may be superior to both autografts and allografts in adaptation, safety, and invasiveness [5].

Ideal characteristics of 3D printed biomaterials include [5, 7, 17]:

• Biocompatibility
• Osteoconductivity
• Porosity for tissue in-growth, blood and nutrient supply to the newly produced tissues
• Customization of shape, size, orientation, and pore connectivity

Objective: Digital Technology and Computer-Guided Alveolar Ridge Augmentation

Alveolar ridge augmentation refers to a variety of procedures designed to correct a deformed alveolar ridge, typically in preparation for dental implant placement. Different techniques and current modalities of alveolar ridge augmentation include the following categories [8, 9]. The current chapter's objective is to expose the contribution of the benefits of digitally guided technology on different techniques of oral regenerative surgery. The bone augmentation techniques described are:

• Guided bone regeneration (GBR) with the use of Ti mesh
• Onlay block grafts
• Ridge split/expansion techniques
• Distraction osteogenesis
• Sinus floor elevation

Computer-Aided Guided Bone Regeneration with Ti Mesh

Guided bone regeneration (GBR) is the most well-established and evidence-based bone augmentation approach with more clinical applications. This technology has the advantages of small surgical trauma and low technical sensitivity. However, the outcome is based upon surgeon's experience and expertise [24]. As mentioned previously, prosthetic-driven guided regeneration may evolve soft and hard tissue augmentation and implant placement according to the ideal location of the prosthesis [8, 24].

In GBR techniques, the bone graft of choice is covered by a membrane that acts as a physical barrier that prevents the migration of epithelial cells and fibroblasts into the defect where augmentation has been performed. This allows the osteoprogenitor cells to reach the site and recreate new bone [4, 13, 34]. However, in vertical bone reconstruction techniques, a space maintenance structure is essential to sustain the mechanical forces and protect the stability of the bone graft [29]. Ti mesh's rigid structure is known to perform successful horizontal and vertical augmentations for alveolar bone in GBR, even though it is most commonly used for vertical bone regeneration [29].

There have been mainly two different options of digital dentistry contribution in the fabrication of a Ti mesh for GBR purposes in the literature. The stereolithographic model (STL) of the operational area provides the option of pre-bending a prefabricated Ti mesh preoperatively according to the existing defect's anatomy. Preforming the Ti mesh in the 3D analogue presurgically may reduce the operation's duration and increase the fitting accuracy [14]. Moreover, it seems to offset some pressure from the soft tissue on the labial side and can also make an adequate amount of bone augmentation volume around the implants [14, 24].

In addition, the superimposition of intraoral scans with the digital planification of the definitive restoration – digital wax-up (STL files) and the cone beam computed tomography images (DICOM files) – provides the opportunity of the virtual design of a customized Ti mesh according to the morphology of the defect. With the contribution of CAD-CAM technology, the virtual Ti mesh model can be produced for regenerative purpose [35]. The advantages of the referred approach are the decrease of surgical time, the accuracy of the mesh over the defect, the simplification of the surgical steps, and the reduction of postoperative morbidity by reaching at the same time similar success rates with the vertical bone regeneration with conventional Ti mesh [10, 11, 35].

Onlay Block Grafts

Autogenous bone block from the mandible has been indicated as one of the most predictable ways to manage horizontal and vertical bone defects [6]. However, regardless of the method or the instruments used, all the osteotomy is outlined without precise reference points that could help the surgeon determine anatomical structure positions [15]. Osteotomies require a great safety margin, reducing the potential dimension of the harvestable bone block, thus hindering graft volume sufficiency at the donor site to treat the defect. Additionally, the risk of anatomical structural damage and postoperative patient morbidity is present [15].

Computer-guided implantation and osteotomies have been more precise than traditional freehand drilling procedures due to the working direction imposed by the surgical guide [15, 22].

The advantages of a computer-guided procedure are controlling the osteotomy lines and drillings and maximizing the harvestable bone block volume to the bone volume needed for defect reconstruction by protecting at the same time the

sensitive anatomical structures, for example, the inferior alveolar nerve. As a result, a digital software program can enhance surgical treatment planning prior to bone transplantation [15, 37].

Computer-Guided Ridge Splitting Technique

Recent but very few studies have proposed a computer-guided, flapless, alveolar ridge splitting technique using customized surgical guides to every step of the surgery, from incision to implant placement. The conclusion is that with guided flapless alveolar ridge splitting:

- The periosteum preservation is effectively achieved, thus maintaining an adequate blood supply to the split buccal plate of bone.
- The split ridge fracture is stabilized.
- The resorption rate of the bony plates is reduced.

offering the advantages of a predictable, less invasive, atraumatic technique and a viable treatment option in cases of immediate implant placement with minimized treatment time [16].

Distraction Osteogenesis

In bone regeneration techniques, distraction osteogenesis seems to be an alternative to bone regeneration with biomaterials or grafts retrieved from distant donor sites [18]. The most common intraoperative risk of the mentioned technique is the prediction of destruction vector and the risk of damaging neighboring anatomical structures [18]. Developments in computerized structural modeling have provided surgeons with a platform to customize the surgical design. This can also be applied in cases where distraction osteogenesis is chosen to rehabilitate defects or deformities.

The concept of guided distraction osteogenesis is the same as in previous guided osteotomies. After medical data processing, virtual surgical planning with the contribution of computer-aided design (CAD) and computer-aided manufacturing (CAM) leads to the fabrication of an individualized surgical template. This surgical guide leads the final position of the screws and the distraction osteogenesis device itself in the recipient site. As a result, the accuracy of the device insertion, the predictability of the treatment outcome, and the protection of neighboring sensitive anatomical structures are increased [12, 26, 33].

Computer-Guided Sinus Floor Elevation

Implant placement in the posterior maxilla many times seems compromised due to the following reasons:

- The alveolar bone quantity might be inadequate due to post-extraction resorption of the alveolar ridge and the maxillary sinus pneumatization.
- The alveolar bone quality is poor in the posterior maxilla.

Computer-guided sinus floor elevation technique was firstly introduced in 2008 by Rosenfeld and Mandelaris [25]. Several studies have supported that CAD/CAM surgical stent might significantly enhance the quality and the results of the sinus floor elevation technique reducing the incidence of rupturing the Schneiderian membrane, thus avoiding postoperative maxillary sinusitis, graft infection, and implant loss.

One of the most significant advantages of this technique is the capacity to avoid cutting through the maxillary sinus septum using a guide that establishes the window design in a reduced operating time. The lateral window's virtula planning allows the operator to identify the exact thickness of the sinus wall and the level of the alveolar antral artery at the lateral osteotomy outline [30].

Proper stabilization of the surgical guide is of crucial importance in order to effectively translate the virtual plan intraoperatively. To achieve this, the guide was tightly fixed using titanium screws to avoid the chance of surgical guide instability, especially at the osteotomy drilling stage. The positions of the fixating screws have to be planned so as not to interfere with the path in cases of immediate implant placement or damage to the adjacent teeth roots [30, 32].

Reliability and Accuracy of Guided Oral Surgery

The execution of an oral surgery procedure is considered more accurate with less intraoperative time than the freehand surgery, especially when the surgeon lacks experience [1, 3, 31]. The guided workflow includes mainly six steps:

1. Patient assessment
2. Data collection
3. Data manipulation
4. Virtual implant planning
5. Guide and prosthesis manufacture
6. Digitally aid-guided operation

Each of the abovementioned steps requires a specific approach. An insufficient completion of one or more of those steps leads to a relative percentage of deviation between the planification and the postoperative result (Al Yafi et al., 2019). A more extended description of possible factors that may decrease digitally guided surgery accuracy rates is mentioned on Chap. 29 "Computer-Guided Implant Dentistry."

Conclusion

The technology of digital dentistry is becoming more pronounced in the field of oral and implant surgery by providing higher intra-surgical accuracy and lower operational time, rates of morbidity, and complications [23, 27]. However, the surgeon should be qualified with the knowledge to execute freehand surgery as well in order to compensate for the possible complications of the digital workflow when they arise.

References

1. Al Yafi F, Camenisch B, Al-Sabbagh M. Is digital guided implant surgery accurate and reliable? Dent Clin N Am. 2019;63:381–97.
2. Bornstein, M. M., Scarfe, W. C., Vaughn, V. M. & Jacobs, R.. Cone beam computed tomography in implant dentistry: a systematic review focusing on guidelines, indications, and radiation dose risks. Inter J Oral Maxillofac Implants. 2014;29.
3. Bover-Ramos F, Viña-Almunia J, Cervera-Ballester J, Peñarrocha-Diago M, García-Mira B. Accuracy of implant placement with computer-guided surgery: a systematic review and meta-analysis comparing cadaver, clinical, and in vitro studies. Int J Oral Maxillofac Implants. 2018;33:101–15.
4. Caballé-Serrano J, Munar-Frau A, Ortiz-Puigpelat O, Soto-Penaloza D, Peñarrocha M, Hernández-Alfaro F. On the search of the ideal barrier membrane for guided bone regeneration. J Clin Exp Dent. 2018;10:e477–83.
5. Ceccarelli G, Prest R, Benedetti L, Cusella De Angelis MG, Lupi SM & Rodriguez Y Baena R.. Emerging perspectives in scaffold for tissue engineering in oral surgery. Stem Cells Inter. 2017. 2017.
6. Chen ST, Beagle J, Jensen SS, Chiapasco M, Darby I. Consensus statements and recommended clinical procedures regarding surgical techniques. Int J Oral Maxillofac Implants. 2009;24(Suppl):272–8.
7. Cheng X, Yoo JJ, Hale RG, Davis MR, Kang H-W, Jin S. 3D printed biomaterials for maxillofacial tissue engineering and reconstruction—A review. Open J Biomed Mater Res. 2014;1:1–7.
8. Chiapasco M, Casentini P. Horizontal bone-augmentation procedures in implant dentistry: prosthetically guided regeneration. Periodontology. 2018;2000(77):213–40.
9. Chiapasco M, Casentini P, Zaniboni M. Bone augmentation procedures in implant dentistry. Inter J Oral Maxillofac Implants. 2009;24.

10. Ciocca L, Lizio G, Baldissara P, Sambuco A, Scotti R, Corinaldesi G. Prosthetically CAD-CAM-guided bone augmentation of atrophic jaws using customized titanium mesh: preliminary results of an open prospective study. J Oral Implantol. 2018;44:131–7.

11. Cucchi A, Bianchi A, Calamai P, Rinaldi L, Mangano F, Vignudelli E, Corinaldesi G. Clinical and volumetric outcomes after vertical ridge augmentation using computer-aided-design/computer-aided manufacturing (CAD/CAM) customized titanium meshes: a pilot study. BMC Oral Health. 2020;20:1–11.

12. Dahake SW, Kuthe AM, Chawla J, Mawale MB. Rapid prototyping assisted fabrication of customized surgical guides in mandibular distraction osteogenesis: A case report. Rapid Prototyp J. 2017.

13. Dahlin C, Linde A, Gottlow J, Nyman S. Healing of bone defects by guided tissue regeneration. Plast Reconstr Surg. 1988;81:672–6.

14. De Moraes PH, Olate S, De Albergaria-Barbosa JR, De Moraes P, Olate S, Albergaria-Barbosa J. Maxillary reconstruction using rhBMP-2 and titanium mesh. Technical note about the use of stereolithographic model. Int J Odontostomat. 2015;9:149–52.

15. De Stavola L, Fincato A, Bressan E, Gobbato L. Results of computer-guided bone block harvesting from the mandible: a case series. Inter J Periodont Restorat Dentistry. 2017;37.

16. Dohiem M, Khorshid HE, Zekry KA. An innovative computer guided ridge splitting flapless technique with simultaneous implant placement: a case report. Fut Dent J. 2018;4:16–22.

17. Fahmy MD, Jazayeri HE, Razavi M, Masri R, Tayebi L. Three-dimensional bioprinting materials with potential application in pre-prosthetic surgery. J Prosthodont. 2016;25:310–8.

18. Hany HE, El Hadidi YN, Sleem H, Taha M, El Kassaby M. Novel technique and step-by-step construction of a computer-guided stent for mandibular distraction osteogenesis. J Craniofac Surg. 2019;30:2271–4.

19. Harris D, Horner K, Gröndahl K, Jacobs R, Helmrot E, Benic GI, Bornstein MM, Dawood A, Quirynen M. EAO guidelines for the use of diagnostic imaging in implant dentistry 2011. A consensus workshop organized by the European Association for Osseointegration at the Medical University of Warsaw. Clin Oral Implants Res. 2012;23:1243–53.

20. Jacobs R, Salmon B, Codari M, Hassan B, Bornstein MM. Cone beam computed tomography in implant dentistry: recommendations for clinical use. BMC Oral Health. 2018;18:1–16.

21. Jamali J, Kolokythas A, Miloro M. 11 clinical applications of digital dental Technology in Oral and Maxillofacial Surgery. Clin App Digital Dent Technol. 2015;207

22. Joda T, Gallucci GO. The virtual patient in dental medicine. Clin Oral Implants Res. 2015;26:725–6.

23. Laleman I, Bernard L, Vercruyssen M, Jacobs R, Bornstein MM, Quirynen M. Guided implant surgery in the edentulous maxilla: a systematic review. Inter J Oral Maxillofac Implants. 2016;31.

24. Li, S., Zhang, T., Zhou, M., Zhang, X., Gao, Y. & Cai, X. A novel digital and visualized guided bone regeneration procedure and digital precise bone augmentation: a case series. Clin Implant Dent Relat Res. 2020.

25. Mandelaris GA, Rosenfeld AL. A novel approach to the antral sinus bone graft technique: the use of a prototype cutting guide for precise outlining of the lateral wall. A case report. Inter J Periodont Restorat Dentistry. 2008;28.

26. Mao Z, Zhang N, Cui Y. Three-dimensional printing of surgical guides for mandibular distraction osteogenesis in infancy. Medicine. 2019;98.

27. Margvelashvili-Malament M, Att W. Current workflows for computer-aided implant surgery: a review article. Curr Oral Health Rep. 2019;6:295–305.

28. Maroulakos M, Kamperos G, Tayebi L, Halazonetis D, Ren Y. Applications of 3D printing on craniofacial bone repair: a systematic review. J Dent. 2019;80:1–14.

29. Merli M, Moscatelli M, Mariotti G, Rotundo R, Bernardelli F, Nieri M. Bone level variation after vertical ridge augmentation: resorbable barriers versus titanium-reinforced barriers. A 6-year double-blind randomized clinical trial. Int J Oral Maxillofac Implants. 2014;29:905–13.

30. Osman AH, Mansour H, Atef M, Hakam M. Computer guided sinus floor elevation through lateral window approach with simultaneous implant placement. Clin Implant Dent Relat Res. 2018;20:137–43.

31. Smitkarn P, Subbalekha K, Mattheos N, Pimkhaokham A. The accuracy of single-tooth implants placed using fully digital-guided surgery and freehand implant surgery. J Clin Periodontol. 2019;46:949–57.

32. Strbac, G. D., Giannis, K., Schnappauf, A., Bertl, K., Stavropoulos, A. & Ulm, C. 2020. Guided lateral sinus lift procedure using 3-dimensionally printed templates for a safe surgical approach: a proof-of-concept case report. J Oral Maxillofac Surg: Off J Am Assoc Oral Maxillofac Surg

33. Tan A, Chai Y, Mooi W, Chen X, Xu H, Zin MA, Lin L, Zhang Y, Yang X, Chai G. Computer-assisted surgery in therapeutic strategy distraction osteogenesis of hemifacial microsomia: accuracy and predictability. J Craniomaxillofac Surg. 2019;47:204–18.

34. Tinti C, Parma-Benfenati S, Polizzi G. Vertical ridge augmentation: what is the limit? Int J Periodontics Restorative Dent. 1996;16:220–9.

35. Tommasato G, Casentini P, Del Fabbro M, Dellavia C, Chiapasco M. GBR of atrophic edentulous ridges with customized CAD-CAM titanium meshes: a prospective study. Clin Oral Implants Res. 2020;31:250.

36. Venkatesh E, Elluru SV. Cone beam computed tomography: basics and applications in dentistry. J Istanbul Univ Facult Dentistry. 2017;51:S102.

37. Verdugo F, Simonian K, Raffaelli L, D'Addona A. Computer-aided design evaluation of harvestable mandibular bone volume: a clinical and tomographic human study. Clin Implant Dent Relat Res. 2014;16:348–55.

Canine Impaction and Fenestration Technique

Amirhossein Moaddabi, Sarah Akbari, and Parisa Soltani

Introduction

An impacted tooth is a tooth that doesn't erupt until its chronological eruption date, even after its root is completed [1].

Canines are one of the last teeth which erupt in the arch. Some factors like overretention of the primary teeth, lack of space, and palatal or labial deviation of the lateral incisor could influence canine impaction [2].

Canine impaction is a common clinical situation that requires interdisciplinary treatment [3]. The maxillary canine impaction incidence is the most common form of impaction after the third molar is more than twice the mandibular canine [3]. Maxillary canine impaction occurs in 2% of the whole population and is more common in women than in men. Eight percent of the impacted maxillary canines are bilateral. One-third of them are located labially, and two-thirds of them are located palatally [3–5].

Etiology

Canine plays an essential role in the esthetic smile and functional occlusion, so we should pay attention to any factors involving the canine's normal eruption [1]. Several factors can cause canine impaction; some of them are systemic, localized, and genetic factors [3]. It was found that 85% of the palatally impacted canines had enough space for the eruption. In contrast, only 17% of the labially impacted canines had enough space for the eruption [6]. Also, there are two major theories for the palatal displacement of maxillary canine, which are "genetic" theory and "guidance" theory [7].

Here we mention them in a short form:

Guidance theory mentions the root of the lateral incisor as a guidance for the canine eruption, so in the absence or malformation of the lateral incisor, the canine will not be able to erupt [8].

Genetic theory mentions genetic as the primary reason for canine impaction and believes that it occurs containing some other problems such as missing or small lateral incisors, enamel hypoplasia, infraocclusion of primary molars, and aplasia of second premolars [3, 9].

Diagnosis of Canine Impaction

Early diagnosis of canine impaction is essential because it can reduce the treatment time, cost, and complication [3]. The most straightforward way for early detection of canine impaction is a clinical and tactile evaluation at the age of 9 to 10 years. Because canine, erupts by the age of 10 to 12 years, and contains a buccal bulge that is palpable 1 year before its eruption.

The final diagnosis of canine impaction is based on both clinical and radiographic examinations [3].

A. Moaddabi (✉)
Assistant professor, Department of Oral and Maxillofacial Surgery, Dental Research Center, Mazandaran University of Medical Sciences, Sari, Iran

Faculty of Dentistry, Mazandaran,University of Medical Sciences, Sari, Iran
e-mail: m.moaddabi@mazums.ac.ir

S. Akbari
Department of Dentistry, Dental student of Mazandaran University of Medical Science, Member of the Student Research Committee, Sari, Iran
e-mail: Sarahakbari1376@yahoo.com

P. Soltani
Department of Oral and Maxillofacial Radiology, Dental Implants Research Center, Dental Research Institute, School of Dentistry, Isfahan University of Medical Sciences, Isfahan, Iran
e-mail: p.soltani@dnt.mui.ac.ir

© The Author(s), under exclusive license to Springer Nature Switzerland AG 2021
M. R. Stevens et al. (eds.), *Innovative Perspectives in Oral and Maxillofacial Surgery*,
https://doi.org/10.1007/978-3-030-75750-2_31

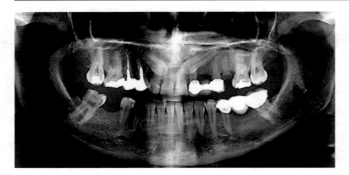

Fig. 31.1 Panoramic view of bilateral maxillary impacted canine

Clinical Evaluation

Points that we should pay attention during the clinical evaluation include the morphology and position of the adjacent teeth, the contour of the bone, the amount of space for eruption, and the mobility of teeth [10].

Here are some clinical situations which might be signs of canine impaction [4]:

1. Absence of a normal labial canine bulge (as we mentioned above, the canine buccal bulge is usually palpable 1 year before its eruption by the age of 9 to 10 years)
2. Delayed eruption of the permanent canine or prolonged retention of the primary canine
3. Presence of a palatal bulge
4. Delayed eruption, distal tipping, or migration of the lateral incisor [10] (Fig. 31.1)

Radiographic Evaluation

Radiographic evaluation is an integral part of diagnosis and treatment planning and evaluates the consequences of the impaction of maxillary and mandibular canines. Two-dimensional radiographs have been traditionally used for the diagnosis and evaluation of impacted canines and their associated effects. These modalities include intraoral periapical and occlusal radiographs as well as extraoral projections, such as panoramic and lateral and posteroanterior cephalometric radiographs. Often a combination of these radiographic examinations must be used to provide the necessary information for diagnosis and treatment planning [11, 12]. The introduction of affordable and accessible three-dimensional imaging into dentistry has been widely used in impacted canines, replacing two-dimensional radiographs in particular applications.

Periapical radiographs can be used for the diagnosis of impacted canines in case of a delayed eruption. In addition, two periapical radiographs obtained with different tube angulations or a periapical image combined with a modality with different x-ray angles may be applied for localization of impacted canines using the buccal object or the same lingual opposite buccal (SLOB) rule [13]. Periapical radiographs can also help in assessing the effects of impacted canines on adjacent teeth. For instance, moderate to severe root resorption of the adjacent lateral incisors can be detected on periapical images. Moreover, periapical radiographs can reveal an enlarged dental follicle around the impacted canine [14]. Occlusal radiographs were also previously used for localization of impacted canines. Although using this approach alone for localizing maxillary canines might be deceptive [15].

Apart from panoramic radiographs that are still routinely used as scout images for canine impaction, obtaining other extraoral two-dimensional radiographs for impacted teeth is no longer common. A panoramic image is useful to provide an overall view of the impacted canine's development and position and its relation with adjacent teeth. However, superimposition and low spatial resolution impair panoramic radiographs' ability to demonstrate details such as root resorption or exact positioning of impacted teeth [11].

The emergence of three-dimensional imaging using cone beam computed tomography (CBCT) has revolutionized the radiographic examination of impacted teeth. CBCT is (Figs. 31.2 and 31.3) considered a cost-effective imaging modality for localization of impacted canines, helping in determining the treatment plan for surgical exposure or extraction. It also helps in the diagnosis of the various consequences of impacted canine teeth, such as root resorption and bone support in the adjacent incisors or cystic degeneration of the dental follicle [11, 16]. In practical scenarios of impacted canines, a single CBCT exposure can replace using a combination of radiographic modalities for diagnostic purposes. Studies have shown that CBCT improves the diagnostic capabilities and treatment outcomes compared to two-dimensional images [17–19]. Three-dimensional data can also be used to replicate prototypes of the dentition which can be used for demonstrational purposes, treatment planning, and fabrication of bonded attachments and other precision accessories [20]. In general, CBCT is strongly recommended for the evaluation of impacted maxillary or mandibular canines.

Radiology for Predictive Diagnosis of Canine Impaction

Impaction is diagnosed when unerupted canine teeth with advanced root development exceeding three-quarters of the final root length are detected on radiographs. Predictive diagnosis of impacted canines is clinically significant because treatment of this condition is challenging. Several investigators have proposed methods to predict canine impaction radiographically. Geometric angular and linear measurements on two-dimensional or three-dimensional images were used

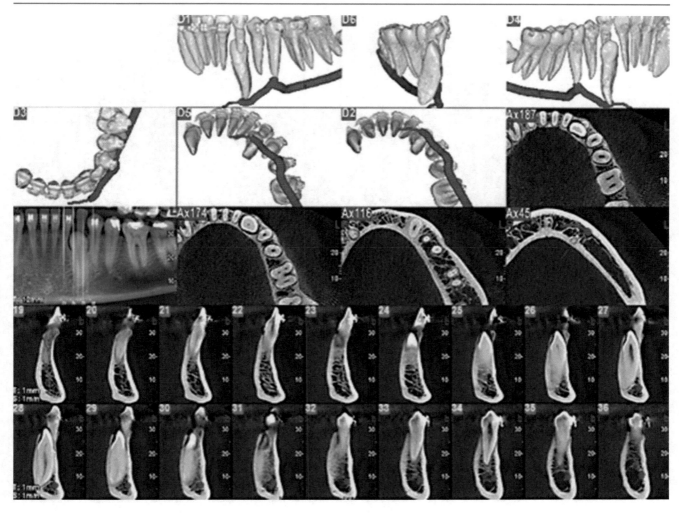

Fig. 31.2 CBCT view of mandibular impacted canine

to detect the eruption's ectopic path in maxillary canines. One of the widely used predictors is identifying the cusp tip of the canine in question concerning the adjacent lateral incisor. This method, which is called sector analysis, was proposed by Ericson and Kurol and modified by other investigators [21]. It has been reported that most eventually impacted canines are the ones with their cusp tip located in more mesial sectors [22, 23]. Other parameters investigated are the canine to midline angle, canine cusp to midline distance, canine cusp to the occlusal plane, and several other angular or linear measurements. The results of multiple studies indicate good predictive values of these measurements in detecting eventual impaction of the maxillary canines [24–26].

Radiology for Localization of Impacted Canines

A combination of two-dimensional images with different x-ray angulations either in the horizontal or vertical plane was traditionally used for localization of impacted canines

using the buccal object or SLOB rule. If the crown of the impacted canine moves in the direction of the tube shift, it is located lingual to the reference object. If it moves in the opposite direction, it is located buccal to the reference structure. As mentioned, occlusal radiographs were used to localize the buccal or lingual position of impacted mandibular canines. Some investigators proposed methods to determine the lingual/palatal or buccal location of impacted canines in a single two-dimensional radiograph, such as a panoramic image [27–29]. However, with the advent and popularity of CBCT in dentistry, these techniques are only reserved for rare occasions. CBCT provides excellent localization information for impacted teeth along with other clinically essential findings [12].

Radiology for Consequences of Impacted Canines

Impacted teeth may lead to several pathologic effects, including root resorption of adjacent teeth and hyperplastic or cys-

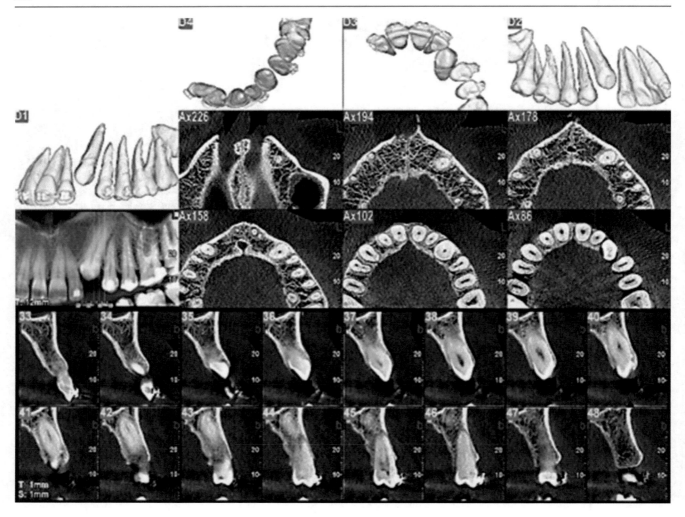

Fig. 31.3 CBCT view of maxillary impacted canine

tic changes in the dental follicle of the impacted teeth. Radiographic modalities can be used for detecting these entities, which may affect the treatment approach for impacted canines.

Treatment

The canine impaction treatment needs cooperation between the orthodontist and the oral and maxillofacial surgeon, which demands the patient's cooperation, high cost, long treatment duration, and chances of damage to the tooth adjacent structures [1, 3]. Early diagnosis with the extraction of the primary canine increases spontaneous eruption and reduces the impaction's severity. Some other stuff helping the canine eruption or improving the treatment prognosis include removing barriers such as a supernumerary tooth, odontoma, fibrous bands, and tooth sac and creating space in the arch by distalization of the molar and maxillary expansion [1]. Surgical exposure and orthodontic management are used when we are extremely sure that the tooth will not erupt spontaneously [30].

Several factors can influence the treatment decision of an impacted maxillary canine, such as:

- Patient's age
- Patient's motivation
- Suitability of the first premolar
- Sufficient space in the arch
- Height of the canine's crown
- Position of the canine tooth
- Anteroposterior position of the root apex of the canine
- Labiopalatal position of the canine
- Canine angulation to the midline
- Overlap and root resorption of the adjacent incisor
- Sufficient width of the attached gingiva [4]

Tips on Local Anesthesia and Homeostasis from the Author's Point of View

Due to the author's experience, the prerequisite for every successful surgery is the achievement of deep local anesthesia, which makes both the patient and the surgeon calm and peaceful. When the patient feels pain, his/her blood pressure will increase, causing bleeding and endangering isolation and homeostasis. The vasoconstrictor inside the anesthetic solution (if it is not contraindicated) provides homeostasis and prevents bleeding. It is helpful, especially in surgeries needing isolation (in this chapter, isolation is needed for the attachment of the orthodontic button to the exposed tooth by composite). On the other hand, when the patient is calm and does not feel pain, his/her blood pressure will not increase, so the possibility of bleeding will decrease, and isolation will be provided.

According to the impacted canine position, the required anesthesia technique differs: In maxillary arch when the canine is impacted palatally, nasopalatine technique is required for both open and close techniques. But when using the close technique, as far as the needle must pass the buccal aspect, the buccal tissue needs to be numbed by infiltration or bilateral ASA. When the maxillary canine is located labially, and an Apically Positioned Flap (APF) technique is used, Anterior Superior Alveolar nerve (ASA) nerve block or infra-orbital (IO) nerve block technique is used. For extra homeostasis, infiltration can be used. When using the close technique, ASA or IO nerve block is used for the buccal mucosa, and a nasopalatine nerve block technique is used for the palatal tissues (to reduce the pain of palatal injection, we can use topical anesthesia agents). When using the open technique (gingivectomy), anesthesia for the buccal mucosa is enough.

Mandibular impacted canines are located labially, palatally, or in the middle of them; anyway, anesthesia for the buccal and lingual soft tissue and mandibular bone is needed, which is provided by the Inferior alveolar nerve block (IAN). The inferior alveolar nerve block numbs the pulp and periodontal ligament of the teeth in the same side of injection, the mandibular bone, the corner of the mouth, the anterior two-thirds of the tongue, and the floor of the mouth. Mental nerve block also numbs the buccal soft tissue of the same side of the injection and is helpful. To enhance the quality of anesthesia and to achieve more homeostasis, infiltration can be helpful, especially in the buccal tissue.

As far as we mentioned above, as the orthodontic chain needs to be attached to the crown by composite and this procedure needs isolation, homeostasis is an important factor to achieve a successful result. In addition to suitable anesthesia, which is done before the operation, some other things need to be done during and after the operation in order to achieve homeostasis. Here we mention them in a short form:

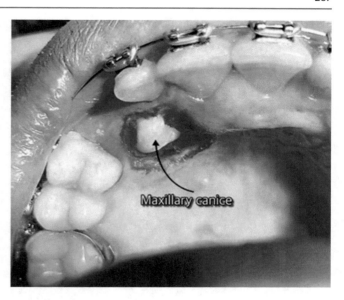

Fig. 31.4 Clinical view of using electrosurgery in open eruption – the technique for palatally impacted maxillary canine

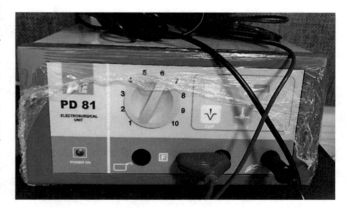

Fig. 31.5 Electrosurgery

During the surgery, we can use two methods to enhance healing and homeostasis:

Electrosurgery and Diode Laser

Due to the author's experience, usage of electrosurgery (Figs. 31.4 and 31.5) during the surgery provides suitable homeostasis, isolation, and healing. This technique is often used in palatal area, as it has adequate keratinized tissues. It is worth mentioned that this technique requires a powerful suction. During using electrosurgery, the surgeon should be careful about patient's lip, not to be burned.

The other method is the usage of the diode laser. This method provides a clean area and increases isolation. We usually use a diode laser (Figs. 31.6 and 31.7. Sobouti) with the wavelength of 980 NM, because in this wavelength, the absorption of hemoglobin is the maximum and provides the best possibility of cutting the soft tissue (Author).

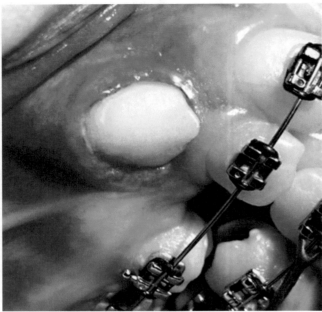

Courtesy of Dr. Farhad Sobouti

Fig. 31.6 Sobouti—clinical view of using diode laser for canine impaction

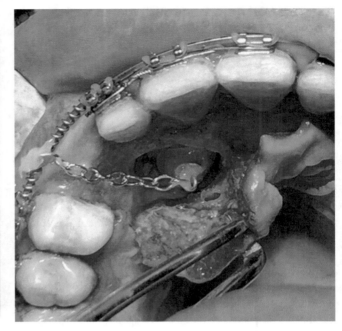

Fig. 31.8 Clinical view of using the close technique for palatally impacted maxillary canine

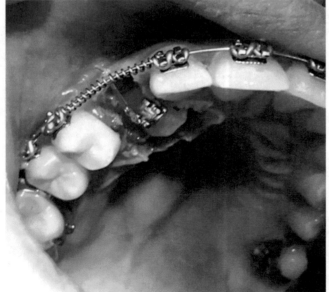

Courtesy of Dr. Farhad Sobouti

Fig. 31.7 Sobouti—clinical view of using diode laser for labially impacted maxillary canine

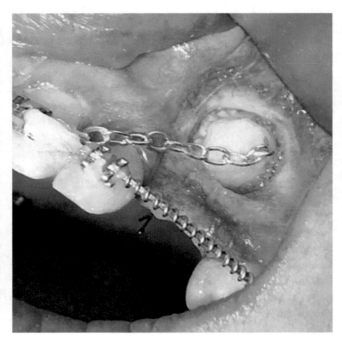

Fig. 31.9 Clinical view of using close technique in labially impacted maxillary canine

Treatment

There are two basic methods for exposure of the impacted canine, open eruption technique and closed eruption technique [1, 31].

In the close technique (Figs. 31.8 and 31.9), the crown of the impacted canine is exposed by a surgical flap, an orthodontic device is attached to the exposed crown, and then the flap is sutured back. In this method, the only part which will stay exposed is the eruption chain (not the

Table 31.1 Canine impaction treatment [32]

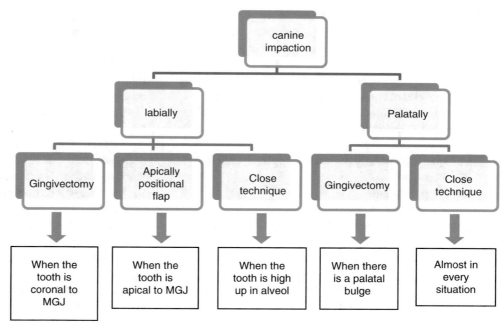

crown) [31]. The close technique can be used in labially impacted canine if the tooth is high up in the alveoli and almost in any situation in palatal impactions (Table 31.1) [32].

Clinical view of using the close technique for labially impacted mandibular canine

Contrary to the close technique, in the open technique, whether there is a flap reflection or a window cut, the crown will stay exposed.

A window cut is called a gingivectomy, and a flap reflected on the apical side is called apically positioned flap (APF) [31].

The APF technique is used in labial impactions, and when the canine is placed apically to the mucogingival Junction (MGJ) but not that apically that it makes it hard for the surgeon to suture the flap [32].

Due to author's experience, in APF technique, after the flap is reflected and the radiographic images (panoramic or CBCT) are evaluated again, for removing the bone, first we use carbide round end bur (number 2) and surgical handpiece (1/1). After that, to expose the crown, the bone which is on the crown is removed near the Cementoenamel Junction (CEJ). To continue bone removal in a more conservative way, we change the bur to a small taper fissure.

After adequate crown exposure for placing the orthodontic buttons, we luxate the tooth by a small elevator for easier movement of the tooth.

Gingivectomy, or window technique which is the title of this chapter, is the easiest and least technique-sensitive method for canine exposure.

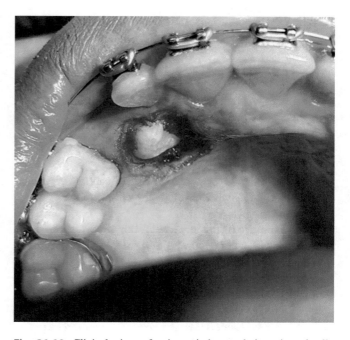

Fig. 31.10 Clinical view of using window technique in palatally impacted maxillary canine

Gingivectomy (Fig. 31.10) can be used in both buccal and palatal impactions of the canine but very special conditions especially when the canine is impacted buccally: The crown of the canine must be coronal to the MGJ, and significant amounts of bone must not cover the canine.

On the palate, if the tooth is identifiable by a bulge, a gingivectomy may be selected [32]. In both buccal and palatal impactions, gingivectomy technique requires the crown to be exposed by removing the overlying bone and gingiva from the crown. After exposure of the labial impacted crown, there should be a 2–3 mm band of keratinized gingiva [31].

In summary, the three basic techniques can be classified according to the labiopalatal location of the impacted canine:

- Techniques for buccally positioned impacted canines
- APF technique
- Closed flap technique
- Gingivectomy technique
- Techniques for palatally positioned impacted canines
- Closed flap technique
- Gingivectomy technique [32]

Although surgical exposure of impacted canines and orthodontic eruptions are the preferred option to achieve a suitable occlusal and esthetic result, they do carry some risks, and some conditions may endanger the success of orthodontic management [32].

When these conditions are present, the extraction of the impacted canine may be indicated. Such conditions include:

- Pathologic changes around the impacted tooth
- Ankylosis of the tooth
- Patient not willing to undergo orthodontic treatment
- Severe root dilaceration
- Severe lack of arch space
- Anatomic considerations (e.g., adjacent to the floor of the nose)
- First premolar in the position of the canine, even with good occlusion and well-aligned teeth [33]

After exposure of the impacted tooth, the overlying bone is removed with a bur or curette, and the follicle is minimally debrided to allow access to the tooth [31].

Homeostasis can be achieved using electrosurgery or by packing cotton pellets soaked in hemostatic agents around the exposed tooth [31]. Depending on the manufacturer's guidelines, the isolated tooth is then etched for the appropriate period of time and rinsed and dried, and the eruption device bonded to the tooth using a light-cured, acid-etch composite material.

Avoidance and Management of Intraoperative Complications

Apart from choosing the right technique for surgical exposure, the surgeon must consider several intraoperative details to obtain the best possible outcome.

1. Flap design. Inappropriate flap design does not prepare suitable access for the surgeon and can cause periodontal problems like loss of keratinized gingiva and attachment. In both labial and palatal impactions, sulcular or crestal incisions are recommended. Placing the incision in the unattached mucosa can make orthodontic chain cause clefting in the labial periodontium when pulling through the keratinized mucosa.
2. Appropriate homeostasis and isolation. Most bonding materials need the liquid to be controlled in the area of working when the bracket is being bonded. If it is ignored, the brackets will be debonded.
3. Tooth exposure. Almost two-thirds of the crown must be exposed to provide sufficient area for the orthodontic chain and bracket to be attached. The surgeon must be careful while removing the bone, not to damage the coronal structures. The surgeon also must be careful not to expose beyond two-thirds of the crown because it can cause external resorption [32].

All Surgeries Require Postoperative Considerations to End Well

We mentioned some of them below:

- Oral hygiene maintenance
- Postoperative pain
- Soft diet
- Surgical site infection
- Failure of the orthodontic bracket to bond to the tooth
- Long-term postoperative considerations
- Periodontal considerations (e.g., dehiscence of the flap, lack of attached gingiva)
- Failure to erupt
- Damage to roots of adjacent teeth
- Devitalization of the pulp [32]

Due to author's experience, after surgeries containing exposure, especially in the palatal aspect of the maxillary canine, the patient does not experience much pain and swelling, but we can reduce the pain by prescribing suitable painkillers before and after the surgery.

We can use routine painkillers, including NSAIDs, before and after the surgery. Using painkillers before the surgery might reduce the need for using painkillers after surgery. We usually prefer to use ibuprofen 400 mg before and after the surgery. Usually, there is no need for prophylaxis of antibiotics before the surgery, and if the surgery is done in a clean way, there is no need for prophylaxis after the surgery.

Conclusion

Impaction of canine is a manageable abnormality in which its treatment prognosis highly depends on localization and timing of the impacted tooth. Each of the open and close techniques has its own indications and should not be used instead of each other. It was found that surgery time is the same in both techniques, but the patient experiences more pain in the open technique. Complications were more severe in bilateral cases.

References

1. Biswas N, Biswas SH, Shahi AK. Maxillary impacted canine: diagnosis and contemporary Ortho surgical management guidelines. Inter J Sci Stud. 2016;3(10):166–70.
2. Vijayalakshmi R, Ramakrishnan T, Nisanth S. Surgical exposure of an impacted maxillary canine and increasing a band of keratinized gingiva. J Indian Soc Periodontol. 2009;13(3):164.
3. Manne R, Gandikota C, Juvvadi SR, Rama HR, Anche S. Impacted canines: etiology, diagnosis, and orthodontic management. J Pharm Bioallied Sci. 2012;4(Suppl 2):S234.
4. Bishara SE, Ortho D. Impacted maxillary canines: a review. Am J Orthod Dentofac Orthop. 1992;101(2):159–71.
5. Littlewood SJ, Mitchell L. An introduction to orthodontics. Oxford University Press; 2019.
6. Jacoby H. The etiology of maxillary canine impactions. Am J Orthod. 1983;84(2):125–32.
7. Richardson G, Russell KA. A review of impacted permanent maxillary cuspids-diagnosis and prevention. J Canadian Dent Assoc. 2000;66(9):497–502.
8. Becker A. The orthodontic treatment of impacted teeth, 2nd edt. London: Informa Healthcare UK Ltd.; 2007.
9. Peck S, Peck L, Kataja M. The palatally displaced canine as a dental anomaly of genetic origin. Angle Orthod. 1994;64(4):250–6.
10. Hsu YC, Kao CT, Chou CC, Tai WK, Yang PY. Diagnosis and management of impacted maxillary canines. J Orthod Repub China. 2019;31(1):4–11.
11. Alqerban A, Jacobs R, Lambrechts P, Loozen G, Willems G. Root resorption of the maxillary lateral incisor caused by impacted canine: a literature review. Clin Oral Investig. 2009;13(3):247–55.
12. Maverna R, Gracco A. Different diagnostic tools for the localization of impacted maxillary canines: clinical considerations. Prog Orthod. 2007;8(1):28–44.
13. Bishara SE, Ortho D. Impacted maxillary canines: a review. Am J Orthod Dentofac Orthop. 1992;101(2):159–71.
14. Chaushu S, Kaczor-Urbanowicz K, Zadurska M, Becker A. Predisposing factors for severe incisor root resorption associated with impacted maxillary canines. Am J Orthod Dentofac Orthop. 2015;147(1):52–60.
15. Jacobs SG. The impacted maxillary canine. Further observations on aetiology, radiographic localization, prevention/intercep-

tion of impaction, and when to suspect impaction. Aust Dent J. 1996;41(5):310–6.
16. Bedoya MM, Park JH. A review of the diagnosis and management of impacted maxillary canines. J Am Dent Assoc. 2009;140(12):1485–93.
17. Alqerban A, Jacobs R, van Keirsbilck P-J, Aly M, Swinnen S, Fieuws S, et al. The effect of using CBCT in the diagnosis of canine impaction and its impact on the orthodontic treatment outcome. J Orthod Sci. 2014;3(2):34–40.
18. De Grauwe A, Ayaz I, Shujaat S, Dimitrov S, Gbadegbegnon L, Vande Vannet B, et al. CBCT in orthodontics: a systematic review on justification of CBCT in a paediatric population prior to orthodontic treatment. Eur J Orthod. 2019;41(4):381–9.
19. Chauhan D, Datana S, Agarwal SS, Vishvaroop VG. Development of difficulty index for management of impacted maxillary canine: a CBCT-based study. Med J Armed Forces India. 2020.
20. Faber J, Berto PM, Quaresma M. Rapid prototyping as a tool for diagnosis and treatment planning for maxillary canine impaction. Am J Orthod Dentofac Orthop. 2006;129(4):583–9.
21. Ericson S, Kurol J. Early treatment of palatally erupting maxillary canines by extraction of the primary canines. Eur J Orthod. 1988;10(4):283–95.
22. Warford JH Jr, Grandhi RK, Tira DE. Prediction of maxillary canine impaction using sectors and angular measurement. Am J Orthod Dentofac Orthop. 2003;124(6):651–5.
23. Lindauer SJ, Rubenstein LK, Hang WM, Andersen WC, Isaacson RJ. Canine impaction identified early with panoramic radiographs. J Am Dent Assoc. 1992;123(3):91–2.
24. Margot R, Maria CDLP, Ali A, Annouschka L, Anna V, Guy W. Prediction of maxillary canine impaction based on panoramic radiographs. Clin Exper Dent Res. 2020;6(1):44–50.
25. Alqerban A, Jacobs R, Fieuws S, Willems G. Radiographic predictors for maxillary canine impaction. Am J Orthod Dentofac Orthop. 2015;147(3):345–54.
26. Schindel RH, Sheinis MR. Prediction of maxillary lateral-incisor root resorption using sector analysis of potentially impacted canines. J Clin Orthod. 2013;47(8):490–3.
27. Chaushu S, Chaushu G, Becker A. The use of panoramic radiographs to localize displaced maxillary canines. Oral Surg Oral Med Oral Pathol Oral Radiol Endodontol. 1999;88(4):511–6.
28. Katsnelson A, Flick WG, Susarla S, Tartakovsky JV, Miloro M. Use of panoramic x-ray to determine position of impacted maxillary canines. J Oral Maxillofac Surg. 2010;68(5):996–1000.
29. Nagpal A, Pai KM, Setty S, Sharma G. Localization of impacted maxillary canines using panoramic radiography. J Oral Sci. 2009;51(1):37–45.
30. Warford JH Jr, Grandhi RK, Tira DE. Prediction of maxillary canine impaction using sectors and angular measurement. Am J Orthod Dentofac Orthop. 2003;124(6):651–5.
31. Beadnell SW. Management of the impacted canine. Curr therapy Oral Maxillofac Surg. 2012;1:135–45.
32. Kademani D, Tiwana P. Atlas of oral and maxillofacial surgery. Elsevier Health Sciences; 2015.
33. Bishara SE. Clinical management of impacted maxillary canines. Semi Orthod. 1998;4(2):87–98. WB Saunders.

Principles of Endodontic Surgery Combined with CAD/CAM Technology

32

Francesc Abella Sans and Ahmed Seyam

Introduction

Endodontic surgery is a procedure to treat apical periodontitis in non-healed endodontically treated teeth by removing the root end of the affected tooth and placing a root-end filling material as an apical seal. This procedure consists of eliminating bacterial organisms and necrotic tissues, which persist in the root canal system and result in apical periodontitis (AP). Moreover, it eliminates persistent bacteria in apical deltas, isthmuses, and canal irregularities.

Apical periodontitis (AP) is defined as an inflammatory lesion in the periradicular tissues that could result from infection of the dental pulp and physical and iatrogenic trauma. Although nonsurgical root canal retreatment is an excellent option with a high success rate, this technique is not flawless and could fail in cases of extraradicular infections, presence of cholesterol crystals, true cysts, or foreign body reactions. In these situations, the clinician should consider endodontic surgery or, in some specific cases, an intentional replantation.

Endodontic surgery was introduced in the mid-800 s when the success rate of traditional endodontic surgery was much lower than at present. Following the operating microscope's introduction, micro-instruments, ultrasonic instruments, and more biocompatible materials, the success rate increased substantially. In 2010, Setzer et al. published a meta-analysis and systematic review. They reported a statistically significant difference in success rates between traditional endodontic surgery and modern endodontic microsurgery (59% vs. 94%, respectively). The relative risk ratio showed that the probability of success for modern endodontic microsurgery was 1.58 times the probability of success for traditional endodontic surgery [1]. Table 32.1 shows

Table 32.1 Comparison between traditional endodontic surgery and modern endodontic surgery

	Traditional endodontic surgery	Modern endodontic surgery
Magnification	Without a microscope	With a microscope
Bone access armamentarium	Standard surgical bur	Bone cutting bur or piezosurgery
Size of osteotomy	Large	Small
Instruments	Large instruments	Small instruments
Bevel angle	Acute with a 45° bevel	0–10° bevel angle
Root-end preparation	With bur	With an ultrasonic tip
The direction of cavity preparation	Off angle	Aligned
Root-end filling material	Amalgam	Biocompatible materials

the principle differences between traditional and modern endodontic surgery.

Cone-beam computed tomography (CBCT) is a valuable diagnostic aid that plays an essential role in planning endodontic surgery. CBCT imaging has various advantages over conventional radiographs as it provides the clinician with a clear view of three-dimensional (3D) objects to show the relationship between the root tips and adjacent vital structures in the maxillary sinus, mandibular nerve, and mental foramen. This radiographic system also eliminates the superimposition of anatomic structures, such as the zygomatic bone and alveolar bone. Moreover, CBCT is particularly useful in detecting early periradicular lesions that do not appear in conventional two-dimensional (2D) radiographs, such as the presence of fenestrations, cortical bone plate thickness, and the actual size and extent of these lesions.

F. A. Sans (✉) · A. Seyam
Department of Endodontics, Universitat Internacional de Catalunya, Sant Cugat del Vallès, Barcelona, Spain
e-mail: franabella@uic.es

© The Author(s), under exclusive license to Springer Nature Switzerland AG 2021
M. R. Stevens et al. (eds.), *Innovative Perspectives in Oral and Maxillofacial Surgery*,
https://doi.org/10.1007/978-3-030-75750-2_32

Indications of Endodontic Surgery

The decision to treat a case surgically or nonsurgically is always challenging for the clinician. The first and most important step in making a treatment decision is to determine the persisting periradicular lesion's main cause. The following points can be used as a guide when considering endodontic surgery:

1. **Pre-treatment condition**: In general, when managing an infected tooth with an adequate root canal filling without a missed canal and there is a well-adapted coronal seal, the clinician could consider endodontic surgery. Figure 32.1

shows a large periradicular lesion with an adequate root canal filling and coronal seal. On the other hand, when managing a tooth with a poor quality root canal filling and coronal restoration, the clinician should always consider nonsurgical retreatment.

2. **Presence of post:** When removing a coronal restoration, such as a well-adapted crown with a large custom-made post, is impractical as in (Fig. 32.2), endodontic surgery becomes a viable alternative.

3. **Technical difficulties:** Complications arising from root canal treatment failures caused by blocked canals, irretrievable separated file in the apical third, nonnegotiable

Fig. 32.1 (**a**) Clinical image showing a sinus tract in tooth #21. (**b**) Initial periapical radiograph showing a large periradicular lesion in tooth #21 and #22. (**c**) Osteotomy and removal of granulation tissue. (**d**) Root-end resection of the apical part of both infected teeth. (**e**) Periapical radiograph at 3-year follow-up showing healing without the need of performing any guided tissue/bone regeneration

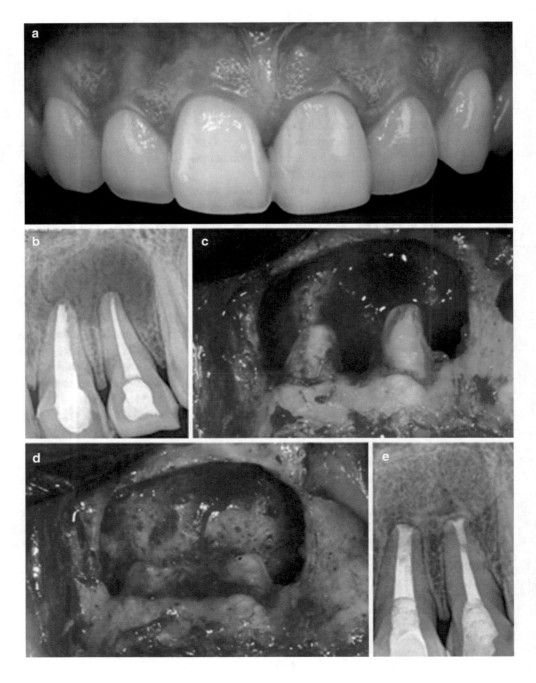

Fig. 32.2 Endodontic surgery was performed after failure of nonsurgical retreatment because post removal was impractical. (**a**) Initial radiograph of tooth #21 with a large custom-made post. (**b**) Submarginal incision was made to preserve the crown margins. (**c** and **d**) Treatment planning using CBCT and digital guides. (**e** and **f**) Bone access and root-end resection using a trephine bur with a digitally guided template. (**g**) Root-end filling material (MTA). (**h**) Postoperative radiograph

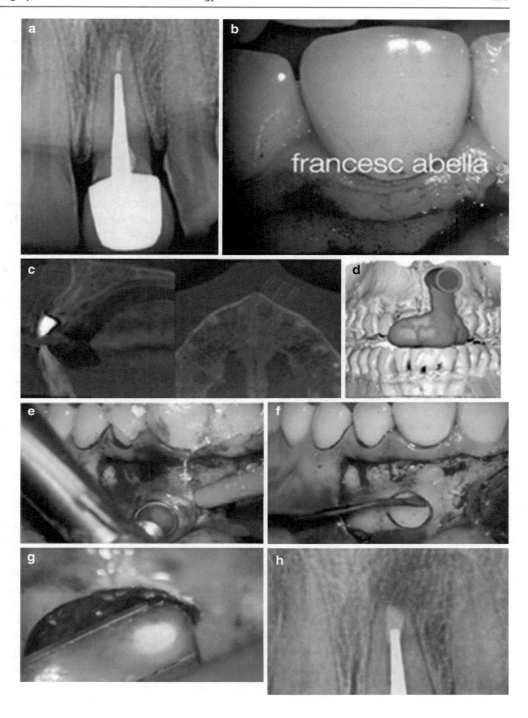

ledges, hard cement filling material, apical transportation, and extremely calcified canal.

4. When **extraradicular infection** cannot be treated with a nonsurgical endodontic approach, the clinician should resort to surgical intervention. Additionally, endodontic surgery is helpful in **histological examinations** when a biopsy is required.

5. **Exploration for vertical root fracture:** Detecting the presence of vertical root fracture using an exploratory flap technique. Although CBCT is a noninvasive technique to detect vertical root fractures, there are some factors that may obscure the fracture line, such as the artifacts caused by the gutta-percha, the size and direction of the fracture line, and also the quality of the CBCT scan.

Contraindications

The clinician should consider the following factors before considering endodontic surgery:

1. **Patient-related factors:** Certain diseases may hamper endodontic surgery, such as heart disease, (infective endocarditis and rheumatic fever), respiratory diseases (chronic bronchitis), hematological disorders (hemophilia A or von Willebrand's disease), and endocrine disorders such as uncontrolled diabetes.
2. **Anatomical factors:** Periradicular lesions that are in close proximity or in contact with vital structures, such as maxillary sinus, mental bundle, mandibular canal, and palatine neurovascular bundle, may complicate the procedure and result in further damages. Moreover, infection of the palatal root will complicate surgery, due to the thickness of the palatal tissues and the greater palatine artery, which may be severed during flap elevation. Moreover, the external oblique ridge in the mandible, combined with lingually oriented infected root tips, encumbers access.
3. **Periodontal factors:** Teeth with poor stability and a crown root ratio of less than (1:1), or whose proportion may be affected, are not candidates for endodontic surgery.
4. **Uncooperative patients**: Patients who are not motivated or do not want to invest in this type of surgery to save a tooth.

Factors Affecting the Outcome of Endodontic Surgery

1. **Magnification and root-end filling material:** Under high magnification and illumination of the operating microscope, detection of root canal irregularities, microcracks, isthmus, and lateral canals has become more productive and effective. In addition, operating microscopes compared with magnifying loupes showed significantly better outcomes [2]. Therefore, it is impossible to perform a high-quality and predictable treatment without using a microscope.

A recent meta-analysis that evaluated different factors that may affect the success rate of endodontic surgery reported that mineral trioxide aggregate (MTA) was significantly associated with better treatment outcomes than with other retro-filling materials such as intermediate restorative material (IRM) and ethoxy benzoic acid (Super EBA) [3]. Recently developed and new bioceramic materials are promising for endodontic surgery, although there is less scientifically based evidence for these materials than there is for MTA.

2. **Gender and tooth type:** Most studies have concluded that female patients have better healing outcomes. Regarding tooth type, these studies reported that anterior teeth, which might be easier to access, have shown higher success rates than in the posterior teeth [4].
3. **Lesion type and bone defect dimensions:** Periodontally involved lesions >4 mm have an adverse effect on the outcome. Song et al. (2013) assessed the influence of bone defects on the outcome of endodontic microsurgery. They concluded that teeth with a buccal bone plate higher than 3 mm presented higher success rates than teeth with a buccal bone plate less than 3 mm in height (94.3% vs. 68.8%, respectively). Tellingly, marginal bone loss was not a significant prognostic factor in the outcome [5].

Technique

Before endodontic surgery, the clinician must perform a comprehensive clinical and radiographic examination. CBCT imaging should be the standard tool for endodontic evaluation and treatment planning. However, the European Society of Endodontology (ESE) position statement recommends that CBCT be used only in complicated cases of endodontic surgery [6]. In contrast, the authors of this chapter recommend using the CBCT in almost all cases because it is hard to predict the difficulty of a case from a surgical point of view.

The choice of the anesthetic solution in endodontic surgery is controversial. Local anesthesia with a vasoconstrictor (for instance, epinephrine 1:50.000 and lidocaine 2%) achieves localized hemostasis, which provides the clinician with a clearer surgical field. Regardless of the injection technique used, infiltration is mandatory to achieve hemostasis. If the patient has a severe cardiovascular disorder, the clinician is required to consult the patient's physician before the administration of anesthesia for endodontic surgery. In order to provide enough time for hemostasis to occur, local anesthesia with a vasoconstrictor should be administered at least 20–30 minutes before flap elevation.

A number of factors, such as the width of the attached gingiva, blood supply, muscle attachments, bony prominence, and crown margins, determine the flap design, which is divided into:

1. Full mucoperiosteal:
   A. Horizontal flap: without vertical releasing incision
   B. Triangular flap: one vertical releasing incision
   C. Rectangular flap: two vertical releasing incisions
   D. Trapezoidal flap: two diverging vertical releasing incisions
2. Limited mucoperiosteal:
   A. Semilunar incision (no longer used because it decreases vascularization, delays healing, hampers reapproximation and suturing, and provides a limited surgical field).
   B. Submarginal incision: This incision is made within the attached gingiva parallel to the gingiva's marginal contour.
   C. Papilla base incision: This technique consisted of two releasing vertical incisions, connected by the papilla base incision and intracellular incision (Fig. 32.3).

Surgical Access

Hard Tissue Access: Osteotomy

After flap elevation, accessing the root tip becomes easier in cases of the non-intact cortical plate (e.g., bone fenestration). If the cortical plate is intact, bone removal can be performed by using piezosurgery or digitally guided splints or with a surgical handpiece with rear air exhaust to avoid emphysema or air embolism. Bone removal is prepared by gently brushing the bone with a surgical handpiece and a coolant to avoid high temperatures (47 to 50 °C), which could cause bone necrosis and irreversible cellular damage. Surgical carbide burs should be preferred over diamond burs because diamond burs can clog with the residual bone tissues and overheat the bone.

The main advantage of piezosurgery is selective cutting, as it cuts only mineralized tissues such as tooth and bone while preserving other vital structures such as blood vessels, nerves, and mucosa. Piezosurgery instruments provide optimal visibility of the surgical site and reduce noise and vibration for patient comfort. These tips work linearly, which provides precise and safe osteotomies. Furthermore, piezosurgery technology also allows for an air-water cavitation effect and constant irrigation, ensuring a clear surgical site. However, the clinician must be aware that despite the latest advances in this technology, piezosurgery may make the procedure longer.

Piezoelectric surgery could currently be used in most stages of endodontic surgery (osteotomy, root-end resection, and root-end preparation) as well as in the enucleation of radicular cysts. Little research has been conducted on the effect of piezosurgery on root-end resection [7].

Localizedhemostasis

One of the keys to successful endodontic surgery is to control bleeding, which should be managed from start to end. Wherever possible, removal of granulation tissues must be taken into account since it enhances bleeding control. Besides, various topical hemostatic agents can be used when bleeding cannot be controlled. These agents are divided into:

1. Chemical agents: epinephrine, ferric sulfate, and aluminum chloride
   A. Epinephrine pellets: Epinephrine cotton pellets are packed into the osteotomy site, and pressure is applied for 2–3 minutes. Then, the pellets are removed one by one, leaving the last one in the bony crypt to maintain hemostasis and avoid reopening the ruptured vessels. In this case, the last epinephrine pellet should be removed before the closure of the surgical site.
   B. Ferric sulfate: Ferric sulfate (e.g., Stasis®) is an excellent hemostatic agent that agglutinates blood proteins to occlude capillary orifices. This agent can be easily applied and removed from the crypt. Ferric sulfate must be thoroughly removed before the closure of the surgical site to avoid bone damage and speed up healing.
   C. Aluminum chloride: This paste is normally used for gingival retraction. However, Von Arx et al. (2006), introducing aluminum chloride (e.g. Expasyl) to secure hemostasis in endodontic surgery, concluded that Expasyl alone or combined with Stasis® appears to be the most efficient agent to control bleeding within the bony defects created in a rabbit calvarium model [8].

Fig. 32.3 A 38-year-old female came to our clinic with a symptomatic apical periodontitis associated with tooth #21. (**a** and **f**) Initial situation. (**b**) Papilla base incision. (**c**) Removal of granulation tissue and osteotomy. (**d**) Root-end preparation using piezosurgery. (**e**) Granulation tissue. (**g**) Post-operative radiograph. (**h**) Periapical radiograph taken at 9 months posttreatment. Collagen membrane was used without guided tissue regeneration

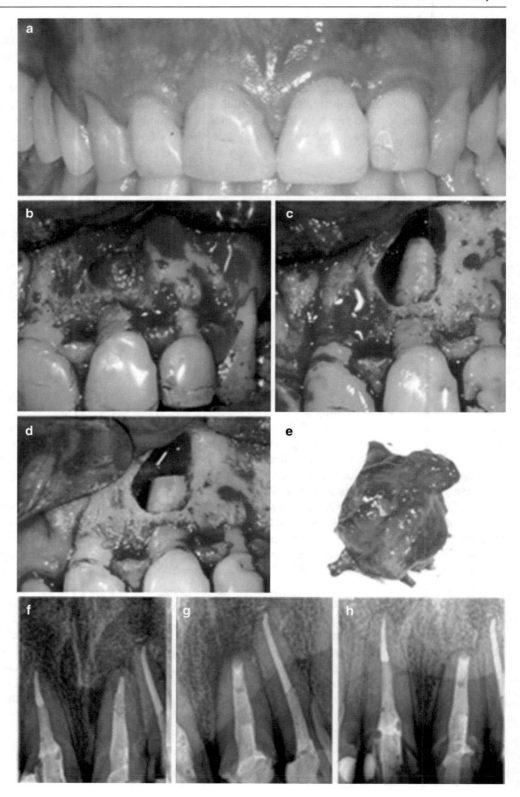

2. Mechanical agents: Bone wax, calcium sulfate, polytetra-fluoroethylene (PTFE)

PTFE is an innocuous material that exerts a mechanical hemostatic barrier effect. PTFE strips are used as an adjunct to epinephrine-impregnated gauze. They leave no hemostatic material traces that might impair postoperative healing and offer a synergistic effect on bleeding control during endodontic surgery.

3. **Biological agents**: Thrombin
4. **Absorbable hemostatic agents**: Gelfoam, Surgicel, calcium sulfate, Surgiplast

Root-End Resection

Aims of root-end resection:

1. Removal of anatomic variations in the apical third, such as apical lateral canals, apical deltas, and calcification. Approximately 75% of teeth have canal aberrations (e.g., accessory or lateral canals) in the apical 3 mm of the tooth [9].
2. Removal of pathological lesions, such as uncleansable contaminated apex, isthmus tissues, fractured root end, and foreign materials such as extruded gutta-percha or a separated file.
3. Creation of apical seal to create an environment conducive to periodontal regeneration.

Angle of Root-End Resection

Traditionally, root-end resection was performed at a 45° angle. Nevertheless, this long bevel technique has some disadvantages, as it removes more root structure, exposes more dentinal tubules, and increases the probability of overlooking important palatal or lingual anatomy, such as lateral canals. The advent of magnification and illumination in endodontic microsurgery has eliminated the concept of bevelling, which is now reduced to 0–10° (Fig. 32.4), which predictably meets the following important criteria:

1. Greater encroachment of the lingual root surface and inclusion of all apical ramifications
2. Shorter cavosurface margin, resulting in a greater better sealing ability

3. Less possibility of incomplete resection
4. Easier root-end resection and easier isthmus preparation
5. Less exposure of dentinal tubules
6. Even distribution of forces in the apical area reduces the likelihood of vertical root fracture

There are different types of instruments to perform root-end resection, such as diamond burs, tungsten carbide burs, and ultrasonic tips.

Root-End Preparation

The concept of microsurgery has revolutionized root-end preparation to an unprecedented extent. Historically, root-end preparation (REP) was performed using burs that could perforate the lingual surface. Thus, with the introduction of ultrasonic instrumentation, it is now possible to carry out this technique parallel to the tooth's long axis and make a proper apical seal (Fig. 32.5). The ideal root-end preparation should measure at least 3 mm in depth and should be performed using ultrasonic or piezosurgery tips. The advantages over the bur preparation technique include less smear layer, deeper cavity preparation to include ramification in the apical part, smaller osteotomy size, and lower risk of perforation of the root's lingual surface.

Ultrasonic or piezosurgery tips are available in various types, lengths, and diameters. They can be coated (diamond coated, or zirconium nitride coated) or non-coated. Coated ultrasonic tips improve cutting efficiency and are faster than non-coated tips in root-end preparations, but the coated type produces more smear layers.

The key to a successful root-end resection and preparation is to apply little pressure over the tip while sufficiently irritating it. Wherever possible, the clinician should always prepare all the non-instrumented areas, such as the isthmus area, which contains contaminated pulp tissues. After completion of the root-end preparation, the cavity could be rinsed with 17% EDTA to remove the smear layer and lastly with chlorhexidine (CHX) to remove bacterial infection.

Root-End Filling

The ideal root-end filling material should be dimensionally stable, provide proper sealing ability, induce regeneration of periodontal ligament, and provoke cementogenesis. In addition, this material should be noncarcinogenic, biocompati-

Fig. 32.4 A patient came to our clinic with a chief complaint of pain on biting. (**a**) Preoperative periapical radiograph of tooth #16 with large periradicular lesion on the mesial root. (**b**) Bone removal using piezosurgery. (**c**) Root-end resection was performed at 0–10° to eliminate apical ramifications. (**d**) Postoperative radiograph and MTA- filled mesial root. (**e**) Radiograph showing healing at 5-year follow-up

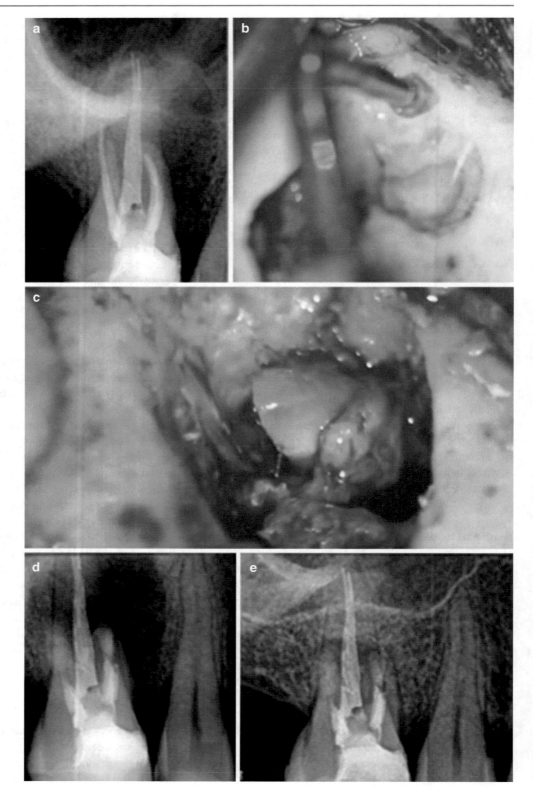

Fig. 32.5 Male patient came to our clinic with a sinus tract and failure of the previous root canal treatment. (**a**) Clinical image of tooth #46 showing submarginal incision. (**b**) Preoperative periapical radiograph showing apical periodontitis in the mesial root. (**c**) Axial view of CBCT indicating a periradicular lesion perforating the buccal cortical plate. (**d** and **e**) Postoperative radiograph showing the healing process at 2-year follow-up. (**f**) Root-end preparation using ultrasonic tips parallel to the long axis of the root

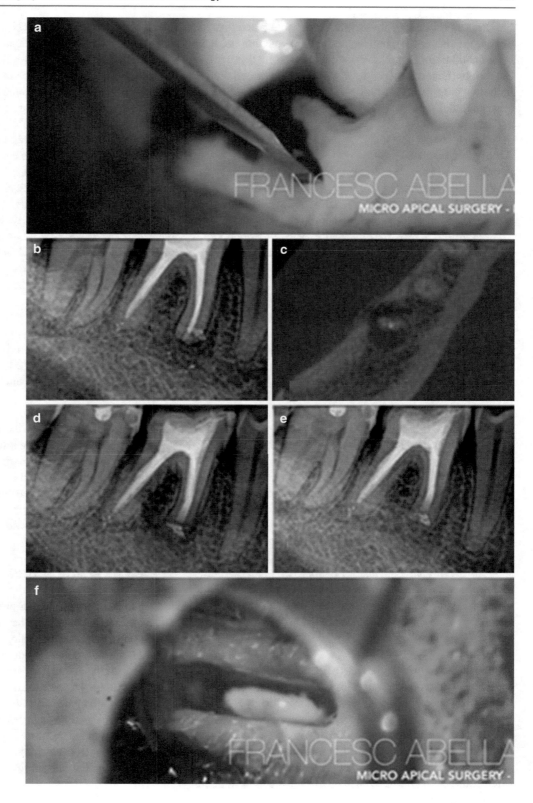

ble, insoluble in tissue fluids, non-resorbable, bacteriostatic or bactericidal, easy to handle, and radiopaque, not not have stain dental tissues, and have a sufficient setting time.

Various materials have been used as a root-end filling, including amalgam, zinc oxide-eugenol (intermediate restorative material and Super-EBA), glass ionomer, composite, and MTA.

Amalgam

Amalgam is no longer used as a root-end filling, mainly due to corrosion resulting in tissue argyria (i.e., amalgam tattoo in the adjacent tissues), its low sealing ability, and failure to induce periodontal ligament regeneration.

In addition, it provokes thermal expansion, which could result in microcracks and leads to failure of the treatment.

Zinc Oxide-Eugenol (ZOE) Cement

ZOE is available in two forms: intermediate restorative material (IRM) and Super-EBA.

Both IRM and Super-EBA have the same favorable properties and are better than amalgam. The main difference between the two is that Super-EBA has a lower amount of eugenol (37.5% eugenol), which causes tissue irritation, and contains ethoxy benzoic acid, which enhances the setting time and strength of basic ZOE cement. Both IRM and Super-EBA are biologically tolerated in the periradicular tissues. However, they have a limited antibacterial effect.

Compomers

Dyract and Geristore are examples of resin-modified glass ionomers. Dyract is a light-cured material, whereas Geristore is a dual-cured material. The seal and marginal adaptation of light-cured glass ionomer cement (GIC) are superior to dual-cured GIC. Dyract and Geristore are shown to be equal or superior to IRM and equivalent to Super-EBA in their ability to reduce apical leakage when used as a root-end filling material [10]. However, contamination with blood may adversely affect the outcome when GIC is used as a REF.

Composite

Composite resin, which has an excellent sealing ability under complete isolation, is superior to amalgam, GIC, and IRM. However, blood contamination during bonding adversely affects its strength and sealing ability. Thus, the composite resin is not recommended for use as a root-end filling material because it is difficult to isolate during endodontic surgery. Composite is a good alternative to be used when complete isolation is easily achieved, such as in intentional replantation.

Mineral Trioxide Aggregate (MTA)

MTA was originally developed from Portland cement by Dr. Torabinejad in 1993 and appeared in the market in 1999 as grey MTA (Pro Root MTA, Dentsply Tulsa Dental Specialties, Johnson City, TN). The main components of grey MTA are tricalcium silicate, tricalcium aluminate, tricalcium oxide, silicate oxide, mineral oxide, and bismuth oxide. Later, the white version of MTA (Angelus MTA, Londrina, Brazil) was introduced to Brazil in 2001. White MTA mainly differs from grey MTA in the absence of iron, which causes discoloration.

MTA is currently considered the gold standard material in endodontic surgery. Given its excellent sealing ability when the proper setting is achieved, this material induces cementoblasts to produce hard tissues. In addition, this MTA shows excellent biocompatibility and bioactivity. A recent meta-analysis reported that MTA was generally associated with better clinical outcomes (90.8% success) compared with other materials such as IRM and Super EBA [3]. (Seung Baek et al. 2010), in a study on periradicular tissues in dogs, reported that MTA showed the most favorable periradicular tissue response. The distance between the MTA and the regenerated bone was similar to that of the average periodontal ligament thickness in dogs [11]. In spite of the outstanding performance of this material, it has some drawbacks, including long setting time (2 hours and 45 minutes), difficult handling, discoloration, and high cost.

Bioceramics

With the aim of overcoming the aforementioned drawbacks and limitations of MTA, new bioactive materials have been developed that stand out for their shorter setting time, easier handling and application, and low cost.

Studies concluded that there are no significant differences between MTA and bioceramics in relation to biocompatibility, antibacterial effect, and sealing ability.

Regenerative Procedures

Endodontic surgery has a poor prognosis in cases with loss of cortical bone plate overlying the root (for example, endo/perio lesions with the communication). In general, when a periodontal defect or denuded root or dehiscence is encountered while performing endodontic surgery, guided tissue regeneration could be implemented. Some studies have reported that periodontally affected teeth and cases with a complicated osteotomy (through and through lesions) could benefit from the application of guided tissue regeneration (GTR) in three ways: higher success rate, accelerated healing process, and non-epithelial migration into the surgical site.

Guided Endodontic Surgery

In 1991, Duet and Preston demonstrated the first dental application of computer-aided design and computer-aided manufacturing (CAD/CAM) technology by introducing a

Fig. 32.6 Step by step in design and production of a 3D printed or milled object

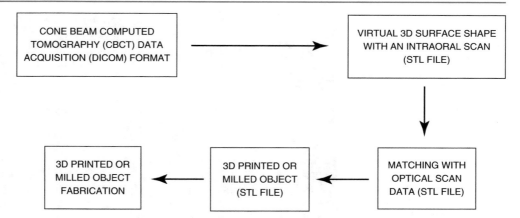

subtractive fabrication-milling machine to realize fixed restorations [12]. Since then, the number of these applications has increased considerably, benefiting the field of endodontics. All CAD/CAM applications involve three steps: digital data acquisition using a CBCT and/or intraoral scanner, data processing and design within a software application, and fabrication by milling or printing (Fig. 32.6).

Over the years, it has been possible to verify the benefit of using 3D printed objects in the different dental disciplines, both in teaching and in managing certain procedures. The field of endodontics is no exception to this, and 3D objects through adequate digital planning allow simpler, minimally invasive, precise treatments that are shorter and, especially, more comfortable for the patient [13].

The main factors that affect the prognosis of endodontic surgery are the type of lesion, the retro-filling material used, and the state of the coronal restoration. To all this, the position of the affected teeth must be taken into account, since various studies have concluded that the mandibular molars have the worst outcome, mainly due to their difficult access (thick cortical bone) and different anatomical obstacles (mental foramen or nerve inferior alveolar). Another factor to consider is the degree of bone destruction at the periapical level since the extent of the osteotomy performed to reach the lesion is associated with the degree of postoperative complications such as pain and swelling. Furthermore, (Gutmann and Harrison 1985) described the extent of the osteotomy tends to increase in cases with an intact buccal cortical plate because the exact location of the affected apex is difficult to locate [14]. Therefore, the objective is to direct the osteotomy in a way that allows the extraction of the last millimeters of the affected apices with the greatest possible precision,

a goal that is extremely difficult to achieve solely by mental navigation.

In this sense, CBCT is considered essential before performing a surgical procedure of these characteristics. Although CBCT is very useful and has an approximate 1: 1 ratio, controlling the procedure depends on the precision with which each clinician can orient themselves three-dimensionally with respect to the corresponding structures' real situation. The problem is that this step is not predictable and continues to leave considerable room for error. More and better aids have been sought to try to solve this phase of endodontic surgery in recent years.

In 2007, Pinsky et al. were the first to design and manufacture CAD/CAM surgical guides for the application of endodontic surgery. When comparing the location of the apices between the guided and the freehand system, they found that the former was significantly superior [15]. In recent years, particularly thanks to the evolution of 3D printing, there has been a renewed interest in surgical guides (templates) for endodontic surgery. The first case that can be considered a truly guided case of endodontic surgery was described in 2018 by Giacomino et al., in which three clinical cases used trephines to perform both the osteotomy and the resection of the root end [15] Fig. 32.7 shows an AP in both the mesial and distal roots, treated with digitally guided endodontic surgery and trephine.

In summary, guided endodontic surgery based on splints (templates) is being recognized as one additional option for these procedures, but it is clear that studies further validating the technique are still lacking. An alternative to take into account in these design and manufacturing processes is the use of a dynamic navigation system, which has a high degree of precision.

Fig. 32.7 A 45-year-old male came to our clinic with a symptomatic apical periodontitis associated with tooth #46. (**a** and **b**) Preoperative radiographs indicating two separated periradicular lesions in both the mesial and distal roots of tooth #46. (**c**) Digital design of the template. (**d**) Trephine was used to perform osteotomy and root-end resection. (**e**) Root-end preparation using ultrasonic tips. (**f**) Root end was filled with MTA material. (**g**) S conservative trephine osteotomy was performed. (**h**) Postoperative radiograph of the outcome

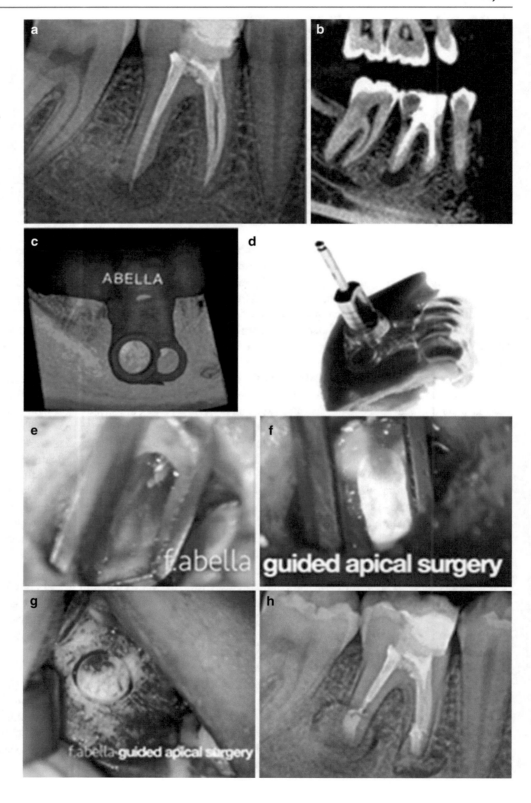

References

1. Setzer FC, Shah SB, Kohli MR, Karabucak B, Kim S. Outcome of endodontic surgery: a meta-analysis of the literature—part 1: comparison of traditional root-end surgery and endodontic microsurgery. J Endod. 2010;36(11):1757–65.

2. Tsesis I, Rosen E, Taschieri S, Strauss YT, Ceresoli V, Del Fabbro M. Outcomes of surgical endodontic treatment performed by a modern technique: an updated meta-analysis of the literature. J Endod. 2013;39(3):332–9.

3. Song M, Jung IY, Lee SJ, Lee CY, Kim E. Prognostic factors for clinical outcomes in endodontic microsurgery: a retrospective study. J Endod. 2011;37(7):927–33.

4. Song M, Kim SG, Shin SJ, Kim HC, Kim E. The influence of bone tissue deficiency on the outcome of endodontic microsurgery: a prospective study. J Endod. 2013;39(11):1341–5.

5. Patel S, Durack C, Abella F, Roig M, Shemesh H, Lambrechts P, Lemberg K. European Society of Endodontology position statement: the use of CBCT in endodontics. Int Endod J. 2014;47(6):502–4.

6. Abella F, de Ribot J, Doria G, Duran-Sindreu F, Roig M. Applications of piezoelectric surgery in endodontic surgery: a literature review. J Endod. 2014;40(3):325–32.

7. Von Arx T, Jensen SS, Hänni S, Schenk RK. Haemostatic agents used in periradicular surgery: an experimental study of their efficacy and tissue reactions. Int Endod J. 2006;39(10):800–8.

8. De Deus QD. Frequency, location, and direction of the lateral, secondary, and accessory canals. J Endod. 1975;1(11):361.

9. Greer BD, West LA, Liewehr FR, Pashley DH. Sealing ability of Dyract, Geristore, IRM, and super-EBA as root-end filling materials. J Endod. 2001;27(7):441–3.

10. Baek SH, Lee WC, Setzer FC, Kim S. Periapical bone regeneration after endodontic microsurgery with three different root-end filling materials: amalgam, SuperEBA, and mineral trioxide aggregate. J Endod. 2010;36(8):1323–5.

11. Duret F, Preston JD. CAD/CAM imaging in dentistry. Curr Opin Dent. 1991;1(2):150–4.

12. Shah P, Chong BS. 3D imaging, 3D printing and 3D virtual planning in endodontics. Clin Oral Investig. 2018;22:641–54.

13. Gutmann JL, Harrison JW. Posterior endodontic surgery: anatomical considerations and clinical techniques. Int Endod J. 1985;18:8–34.

14. Pinsky HM, Champleboux G, Sarment DP. Periapical surgery using CAD/CAM guidance: preclinical results. J Endod. 2007;33:148–51.

15. Giacomino CM, Ray JJ, Wealleans JA. Targeted endodontic microsurgery: a novel approach to anatomically challenging scenarios using 3-dimensional-printed guides and trephine burs- a report of 3 cases. J Endod. 2018;44:671–7.

Posterior Iliac Crest Harvest

33

Mark R. Stevens and Chris Ibrahim

History

Bone grafting dates back to the prehistoric era. Paleopathologic research has records of surgical intervention of fractures and drilled skull defects that have shown a process of bone regeneration [1]. Previous evidence shows accounts of the primordial people treating bone fractures by realigning the parts perfectly and splinting. If the fracture repair was a failure they would insert a wooden stick into the medullary canal [2]. Prehistoric people known as the Khuritis in 2000 BC were amongst the first to use a piece of animal bone as a donor graft to a 7 mm defect in a skull secondary to injury. The cranium examined 1000 years later showed regrowth around the grafted bone, thus showing this individually survived after the implanting of xenograft [3, 4].

Indications and Contraindications

The posterior iliac crest is the preferred donor site when bone defects require between 40 and 120 ml of uncompressed autogenous cancellous marrow or when a large corticocancellous block up to 5x5cm is desired (Fig. 33.8). A combination of uncompressed autogenous cancellous marrow with corticocancellous block may also be used (Fig. 33.9). Common indications for posterior iliac crest harvest are for large defects usually in the maxillofacial area especially the mandible (Fig. 33.7). They are also useful when larger voids cannot be addressed by regional tissue-grafting techniques. The posterior iliac crest is especially helpful when there is a need for osteo-competent cells, such as fibrous fractures or osteotomy sites with large gaps. Frequently, the posterior iliac is utilized when there is a need for additional osseous structural stability within large traumatic or oncologic defects [5, 6].

Posterior iliac crest harvest is indicated for bony defects that range between four and twelve centimeters. Common examples that require planning posterior iliac crest grafts include hemi-maxillary defects, total alveolar ridge augmentation of the jaws, and mandibular defect greater than 6 cm large down-fractures, for edentulous Le Fort I [7].

Many advantages to a posterior iliac versus anterior iliac crest bone graft harvest are illustrated in Box 1. A major consideration when considering the harvest of the posterior ilium to that of the anterior ilium is additional operating time. The posterior iliac crest harvest requires on average a minimum of two additional hours. This is due to a prone position for surgical access. The table should also have a 210° of reverse hip flexion. The prone or lateral position will also delay the operation due to the fact that the harvest and reconstruction surgical teams cannot operate simultaneously. Further special attention is required in maintaining the endotracheal tube position when flipping the patient back and forth between supine and prone, as well as the redraping and maintenance of a strict sterile technique

---

Box 1

Advantages to posterior iliac crest bone graft harvest versus anterior iliac crest bone graft harvest [15]

Posterior approach
- Shorter surgical time
- Less blood loss
- Yield more bone
- Quicker return to ambulation
- Less seromas/hematoma
- Less subjective pain
- Less gait disturbance

M. R. Stevens (✉)
Department of Oral and Maxillofacial Surgery, Augusta University, Augusta, GA, USA
e-mail: MASTEVENS@augusta.edu

C. Ibrahim
Resident of Oral and Maxillofacial Surgery, Dental College of Georgia at Augusta University, Augusta, GA, USA
e-mail: Cibrahim@augusta.edu

© The Author(s), under exclusive license to Springer Nature Switzerland AG 2021
M. R. Stevens et al. (eds.), *Innovative Perspectives in Oral and Maxillofacial Surgery*,
https://doi.org/10.1007/978-3-030-75750-2_33

[6, 7]. Surgeons should also take into account and document the body mass index of a patient. There may be a need to adjust for ventilation needs upper arm and head positions, as well as the prevention of pressure spots in the pelvis and genitalia.

The contraindications are few, but patients with previous pelvic fractures, osteomyelitis, and local radiation to harvest site are not candidates for posterior iliac harvest. Relative contraindications should include current and past use of oral and intravenous bisphosphonates, history of chemotherapy, and long-term use of steroid or methotrexate. With respect to the surgical contraindications, the surgeon must include the risks that would not be unsuitable for general anesthesia [5–7].

Anatomy

The pelvic bone supports the spinal column and protects the abdominal organs. This unique skeletal apparatus consists of three relatively large bony structures, sacrum, coccyx, and bilateral anterolateral iliac bones. The ilium of the pelvic girdle individually is further divided into regions labeled the ilium, ischium, and pubis. All are separate bones during childhood and joined by the triradiate cartilage. During puberty, these structures fused together to form a single bony component. The ilium is suitable as a donor site for bone harvesting from its anterior and posterior regions.

The inferior iliac spine (AIIS) in a lateral view is the most anterior and inferior bony eminence. Superiorly on the iliac crest is the anterior superior iliac spine (ASIS). Posteriorly is the iliac crest that has a posterolateral prominence which forms the iliac tubercle and a site for bone harvest. The posterior ilium borders are the iliac crest superiorly, posterior superior iliac spine (PSIS) posteriorly, and the greater sciatic notch inferiorly. The posterior ilium is slightly concave on the lateral surface with three distinct ridges: the posterior, anterior, and inferior gluteal lines. These bony ridges signify the origin of the gluteus muscles [6].

The ilium is an extensive attachment site for the muscles that are involved in hip abduction. These muscles include the gluteus medius and gluteus minimus. The gluteus maximus also attaches to the ilium and is responsible for extension and lateral rotation of the hip joint as well as the upper fibers being involved in the abduction and lower fibers in adduction. The gluteus maximus is innervated by the inferior gluteal nerve, which is a branch of the sciatic plexus that derives

from L4 to S3. The lumbodorsal fascia is attached to the medial aspect of the posterior iliac crest. This fascia serves to bind down the extensor muscles of the vertebral column and divide them from the muscles connecting the vertebral column to the upper extremity [5–7].

The abdominal aorta artery bifurcates at the level of L5-S1 in which two common iliac artery vessels span ~4 cm and terminate in front of the sacroiliac joint. The common iliac artery then divides into the external and internal iliac arteries. The internal iliac artery is the major arterial supply of the pelvis and divides into the anterior and posterior division.

The superior gluteal artery (SGA) is a branch of the posterior division of the internal iliac artery. It reaches the gluteal region through the greater sciatic notch above the piriformis muscle. The SGA divides into superficial and deep branches. The superficial division enters between the gluteus maximus and medius. The deep division passes through the gluteus medius and minimus. The inferior gluteal artery is a branch of the anterior division of the internal iliac artery. It enters the pelvis through the greater sciatic notch below the piriformis muscle. It supplies the gluteus maximus and also gives rise to the sciatic artery and anastomotic branch. Important clinical facts about the superior gluteal artery are that the surgeon should be aware of its proximity when harvesting bone from the posterior iliac crest. Surgeons should avoid the sciatic notch since both the sciatic nerve and superior gluteal artery are contained within the notch. Thus, the landmark of PSIS should be identified. On average, the arterial supply of the gluteal muscles lies ~63 mm anterior-inferiorly from PSIS and ~ 37 mm inferior to a line drawn perpendicular to the vertical axis at the level of the PSIS.

The neurological structures that should be highlighted are the superior cluneal nerves which originate from L1-L3 and cross over the posterior iliac crest. These nerves supply sensory innervation to the superior two/thirds of the buttocks and are located on average ~ 68 mm anterosuperiorly from the PSIS (Box 2). Middle cluneal nerves originate from the S1-S3. This nerve is the sensory innervation into the medial buttocks. This nerve course the sacrum foramen laterally. Surgical awareness of excessive periods of retraction of the soft tissue may lead to either the superior or middle cluneal nerve dysthesia and or possible symptomatic neuromas [6]. Box 2 Illustrates a summary of the notable bones, nerves, fascia, muscles, and vessels that should be identifiable during a posterior iliac crest bone harvest.

Box 2

Notable Anatomy Associated with the Posterior Iliac Crest Bone Harvest [16]

<u>Bones</u>
- Pelvis
  – Ilium
     Posterior iliac crest
     Posterior tubercle
     Posterior superior iliac spine
     Greater sciatic notch

<u>Nerves</u>
- Superior cluneal n. (sensory to superior 2/3 of the buttocks)
- Middle cluneal n. (sensory to the middle of the buttocks)

<u>Fascia</u>
- Thoracolumbar fascia

<u>Muscles</u>
- Gluteus maximus m.
- Gluteus medius m.
- Gluteus minimus m.

<u>Vessels</u>
- Internal iliac artery
  – Anterior div.
     Inferior gluteal artery (supplies gluteus maximus)
  – Posterior div.
     Superior gluteal artery
     • Superficial branch (supplies gluteus maximus)
     • Deep branch (supplies gluteus medius, minimus)

Surgical Technique

The harvest is usually performed first to minimize repositioning time and the risk of surgical site contamination. The patient is placed in a prone jackknife position with the table flexed at 210 degrees with lateral decubitus to facilitate the approach. Appropriate padding to extremities with an extension of the arms lateral and superior with shoulders abducted 90 degrees. A roll can be placed to the anterior pelvic region to take weight and pressure off the anterior ilium, and a larger support roll can be placed under the anterior thighs to the pubic area [6].

Positioning of the patient is critical. Minimizing surgical time, displaying the identifying structures, such as the triangular tubercle for easier palpation, and reduction of blood loss due to reduction of the local venous pressure are all a result of good positioning [7].

When preparing and draping the surgical site, it is wise to include both of the posterior ilium sites even if bone harvesting is planned for only one site. Prepping a wider surgical site will help the surgeon have a reference of bodily orientation. Anatomical landmarks are palpated and marked with a surgical pen. Due to a large amount of soft tissue thickness,

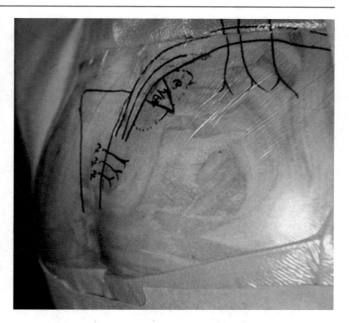

Fig. 33.1 The posterior iliac crest prepped and surgically marked with superior and middle cluneal nerves outlined [16]

structures often need to be reidentified by palpation and marked such as the posterior iliac crest, the posterior superior iliac spine (PSIS), and the midline of the sacrum [6].

Typically, lidocaine with 1:100,000 epinephrine is injected into the surgical site. A curvilinear incision is made approximately 6-8 cm in length illustrated in Fig. 33.1. The center of the incision should be made over the palpable triangular bony prominence and the origin of the gluteus maximus muscles. Doing so will also place the incision between the main sensory branches of the superior and middle cluneal nerves. The incision is carried through the dermis, subcutaneous tissue, variable amounts of fat, the thoracolumbar fascia, and finally the periosteum over the posterior iliac crest. Electrocautery is recommended for a sharp reflection of the gluteus maximus muscle due to its dense sharp fiber attachment. The reflection should be adequate enough to visualization of a 5x5-cm portion of the lateral cortex. Obtaining a graft larger than 5x5cm increases the risk of fracture [5]. Dissection should be at least 1 cm from the (PSIS) to avoid disturbing the sacroiliac ligament.

Prior to surgery, the surgeon has estimated the size and type of graft (cancellous, corticocancellous block for the reconstruction) [5]. It is recommended the harvest site outline be 1 cm lateral from PSIS, and not extended more than 5 cm inferior from the crest. The surgeon should direct the line so that is perpendicular to the crest rim to avoid undermining the PSIS. Box 3 illustrates average distances between PSIS and vital structures. A total of four cuts that follow the square outline is performed with a reciprocating saw fol-

Box 3

Distances between the posterior superior iliac spine (PSIS) and vital structures measured from six cadavers [10]

Measurement line	Average (mm)
PSIS, superior cluneal nerve	68.8
PSIS, gluteal line	26.6
PSIS, superior gluteal vessels	62.4

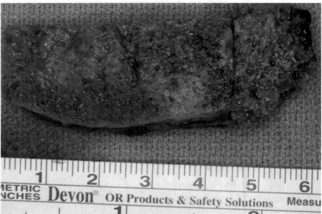

Fig. 33.3 A corticocancellous block is removed from the posterior ilium crest [16]

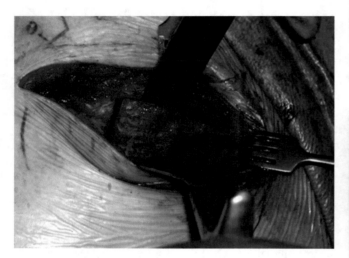

Fig. 33.2 The posterior iliac crest is exposed; osteotomies are made. And curved osteotome is used gradually to remove a corticocancellous block from the hip [16]

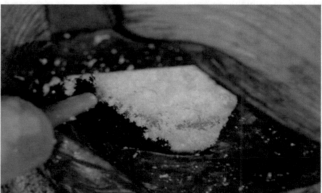

Fig. 33.4 A corticocancellous block is removed from the posterior ilium crest, and microfibrillar bovine collagen is added to the donor site [16]

lowed by curved osteotomes. The first cut is the posterior wall of the outline and starts in an inferior direction at the center of the crest of this triangular ridge. The second cut which is the superior portion of the outline will start at the ridge and go in a superior to anterior direction. The third cut which is the anterior wall of the outline is in a superior to anterior direction followed by the fourth cut which is the inferior wall of the outline proceeding in the anterior to posterior direction. All walls have not connected; the cortical cancellous block is then separated using a 1-inch (2.54 cm) curved osteotome. The separation of this cortical cancellous block should be done with great care as the ilium is at risk for fracture. Figure 33.2 demonstrates the use of a curved osteotome to gradually remove the corticocancellous block from the hip. It is advised to first mallet the curved osteotome in a superior and inferior direction along the superior wall of the block. The direction of the osteotome should then be directed from the most posterior-superior aspect of the block towards the most anterior-inferior facet. When all sides of the block are mobile, the bone graft is removed from the surgical site and stored in saline. Figure 33.3 demonstrates a corticocancellous block [5, 7, 8].

The cancellous marrow is exposed, and the surgeon may use bone curettes or a 3/8-inch bone gouge by rotating the wrist in a clockwise fashion. This motion will harvest large coils of cancellous bone. Once the marrow is not able to be obtained with the bone gouge, then the back action and straight curettes are utilized. The goal of harvesting the cancellous marrow (Fig. 33.6) should be to obtain the greatest number of stem cells which are concentrated in the medial cortex. Harvesting of 8 to 10 ml of uncompressed cancellous bone is required for every 1 cm of defect. Once harvest is completed, a bone rasp is used to remove sharp bony edges. Hemostasis should be achieved at this time prior to drain placement. Bone wax, platelet-poor plasma, or bovine collagen (Fig. 33.4) can be used to help control hemorrhage. The 7 mm suction drain is applied to the donor site (Fig. 33.5). Attention to drain exiting anterior should be taken so that patient does not lie directly on it [7].

Closure of the surgical site should begin with repositioning of the gluteus maximus and medius muscles. Use of 2–0

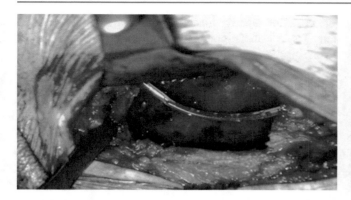

Fig. 33.5 Donor site with JP placed [16]

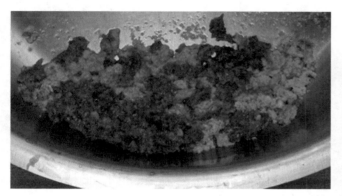

Fig. 33.6 Harvesting of the cancellous marrow [16]

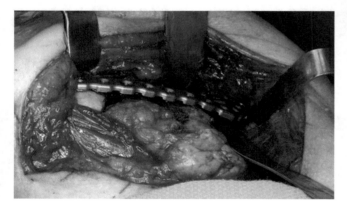

Fig. 33.7 A large 7 cm continuity defect of the right mandible with reconstruction plate placed [16]

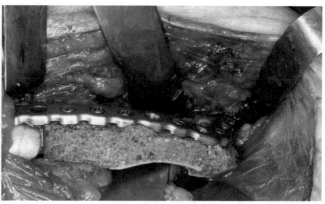

Fig. 33.8 A corticocancellous block from the posterior iliac crest has been placed in this 7 cm continuity defect and secured to the reconstruction plate with screws [16]

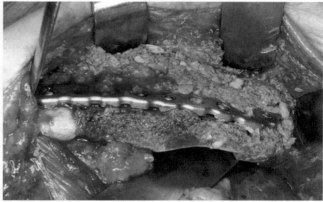

Fig. 33.9 Additional cancellous graft disturbed evenly around the corticocancellous block prior to closure [16]

or 3–0 vicryl resorbable sutures to suspend these muscles to the thoracolumbar fascia at the ridge is recommended. The subcutaneous layers are closed with 3–0 vicryl resorbable sutures; superficial dermal layers can be closed with a 4–0 monocryl resorbable suture in a running subcuticular fashion or with small skin staples. Pressure dressing with gauze and silk or foam tape should be applied to make sure the drain is exiting anteriorly [7].

Complications

Although the posterior iliac crest bone harvest technique is one that has been used for over 100 years and still used today, it's a known fact that no surgery exists without the risk of the dreaded complications. The list of eventful healing reasons can range from donor site pain, infection, seromas, hematoma or acute bleeding, nerve injury, muscle weakness, fractures, gait disturbances, and vessel injury [6, 7].

Donor site pain is common if not the most common grievance after surgery, followed by immobilization. The pain can be caused by numerable reasons but very difficult to isolate the etiology. A seroma can be a very common cause of pain that is usually treated with aspiration of the fluid collection and placement of drain. Yet the precise cause of donor site pain not related to seroma can be difficult to identify. Donor site pain is not well understood, but it may be directed towards muscular stripping of the abductors from the ilium or even injury to the superior/middle cluneal nerves [9, 10].

The pain from nerve injury is often characterized as paresthesia, anesthesia dolorosa, or dysesthesia. The superior cluneal nerves are most vulnerable to injury during harvesting of the posterior iliac crest [9, 10].

Vascular injuries are rare but can be the most serious of all complications. The main reasons for vascular injury can be that the harvesting site is too close to the greater sciatic notch as well as the improper placement of retractors. Any vascular injury must be explored, and the vessel in question must be ligated or undergo embolization [11].

Fractures of the posterior ilium are not only rare but are usually results of preexisting risk factors. Previous surgery to the harvest site, metabolic disease, smoking, and of course an unfavorable ostectomy that undermines the posterior ilium and sciatic notch, thus weakening the unique skeletal apparatus of the pelvic bone [7].

Gait disturbance is not common but may be a suspicious sign for a sequela of issues that may arise such as a fracture or malposition when suspending the gluteal muscles [7].

Innovations

Due to the morbidity of harvesting large amounts of autogenous bone from the posterior iliac crest, advances using autologous bone marrow aspirate concentrate (BMAC) with recombinant human bone morphogenetic protein-2 (rhBMP-2) and allograft have achieved similar results. Both innovative biomaterials have given the opportunity for the surgeon and patient to achieve the desired surgical outcome of bony growth in the osseous defects with the addition of the (PICBG) or without.

Bone Marrow Aspirate Concentrate (BMAC)

Bone marrow aspirate concentrate is obtained by iliac crest aspiration, and it exemplifies the few alternatives for acquiring progenitor cells and growth factors. A high concentration of growth factors such as platelet-derived growth factor (PDGF), transforming growth factor- β (TGF-β), interleukin-1 receptor antagonist (IL-1RA), and (rhBMP-2,7) are conveyed to have anabolic and anti-inflammatory effects which would be very beneficial for postoperative healing or regenerative medicine [12].

The surgical technique and processing method for obtaining BMAC is a minimally invasive procedure with low risk of postoperative complications. The patient is positioned either supine or prone; if the patient is supine, then the harvest site will be the anterior superior iliac spine or the iliac crest. Inversely, if the patient is in the prone position, then

the posterior superior iliac crest region will be the yielding site. The anesthetic options range from conscious sedation, local anesthesia, or general anesthesia. Once bony landmarks are palpated and identified, the patient is then sterilized and surgically draped. The dermis is injected down to the periosteum with 1% lidocaine without epinephrine in between the posterior iliac crest and sacroiliac joint [12].

A bone marrow aspiration kit is utilized; within the kit is a bone aspirating needle trochar, a 30-mL syringe, and the anticoagulant citrate dextrose solution, formula A (ACD-A). The bone aspirating needle trochar is percutaneously inserted through the dermis until it reaches the posterior iliac crest. Manual pressure is used to position the trochar against the dense cortical bone in the middle of the posterior crest. The needle should be parallel to the iliac crest or perpendicular with (PSIS) assuming the harvest site is from the posterior superior iliac crest. The battery-powered instrument is applied against the cortical bone so that the trochar and needle can enter the medullary cavity of the posterior iliac crest. After the trochar is in the medullary cavity, the 1 ml of heparin (1000 U/mL) is preloaded in the aspiration needles to prevent clot formation and coagulation. Bone marrow aspirate can vary from 30–90 mL[12].

The sample that has been aspirated is now processed; the BMA is filtered through a 200-mm-mesh filter into 50-mL conical tubes. Then 1 to 1.5 mL of the filtered BMA is pipetted into a centrifuge tube that can hold a minimum of 2 ml in which is sent for hemanalysis and complete blood count with differential. Afterwards, 30 to 90Ml of BMA is transferred into 2 x 50 mL conical tubes and centrifuged at 2400 rpm for 10 minutes, the surgeon will now start to see a buff coat and platelet-poor plasma (PPP) layer that is discarded. The aspirate is then centrifuged again at 3400 rpm for 6 minutes. The BMAC/white cell pellet is resuspended in (PPP) and hemanalysis (including monocyte count) is recorded to determine the assay of the leftover remnants [12].

Recombinant Human Bone Morphogenetic Protein-2

Recombinant human bone morphogenetic protein-2 (rhBMP-2) was discovered in 1965 by Marshall R. Urist, an orthopedic surgeon. Bone morphogenetic proteins belong to a group of growth factors known as transforming growth factor beta (TGF-β), a group of biologic molecules that are involved in osteoblastic differentiation and osteogenesis. Commercially available BMP is now produced in mass quantities with the use of transplantation of human BMP genes into bacterial cells which is regulated to produce protein products; this process is called recombinant human BMP (rhBMP) [13].

The bone morphogenetic protein types that have shown osteogenic properties have been BMP-2, -4, -6, -7, -9, and −14. BMP-2 and -7 have validated the direct promotion of local neovascularization. BMPs require a molecular carrier in the form of an acellular sponge (ACS) in order to the delivered and maintained to a recipient site intended for osseous targets [13]. One study revealed that bony regeneration in humans concluded using rhBMP-2/ACS is a complete osseous regeneration alternative to conventional iliac particular marrow cancellous bone grafts. The rhBMP-2 also showed great results in the reconstruction of large defects occurring in the mandible after tumor resection and osteonecrosis treatment [14].

Conclusion

The posterior iliac crest bone harvesting technique can provide a large amount of cortical and cancellous bone that is desirable for osseous defects. The surgeon should educate the patient on all the risks that could and may happen such as donor site pain. Consultation with physical therapy and pain management service should not be overlooked, as they can provide a quality of service for a procedure such as this. With the new innovative applications of biomaterials and autologous harvesting techniques, the option of posterior iliac crest bone graft harvest may become a lower priority procedure for the surgeon for bone grafting yet should still be learned and utilized when a proper opportunity arises.

References

1. (History) Bone grafting historical and conceptual review starting with an old manuscript by Vittorio Putti.
2. Urist MR, O'Connor BT, Burwell RG. Bone graft, derivatives & substitutes. Cambridge: Butterworth-Heinemann; 1994. p. 3–102.
3. Flati G, Di Stanislao C. Chirurgia nella preistoria. Parte I Provincia MedAquila. 2004;2:8–11.
4. Hamada G, Rida A. Orthopaedics in ancient and modern Egypt. Clin Orthop. 1972;89:253–68.
5. "Posterior iliac crest bone grafting." Atlas of oral and maxillofacial surgery, by Paul Tiwana, Elsevier - Health Sciences Div, 2015, pp. 1270–1274.
6. Haggerty CJ, Laughlin RM. Chapter 54 posterior iliac crest bone graft. In: Morrissey PB, Nadeau RA, Hoffmeister EP, editors. Operative atlas of oral and maxillofacial surgery. Wiley-Blackwell; 2015.
7. Marx R, Stevens M. Atlas of oral and extraoral bone harvesting, chapter 3: posterior ileum. Hanover Park, Ill: Quintessence Publishing; 2010.
8. Zouhary KJ. Bone grafting from distant sites: concepts and techniques. Oral Maxillofac Surg Clin North Am. 2010;22:301.
9. Lu J, Ebraheim NA, Huntoon M, Heck BE, Yeasting RA. Anatomic considerations of superior cluneal nerve at posterior iliac crest region. Clin Orthop. 1998;347:224–8.
10. Xu R, Ebraheim NA, Yeasting RA, Jackson WT. Anatomic considerations for posterior iliac bone harvesting. Spine. 1996;21:1017–20.
11. Ebraheim NA, et al. Bone-graft harvesting from iliac and fibular donor sites: techniques and complications. J Am Acad Orthopaed Surg. 2001;9(3):210–8. https://doi.org/10.5435/00124635-200105000-00007.
12. Chahla J, et al. Bone marrow aspirate concentrate harvesting and processing technique. Arthroscopy Techn. 2017;6(2) https://doi.org/10.1016/j.eats.2016.10.024.
13. Roberts TT, Rosenbaum AJ. Bone grafts, bone substitutes and Orthobiologics. Organogenesis. 2012;8(4):114–24. https://doi.org/10.4161/org.23306.
14. Herford AS. The use of recombinant human bone morphogenetic protein-2 (rhBMP-2) in maxillofacial trauma. Chinese J Traumatol - English Ed. Published online 2017. https://doi.org/10.1016/j.cjtee.2016.05.004.
15. Marx RE, Morales MJ. Morbidity from bone harvest in major jaw reconstruction: a randomized trial comparing the lateral anterior and posterior approach to the ilium. J Oral Maxillofac Surg. 1988;48:196–203.
16. Oral and Maxillofacial Surgery, Dental College of Georgia at Augusta University, Augusta, Georgia, USA.

Anterior Iliac Crest Graft Technique

34

Kyle Frazier and Mark R. Stevens

History

The use of the ilium for autogenous bone harvest is one of the earliest innovations in oral and maxillofacial surgery. This technique dates to the late 1800s when orthopedic surgeons first used iliac harvesting for grafting into the lumbar spine and for consolidation of pseudoarthroses of limbs. Maxillofacial surgeons adopted this procedure in the second decade of the twentieth century. In 1915, Klapp and Schroeder reported they used an iliac graft to reconstruct a mandibular defect. The next year, Lindermann reported he had already used this technique in 160 cases for mandibular reconstruction. Ilium bone harvesting continued to be used extensively in maxillofacial surgery in World War II [1]. At that time, the anterior ilium was the only site considered for bone harvest.

It was not until 1946 that the posterior iliac crest was utilized for bone grafting [2]. Dingman quickly introduced the posterior approach to craniomaxillofacial surgery 4 years later in 1950 [3]. Today, both techniques are widely used in oral and maxillofacial surgery. Although vascularized free tissue transfer is being used more widely now than in previous times, the ilium still provides oral and maxillofacial surgeons with an excellent source of nonvascularized bone for a variety of uses within the specialty.

All figures/boxes contained in this manuscript are original and the property of the authors.

K. Frazier
Augusta University Medical Center, Dental College of Georgia
Oral & Maxillofacial Surgery, Augusta, GA, USA
e-mail: kyfrazier@augusta.edu

M. R. Stevens (✉)
Department of Oral and Maxillofacial Surgery, Augusta University, Augusta, GA, USA
e-mail: MASTEVENS@augusta.edu

Indications and Contraindications

The anterior iliac crest bone harvest technique can be utilized in any surgery in which a nonvascularized bone graft of up to 50 cc is required. Both cancellous and corticocancellous bone can be harvested, depending on the need at the recipient site. Anterior iliac crest bone grafts are commonly indicated in post-traumatic defects, post-ablative defects (from both benign and malignant pathology), alveolar cleft bone grafting, and alveolar ridge augmentation prior to dental rehabilitation.

Different potential volumes of bone harvest are listed in the literature, but there is consensus that no more than 50 cc can be expected from a single anterior iliac crest site. It is generally assumed when reconstructing a mandibular defect that every 1 cm needed for reconstruction will require around 10 cc of bone graft. Thus, a single anterior iliac crest site should not be utilized for mandibular reconstruction greater than five centimeters [4]. If greater than 50 cc of bone is necessary, the surgeon should consider bilateral anterior iliac crest sites or a posterior iliac crest bone harvest, instead.

It is important for the surgeon to consider the recipient site when deciding which grafting technique to use. Bone removed from the ilium is nonvascularized and should therefore be placed into a non-contaminated site [4]. Since the graft has no vascularization itself, it relies on a vascular tissue bed from the recipient site for nutrients. It is not surprising, then, that nonvascularized grafts were found to have higher failures compared to vascularized bone grafts in reconstructing sites resected due to malignancies, likely secondary to the radiation these patients received [5].

Considering the donor site is also important when treatment planning. Patients with previous hernia repairs may have a greater risk of abdominal perforation. Obesity complicates the surgical approach, as the thickness of soft tissue overlying the anterior iliac crest is much greater and retraction is more difficult after reaching the donor site. The surgeon should inquire as to whether the patient has any history

© The Author(s), under exclusive license to Springer Nature Switzerland AG 2021
M. R. Stevens et al. (eds.), *Innovative Perspectives in Oral and Maxillofacial Surgery*, https://doi.org/10.1007/978-3-030-75750-2_34

of pelvic fractures, pelvic osteomyelitis, bony metastasis, or radiation to the site.

Systemic conditions should also be considered. Anterior iliac crest bone harvest is contraindicated when the patient has a history of metabolic bone diseases (e.g., osteogenesis imperfecta). The use of bisphosphonates, chemotherapy, and long-term steroids are relative contraindications for the procedure [4].

Anatomy

The bony pelvis comprises the sacrum, the coccyx, and a pair of hip bones anterolaterally. The two hip bones are comprised of three parts each: the ilium, ischium, and pubis. The ilium is suitable for bone harvesting from the anterior and posterior portions. The crest of the ilium stretches from the anterior superior iliac spine (ASIS) to the posterior superior iliac spine (PSIS). The crest bulges posterolaterally from the ASIS and forms the iliac tubercle.

Several different muscles find their origins and insertions on the ilium, and the bone also has multiple ligamentous attachments. The iliacus overlies the iliac fossa and must be reflected during the harvest. The tensor fascia lata has its origin at the anterior superior iliac spine and the anterolateral portion of the anterior iliac crest. It is contiguous with the iliotibial tract, which inserts in the lateral condyle of the tibia. Damage to this muscle will result in postoperative gait disturbances [6]. Scarpa's fascia, the deep membranous layer of the superficial fascia of the abdomen, is also encountered during the approach.

Multiple nerves deserve special attention in the anterior approach to the ilium. The lateral femoral cutaneous nerve lies medial to the subcostal nerve and between the psoas and iliacus muscles. It provides sensation to the skin of the anterior and lateral thigh. Murata et al. performed a cadaver study in which the bilateral lateral femoral cutaneous nerves of 108 specimens were examined. They identified four variants of the nerve: type A (crossing over the iliac crest more than two centimeters posterior to the anterior superior iliac spine), type B (crossing over the iliac crest within two centimeters posterior to the anterior superior iliac spine), type C (crossing at the anterior superior iliac spine), and type D (crossing under the inguinal ligament and anterior to the anterior superior iliac spine) [7]. In addition, in about 2.5% of patients, the nerve courses anterior to the inguinal ligament, putting it at risk for injury when the incision is extended over the anterior iliac spine. The anatomical variation of this nerve is significant due to the risk of damaging the nerve during the approach to the anterior iliac crest, with the possible sequela of meralgia paresthetica (see "Complications" below).

The iliohypogastric nerve overlies the iliac tubercle and provides sensory innervation to the skin of the lateral aspect of the buttock and the pubis. It is the most commonly injured nerve during anterior iliac crest bone harvesting. The lateral branch of the subcostal nerve also provides sensation to the lateral buttock and can be affected in this approach.

Box 34.1 summarizes the key anatomical structures related to the anterior iliac crest bone harvesting technique.

Box 34.1 Notable anatomy associated with the anterior iliac crest bone harvest
Bones

- Pelvis
  - Sacrum
  - Coccyx
  - Hip bones (2)
    Pubis
    Ischium
    Ilium
    - Anterior iliac crest
    - Anterior tubercle
    - Anterior superior spine

Nerves

- Lateral femoral cutaneous nerve
- Iliohypogastric nerve
- Lateral branch of the subcostal nerve

Muscles

- Iliacus
- Tensor fascia lata
- External abdominal oblique
- Internal abdominal oblique
- Transversus abdominis

Surgical Technique

Due to the need for excellent anesthesia and a strict sterile technique, the anterior iliac crest bone harvest is performed in the operating room setting. The patient is induced into the general anesthetic state and intubated. By virtue of the anterior approach, the patient can be placed in a supine position, generally allowing for a second maxillofacial team to cooperate at the head simultaneously. A hip roll is placed beneath the pelvis for the accentuation of the anterior iliac crest anatomy. The anterior superior iliac spine, iliac tubercle, and anterior iliac crest are palpated and marked. The proposed incision line is then marked 2–4 cm lateral to the height of the anterior iliac crest, starting 1 cm posterior to the ASIS and extending 1–2 cm anterior to the iliac tubercle (~4–6 cm in total length). Local anesthesia is administered, and the patient is prepped and draped in a sterile fashion. The abdominal skin is then pulled medially to orient the incision line over the anterior iliac crest. A 10 blade is used to incise through the skin, and electrocautery is used through subcutaneous tissue until Scarpa's fascia is reached. The overlying fat can be cleaned off of Scarpa's fascia using a surgical sponge. Scarpa's fascia is then sharply dissected. At this point, the external abdominal oblique muscle is seen coursing from the medial to the iliac crest, and the tensor fascia lata muscle is seen coursing from the lateral to the iliac crest. A periosteal incision is made between the two attachments.

At this point, the surgeon must decide what type of harvest technique will be utilized. If cortical bone is not required at the donor site, then a cancellous-only harvest can be performed. The clamshell approach utilizes an osteotome with or without a reciprocating saw to make a mid-crestal split, resulting in greenstick fractures of the medial and lateral cortices. The marrow is then exposed, which can be harvested with curettes and gouges. The medial trap door and bilateral trap door approaches are similar, but they add medial or bilateral cortical plate osteotomies (respectively) for better access and more complete marrow harvesting. The muscle attachments are left intact, and vertical cortical osteotomies are made through the muscle fibers overlying the medial and lateral cortical plates. In all instances, the cortices are reduced after harvesting and fixated with either sutures or wires.

For cases requiring cortical bone in addition to cancellous bone, a medial approach is preferred. The iliacus is reflected about 5–7 cm from the crest. An outline is marked for the desired osteotomy, keeping the anterior vertical osteotomy at least 2 cm posterior to the anterior superior iliac spine. The osteotomies are then accomplished with a reciprocating saw, and an osteotome is used approximating the lateral wall in order to maximize the amount of cancellous bone connected to the cortical graft. The osteotome is then levered medially, releasing the corticocancellous block (Figs. 34.1 and 34.2). Curettes and gouges are used to remove any additional marrow still attached to the lateral cortex.

Hemostasis can be achieved with various local measures (e.g., microfibrillar collagen, thrombin). Drains may be placed to prevent hematoma/seroma formation but are not necessary in every case. A layered closure is accomplished,

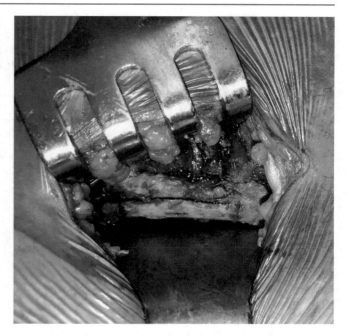

Fig. 34.1 The anterior iliac crest is exposed, and osteotomies are made to remove a corticocancellous block

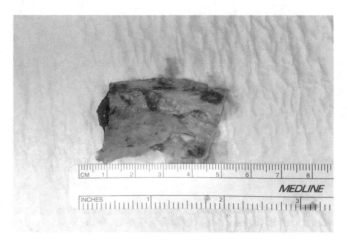

Fig. 34.2 A corticocancellous block is removed

and an appropriate pressure dressing is placed. The bone graft is then taken to the recipient site to be utilized for its indication. (Figs. 34.3, 34.4, and 34.5).

Anterior iliac crest bone harvesting is nearly identical in the pediatric population with the exception that there is a cartilaginous cap over the iliac crest. Disruption of the cap may result in a contour deformity due to an alteration of growth at the crest itself. However, it is safe to harvest below the cap, so it is reflected during surgery for protection, and then, surgery proceeds as described above [4, 6].

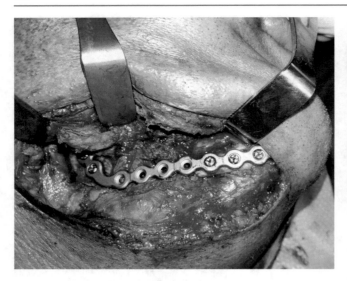

Fig. 34.3 A large continuity defect of the right mandible with reconstruction plate placed

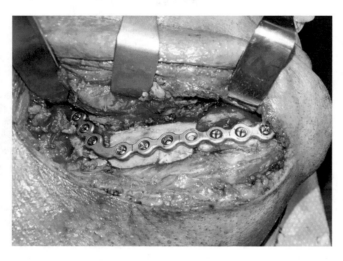

Fig. 34.4 A corticocancellous block from the anterior iliac crest has been placed in the continuity defect and secured to the reconstruction plate with screws

Complications

While the anterior iliac crest bone harvest technique is a well-accepted and commonly used technique, it does carry the risk of multiple complications. However, the vast majority of complications are minor and short-term in duration. Fawzi et al. performed a retrospective review of 180 patients that had received bone harvests from either the iliac crest or the calvarium. The results showed that the iliac crest harvest had a 5.6% risk of a major complication, whereas the calvarial harvest had a 14.5% risk of major complication ($p = 0.08772$). Major risks included in the study for iliac crest grafts were hematoma (4%), infection (0.8%), and hemorrhage (0.8%). Fracture was also included as a potential major complication,

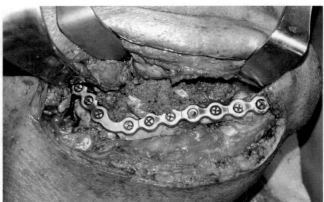

Fig. 34.5 Additional cancellous graft spackled around the corticocancellous block prior to closure

but no patients experienced this sequela. However, the iliac crest harvest had a 60.8% risk of a minor complications, whereas the calvarial harvest had only a 25.4% risk of minor complications (P < 0.0001). Of the minor complications, pain was by far the most common problem, with a 42% incidence in the iliac crest group. Other minor complications included edema (7%) and gait disturbance (12%) [8].

Barone et al. designed a prospective study involving 235 patients receiving an anterior iliac crest bone harvest over a 10-year period. Only two patients had a complication other than pain or paresthesia (one fracture of the anterior iliac crest and two hematomas). Postoperative pain was experienced by 99% of patients 1 week after surgery, but this had reduced to 1% at 28 days and 0% at 6 weeks. Similarly, 100% of patients reported difficulty walking during the first week after surgery, but only 1 patient still experienced this problem after 5 weeks. Half of the patients experienced hypoesthesia 1 week after surgery, but no patients still experienced hypoesthesia after 4 months [9]. Meralgia paresthetica, characterized by paresthesia and disturbances of sensation in the anterolateral surface of the thigh in the area supplied by the lateral cutaneous femoral nerve, appears to be a rare complication [10]. However, meralgia paresthetica has been reported up to 40 years after anterior iliac crest bone harvesting, thought to be secondary to heterotopic ossification on the anterosuperior iliac spine [11].

Cosmetic deformities may result from either full-thickness bone harvesting (removing the medial cortex, lateral cortex, and crest) or, in the case of children, disruption of the cartilaginous cap. Full-thickness bone harvesting is usually not performed for maxillofacial bone grafting, and careful attention in maintaining the superolateral rim of the crest should minimize a cosmetic problem. As stated in the technique section above, retraction of the cartilaginous cap in children will minimize the risk of subsequent deformity. Peritoneal perforation can also occur, but the risk is minimized with a careful surgical technique [6].

Innovations

Anterior iliac crest bone harvesting has been a mainstay of maxillofacial surgery for a century, with most of the innovation occurring in the early 1900s. It was not until the start of the twenty-first century that significant advances were made to enhance this technique. Specifically, the use of bone marrow aspirate concentrate (BMAC) and recombinant human bone morphogenetic protein-2 (rhBMP-2) have given surgeons tools to add to, or in many instances to replace, traditional iliac crest harvesting.

Bone Marrow Aspirate Concentrate (BMAC)

Bone marrow aspirate concentrate is a technique of obtaining cancellous bone from a donor site and then concentrating the specimen such that there is a four- to sevenfold increase in available osteocompetent cells per volume. The concentrate can then be added to allogeneic or autogenous grafts and used for a variety of purposes such as continuity defects, ridge augmentations, and sinus lifts. Multiple donor sites can be used, but often, the bone marrow is taken from the anterior or posterior ilium. The major advantages of this technique over the open iliac crest harvest are the minimally invasive surgical approach and the concentration of the osteocompetent cells obtained. However, unlike the open iliac crest harvest, the BMAC system cannot supply the surgeon with cortical bone. That being said, the technique can be combined with allogeneic cortical bone grafts when necessary.

Obtaining BMAC is relatively straightforward. When harvesting from the anterior ilium, two separate 2 mm incisions are made in the skin 2 cm and 6 cm posterior to the anterior superior iliac spine, and a hemostat is used to bluntly dissect down to the iliac cortex. A trocar that has been wetted with heparin 1000 U/mL is then inserted through the tract, avoiding contact with subcutaneous fat, as the thromboplastin in the fat may initiate clotting. The trocar is pressed through the cortex into the marrow space, and the plunger is aspirated. The surgeon continues to aspirate as the marrow is drawn into the syringe, and the syringe is rotated a full 360 degrees over every 5 mL of aspirate. Once 5 mL is obtained, the trocar is repositioned, and aspiration continues in the same fashion. A goal of 30 mL of bone marrow from each site is reasonable. The bone marrow aspirate is placed into a bag containing an anticoagulant solution until the entire volume needed is collected, at which time it is filtered and placed into a chamber that is double spun in a centrifuge. The layered product contains the BMAC as its bottom layer, which is then collected and added to whatever carrier the surgeon desires (e.g., allogeneic bone particulate). The puncture sites are closed with single interrupted sutures [4].

Recombinant Human Bone Morphogenetic Protein-2

Recombinant human bone morphogenetic protein-2 (rhBMP-2) is one of several proteins known for its osteoinductive properties. Bone morphogenetic proteins (BMPs) are members of the transforming growth factor-beta group. There are nearly 20 known BMPs currently, but only BMP-2, -4, -6, and -7 are known to have osteoinductive properties [12]. Unlike traditional bone grafts, rhBMP-2 is not derived from bony structure (e.g., the iliac crest of an autograft or donor bone from an allograft). Instead, it is a protein isolated and cloned using recombinant gene technology. It is then placed onto an acellular collagen sponge (ACS) and delivered to the recipient to induce the production of bone de novo. (Fig. 34.6).

In the late 1990s and early 2000s, following successful animal studies, a series of human studies were published demonstrating the safety of using rhBMP-2 for alveolar ridge preservation/augmentation as well as maxillary sinus floor augmentation [13–15], which are currently the two FDA-cleared uses for rhBMP-2/ACS. For these smaller applications, the acellular collagen sponge soaked with rhBMP-2 can be placed directly into the recipient site (e.g., maxillary sinus or tooth extraction socket). However, there are also several off-label uses for which rhBMP-2/ACS is commonly used in oral and maxillofacial surgery, such as grafting nonunions, craniofacial defects, and mandibular continuity defects. In these instances, the bony gap may be large enough such that the rhBMP-2/ACS is best used in conjunction with cancellous allografts. The rhBMP-2 soaked collagen sponge is cut into pieces and mixed in a 1:1 ratio with the bone allograft and placed into the defect [4].

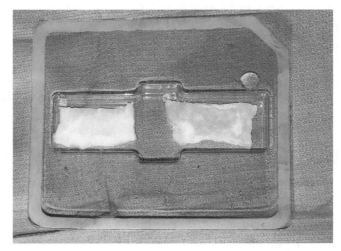

Fig. 34.6 Two acellular collagen sponges after reconstitution with rhBMP-2

The patient must be made aware that significant edema can result from the use of rhBMP-2/ACS due to its chemotactic action and hypertonicity. The surgeon should also consider this if being used in areas that significant edema could compromise the surgical site. Other untoward side effects include ectopic bone formation, osteoclast-mediated bone resorption, and inappropriate adipogenesis [16]. In addition, the possibility of rhBMP-2 as a carcinogen is controversial. BMP-2 is upregulated in several tumors, including prostate, breast, oral mucosa, pleura, and bone. One study did find an increase in cancer among patients that received rhBMP-2 in a compression-resistant matrix [17], but other studies have failed to show the same results [16]. Kelly et al. performed a retrospective review of the incidence of cancer in 467,916 Medicare patients undergoing spinal arthrodesis from 2005 to 2010 and found that the use of BMP was not associated with an increase in the risk of cancer within a mean 2.9-year time window [18]. Furthermore, Schmidt et al. found no increase in the risk of new cancer in a pediatric population receiving rhBMP-2 for alveolar cleft grafts at their institution with follow-up ranging from 2–11 years [19]. More research is needed to determine the risk (if any) associated with the use of rhBMP-2 as it relates to cancer formation. Nevertheless, rhBMP-2 has been proven an effective means of osteogenesis. In many cases, it obviates the need for autogenous bone harvesting, saving the patient from postoperative complications associated with the donor site. Other times, it can be used in combination with autogenous or other types of bone grafts to further enhance osteogenesis.

Conclusion

The anterior iliac crest bone harvesting technique has been used in oral and maxillofacial surgery for over 100 years and today remains an invaluable tool in the armamentarium of surgeons. In general, the surgery is highly successful, is well-accepted by patients, and has a low risk of major complications. Although it is likely that as vascular free tissue transfer and tissue regeneration techniques advance, the use of AICBH will become utilized less than it previously was, it is unlikely that this technique will ever be completely supplanted.

References

1. Tessier P, Kawamoto H, Matthews D, et al. Taking bone grafts from the anterior and posterior Ilium – tools and techniques: II. A 6800-case experience in maxillofacial and craniofacial surgery. Plast Reconstr Surg. 2005;116(Supplement):25S–37S. https://doi.org/10.1097/01.prs.0000173951.78715.d7.
2. DICK IL. Iliac-bone transplantation. J Bone Joint Surg Am. 1946;28:1–14.
3. Dingman RO. The use of iliac bone in the repair of facial and cranial defects. Plast Reconstr Surg. 1950;6(3):179–95. https://doi.org/10.1097/00006534-195009000-00001.
4. Marx R, Stevens M. Atlas of oral and extraoral bone harvesting. Hanover Park: Quintessence; 2010.
5. Akinbami B. Reconstruction of continuity defects of the mandible with non-vascularized bone grafts. Systematic literature review. Craniomaxillofac Trauma Reconstr. 2016;9(3):195–205. https://doi.org/10.1055/s-0036-1572494.
6. Haggerty CJ, Laughlin RM. Atlas of operative oral and maxillofacial surgery. Chichester: Wiley-Blackwell; 2015. https://doi.org/10.1002/9781118993729.
7. Murata Y, Takahashi K, Yamagata M, Shimada Y, Moriya H. The anatomy of the lateral femoral cutaneous nerve, with special reference to the harvesting of iliac bone graft. J Bone Jt Surg Ser A. Published online. 2000; https://doi.org/10.2106/00004623-200005000-00016.
8. Riachi F, Naaman N, Tabarani C, Berberi A, Salameh Z. Comparison of morbidity and complications of harvesting bone from the iliac crest and calvarium: a retrospective study. J Int oral Heal JIOH. 2014;6(3):32–5. http://www.ncbi.nlm.nih.gov/pubmed/25083030. Accessed 30 Sept 2020.
9. Barone A, Ricci M, Mangano F, Covani U. Morbidity associated with iliac crest harvesting in the treatment of maxillary and mandibular atrophies: a 10-year analysis. J Oral Maxillofac Surg. 2011;69(9):2298–304. https://doi.org/10.1016/j.joms.2011.01.014.
10. Weikel AM, Habal MB. Meralgia paresthetica: a complication of iliac bone procurement. Plast Reconstr Surg. Published online. 1977; https://doi.org/10.1097/00006534-197710000-00012.
11. Yamamoto T, Nagira K, Kurosaka M. Meralgia paresthetica occurring 40 years after iliac bone graft harvesting: case report. Neurosurgery. 2001;49(6):1455–7. https://doi.org/10.1097/00006123-200112000-00028.
12. Herford AS. The use of recombinant human bone morphogenetic protein-2 (rhBMP-2) in maxillofacial trauma. Chinese J Traumatol - English Ed. Published online. 2017; https://doi.org/10.1016/j.cjtee.2016.05.004.
13. Boyne PJ, Marx RE, Nevins M, et al. A feasibility study evaluating rhBMP-2/absorbable collagen sponge for maxillary sinus floor augmentation. Int J Periodontics Restorative Dent. Published online. 1997;
14. Howell TH, Fiorellini J, Jones A, et al. A feasibility study evaluating rhBMP-2/absorbable collagen sponge device for local alveolar ridge preservation or augmentation. Int J Periodontics Restorative Dent. Published online. 1997;
15. Cochran DL, Jones AA, Lilly LC, Fiorellini JP, Howell H. Evaluation of recombinant human bone morphogenetic Protein-2 in Oral applications including the use of endosseous implants: 3-year results of a pilot study in humans. J Periodontol. Published online. 2000; https://doi.org/10.1902/jop.2000.71.8.1241.
16. James AW, LaChaud G, Shen J, et al. A review of the clinical side effects of bone morphogenetic protein-2. Tissue Eng - Part B Rev. Published online. 2016; https://doi.org/10.1089/ten.teb.2015.0357.
17. Carragee EJ, Chu G, Rohatgi R, et al. Cancer risk after use of recombinant bone morphogenetic protein-2 for spinal arthrodesis. J Bone Jt Surg - Ser A. Published online. 2013; https://doi.org/10.2106/JBJS.L.01483.
18. Kelly MP, Savage JW, Bentzen SM, Hsu WK, Ellison SA, Anderson PA. Cancer risk from bone morphogenetic protein exposure in spinal arthrodesis. J Bone Jt Surg - Am Vol. Published online. 2014; https://doi.org/10.2106/JBJS.M.01190.
19. Schmidt C, Patel S, Woerner J, Ghali G. Does RHBMP-2/ACS use result in an increased incidence of cancer formation in pediatric patients. Int J Oral Maxillofac Surg. Published online. 2019; https://doi.org/10.1016/j.ijom.2019.03.598.

SARPE and MARPE

Federico Hernández-Alfaro and Adaia Valls-Ontañón

Introduction

Transverse maxillary deficiency is a relatively common type of malocclusion in the primary and early mixed dentition, occurring in 8–22% of this population [1]. Its underlying cause is unclear, although some causative factors have been reported, such as upper airway obstruction, mouth breathing, habits as thumb sucking, or alterations in skeletal, dental, or soft tissues. If left untreated during the primary dentition, it will probably affect permanent dentition, leading to a narrow maxilla, deep palatal vault, and posterior crossbite. Subsequently, asymmetric mandibular growth and facial disharmony may arise, functional changes in the masticatory muscles and the temporomandibular joint [2]. Thus, several treatments have been proposed in order to correct this malocclusion.

Small transverse discrepancies can be managed by dental orthodontic traction. However, when the transverse dentoalveolar discrepancy is greater than 4 mm (measured at the skeletal level), it requires some skeletal palatal transverse expansion utilizing an orthopedic or a surgical approach, as further detailed thereunder.

Rapid palatal expansion (RPE) has been widely used to address the maxilla's transverse dimension in growing patients by remodeling the midpalatal suture and intermaxillary sutures [3]. However, separation of the midpalatal suture with aging becomes gradually more difficult, as the ossification of the midpalatal suture starts around 11 years old. Afterward, calcification and interdigitation of the suture increases. At the same time, the sutural gap decreases pro-

gressively throughout life [4]. Also, there is a complex three-dimensional articulation using sutures between palatal bones with zygomatic and sphenoid bones posteriorly and maxillary bone anteriorly.

Therefore, in adult patients with a fused midpalatal suture, RPE becomes useless. Even more, undesired dental effects such as buccal tipping of posterior teeth, decreased buccal bone thickness, and buccal root resorption might occur when tooth-borne devices are used. Thus, in nongrowing patients, a surgical reopening of the midpalatal suture is required, which is well-known as surgically assisted rapid palatal/maxillary expansion (SARPE or SARME, respectively). It has been classically postulated that the age limit for performing orthopedic disjunction without the need for surgical intervention is 15 years of age [5]. However, there is controversy about it, and nowadays, several authors have reported orthopedic expansion in older patients since chronological age is not a valid indicator of bone maturation age.

In this context, the literature reveals the following anatomical development key features of the midpalatal suture: (a) although it may show obliteration during the juvenile period, it rarely has a marked degree of closure until the third decade of life; (b) it starts to obliterate earlier in its posterior area than in its anterior region; (c) suture closure progresses more rapidly in the oral than in the nasal side of the palatal vault; and (d) in palate splitting with RPE devices, most of the resistance to separation is due to circummaxillary sutures [6]. Therefore, assessment of the midpalatal suture maturation stage by way of CBCT is considered an essential clinical tool for treatment choice between RPE and SARPE [4]. However, it is not without clinical risk error [7].

On that basis and to avoid surgical invasiveness, some researchers have looked for nonsurgical alternatives for maxillary expansion in young adults. Thus, the use of bone-supported orthopedic miniscrews has been proposed as anchorage devices for applying mechanical forces around the midpalatal suture in late adolescents to avoid surgical osteotomies [8, 9]. This technique, known as miniscrew assisted rapid

F. Hernández-Alfaro
Department of Oral and Maxillofacial Surgery, International University of Catalonia, Barcelona, Spain

Teknon Medical Center, Barcelona, Spain
e-mail: director@institutomaxilofacial.com; h.alfaro@uic.es

A. Valls-Ontañón (✉)
Department of Oral and Maxillofacial Surgery, Teknon Medical Center, Barcelona, Spain
e-mail: avalls@institutomaxilofacial.com; avalls@uic.es

palatal expansion (MARPE), aims to expand the palate in final-growing patients with skeletal expanders, thus enhancing orthopedic forces while avoiding side effects SARPE.

In front of such a diversity of treatments and the extensive published literature, there is currently controversy about each one's indications and the best choice treatment.

Expansion Devices: From Tooth-Borne to Hybrid and Bone-Borne Appliances

Conventional expanders are tooth-supported appliances. However, its dental support has been related to detrimental periodontal consequences with buccal tipping, decreased buccal bone thickness while increasing palatal bone thickness, and buccal root resorption of the posterior teeth from limited skeletal movements and lack of long-term stability. So, two extra different expander designs have been described in the literature. First, the hybrid expanders are a combination of tooth- and bone-borne devices. Although dental side effects have been reduced, they still may arise. Therefore, full bone-borne expanders have been designed, which comprise a palatal jackscrew anchored bicortically to the cortical bone of the palate and of the nasal floor with four miniscrews (Figs. 35.1 and 35.2).

Regarding its clinical application, tooth-borne devices are used for RPE since proper palatal expansion can be achieved in growing patients with an open palatal suture without further bone invasiveness and children's need to undergo procedures under anesthesia. On the other hand, concerning appliances used in SARPE and MARPE, both hybrid or bone-borne expanders have been used, although currently, the latest is advisable to avoid dental side effects.

Surgical Technique: SARPE and MARPE

Several SARPE techniques have been proposed since Brown first described it in 1938, attending to where osteotomies should be placed, its approach, and the type of expander device, among others (Figs. 35.3, 35.4, and 35.5).

First, planning extension and placement of osteotomies is a patient-tailored procedure, as it depends on the skeletal and dental particularities of each patient and stated objectives.

The classical two-segment transpalatal osteotomy procedure involves, in addition to a vertical midpalatal suture cut between both central incisors, a horizontal LeFort I osteotomy (Fig. 35.4). On the other hand, the three-segment transpalatal SARPE design requires two vertical osteotomies from both lateral pyriform rims through the apexes of lateral

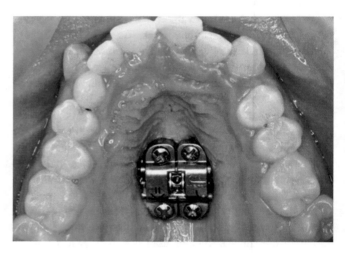

Fig. 35.2 Bone-borne device

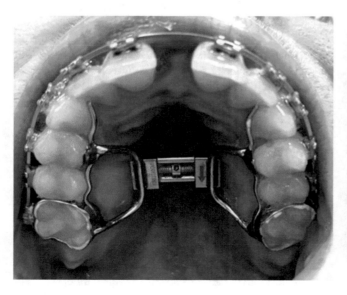

Fig. 35.1 Hybrid device

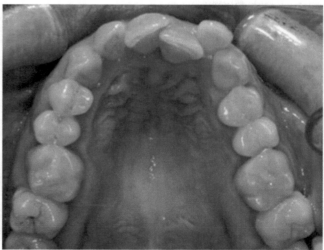

Fig. 35.3 Transverse maxillary hypoplasia: preoperative clinical picture

incisors and canines that run backward parallel to the mid-palatal suture. Similarly, four-segment transpalatal osteotomy adds an extra osteotomy behind the premaxilla that connects both vertical osteotomies from lateral pyriform rims, which enables complete mobilization of the anterior segment containing the incisors. Finally, asymmetric designs can be carried out when required. The pterygomaxillary disjunction or maxillary downfracture is performed when a significant posterior maxillary expansion is needed; otherwise, it leads to a V-shaped expansion of the maxilla in the transversal plane [10].

Moreover, maxillary downward movement can be easily achieved in the context of SARPE by placing two-hole miniplates from both lateral pyriform rims medially to the level of the upper incisor's apexes, following a medial direction (Fig. 35.6). Therefore, when transverse distraction is carried out, the miniplates placed diagonally serve as a pulley and provide an additional downward movement. Similarly, for-

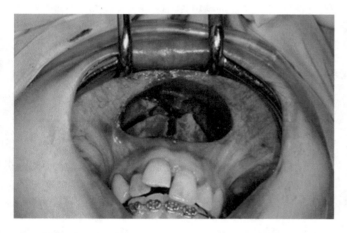

Fig. 35.4 Intraoperative picture of a SARPE with a vertical midpalatal osteotomy and through a minimally invasive approach

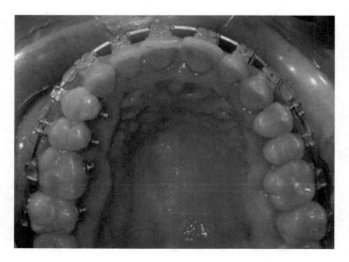

Fig. 35.5 Final surgical and orthodontic treatment picture

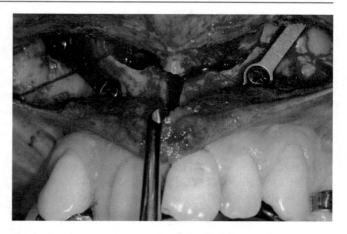

Fig. 35.6 Two segment SARPE with two additional oblique miniplates to promote downward movement

ward movement can also be obtained in the context of SARPE by placing two miniplates or miniscrews at the apical level of molars of the upper jaw and two miniplates or miniscrews at the apical level of lower canines and then using elastic bands.

It is recommended to activate the device intraoperatively to check the symmetrical and complete expansion of both sides, and one-millimeter expansion remains at the time of surgery. Afterward, a latency period of 5–7 days is required for bony callus formation, which is followed by the expander activation period, which ranges from 0.25 to 1 millimeter per day, depending on the patient's age (the pace can be faster for younger patients) and author's preferences. Distraction is continued until the desired correction is achieved, and finally, the contention period with the expander in place is required for proper ossification while avoiding relapse. It ranges between 8 and 20 weeks, depending on each author's preferences.

Although this technique has been classically related to increased patient's morbidity, the need for general anesthesia, and the inherent hospital admission, nowadays, it is usually performed through a minimally invasive approach that takes around 30 minutes and entails low morbidity, which allows the procedure to be carried out on an outpatient basis (Fig. 35.4) [11]. Similarly, other authors have proposed an endoscopically-assisted SARPE [12]. In the end, the minimal approach reduces postoperative swelling and discomfort and guarantees vascular support to the maxilla via the vestibular corridors.

On the other hand, the MARPE technique is carried out under local anesthesia and comprises the insertion of four bicortical miniscrews adjacent to the midpalatal suture, being two mesial and two distal to the expanding tool. The fixation in both cortical plates is fundamental to aid the anchorage during expansion and to surpass the resistance of maxillary bones to separation. Therefore, correct selection of miniscrew length is mandatory, assessed by CBCT by measuring the thickness of soft and bone tissue where miniscrews are placed. Nowadays, specific software and CAD/CAM technology allow for manufacturing surgical guides and customized devices, which enable a flapless surgery and a perfect fit of the expander, respectively.

Additional minimally invasive surgical techniques have been described in the context of MARPE to overcome areas of resistance. Since regional acceleratory phenomenon (RAP) induced by surgical trauma has been demonstrated as an effective method for accelerating tooth movement, it has been implemented for corticotomy-assisted expansion, where the alveolar's bilateral decortication of buccal and palatine bones is carried out in order to reduce expansion resistance [13]. Similarly, corticopuncture facilitated MARPE [14] consists of performing bone perforations every 2 millimeters along the midpalatal suture. They can be done manually by inserting and removing a titanium miniscrew or with a burr and a screwdriver. Finally, some authors advocate for a surgically assisted MARPE by performing a minimally invasive midpalatal suture surgical separation, which is carried out on an outpatient basis [15].

Dentoalveolar and Skeletal Changes and Stability after SARPE and MARPE

As previously mentioned, RPE induces buccal tipping of the supportive teeth at the dentoalveolar level, apart from alveolar thickness decreases on the buccal side but increases on the palatal side. The literature suggests that MARPE produces less loss of buccal alveolar bone than conventional RPE protocols [16, 17].

Focusing on skeletal changes, it has been reported that during RPE treatment, the skeletal structure of the middle third of the face separates into a pyramidal shape when viewed from the coronal plane [18]. In other words, the amount of expansion decreases upwards. Likewise, such changes can also be observed in patients undergoing treatment with MARPE [17], where bone bending occurs in the zygomatic process of the temporal bone [19]. Conversely, in patients undergoing SARPE, a pure lateral movement is observed, while no skeletal changes are observed beyond the LeFort I osteotomy. However, it is important to highlight that SARPE without pterygomaxillary disjunction leads to a V-shaped transverse expansion with a wider expansion in the anterior nasal spine than in the posterior nasal spine. In contrast, its disconnection leads to a parallel opening of the midpalatal suture [10]. Similarly, MARPE procedures also induce a V-shaped transverse expansion with a wider expansion in the anterior nasal spine because of the pterygomaxillary suture rigidity and the intermaxillary suture obliterates earlier in its posterior part.

All described procedures present stable skeletal changes, and no transpalatal arch retainers are recommended, although they are not exempt from some dental relapse.

Impact of SARPE and MARPE on Upper Airway and Facial Soft Tissue

Several investigations support that maxillary expansion through RPE, SARPE [20], and MARPE [21], has beneficial effects at the level of the maxillary bone and the nasal cavity width, promoting its expansion and the consequent improvement on upper airway resistance. Moreover, transverse maxillary width correction allows tongue reposition, which releases oropharyngeal collapse. However, maxillary expansion does not produce a large enough widening of the airway to be considered a form of treatment for obstructive sleep apnea.

Perinasal soft tissue sustain changes after MARPE: the nose tends to widen and move forward and downward, leading to increased nasal volume [22]. Likewise, alar width could also increase in patients submitted to SARPE [23, 24]. However, perinasal soft tissue reconstruction using an alar cinch (Fig. 35.7) and minimally invasive approaches should be able to control alar base widening.

Recommended Treatment Algorithm

In conclusion, patient-tailored treatment is mandatory. After a thorough evaluation of the patient and setting treatment targets, a CBCT is recommended in order to assess the suture maturation stage. In young adults with a potential suture opening, MARPE can be attempted unless in the following situations, where SARPE is advisable: large expansions

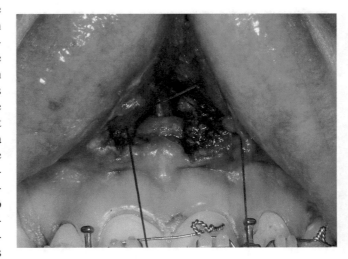

Fig. 35.7 Crossed alar cinch suture sequence

(>5 mm) and the necessity of additional maxillary forward or downward movement.

Secondly, whatever the used technique (MARPE or SARPE), bone-borne devices are advisable in order to avoid dental side effects.

Finally, clinicians should thoroughly explain the related potential complications to patients before MARPE or SARPE initiation, being expansion failure and bleeding the most common, respectively. Likewise, anticipated changes in the paranasal area should be as well highlighted.

References

1. Agostino P, Ugolini A, Signori A, Silvestrini-Biavati A, Harrison JE, Riley P. Orthodontic treatment for posterior crossbites. Cochrane Database Syst Rev. 2014;(8):CD000979.
2. Ugolini A, Doldo T, Ghislanzoni LT, Mapelli A, Giorgetti R, Sforza C. Rapid palatal expansion effects on mandibular transverse dimensions in unilateral posterior crossbite patients: a three-dimensional digital imaging study. Prog Orthod. 2016;17:1.
3. Lin L, Ahn HW, Kim SJ, Moon SC, Kim SH, Nelson G. Tooth-borne vs bone-borne rapid maxillary expanders in late adolescence. Angle Orthod. 2015;85(2):253–62.
4. Angelieri F, Franchi L, Cevidanes LHS, Gonçalves JR, Nieri M, Wolford LM, et al. Cone beam computed tomography evaluation of midpalatal suture maturation in adults. Int J Oral Maxillofac Surg. 2017;46(12):1557–61.
5. Bell RA. A review of maxillary expansion in relation to rate of expansion and patient's age. Am J Orthod. 1982;81(1):32–7.
6. Persson M, Thilander B. Palatal suture closure in man from 15 to 35 years of age. Am J Orthod. 1977;72(1):42–52.
7. Barbosa NMV, Castro AC, Conti F, Capelozza-Filho L, Almeida-Pedrin RR, Cardoso MA. Reliability and reproducibility of the method of assessment of midpalatal suture maturation: a tomographic study. Angle Orthod. 2019;89(1):71–7.
8. Pulver RJ, Campbell PM, Opperman LA, Buschang PH. Miniscrew-assisted slow expansion of mature rabbit sutures. Am J Orthod Dentofac Orthop. 2016;150(2):303–12.
9. Lee KJ, Park YC, Park JY, Hwang WS. Miniscrew-assisted nonsurgical palatal expansion before orthognathic surgery for a patient with severe mandibular prognathism. Am J Orthod Dentofac Orthop. 2010;137(6):830–9.
10. Möhlhenrich SC, Modabber A, Kamal M, Fritz U, Prescher A, Hölzle F. Three-dimensional effects of pterygomaxillary disconnection during surgically assisted rapid palatal expansion: a cadaveric study. Oral Surg Oral Med Oral Pathol Oral Radiol. 2016;121(6):602–8.
11. Hernandez-Alfaro F, Mareque Bueno J, Diaz A, Pagés CM. Minimally invasive surgically assisted rapid palatal expansion with limited approach under sedation: a report of 283 consecutive cases. J Oral Maxillofac Surg. 2010;68(9):2154–8.
12. Li K, Quo S, Guilleminault C. Endoscopically-assisted surgical expansion (EASE) for the treatment of obstructive sleep apnea. Sleep Med. 2019;60:53–9.
13. Echchadi ME, Benchikh B, Bellamine M, Kim SH. Corticotomy-assisted rapid maxillary expansion: a novel approach with a 3-year follow-up. Am J Orthod Dentofac Orthop. 2015;148(1):138–53.
14. Suzuki SS, Braga LFS, Fujii DN, Moon W, Suzuki H. Corticopuncture facilitated microimplant-assisted rapid palatal expansion. Case Rep Dent. 2018;2018:1392895.
15. Lee SC, Park JH, Bayome M, Kim KB, Araujo EA, Kook YA. Effect of bone-borne rapid maxillary expanders with and without surgical assistance on the craniofacial structures using finite element analysis. Am J Orthod Dentofac Orthop. 2014;145(5):638–48.
16. Copello FM, Marañón-Vásquez GA, Brunetto DP, Caldas LD, Masterson D, Maia LC, et al. Is the buccal alveolar bone less affected by mini-implant assisted rapid palatal expansion than by conventional rapid palatal expansion?-a systematic review and meta-analysis. Orthod Craniofac Res. 2020;23(3):237–49.
17. Park JJ, Park YC, Lee KJ, Cha JY, Tahk JH, Choi YJ. Skeletal and dentoalveolar changes after miniscrew-assisted rapid palatal expansion in young adults: a cone-beam computed tomography study. Korean J Orthod. 2017;47(2):77–86.
18. Corbridge JK, Campbell PM, Taylor R, Ceen RF, Buschang PH. Transverse dentoalveolar changes after slow maxillary expansion. Am J Orthod Dentofac Orthop. 2011;140(3):317–25.
19. Cantarella D, Dominguez-Mompell R, Moschik C, Sfogliano L, Elkenawy I, Pan HC, et al. Zygomaticomaxillary modifications in the horizontal plane induced by micro-implant-supported skeletal expander, analyzed with CBCT images. Prog Orthod. 2018;19(1):41.
20. Nada RM, van Loon B, Schols JG, Maal TJ, de Koning MJ, Mostafa YA, et al. Volumetric changes of the nose and nasal airway 2 years after tooth-borne and bone-borne surgically assisted rapid maxillary expansion. Eur J Oral Sci. 2013;121(5):450–6.
21. Hur JS, Kim HH, Choi JY, Suh SH, Baek SH. Investigation of the effects of miniscrew-assisted rapid palatal expansion on airflow in the upper airway of an adult patient with obstructive sleep apnea syndrome using computational fluid-structure interaction analysis. Korean J Orthod. 2017;47(6):353–64.
22. Lee SR, Lee JW, Chung DH, Lee SM. Short-term impact of microimplant-assisted rapid palatal expansion on the nasal soft tissues in adults: a three-dimensional stereophotogrammetry study. Korean J Orthod. 2020;50(2):75–85.
23. Magnusson A, Bjerklin K, Kim H, Nilsson P, Marcusson A. Three-dimensional computed tomographic analysis of changes to the external features of the nose after surgically assisted rapid maxillary expansion and orthodontic treatment: a prospective longitudinal study. Am J Orthod Dentofac Orthop. 2013;144(3):404–13.
24. Lee KC, Perrino M. Alar width changes due to surgically-assisted rapid palatal expansion: a meta-analysis. J Orthod Sci. 2017;6(4):115–22.

Nerve Involvement in Oral Surgery

36

Kristopher L. Hasstedt, Roger A. Meyer, and Shahrokh C. Bagheri

The most commonly injured TN5 branches are the inferior alveolar nerve (IAN) and the lingual nerve (LN), both of which are branches of the mandibular/third division (V3) of the TN5. Others such as the mental nerve (MN), long buccal nerve (LBN), both of which are part of V3, and the infraorbital nerve (ION), from the maxillary/second division (V2) of the TN5, are less common, but they can also cause untoward sensory symptoms (neurosensory dysfunction/NSD). Such injuries cause altered sensation (paresthesia/decreased or loss of sensation, pain, hypersensitivity), which may seriously interfere with the performance of normal orofacial activities (Table 36.1), and if they fail to resolve and become persistent or permanent, it will most likely adversely affect the quality of life in afflicted patients.

Treatment of TN5 injuries requires a number of steps, beginning with a nerve injury evaluation. Based on the nerve evaluation findings, continued monitoring versus nerve repair, nerve gap reconstruction, and/or sensory rehabilitation is performed.

Incidence and Etiology

Out of all TN5 injuries, the incidence of permanent nerve dysfunction is low. The most common cause of mandibular nerve injury remains third molar extractions. The rate of permanent injury following third molar extraction is 0.04–0.6%

K. L. Hasstedt (✉) · S. C. Bagheri
Georgia Oral and Facial Reconstructive Surgery,
Atlanta, GA, USA
e-mail: kristopher0930@gmail.com

R. A. Meyer
Department of Surgery, Northside Hospital, Atlanta, GA, USA

Maxillofacial Consultations, Ltd., Greensboro, GA, USA

Medical College of Georgia, August, GA, USA

Private Practice: Georgia Oral and Facial Reconstructive Surgery,
Marietta, GA, USA

Table 36.1 Normal orofacial activities adversely affected by TN5 injuries

Chewing food	Face washing
Drinking liquids	Shaving
Swallowing	Applying facial make-up
Toothbrushing	Playing wind instruments
Singing	Taste sensation

Table 36.2 Incidence of TN5 injury based on procedure

Procedure	Permanent NSD (%)
Local anesthetic injection	0.54
M3 removal	0.001–0.040
Genioplasty	3.33–10.0
Mandibular SSRO	12.8–39.0
SSRO + genioplasty	66.6
Mandibular IVRO	0.01
Mandibular DO	<5.0
Mandible fracture	38.8
ZMC fracture	37.0
Mandibular vestibuloplasty	50–100
Dental implant	0–15

Modified with permission from Meyer and Bagheri [17], pp. 37
TN5 trigeminal nerve, *M3* mandibular third molar tooth, *SSRO* sagittal split ramus osteotomy, *IVRO* intraoral vertical ramus osteotomy, *DO* distraction osteogenesis
Permanent NSD (%) sensory aberration (moderate hypoesthesia to anesthesia +/− hyperesthesia) that persists beyond 3 months post-injury

for LN and 0.1–1% for the IAN (Table 36.2). Injuries to the inferior alveolar nerve (IAN) and lingual nerves (LNs) have long been known complications of the mandibular sagittal split ramus osteotomy (SSRO). Most postoperative paresthesias resolve without treatment. However, microsurgical exploration of the nerve may be indicated in cases of significant persistent sensory dysfunction associated with observed or suspected localized IAN or LN injury. The two most common surgical treatments for mandibular deformities still remain the bilateral sagittal split ramus osteotomy (SSRO) and the intraoral vertical ramus osteotomy (IVRO). Since the

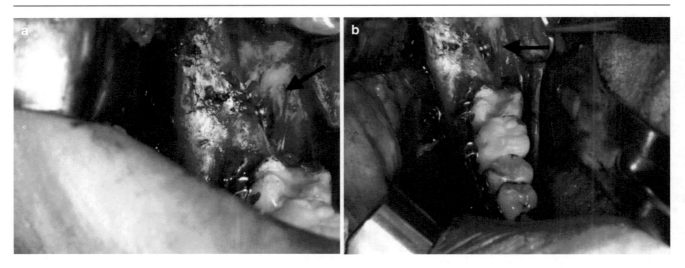

Fig. 36.1 Potential mechanism of LN injury during fixation of SSRO: (**a** and **b**) fixation screw passing into the lingual soft tissues (black arrows)

SSRO was first described in 1942 by Schuchardt, multiple modifications have been developed in order to decrease the risk of injury to the TN5. Injury to the LN during SSRO procedures is most likely due to the fixation technique using bicortical screws than the surgical procedure itself (see Fig. 36.1) [5].

In 2010, Bagheri and associates reported on the incidence and repair of nerve injury following sagittal split osteotomies from 1986 to 2005. They found that the IAN was injured in 39 out of 54 patients, while the LN was injured in 14 out of the 54 patients [5]. In this review, 33.3% of the injuries were noted to be a discontinuity defect, while 27.8% were a partial nerve severance. Al-Moraissi and Ellis studied the difference in NSD between SSRO and IVRO. This study showed results consistent with previous studies, in which the risk of IAN NSD was significantly decreased with IVRO when compared to that of SSRO [1].

Maxillofacial trauma can also be a cause of TN5 injury. The most common cause of an IAN injury following trauma is due to a mandibular angle fracture, whereas the MN is most likely damaged in the presence of a parasymphyseal fracture (Fig. 36.2) [6]. The infraorbital nerve is most commonly injured in conjunction with a zygomaticomaxillary (ZMC) fracture and the LN with a mandibular body fracture [6]. Bagheri et al. reviewed 42 patients that had TN5 injuries associated with facial fractures, with the most common finding being pain with or without numbness, or numbness alone. In this review, compression injuries were the most commonly seen, followed by partial nerve tran-

section [6]. Bagheri et al. 1 noted that 36 (86%) of the patients who had TN5 nerve repairs developed "functional sensory recovery" (FSR) while 6 (14%) showed an MCRS score of 2+ or less [6].

Trigeminal Nerve Anatomy

The trigeminal nerve is divided into three parts: the ophthalmic nerve (V1), maxillary nerve (V2), and mandibular nerve (V3) (Fig. 36.3). The mandibular division of the TN5 leaves the skull through the foramen ovale where it enters the infratemporal fossae. At this junction, the lingual nerve and inferior alveolar nerves are within the same stem and later separate anteriorly in the pterygomandibular space (Fig. 36.4). Sittitavornwong et al. developed a new description of the LN location, dividing its course into three "zones." Zone 1 extends from the skull base to the lingula inferiorly. Zone 2 extends from the lingula to the junction of the internal oblique ridge and mylohyoid line. Zone 3 extends from the inferior extent of zone 2 to the tongue inferiorly. The purpose of this "zoning" of the LN was to identify procedures that would be high risk for LN injury and aid in the identification of the level of LN injury and the prognosis of such injuries [25].

In 1984, Kiesselbach and Chamberlain published a landmark study on the anatomy of the LN in the third molar site. Kiesselbach and Chamberlain showed that the LN was approximately 0.58 ± 0.9 mm lateral to the lingual plate;

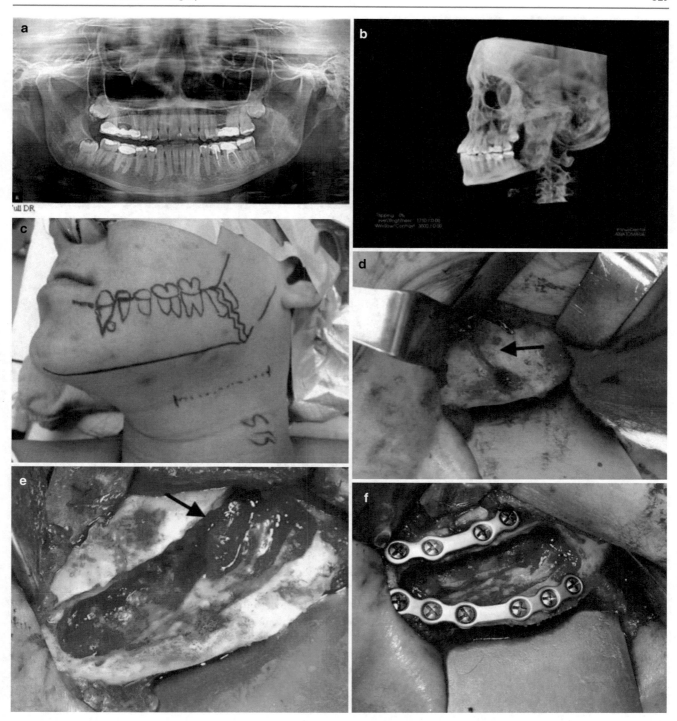

Fig. 36.2 35-year-old woman s/p extraction of tooth #17 with a subsequent left mandibular angle fracture and left IAN neurosensory dysfunction (pain and numbness): (**a**) Postoperative panoramic image following extraction of tooth #17; (**b**) 3-D replication of CT scan showing left mandibular angle fracture (red arrow); (**c**) preoperative mark-ings showing outline of mandible with fracture and incision line (Risdon approach); (**d**) left mandibular angle fracture (black arrow); (**e**) left IAN exposed showing transection injury with proximal stump neuroma (black arrow); (**f**) ORIF of the left mandibular angle fracture with repair of IAN using autologous nerve graft and nerve wrap

Fig. 36.3 Sensory innervation of the face via branches of the three major divisions of the trigeminal nerve. *V1* ophthalmic division, *V2* maxillary division, *V3* mandibular division. (Reproduced with permission from Meyer and Bagheri [17])

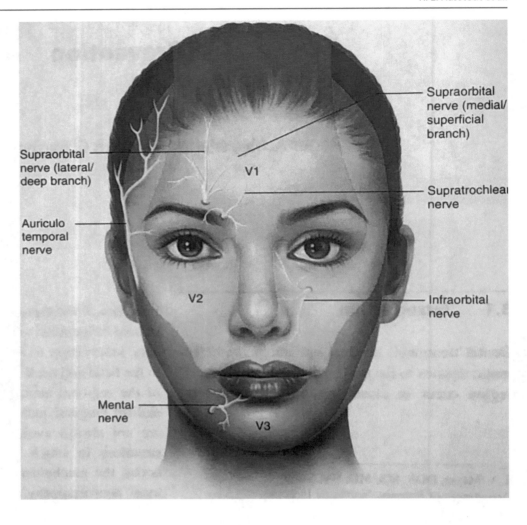

however, in 62% of cadaveric specimens, the LN was in direct contact with the lingual plate [13]. Vertically, the LN was 2.28 ± 1.96 mm below the alveolar crest. In 17.6% of cadaveric specimens, the LN was at or above the alveolar crest level [13]. Kiesselbach's and Chamberlain's work and other studies on LN anatomy document that the location of the LN is highly variable from patient to patient and that "classical" anatomy as depicted in anatomy textbooks and atlases is merely an average position of each anatomic part, which may vary little or a lot in any individual patient.

Behnia and associates performed a large study in 2000, in which 669 LNs from 430 fresh cadavers were examined. In 94 cases (14.05%), the LN was above the lingual crest, and in 1 case (0.15%), the nerve was in the retromolar pad region [8]. In the remaining 574 cases (85.80%), the mean horizontal and vertical distances of the nerve to the lingual plate and the lingual crest are 2.06 ± 1.10 mm (range, 0.00–3.20 mm) and 3.01 ± 0.42 mm (range, 1.70–4.00 mm), respectively [8]. In 149 cases (22.27%), the nerve was in direct contact with the alveolar process's lingual plate [8]. The Behnia study confirms Kiesselbach and Chamberlain's work, which shows

the variation in LN position from patient to patient and re-emphasizes the importance to the surgeon of knowing this anatomical variability.

Once the LN and the IAN separate in the pterygomandibular space, the IAN enters the mandible on the medial aspect through the lingula. The IAN then passes within the mandibular canal and exits through the mental foramen on the lateral mandibular body. The position of the IAN varies from patient to patient in its supero-inferior or mediolateral dimension.

Diagnosis

The most important aspect of the treatment of TN5 injury is establishing the correct diagnosis [16]. In order to do this, it is important to garner a complete history of the injury. How did it happen, did the symptoms change throughout the post-incident course, and was any treatment given at any point following the inciting incident? What are the symptoms that the patient is experiencing? Pain, loss of sensation, or both?

Fig. 36.4 Important sensory branches of the trigeminal nerve in the oral cavity: (**a**) labio-buccal aspect of the maxilla and mandible; (**b**) lingual area of the mandible. (Reproduced with permission from Meyer and Bagheri [17])

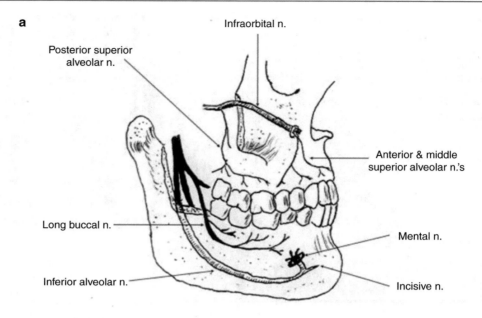

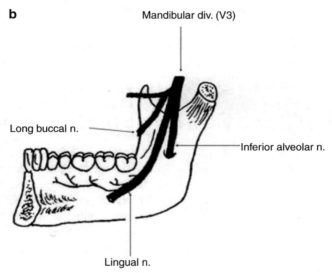

What exacerbates the pain if anything? (Table 36.3) If the patient is experiencing pain, obtain a measure of pain intensity using the visual analogue scale (VAS) estimate. This pain estimate helps compare it to subsequent patient visits to assist in assessing any progress (worsening or improving).

After obtaining a subjective evaluation from the patient, an objective assessment is necessary. A screening evaluation of cranial nerves II-XII is performed and documented. Generally, cranial N I (olfactory nerve) is not evaluated clinically. A neurosensory testing (NST) protocol was developed by Zuniga et al. and has been used for many years to assess the sensory response of nerves to multiple types of stimuli. This NST protocol includes responses to painful stimuli, static light touch, and two-point discrimination [30]. First, the area of altered sensation is mapped out using the "march-

ing needle" technique, in which a 27-gauge needle is placed in an area of normal skin or mucosal sensation and moved every 1–2 mm until the sensation changes. This is repeated until the borders of the affected areas are mapped out. Once the area has been properly identified and marked, NST can begin, starting on the normal side first (Fig. 36.5).

NST is broken down into levels A, B, and C, in which different nerve fibers are evaluated. Level A uses directional discrimination, static two-point discrimination, and stimulus localization to evaluate the A-alpha sensory nerve fibers. Level B uses contact detection with the wooden end of a cotton-tipped applicator or Semmes-Weinstein monofilaments to evaluate the A-beta nerve fibers, which are medium in size. Finally, Level C testing measures nociception using a 27-gauge needle to make light touch to the skin without

Table 36.3 Pain terms adapted from the definitions of the International Association for the Study of Pain

Paresthesia	Abnormal sensation whether spontaneous or evoked and is not unpleasant
Dysesthesia	An unpleasant abnormal sensation, whether spontaneous or evoked. Special cases of dysesthesia include hyperalgesia and allodynia
Anesthesia	It is a pharmacologically induced and reversible state of amnesia, analgesia, loss of responsiveness, loss of skeletal muscle reflexes or decreased stress response, or all simultaneously
Hyperesthesia	Increased sensitivity to stimulation, excluding the special senses. The stimulus and locus should be specified. *Hyperesthesia* may refer to various moms of cutaneous sensibility including touch and thermal sensation without pain, as well as to pain. The word is used to indicate both diminished threshold to any stimulus and an increased response to stimuli that are normally recognized
Hypoesthesia	Decreased sensitivity to stimulation, excluding the special senses. Stimulation and locus to be specified
Synesthesia	A neurological condition in which stimulation of one sensory or cognitive pathway leads to automatic, involuntary experiences in a second sensory or cognitive pathway
Allodynia	Pain due to a stimulus that does not normally provoke pain. The stimulus leads to an unexpectedly painful response. This is a clinical term that does not imply a mechanism. Allodynia may be seen after different types of somatosensory stimuli applied to many different tissues
Sensitization	Increase responsiveness of nociceptive neurons to their normal input and/or recruitment of a response to normally subthreshold inputs. Sensitizations can include a drop in threshold and an increase in suprathreshold response. Spontaneous discharges and increases in receptive field size may also occur

Reproduced with permission from Zuniga and Radwan [31]

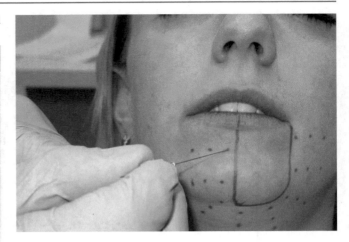

Fig. 36.5 The "marching needle" technique is used to determine the boundaries of the area of altered sensation in a patient with complaints of left lower lip and chin numbness after lower third molar removal. A 27-gauge needle is used beginning in an area of normal sensation, and multiple contacts are made (*red dots*) every few millimeters until the patient reports a change in the sensation (e.g., "sharp" changes to the "dull"). After these determinations have been made from the left to right and inferior to superior, the border of the affected area can be delineated (*solid red line*). (Reproduced with permission from Meyer and Bagheri [16])

indentation. If the patient responds, this is recorded as "response to normal threshold." If no response is appreciated, the needle is used to make an indentation in the skin, but not to break the skin surface. If the patient responds, this is a "response at increased threshold." If the patient still fails to respond, this is "no response." Alternately, pain response can be determined more accurately with an algometer. The results of NST are documented in the patient's chart (Fig. 36.6).

The TN5 sensory function level is unable to be assessed directly; therefore, an indirect method has been developed in order to determine the status of its neurosensory function. The Medical Research Council Scale (MRCS, which originated in the United Kingdom) was originally used to grade and monitor brachial plexus injuries (Table 36.4). This was modified in order to assess the function of the TN5. Using this grading scale, the TN5 function ranges from S0 (no sensation) to S4 (normal). This scale uses two-point discrimination, superficial pain, and touch sensations in order to assess

the sensory function of the TN5. If the patient is being followed periodically because it is hoped that the nerve will recover over time ("expectant observation"), it is advised to document and map the objective findings at each appointment. This will show any changes or improvement from one assessment to another. A grade of S3 or greater is termed "functional sensory recovery" (FSR), which indicates satisfactory responses to superficial pain and static light touch sensation without hyperesthesia and static two-point discrimination of 15 mm [24].

Zuniga et al. studied the relationship of neurosensory testing (NST) to the degree of TN5 injury, finding that there was a significant positive relationship between the sensory impairment score and the degree of nerve injury. In this study, the evaluation of the LN was slightly more accurate than that of the IAN, which had more false negatives and false positives [30]. However, it was concluded that NST is a useful and reasonably accurate clinical method of evaluating the level of function of an injured TN5.

Imaging modalities can be helpful in the diagnosis of TN5 injuries. Computerized tomography (CT) identifies the position of the IAN canal in relation to the third molars. Still, this imaging technique does little to evaluate the condition of the nerve and vascular bundle. When a practitioner is trying to evaluate the nerves themselves, magnetic resonance imaging (MRI) is the choice method. Miloro et al. used MRI to ascertain the position of the LN in a series of patients. Miloro and

Kolokythas found that the LN was above the lingual crest 10% of the time and was in direct contact with the lingual plate 25% of the time [19]. MRI of the LN (now termed *magnetic resonance neurography*, MRN) is helpful in evaluating the status of the LN in suspected injury. This information can be determined if the LN has a discontinuity defect, which would indicate prompt and timely surgical intervention rather than further serial "expectant" clinical evaluations.

The treatment of TN5 injuries depends on the diagnosis of the injury. In 1942, Seddon developed a classification to grade nerve injuries and divided them into three categories: neuropraxia, axonotmesis, and neurotmesis (Table 36.5).

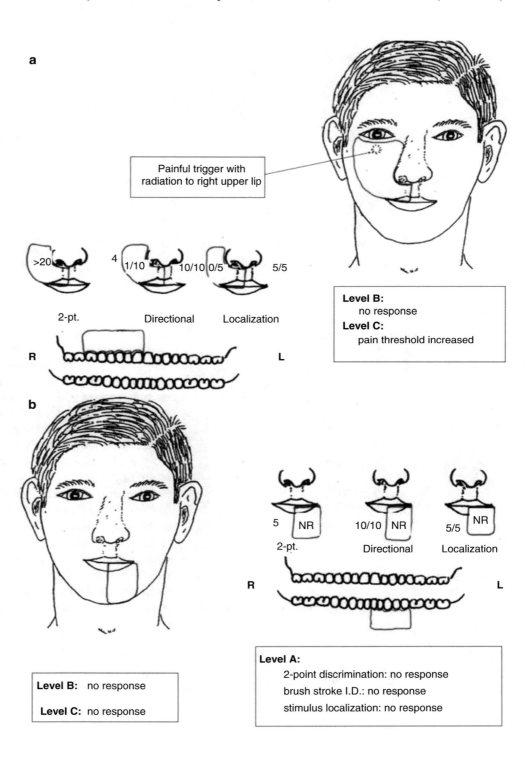

Fig. 36.6 The area of altered sensation and the results of NST are entered into the patient's record. (**a**) Patient with numbness and pain in the right face 6 months following a right ZMC fracture involving the right orbital floor and the inferior orbital rim. Affected areas of face and mouth contained within the *solid black line*, and there is severe hypoesthesia of the right infraorbital nerve. (**b**) Patient with loss of sensation in the left lower lip, chin, and left mandibular gingiva (affected areas contained within the *solid black line*) 4 months after BSSO. Immediate postoperative sensory loss on the right side has resolved. There is the anesthesia of the left IAN. (**c**) Patient with numbness of the right tongue 3 months after the removal of the mandibular third molar. There are also complaints of pain in the right tongue and lingual gingiva when chewing food and brushing the right lower teeth. Affected areas contained with the *solid black line*. Note the trigger area on the lingual aspect of the right mandible. The patient has anesthesia of the right lingual nerve. *NR* no response. (Reproduced with permission from Meyer and Bagheri [16])

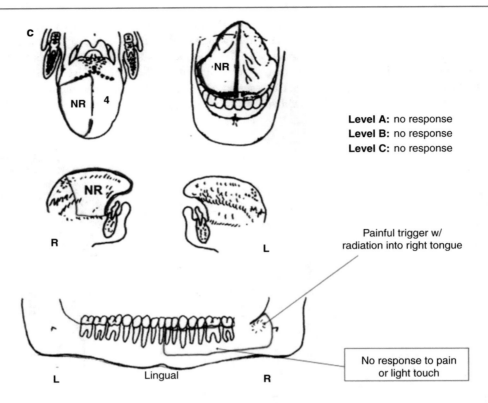

Level A: no response
Level B: no response
Level C: no response

Painful trigger w/
radiation into right tongue

No response to pain
or light touch

Fig. 36.6 (continued)

Table 36.4 Modified MRCS (Medical Research Council Scale)

Grade	Description
S0	No sensation
S1	Deep cutaneous pain in the autonomous zone
S2	Some superficial pain and touch
S2+	Superficial pain and touch plus hyperesthesia
S3	Superficial pain and touch without hyperesthesia and static two-point discrimination >15 mm. Indicates useful sensory function (USF)
S3+	Same as S3 with good stimulus localization and static two-point discrimination of 7–15 mm. Indicates USF
S4	Same as S3 and static two-point discrimination of 2–6 mm. Indicates complete sensory recovery (CSR)

Reproduced with permission from Zuniga and Radwan [31]

Table 36.5 Nerve injury classification with prognosis and need for surgical intervention

Seddon	Sunderland	Prognosis	Need for surgery
Neuropraxia	S1	Good	(−)
Axonotmesis	S2	Unpredictable	(−/+)
	S3	Unpredictable	(−/+)
	S4	Unpredictable	(−/+)
Neurotmesis	S5	Poor	(+)

Neuropraxia describes a "transient block" in which neither the nerve nor the sheath is disrupted [23]. This injury typically results in complete recovery, usually within 4 weeks of injury without treatment. In *axonotmesis*, neuronal axons are disrupted; however, the epineurium is maintained [23]. In the axons distal to the area of injury/discontinuity, Wallerian degeneration occurs and a prolonged neurosensory deficit occurs. Recover from this type of injury takes anywhere from weeks to months, and complete recovery may not occur. In addition to lost sensation (hypoesthesia or anesthesia), painful sensations (dysesthesia) or hypersensitivity (hyperesthesia) may develop within days, weeks, or months of the injury. *Neurotmesis* is due to a partial or complete severing of the nerve or a thermal or chemical injury, either of which produces a sensory impulse conduction block [23]. If there is a partial or complete severance of the nerve, a neuroma (often painful) typically forms on the proximal nerve stump. This neuroma is frequently the cause of pain, either spontaneous or in response to the stimulus (Fig. 36.7), and the pain may become chronic and intractable. Recovery of FSR or resolution of the pain seldom, if ever, occurs with this injury in the absence of microsurgical nerve repair.

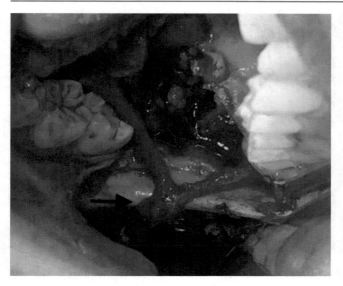

Fig. 36.7 Lingual nerve exposed with neuroma (black arrow)

Microsurgical Treatment and Access

The LN, MN, and LBN are easily accessed intraorally, while the IAN, depending on the suspected location of its injury, may be exposed via a transoral incision (most often for those injuries occurring anterior to the mandibular third molar, M3M) or a submandibular skin incision to provide better access and visualization for an injury that is more posterior. The surgeon may elect to expose the IAN in some patients by using a sagittal split mandibular ramus osteotomy. Exposure of the ION might be done intraorally. However, access and visualization are more satisfactory through a subciliary skin incision, especially when necessary to explore and repair the ION within the infraorbital canal.

Lingual Nerve

The lingual nerve (LN) can be accessed via a typical BSSRO incision on the buccal aspect of the mandible. This incision can be joined at the most posterior tooth's distobuccal line angle with an incision along the lingual gingival sulci of the mandibular teeth. Elevation of a mucoperiosteal flap on the mandible's buccal and lingual aspects will aid in the placement of a self-retaining retractor. Once the LN is visualized in the adjacent soft tissue, it can be dissected out to observe its proximal and distal ends. Depending on the nerve's clinical evaluation, once adequately exposed, the appropriate

repair of the injured nerve can be carried out. If there is a discontinuity defect in the LN, the proximal and distal nerve limbs are dissected free of surrounding connective and/or scar tissue for maximum mobilization. This was having been done; a preexisting "nerve gap" can often be closed without the need for a nerve graft, the two LN stumps after mobilization having been brought together without tension.

Inferior Alveolar Nerve

The IAN has a much longer course of exposure to injury than does the LN. Thus, multiple incisions might be considered to provide adequate access and visualization of the nerve. For those nerve injuries located posterior to the third molar area, a sagittal split ramus osteotomy (SSRO) may be required to fully visualize the injury in the posterior mandible and/or pterygomandibular fossa. However, for injuries to the IAN at or anterior to the third molar area, access can be obtained via intraoral and/or transcutaneous incisions, depending on the individual patient and the surgeon's judgment. An intraoral incision can be performed by making an SSRO incision and elevating a full-thickness mucoperiosteal flap on the buccal aspect. Access to the nerve can then be made by removing the overlying bone. This approach's benefits are the lack of an extraoral scar; however, there might be limited access and visualization with this technique in some patients.

A Risdon approach is used for transcutaneous access (Fig. 36.8). In this technique, the nerve can be accessed from where it enters the mandibular canal to where it exits through the mental foramen. This technique's benefits are increased visualization; however, the patient will always have a scar from the incision on the neck, and there is a small chance of injury to the marginal mandibular branch of the facial nerve (FN7). Careful attention to the local anatomy of the FN7, use of magnification during soft tissue dissection, and a meticulous closure of the incision will mitigate these risks.

Treatment

After the injured nerve has been fully exposed, debrided, and mobilized (decompression procedure), one or more of the following steps are performed in order until the surgeon is satisfied with the result: internal neurolysis, excision of a neuroma or other pathologic tissue, mobilization of proximal and distal nerve stumps, neurorrhaphy without tension, reconstruction of a nerve gap, or a nerve-sharing procedure,

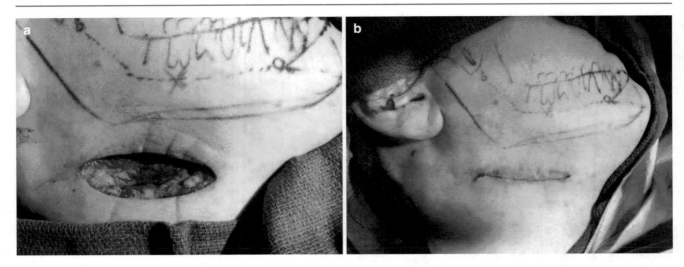

Fig. 36.8 (**a**) Risdon approach incision made in a natural crease line to decrease the visibility of postoperative scar; (**b**) Risdon approach closure, maintaining natural crease line

nerve redirection, or nerve capping. Nerve-sharing and nerve-capping procedures are rarely used anymore in peripheral nerve repairs.

Neurorrhaphy

If the proximal and distal ends of the nerve are able to be re-approximated without tension, then neurorrhaphy is the best option for nerve repair. This is performed by re-approximating the proximal and distal nerve ends together and suturing them with a fine, nylon suture that secures only the epineurium (Fig. 36.9). Usually, four sutures "around the clock" are sufficient for this maneuver. If a tension-free neurorrhaphy is not possible, then a nerve graft will be needed to reconstruct the nerve's continuity.

Nerve Grafting

The purpose of nerve grafting is to reconstruct nerve continuity across a nerve gap when neurorrhaphy cannot be done without creating tension across the repair. A nerve graft is used as an interpositional bridge. When the gap is less than 1.0 cm, repair of an LN is often possible by extensive mobilization of the proximal and distal nerve stumps because the LN has a tortuous course, especially in its distal extension in the floor of the mouth. On the other hand, the IAN is not as equally able to be mobilized, straightened, and extended due to its relatively straight course within the inferior alveolar canal. In some patients, resection of the incisive nerve allows

the mobilization of the IAN sufficient to allow a tension-free neurorrhaphy. However, this is less often possible than is the case with the LN. Processed human nerve grafts are commercially available (Axogen, Alachua, FL), and results of these allografts (AGs) in the repair of TN5 injury have been promising [27]. Yampolsky and associates performed a study on nerve repair using processed nerve AGs and an AG conduit in nerve injuries with a gap of less than 2 cm. Of the 16 patients that met their inclusion criteria, 15 (93.75%) achieved a score of at least S3 (FSR) on the MCR scale [28]. Most recently, Salomon et al. [22], Zuniga et al. [32], Miloro and Zuniga [20], and Callahan et al. [9] have reported on the successful use of nerve AGs in the reconstruction of TN5 nerve gaps created by ablative oncologic surgery in the maxilla and mandible.

Autogenous nerve grafts (ANGs) were, for many years, the "gold standard" for the reconstruction of nerve gaps [14]. The greater auricular nerve (GAN) and the sural nerve (SN) were the most common ANGs used for reconstructing the nerve gap. The SN is harvested via an incision superiorly and posterior to the ankle's lateral malleolus (Fig. 36.10). This nerve supplies sensation to the lateral foot. The SN is longer in length and larger in diameter than the GAN. The GAN is harvested via an incision in a natural skin crease, lateral to the sternocleidomastoid muscle and approximately 6 cm inferior to the earlobe. The GAN has a shorter length and a smaller diameter than the SN. Because of the size discrepancy, a cable graft may need to be placed using the GAN in which two or more parallel nerve grafts are placed within the nerve gap and sutured to the proximal and distal ends of the TN5. The harvesting of an ANG has risks that may be unacceptable to some patients. The GAN harvest results in loss of skin sensation to the lower portion of the ear lobe and skin at the mandible angle. The SN harvest leaves the patient with a loss of sensation to the lateral aspect of the foot. This may be a problem for patients who rely on position sense in their foot, such as rock climbers, basketball players, or other physically active persons. All nerve graft harvest sites are at risk of the development of a neuroma or other painful sequel, which may be difficult to resolve or tolerate. The recent availability of processed nerve allografts has eliminated these concerns for most patients [15].

Nerve Cuff

When the gap is less than 1.0 cm, placement of a nerve cuff (Neuragen, Integra LifeSciences, Plainsboro, NJ) may be considered. This will eliminate the risk of morbidity associated with the harvesting of an autogenous nerve graft. A collagen or polyglycolic acid nerve cuff is placed around the nerve, with the proximal and distal ends of the nerve stumps being secured to the cuff with a suture. It is thought that the nerve cuff acts as a conduit for the axons from the proximal stump to grow, traverse through the nerve gap, and re-

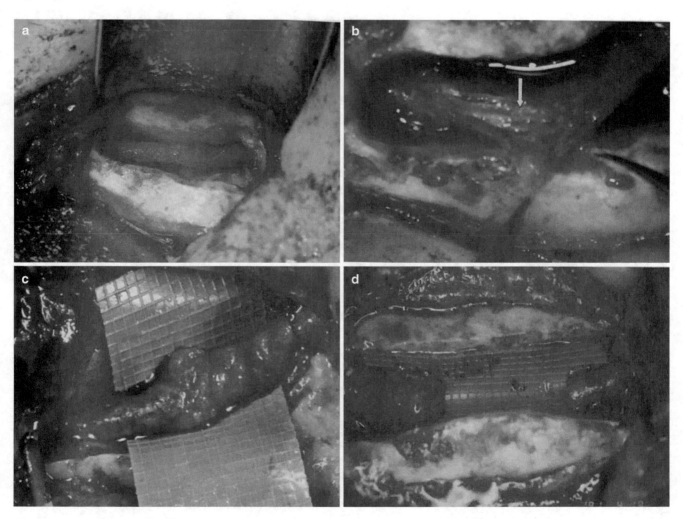

Fig. 36.9 Microneurosurgical procedures: (**a**) external decompression of the IAN. (**b**) Internal neurolysis of IAN. *Arrow* shows intact fascicles. (**c**) Neuroma-in-continuity of the IAN. (**d**) IAN after excision of a neuroma-in-continuity. (**e**) Diagram of a direct neurorrhaphy. (**f**) Sural nerve graft for IAN reconstruction. Areas of microanastamosis (*arrows*). (**g**) Decellularized human nerve graft (Axogen Avance, Alachua, FL) for IAN reconstruction. (**h**) Diagram of guided tissue regeneration with conduit repair (entubulation). (**i**) Neurectomy and epineural nerve capping. (**j**) Nerve redirection procedure. (Reproduced with permission from Bagheri and Meyer [2])

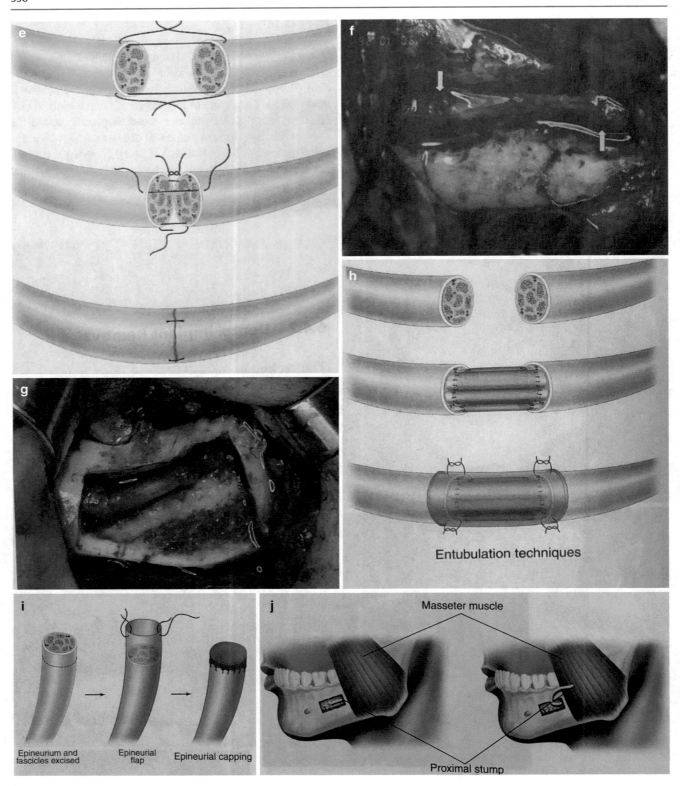

Fig. 36.9 (continued)

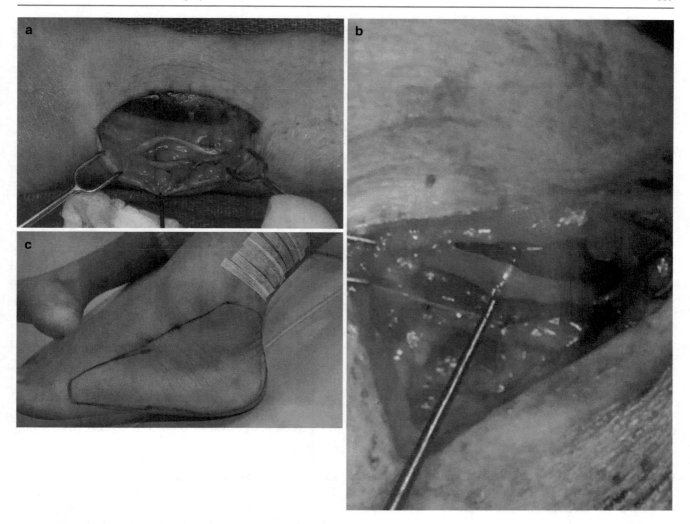

Fig. 36.10 (**a**) Sural nerve graft harvest. (**b**) Greater auricular nerve harvest. (**c**) Resulting area of anesthesia following sural nerve harvest. (Reproduced with permission from Bagheri and Meyer [2])

cannulate the endoneurial tubes within the distal stump of the nerve. Farole studied the effectiveness of placing a Neuragen nerve cuff on nine nerves (6 LN and 3 IAN). Results of this study showed that eight out of the nine showed improvement in symptoms, and none showed any worsening of symptoms [12].

Wilson et al. studied whether patients undergoing LN repair using a Type 1 collagen conduit (NeuraGen) versus a porcine-derived submucosal extracellular matrix (AxoGuard) had similar results. In this study, all patients developed FSR, and no differences were found between the two substrates [26]. Some surgeons, including the authors, place a conduit around ALL nerve repairs. Supposedly, the conduit prevents the inflow of blood or serum onto the repair site and the addi-

tional scarring that might interfere with the passage of new axons across the repair site.

Nerve-Sharing Procedure

The LN or IAN proximal stump may be absent or impossible to expose because of the avulsive results of missile injury or other trauma, infection, ablative oncologic surgery, or anatomic variation, and, therefore, unavailable for repair. If the distal limb of the injured nerve is able to be exposed and it appears to be viable, the nerve can be reconstructed by a *nerve-sharing procedure*. An ANG using the sural nerve from the lower extremity as a donor is used as a bridge between the injured nerve's distal limb and the ipsilateral GAN.

Results

The microsurgical nerve repair results depend on several variables, including time from injury to nerve repair, the type or severity of the nerve injury, age and general health status of the patient, and experience and skill of the surgeon. The sooner that the nerve is repaired, the more likely the patient will eventually recover FSR. Suppose a nerve is known to be transected by direct visualization ("open injury") or strongly suspected (e.g., brisk bleeding from a violated inferior alveolar canal) at the time of a procedure. In that case, the best time to repair it is at the time of the injury if the original practitioner is trained in microneurosurgery. If not, the patient is referred to a nerve injury specialist for the repair within a few days [3]. In cases where the nerve is not visibly transected ("closed injury"), a regimen of "expectant observation" is followed. The patient is re-evaluated every 2–4 weeks, as long as the sensory function continues to improve, as shown by history and NST. If a sensory plateau is seen and no further improvement occurs compared to the previous visit, no further improvement is likely to occur, and further observation will be fruitless. Then it is time to discuss surgical options if the patient is interested in potentially gaining improved neurosensory function. Bagheri et al. define "early repair" as less than 6 months [4]. Bagheri showed that patients who had surgical repair within 6 months of the injury were more likely to develop FSR than patients who were treated more than 6 months after the injury [4]. When a nerve injury is not directly visualized (closed injury) or strongly suspected at the time of the responsible procedure but fails to resolve or improve to the patient's satisfaction as documented by serial NST, nerve repair within 3 months of nerve injury results in better outcomes. Susarla et al. showed that 93% of patients had FSR within 1 year if their nerve injury was repaired within 90 days, compared to 62% of those having repair after 90 days [24]. Bagheri et al. found that patients were much more likely to achieve FSR if nerve injuries caused by maxillofacial trauma were repaired within a nine-month period from the time of injury [6].

Studies have also shown that the preoperative neurosensory function of the injured nerve plays a role in the prognosis. In general, the better the preoperative neurosensory function, the better the outcome following surgical repair. It has been well-documented that patients who do not develop neuropathic pain following their sensory nerve injury are very unlikely to develop it after repair of the nerve injury [33]. On the other hand, if a patient develops a pain syndrome after the nerve injury, there is a significantly less chance of gaining even partial pain relief following repair of the injury [33].

In general, younger patients achieve better functional results than elderly patients. Bagheri et al. showed that for every year over the age of 45 years old, there was a 5.5% decrease in achieving FSR [4]. Pogrel found that patients less than 40 years old were much less likely to develop long-term neurosensory dysfunction [21]. Miloro evaluated the effect of immediate nerve repair with decellularized nerve graft in pediatric patients (age < 18 years) following ablation of mandibular pathology. Miloro found that 100% of pediatric patients developed FSR at one year, whereas none of the patients without immediate repair developed FSR [20]. In a similar study with adults, only 85.7% of patients developed FSR at one year [22]. There was also a difference in the amount of time it took for the patients to score at a minimum of S3. Pediatric patients, on average, developed FSR at 75 days postoperatively compared to 110 days in the adult study [20].

The patient's general health can influence healing and thus the results of nerve repair. Conditions that compromise the immune system or the peripheral vascular system, such as diabetes mellitus, various connective tissue diseases (such as lupus erythematosus), cancer chemotherapy, or chronic tobacco smoking, undoubtedly adversely affect the healing of nerve tissues.

There is a "learning curve" in microneurosurgery. Practice on laboratory animals and assisting in nerve repairs on human patients are prerequisites to becoming an independent operator. It is estimated that between 50–100 "supervised" microsurgical repairs of peripheral nerve injuries on human patients are necessary to attain an acceptable clinical skill level. In the future, it is speculated that such experience will be achieved in a fellowship program ([29], unpublished).

The most commonly injured nerve during sagittal split osteotomies is the IAN. Bagheri and associates studied the repair of the TN5 after injury following SSRO procedures. In their study of 54 patients, 39 patients had an injury to the IAN, whereas 14 had injuries to the LN and 1 had an injury to the buccal branch [5]. The most common intraoperative finding was a discontinuity defect ($n = 18$, 33.3%), followed by partial nerve severance ($n = 15$, 27.8%), neuroma-in-continuity ($n = 11$, 20.3%), and compression injury ($n = 10$, 18.5%) [5]. The most frequent surgical procedure was autogenous nerve graft reconstruction of the IAN using the SN or GAN ($n = 22$, 40.7%), followed by excision of a neuroma with or without neurorrhaphy ($n = 13$, 24.1%). All the LN injuries ($n = 14$) were partial or complete severances, of which 2 were reconstructed with autogenous nerve grafts and the other 12 underwent neurorrhaphy. The long buccal nerve injury required excision of a proximal stump neuroma without neurorrhaphy. After a minimum of 1-year follow-up, NST showed that 8 nerves (14.8%) showed no sign of recovery, 19 nerves (35.2%) had regained FSR, and 27 nerves (50%) showed full recovery as described by the MRCS [5].

In 2009, Bagheri and associates studied the repair of 222 LN injuries. In this study, the most common cause of injury was the removal of third molars (86%), with SSROs being the second most common cause (6.3%) [4]. Out of the 222 nerves repaired, 201 (90.5%) had a recovery from neurosensory dysfunction of at least FSR (MRCS score of S0) or "complete return of sensation" (MRCS score of S4) [4].

Postoperative Care and Rehabilitation

Following a nerve injury's surgical repair, the patient is followed for the usual postoperative care and incision healing enhancement (if a skin incision was made). Beginning at 1 month after surgery, the patient is seen at monthly intervals at which time NST is done of the distribution of the repaired nerve. Once the patient has regained responses to painful stimuli and static light touch, sensory reeducation (SensReed) is begun. If hyperesthesia is a bothersome side effect, this is controlled with neurotropic medication (e.g., gabapentin, pregabalin, clonazepam).

SensReed is a cognitive behavioral therapy that uses repetitive exercises that can cause changes in the somatosensory cortex which can then compensate for some of the impairments caused by the initial nerve injury [11, 18]. It was initially shown to be effective in rehabilitating patients with sensory injuries in hand. These techniques were then adapted to TN5 injuries in the oral and maxillofacial regions. These exercises are helpful to nerve-injury patients, whether or not they have had microsurgical repair of the injured nerve. SensReed exercises include the patient watching him/ herself in a mirror while lightly stimulating first the contralateral normal side followed by the ipsilateral area of the face with the neurosensory dysfunction. Objects of variable consistency, such as a cotton swab, toothbrush, and bi-pronged hairpin or paper clip, are used. Watching in the mirror enhances tactile perception and the touch and varying qualities (moving or stable, sharp or dull, forceful or light touch, size of contact area, location of the touch, etc.). The exercises are then repeated with the patient's eyes closed. During all these maneuvers with eyes open or closed, the patient is advised to concentrate on the normal area's responses and retain this information while stimulating the area supplied by the injured/recovering nerve. The patient is encouraged to perform these exercises for 3–5 minutes three times each day. The more frequent practice may cause skin or mucosal irritation and is inadvisable.

These exercises are continued daily for at least 1 year or until the patient is satisfied with the injured/repaired nerve's sensory function. During this time, the patient is evaluated every 2–3 months, and NST is repeated to assess for progress. While the objective results of NST (per the MRCS) may or may not improve, the goal is for the patient to have a subjective sense of improvement of sensory nerve function due to central nervous system plasticity (i.e., learning and adaptation), in addition to any concurrent healing of the injured nerve (neurotization, increased conduction speed).

Conclusions

There are well-known and documented risks of injury to the peripheral branches of the TN5 during oral and maxillofacial surgery operations and other dental treatments. The risk of injury to the TN5 should be included in the pre-surgical consent discussion with each patient. If a nerve injury is known to have occurred, it is imperative to evaluate and treat the patient promptly in order to have the best chance of a recovery of FSR.

References

1. Al-Moraissi EA, Ellis E. Is there a difference in stability of neurosensory function between bilateral sagittal Split ramus osteotomy and intraoral vertical ramus osteotomy for mandibular setback? J Oral Maxillofac Surg. 2015;73(7):1360–71.
2. Bagheri SC, Meyer RA. Dental implant-related injuries of the trigeminal nerve. In: Miloro M, editor. Trigeminal nerve injuries. New York City: Springer-Verlag; 2013. p. 87–107.
3. Bagheri SC, Meyer RA. When to refer a patient with a nerve injury to a specialist. J Am Den Assoc. 2014;145:859.
4. Bagheri SC, Meyer RA, Khan HA, et al. A restrospective review of microsurgical repair of 222 lingual nerve injuries. J Oral Maxillofac Surg. 2009;68(4):715–23.
5. Bagheri SC, Meyer RA, Ali Khan H, et al. Microsurgical repair of the peripheral trigeminal nerve after mandibular sagittal split ramus osteotomy. J Oral Maxillofac Surg. 2010;68(11):2770–82.
6. Bagheri SC, Meyer RA, Khan HA, Steed MB. Microsurgical repair of peripheral trigeminal nerve injuries from maxillofacial trauma. J Oral Maxillofac Surg. 2009;67(9):1791–9.
7. Bagheri SC, Meyer RA, Khan HA, et al. Microsurgical repair of the inferior alveolar nerve: success rate and factors that adversely affect outcome. J Oral Maxillofac Surg. 2012;70(8):1978–90.
8. Behnia H, Kheradvar A, Shahrokhi M. An Anatomic study of the lingual nerve in the third molar region. J Oral Maxillofac Surg. 2000;58(6):649–51.
9. Callahan N, Miloro M, Markiewics MR. Immediate reconstruction of the infraorbital nerve after maxillectomy: is it feasible? J Oral Maxillofac Surg. 2020;78(12):2300–5.

10. Ehland EL, Meyer RA, Bagheri SC. Trigeminal nerve injuries. In: Bagheri SC, Khan HA, Stevens MR, editors. Complex dental implant complications. New York City: Springer-Verlag; 2020. p. 217–37.

11. Essick GK, Blakey G, Phillips C. Neurosensory rehabilitation. In: Miloro M, editor. Trigeminal nerve injuries. New Yrok City: Springer; 2013. p. 167–98.

12. Farole A, Jamal B. A bioabsorbable collagen nerve cuff (NeuraGen) for repair of lingual and inferior alveolar nerve injuries: a case series. J Oral Maxillofac Surg. 2008;66(10):2058–62.

13. Kiesselbach JE, Chamberlain JG. Clinical and anatomic observations on the relationship of the lingual nerve to the mandibular third molar region. J Oral Maxillofac Surg. 1984;42(9):565–7.

14. Meyer RA. Nerve harvesting procedures. Atlas Oral Maxillofac Surg Clin N Am. 2001;9:77–91.

15. Meyer RA. Immediate inferior alveolar nerve gap reconstruction. J Oral Maxillofac Surg. 2021;79(3):509.

16. Meyer RA, Bagheri SC. Clinical evaluation of nerve injuries. In: Miloro M, editor. Trigeminal nerve injuries. New York City: Springer-Verlag; 2013. p. 167–98.

17. Meyer RA, Bagheri SC. Etiology and prevention of nerve injuries. In: Miloro M, editor. Trigeminal nerve injuries. New York City: Springer-Verlag; 2013. p. 27–61.

18. Meyer RA, Rath EM. Sensory rehabilitation after trigeminal nerve injury or nerve repair. Atlas Oral Maxillofac Surg Clin North Am. 2001;13:365.

19. Miloro M, Kolokythas A. Imaging of the trigeminal nerve. In: Miloro M, editor. Trigeminal nerve injuries. New York City: Springer-Verlag; 2013. p. 199–212.

20. Miloro M, Zuniga JR. Does immediate inferior alveolar nerve allograft reconstruction result in functional sensory recovery in pediatric patients? J Oral Maxillofac Surg. 2020;78(11):2073–9.

21. Pogrel MA. The results of microneurosurgery of the inferior alveolar and lingual nerve. J Oral Maxillofac Surg. 2002;60(5):485–9.

22. Salomon D, Miloro M, Kolokythas A. Outcomes of immediate allograft reconstruction of long-span defects of the inferior alveolar nerve. J Oral Maxillofac Surg. 2016;74(12):2507–14.

23. Seddon HJ. A classification of nerve injuries. Br Med J. 1942;2(4260):237–9.

24. Susarla SM, Kaban LB, Donoff RB, Dodson TB. Does early repair of lingual nerve injuries improve functional sensory recovery? J Oral Maxillofac Surg. 2007;65(6):1070–6.

25. Sittitavornwong S, et al. Clinical anatomy of the lingual nerve: a review. J Oral Maxillofac Surg. 2017;75(5):926e.1–9.

26. Wilson M, Chuang S, Ziccardi V. Lingual nerve microsurgery outcomes using 2 different conduits: a retrospective cohort study. J Oral Maxillofac Surg. 2016;75(3):609–15.

27. Wolford LM, Rodrigues DB. Nerve grafts and conduits. In: Miloro M, editor. Trigeminal Nerve Injuries. New York City: Springer-Verlag; 2013. p. 271–89.

28. Yampolsy A, Ziccardi V, Chuang SK. Efficacy of acellular nerve allografts in trigeminal nerve reconstruction. J Oral Maxillfac Surg. 2007;75(10):2230–4.

29. Zuniga JR. Possible microneurosurgery fellowship, unpublished comments, 2020.

30. Zuniga JR, Meyer RA, Gregg JM, et al. The accuracy of clinical neurosensory testing for nerve injury diagnosis. J Oral Maxillofac Surg. 1998;56:2.

31. Zuniga JR, Radwan AM. Classification of nerve injuries. In: Miloro M, editor. Trigeminal nerve injuries. New York City: Springer-Verlag; 2013. p. 17–25.

32. Zuniga JR, Williams F, Petrisor D. A case-and-control, multisite, positive controlled, prospective study of the safety and effectiveness of immediate inferior alveolar nerve processed nerve allograft reconstruction with ablation of the mandible for benign pathology. J Oral Maxillofac Surg. 2017;75(12):2669–81.

33. Zuniga JR, Yates DM, Phillips CL. The presence of neuropathic pain predicts postoperative neuropathic pain following trigeminal nerve repair. J Oral Maxillofac Surg. 2014;72(12):2422–7.

Hamidreza Moslemi and Zahra Sadat Torabi

Introduction

Dental implants have been used successfully in oral rehabilitation for many years. Achieving adequate osseointegration is required before implant loading [1], and it depends on several factors. Albrektsson et al., in 1981[2], explained the criteria for implant success, including implant-related factors, host-related factors, surgical factors, biomechanical factors, and systemic factors (Box 37.1). Primary stability is one of the most important factors for successful osseointegration. Ottoni et al. [3] reported that a 9.8 N/cm increase in the insertion torque could lead to a 20% reduction in failure rate. Primary stability is achieved during implant insertion by mechanical friction between the osteotomy site's implant surface and walls. It is affected by bone quality and quantity [4] as well as macro geometric parameters of the implant [5].

Lekholm and Zarb [6] classified bone density based on morphology and distribution of cortical and trabecular bones (D1–D4). It is difficult to achieve adequate primary stability in low-density bone (D3–D4), such as in upper jaws. Many techniques have been attempted to increase the implants' primary stability inserted in these regions, including bi-cortical fixation, under preparation of the implant bed, and the use of osteotomes and condensers. All of these techniques had their own disadvantages. Increased stress and bending forces resulted in a higher fracture rate in bi-cortical fixated implants. Underpreparation may cause the loss of a healing chamber between implant and bone, decreasing the woven bone formation required for osseointegration. Using osteotomes also has its own drawbacks. It is demonstrated that osteotomes condensed the bone in periapical areas rather than lateral walls. Also, using mallet during condensing osteotomy is traumatic and may cause unintentional displacement, fracture, or vertigo. Moreover, micro-fractures in trabecular bone following this procedure can negatively affect and delay the osseointegration.

Huwais et al. [7] introduced a novel approach to implant site preparation to improve implants' primary stability by increasing surrounding bone density. Osseodensification technique can condense the bone along with the osteotomy site. It is the opposite of the conventional drilling method for implant site preparation, a subtractive method that excavates the bone.

Box 37.1 Criteria for implant success. (Adapted from Albrektsson et al. [2])

Implant-related factors	Biocompatibility Surface topography Composition Shape, design, dimensions
Host-related factors	Bone quality, density, volume
Surgical factors	Achieving primary stability Infection Mechanical and thermal trauma
Biomechanical factors	Loading conditions
Systemic factors	Systemic diseases Medications Parafunctional habits

Osseodensification

Rational and Advantages

Osseodensification is a novel implant site preparation technique developed by Salah Huwais in 2013. He invented Densah burs (Versah LLC: The Osseodensification company). These burs were able to densify the bone along the

H. Moslemi (✉) · Z. S. Torabi
Department of Oral and Maxillofacial Surgery, School of Dentistry, Shahid Beheshti University of Medical Sciences, Tehran, Iran
e-mail: hmoslemi71@sbmu.ac.ir

osteotomy walls by their special design. The inventor claimed that the osseodensification method could increase the insertion torque from 25 Ncm for implants placed using the conventional osteotomy preparation technique to 49 Ncm in low-density bone [7].

Osseodensification concept relies on the special design of Densah burs that are used in the counterclockwise direction. Osseodensifying bur is a conically tapered designed bur that can control the expansion process as the bur enters deeper into the bone. The apical end includes at least one lip to grind bone when rotating in the counterclockwise or non-cutting direction and cut bone-in clockwise or cutting direction. The body consists of helical flutes and interposed lands. Each flute has a burnishing face to burnish bone in the counterclockwise direction and an opposing cutting face to cut bone when turned in the clockwise direction. These characteristics are shown in Fig. 37.1.

This special design of Densah burs compacts the drilled bone around the implant osteotomy site. Compacted bone increases the implant's primary stability due to physical interlocking between the bone and the implant threads.

Huwais et al. reported that during osteotomy preparation, the viscoelastic deformation causes the spring-back effect of the compacted bone. When you let the osteotomy site remain empty, the diameter of the osseodensified osteotomy site reduces by 91% of the bur diameter [7]. This spring-back effect creates compressive forces against the implant, thereby enhancing the primary stability, promoting osteogenic activity through a mechanobiologic healing process. High insertion torque is also important for achieving an excellent clinical outcome with early or immediate loading.

Another claimed aspect of the osseodensification technique is that the compacted bone works as an autografted layer that can facilitate the osseointegration because of the high concentration of osteoblasts nucleating in close proximity implant surface.

Studies have been done to investigate the effect of this technique on implant insertion. Lahens et al. [8], in their study on iliac bone in sheep models, concluded that in low-density bone, higher insertion torque levels could be achieved for implants by using the osseodensification technique without impairing osseointegration. The sheep hip model was selected due to its low-density bone configuration. Trisi et al. [9] also conducted a study on sheep models and showed that a 30% increase in bone volume could be achieved using the osseodensification technique in inserting endosteal implants. Huwais et al. [7] reported increased insertion torque using the osseodensification technique in 72 implants inserted in porcine tibial plateau bone samples. They also confirmed the

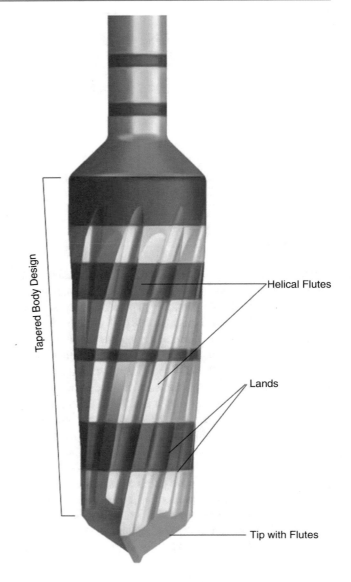

Fig. 37.1 Characteristic of an osseodensification bur

hypothesis that this technique increases bone mineral density and the percentage of bone at the implant surface.

Hindi and Bede [10] evaluated the osseodensification drilling method in the clinic in their prospective observational study. A total of 46 implants were inserted in low-density bone (bone density less than 850 Hounsfield units corresponds to D3–D4) using this method. They reported higher primary stability and increased peri-implant bone density. In the study of Hofbauer and Huwais [11] in which a single implant was placed in a premolar region having

3-mm buccolingual bone width using osseodensification drilling, an insertion torque of more than 50 Ncm was achieved. The advantages of the osseodensification technique are presented in Box 37.2..

Contraindications of osseodensification

Osseodensification is contraindicated in high-density bone (D1–D2) as it is a non-dynamic tissue and lacks plasticity which is required for densification. Also, densification of xenografts should be avoided because they have only inorganic materials with no viscoelasticity.

Box 37.2. Advantages of osseodensification

Increased primary stability
Compaction autografting
Enhanced bone density
Residual ridge expansion
Reduce healing time before implant loading

Osseodensification procedure

Osseodensifying burs can be used with standard surgical engines (800–1200 rpm). To densify bone, the bur rotates in a counterclockwise, non-cutting direction. If it is needed to cut the bone, the bur should turn in clockwise, cutting direction (Fig. 37.2).

In the counterclockwise, non-cutting direction, downward pressure and profuse saline irrigation create a compression wave inside the osteotomy that densify the bone and expand the bony ridge at the same time. A lubrication film is made from the irrigation fluid and the fluid content of the bone and placed between the implant surface and the host bone to reduce friction and more evenly distribute the compressive forces.

Bouncing motion of the bur (in and out of the osteotomy) is recommended, to produce a rate-dependent strain following a rate-dependent stress. This action coupled with the saline irrigation can gently pressurize the bone walls and facilitates increased bone plasticity and bone expansion.

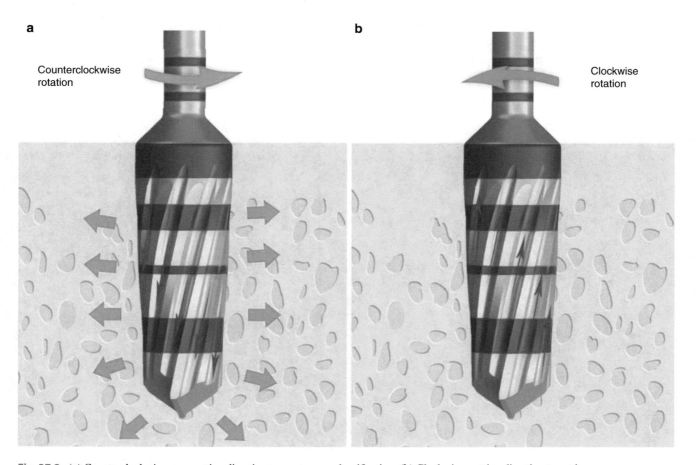

a

Counterclockwise rotation

b

Clockwise rotation

Fig. 37.2 (**a**) Counterclockwise, non-cutting direction to create osseodensification. (**b**) Clockwise, cutting direction to cut bone

Conclusion

Osseodensification has changed the paradigm of implant site preparation. As a novel method for implant insertion, it can be used in low-density bone (D3–D4), such as the upper jaw, to increase primary stability, bone mineral density, and bone volume at the implant surface and reduce the healing time before implants' loading. Also, this technique can be used for ridge expansion in narrow ridges for placement of larger diameter implants. It should be noted that using this method in high-density bone (D1-D2) and xenografts is contraindicated. Well-designed human studies with longer follow-ups are recommended for a higher level of evidence regarding this technique.

References

1. Brånemark PI. Osseointegration and its experimental background. J Prosthet Dent. 1983;50(3):399–410.
2. Albrektsson T, Brånemark PI, Hansson HA, Lindström J. Osseointegrated titanium implants. Requirements for ensuring a long-lasting, direct bone-to-implant anchorage in man. Acta Orthop Scand. 1981;52(2):155–70.
3. Ottoni JM, Oliveira ZF, Mansini R, Cabral AM. Correlation between placement torque and survival of single-tooth implants. Int J Oral Maxillofac Implants. 2005;20(5):769–76.
4. Yoon HG, Heo SJ, Koak JY, Kim SK, Lee SY. Effect of bone quality and implant surgical technique on implant stability quotient (ISQ) value. J Adv Prosthodont. 2011;3(1):10–5.
5. Coelho PG, Jimbo R, Tovar N, Bonfante EA. Osseointegration: hierarchical designing encompassing the macrometer, micrometer, and nanometer length scales. Dent Mater. 2015;31(1):37–52.
6. Lekholm U, Zarb G. Patient selection and preparation. In: Brånemark P, Zarb G, Alberktsson T, editors. Tissue Integrated prostheses: osseointegration in clinical dentistry. Chicago: Quintessence; 1985. p. 199–209.
7. Huwais S, Meyer EG. A novel osseous densification approach in implant osteotomy preparation to increase biomechanical primary stability, bone mineral density, and bone-to-implant contact. Int J Oral Maxillofac Implants. 2017;32(1):27–36.
8. Lahens B, Neiva R, Tovar N, Alifarag AM, Jimbo R, Bonfante EA, et al. Biomechanical and histologic basis of osseodensification drilling for endosteal implant placement in low density bone. An experimental study in sheep. J Mech Behav Biomed Mater. 2016;63:56–65.
9. Trisi P, Berardini M, Falco A, Vulpiani MP. New osseodensification implant site preparation method to increase bone density in low-density bone: In vivo evaluation in sheep. Implant Dent. 2016;25(1):24–31.
10. Hindi AR, Bede SY. The effect of osseodensification on implant stability and bone density: a prospective observational study. J Clin Expe Dent. 2020;12(5):e474.
11. Hofbauer A, Huwais S. Osseodensification facilitates ridge expansion with enhanced implant stability in the maxilla: Part II case report with 2-year follow-up. Implant Pract. 2015;8(2):14–21.

Soft Tissue Plastic Surgery

38

Lory Abrahamian, Pilar Golmayo, and Reem Kheirallah

Gingival Recessions: Etiology and Classification

Gingival recessions are defined as the displacement of the soft tissue margin apical to the cementoenamel junction (CEJ), and they constitute a frequent clinical feature in the general population. Evidence suggests that the predominant cause for localized recessions in young individuals is toothbrushing trauma, while periodontal disease may be the primary cause in older adults. Some predisposing and precipitating factors can be identified.

Predisposing factors:

- Insufficient attached gingiva
- Aberrant frenulum
- Decreased vestibular depth
- Thin phenotype
- Root prominence
- Tooth malposition causing bone dehiscence or fenestration

Precipitating factors:

- Plaque-induced inflammation
- Traumatic brushing/flossing
- Iatrogenic factors
- Occlusal trauma (controversial)
- Habits/piercings

It is of primary importance to diagnose the etiology of the recession to halt its progression. In contrast, a proper classi-

Table 38.1 The Miller classification for gingival recessions

Class I	Doesn't extend to the MGJ; no periodontal loss in the interdental area	100% root coverage
Class II	Extends to or beyond the MGJ; no periodontal loss in the interdental area	100% root coverage
Class III	Extends to or beyond the MGJ; bone or soft tissue loss in the interdental area or malposition of the teeth	Partial root coverage can be anticipated
Class IV	Extends to or beyond the MGJ; severe bone or soft tissue loss in the interdental area and/or malposition of the teeth	Root coverage cannot be anticipated

fication could help the practitioner to decide the correct treatment for the recession. Thus, many classifications have been used for this purpose. Miller in 1985 [1] described one of the most frequently used classifications of recessions (Table 38.1). It is based on the mucogingival junction (MGJ) position, mesial and distal periodontal loss (bone or soft tissue), and tooth malposition. It also assesses how predictable the mucogingival procedures are in terms of root coverage depending on each recession (Fig. 38.1).

The classification of Cairo 2011 [2] is based on the interproximal attachment loss. Since the World Workshop of 2017, this classification was stated as the main instrument to name gingival recessions (Table 38.2) (Fig. 38.2).

Historical Timeline of Soft Tissue Plastic Surgery

Originally proposed by Friedman in 1957 [3], "mucogingival surgery" was defined as any surgery designed to preserve attached gingiva, remove frena or muscle attachment, and increase the depth of the vestibule. Back then, it was believed that a minimum amount of attached gingiva was needed for the maintenance of gingival health around teeth. Multiple studies [4–6] showed that gingival health could be maintained independently of its dimensions and that there was a lack of association between the width of the attached gingiva

L. Abrahamian (✉) · P. Golmayo
Department of Periodontology, Universitat Internacional de Catalunya, Barcelona, Spain
e-mail: lory.abrahamian@uic.es; pilarg_86@hotmail.com

R. Kheirallah
Faculty of Dentistry, Universitat Internacional de Catalunya, Barcelona, Spain
e-mail: reemkhairallah@gmail.com

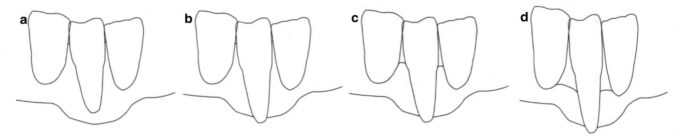

Fig. 38.1 The Miller classification for gingival recessions. (**a**) Class I, (**b**) Class II, (**c**) Class III, (**d**) Class IV

Table 38.2 The Cairo classification for gingival recessions

RT1	No loss of interproximal attachment; interproximal CEJ not detectable mesially and distally	100% root coverage
RT2	Loss of interproximal attachment; the amount of interproximal attachment loss less or equal to the buccal attachment loss	100% root coverage, different procedures
RT3	Loss of interproximal attachment; the amount of interproximal attachment loss is greater than the buccal attachment loss	Full root coverage not achieved

and the development of soft tissue recession in the presence of adequate oral hygiene measures [7]. With time, one important application of this type of surgery became treating gingival recessions. The term "mucogingival surgery" was thus replaced by "soft tissue plastic surgery" by the American Academy of Periodontology [8] since it englobed treating defects in the morphology, position, or amount of gingiva.

This chapter will showcase the most important soft tissue plastic surgery techniques.

Sullivan and Atkins in 1968 [9] explained how to prepare the recipient and donor sites while performing an autogenous free gingival graft (Fig. 38.3). The recipient site preparation procedure includes a horizontal incision at the level of the mucogingival junction extending mesially and distally to the concerned tooth and two vertical incisions connecting the horizontal incision. Sharp dissection of the epithelium, connective tissue, and muscle fibers is then performed down to the periosteum. The recipient bed's surface should be smooth to prevent clot formation in irregularities, which could prevent graft survival in the plasmatic stage. The donor site preparation consists of harvesting an autogenous graft from the palate, which is then immobilized on the recipient bed with sutures. This palatal graft is then closely secured to the recipient bed by interrupted sutures and a sling suture anchoring into the apical periosteum and aiding in the compression of the graft to prevent any movement and the forma-

tion of a coagulum separating the graft from the recipient bed.

The graft's thickness will determine its behavior during healing and its ultimate character; thick grafts having more primary contraction and less secondary contraction than thin grafts.

Tips and tricks for a free gingival graft procedure:

- The recipient bed should be thin in order to prevent mobility and thus necrosis.
- To make sure the recipient bed is not mobile, grab the lower lip and move it laterally: if mobility is seen, dissect the remaining muscle attachments.
- Although it is generally used for increasing the amount of keratinized tissue, a free gingival graft can also be used to partially cover recessions; in that scenario, the horizontal incision is made more coronally than usual.

Pedicle flaps consist of the repositioning of a flap either laterally or coronally. Grupe and Warren proposed laterally positioned flaps in 1956 [10]. This technique is indicated to treat single tooth recessions in cases where sufficiently high and thick keratinized tissue is available from the adjacent area. The recipient site preparation consists of performing a horizontal incision at the level of the CEJ of the concerned tooth, connected to a vertical incision that is parallel to the mesial gingival margin of the recession extending in the alveolar mucosa. The area marked by these incisions is then de-epithelized. The flap preparation consists of a beveled intrasulcular incision along the distal gingival margin of the recession defect and extending in alveolar mucosa, connected to a submarginal horizontal incision at the donor tooth site, preserving at least 1 mm of attached gingiva, followed by an oblique vertical incision extending into alveolar mucosa. Flap elevation is performed by a split-thickness approach ensuring passive placement of the flap laterally on the exposed root surface. Interrupted sutures are then used to

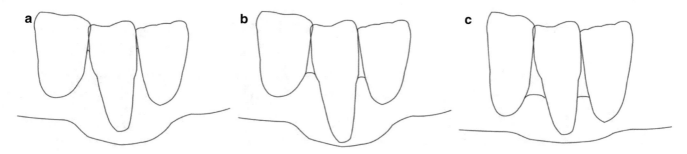

Fig. 38.2 The Cairo classification for gingival recessions. (**a**) RT1, (**b**) RT2, (**c**) RT3

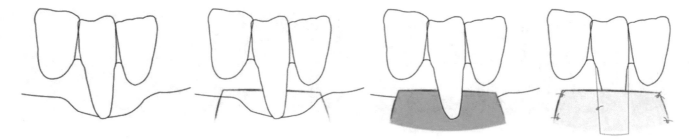

Fig. 38.3 The free gingival graft procedure

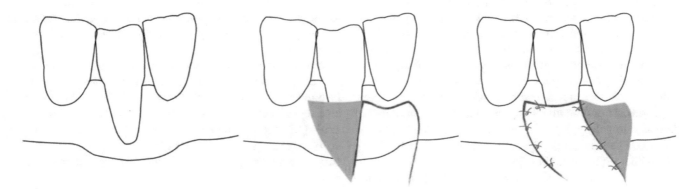

Fig. 38.4 The laterally positioned flap

secure the flap in the desired position mesially and distally, followed by a marginal sling suture in order to advance the flap (Fig. 38.4) coronally.

Tips and tricks for a laterally positioned flap procedure:

– The horizontal incision in the recipient site should be 3 mm, while the submarginal horizontal incision should be 6 mm more than the recession width measured at the CEJ.

– Start performing the interrupted sutures from the most apical extension of the vertical releasing incisions, proceeding coronally, in order to shift the flap coronally and to release tension.

Coronally advanced flaps were first proposed by Allen and Miller in 1989 [11] to treat shallow recessions. The technique consists of performing two vertical incisions at the concerning tooth's line angles and raising a split-thickness

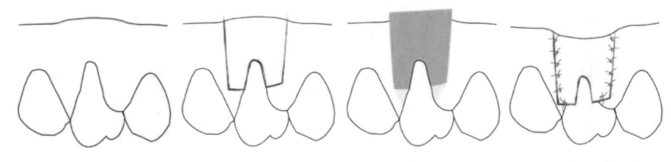

Fig. 38.5 The trapezoidal flap for single recessions

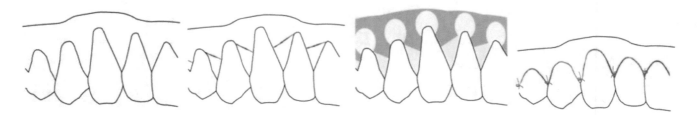

Fig. 38.6 The envelope flap for multiple recessions

flap, which is then coronally advanced and secured at the cementoenamel junction (CEJ) with sutures. This technique was further developed by de Sanctis and Zucchelli in 2007 [12]. It included two horizontal beveled incisions, mesial and distal to the recession defect, and two beveled oblique incisions coming from these, extending to the alveolar mucosa. The flap is then raised with a split–full–split-thickness approach. After de-epithelizing the anatomical papillae, the flap is coronally advanced, and the vertical incisions are sutured. The surgical papillae are secured to the underlying bed with a sling suture (Fig. 38.5).

The same concept may be applied to multiple recessions, using a flap design to cover all recessions in the same session. The envelope flap by Zucchelli and De Sanctis [13] consists of creating submarginal and intrasulcular incisions, going from the tooth that is considered the center of rotation in the surgical papilla rotating towards the ends of the flap during the coronal advancement (Fig. 38.6).

Tips and tricks for a coronally advanced flap procedure:

– Make sure the flap is completely passive and is stable in its final position even without the sutures.
– Perform two types of split incisions apically: a deep one parallel to the bone and a superficial one parallel to the flap where the blade is seen by transparence. This permits to advance the flap coronally.

The coronally advanced flap yields good clinical outcomes in terms of complete root coverage; however, more stability is achieved by combining it with a connective tissue

graft. These are called bilaminar techniques and can be used for single or multiple recessions, using the same flap designs and only adding a connective tissue graft that is sutured to the prepared recipient bed.

One of the most important techniques that combine the use of a connective tissue graft is the tunnel technique. Inspired by Raetzke, who published in 1985 [14] his "envelope technique" for single recessions, and by Zabalegui in 1999 [15] for multiple recessions, the technique further evolved with Aroca in 2010 [16] to include a coronal advancement and permit better root coverage and aesthetic outcomes.

This modified tunnel technique consists of performing intrasulcular incisions without reaching the papillae, followed by a mucoperiosteal dissection extending beyond the mucogingival junction and under each papilla so that the flap can be moved in a coronal direction without tension. Muscle fibers and any remaining collagen bundles on the inner aspect of the flap alveolar mucosa are cut using specific tunnel instruments with extreme care to avoid perforation of the flap and obtain a passive coronal positioning of the flap and the papilla. The harvested connective tissue graft is then inserted in the prepared tunnel and sutured at the level of the CEJ, followed by a coronal advancement of the "flap" and suturing with a sling or horizontal mattress sutures around the contact points aided by composite stops (Fig. 38.7).

Tips and tricks for a tunnel procedure:

– Make sure the "flap" is completely passive before inserting the connective tissue graft.

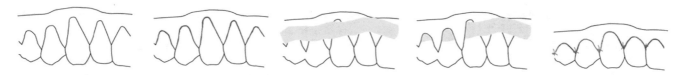

Fig. 38.7 The tunnel procedure

– When placing the graft, make sure to place it at the level of the CEJ and prevent its apical migration by suturing each edge.

Basic Principles of Mucogingival Surgery

Irrespective of the differences in techniques, indications, and surgical designs, there are some basic principles that should be respected in every soft tissue plastic surgery to ensure successful healing and optimal treatment outcomes and prevent undesired complications.

Preoperative Phase

When deciding if the patient is a good candidate for soft tissue plastic surgery, the most important factors to consider are plaque control and tobacco habit. If not controlled, these two factors will severely affect the optimal outcome of any surgical technique.

Flap Preparation

According to Burkhardt 2014 [17], some recommendations related to an ideal flap preparation can be made:

• Incise the sulcular area around teeth and avoid marginal and paramarginal incisions.
• Place midcrestal incisions in edentulous areas.
• Avoid releasing incisions.
• If a releasing incision is required, carry it out as short and as medially as possible.
• Do not place releasing incisions on the buccal root prominences.

It is also important to use a microsurgical approach, minimally elevating the flaps and ensuring a primary closure in the interdental area.

The flap thickness is an essential factor to consider since thick gingival tissue eases manipulation, maintains vascularity, and promotes wound healing during and after surgery.

Moreover, thinner flaps are associated with inferior root coverage outcomes.

Flap Mobilization

Flap tension and the precision of flap margin adaptation influence the extension and severity of scar formation due to primary or second intention healing. Buccal releasing incisions impair the blood supply of the flap and decrease its stability.

Flap Adaptation

Stabilization of the soft tissues covering the wound area with appropriate suturing appears to be a key prerequisite for optimal surgical outcomes. Thinner sutures (6-0 or 7-0) are preferred since they do not lead to tissue tear. Sutures should remain as little as needed to assure the healing wound's stability, depending on the individual situation rather than a stereotype regime.

Postoperative Care

The use of chlorhexidine following periodontal surgery represents a fundamental concept contributing to the reduction of the infective burden in the oral cavity and, hence, the promotion of oral postsurgical health. Moreover, optimal oral hygiene standards are even more important in periodontal plastic surgery.

Autologous Grafts vs. Substitutes

As mentioned above, bilaminar techniques, combining a connective tissue graft, compared to pedicle flaps alone, result in better stability of the gingival margin over time. The connective tissue graft can be harvested from various donor sites, most frequently the palate and the maxillary tuberosity area, and this results in different clinical and histological characteristics of the grafts. The main differences are shown in the table below (Table 38.3).

Table 38.3 Main histological and clinical characteristics of connective tissue grafts harvested from the palate and the tuberosity

	Palate	Tuberosity
Histological characteristics	Lamina propria is loose and more vascularized	Lamina propria is denser and poorly vascularized
	More submucosa	Less submucosa
Clinical characteristics	Higher primary contraction	Hyperplastic tendency

It is also noteworthy to consider the morbidity of the surgery since harvesting a graft from the palate results in higher postoperative pain and anti-inflammatory consumption, along with higher chair time. Regarding the different graft donor sites, better esthetic outcomes in terms of color blending, volume, and texture have resulted from a connective tissue graft harvested from the palate.

Various techniques exist to harvest a connective tissue graft from the palate; the most important ones are the de-epithelized free gingival graft and the subepithelial connective tissue graft. With the first technique, a free gingival graft is harvested traditionally and de-epithelized outside of the mouth. This procedure yields higher tissue quality since the part directly in contact with the epithelium has the highest connective tissue quality. Care must be taken to completely remove the epithelium in order to prevent the formation of epithelial cysts. This harvesting technique results in secondary intention healing at the palate and might lead to higher postoperative pain and bleeding. On the other hand, the subepithelial connective tissue graft harvesting technique consists of directly harvesting the connective tissue beneath the epithelium, also known as lamina propria. With this method, we aim for a primary intention healing at the palate and consequently less patient morbidity.

The use of an autogenous connective tissue graft harvested from the palate or the tuberosity constitutes the "gold standard" for optimal root coverage outcomes. However, it entails a second surgical site and higher patient morbidity. The use of substitutes may counteract this limitation. Allogenic and xenogeneic grafts have been used in root coverage procedures. Acellular dermal matrix grafts primarily and xenogeneic collagen matrix secondly may be considered as alternatives in cases where subepithelial connective tissue grafts harvested from the palate could not be used. In terms of complete root coverage percentage, they yield inferior treatment outcomes.

Surgery on Teeth vs. Implants

Similar soft tissue plastic surgery techniques can be performed on implants aimed mainly at increasing the amount of keratinized mucosa, increasing the thickness of the soft

tissues around implants, and treating buccal soft tissue deficiencies.

The main anatomical difference between teeth and implants affecting the soft tissue healing is the vascularization: around teeth, the vascularization of the gingiva is ensured by the periodontal ligament, the supra-periosteal vessels, and the alveolar bone blood vessels, while around implants, since there is no periodontal ligament, the mucosa receives its blood supply only from the supra-periosteal vessels and the alveolar bone blood vessels.

This difference in the vascularization might be the origin of the frequently observed higher contraction rate of free gingival grafts around implants compared to teeth.

Some clinicians recommend using connective tissue grafts harvested from the tuberosity to counteract this contraction when performing a soft tissue augmentation around implants.

Conclusion

Performing soft tissue plastic surgery around teeth and implants needs a correct diagnosis, an adequate decision-making process to choose the indicated root coverage procedure and proper surgical know-how. With the advancement of technology, a shift will be witnessed towards more minimally invasive techniques using specialized microsurgical instruments. Site-specific and technique-related characteristics are of utmost importance. However, patient-related outcomes should not be forgotten. In fact, periodontal plastic surgery's objective is achieving patient aesthetics with the least morbidity possible and the best prognosis.

References

1. Miller PD. A classification of marginal tissue recession. Int J Periodontics Restorative Dent. 1985;5(2):8–13.
2. Cairo F, Nieri M, Cincinelli S, Mervelt J, Pagliaro U. The interproximal clinical attachment level to classify gingival recessions and predict root coverage outcomes: an explorative and reliability study. J Clin Periodontol. 2011 Jul;38(7):661–6.
3. Friedman N. Mucogingival surgery. Tex Dent J. 1957;75:358–62.
4. Miyasato M, Crigger M, Egelberg J. Gingival condition in areas of minimal and appreciable width of keratinized gingiva. J Clin Periodontol. 1977;4(3):200–9.
5. Wennström J, Lindhe J. Role of attached gingiva for maintenance of periodontal health. Healing following excisional and grafting procedures in dogs. J Clin Periodontol. 1983;10(2):206–21.
6. Wennström J, Lindhe J. Plaque-induced gingival inflammation in the absence of attached gingiva in dogs. J Clin Periodontol. 1983;10(3):266–76.
7. Wennström JL. Lack of association between width of attached gingiva and development of soft tissue recession. A 5-year longitudinal study. J Clin Periodontol. 1987;14(3):181–4.

8. American Academy of Periodontology. Glossary of periodontal terms. 3rd ed. Chicago: American Academy of Periodontology; 1992. p. 1.

9. Sullivan HC, Atkins JH. Free autogenous gingival grafts. I. Principles of successful grafting. Periodontics. 1968;6(3):121–9.

10. Grupe HE, Warren RF. Repair of gingival defects by a sliding flap operation. J Periodontol. 1956;27(2):92–5.

11. Allen EP, Miller PD. Coronal positioning of existing gingiva: short term results in the treatment of shallow marginal tissue recession. J Periodontol. 1989;60(6):316–9.

12. de Sanctis M, Zucchelli G. Coronally advanced flap: a modified surgical approach for isolated recession-type defects: three-year results. J Clin Periodontol. 2007;34(3):262–8.

13. Zucchelli G, De Sanctis M. Treatment of multiple recession-type defects in patients with esthetic demands. J Periodontol. 2000;71(9):1506–14.

14. Raetzke PB. Covering Localized Areas of Root Exposure Employing the 'Envelope' Technique. J Periodontol. 1985;56(7):397–402.

15. Zabalegui I, Sicilia A, Cambra J, Gil J, Sanz M. Treatment of multiple adjacent gingival recessions with the tunnel subepithelial connective tissue graft: a clinical report. Int J Periodont Restor Dent. 1999;19(2):199–206.

16. Aroca S, Keglevich T, Nikolidakis D, Gera I, Nagy K, Azzi R, Etienne D. Treatment of Class III multiple gingival recessions: a randomized-clinical trial. J Clin Periodontol. 2010;37(1):88–97.

17. Burkhardt R, Lang NP. Fundamental principles in periodontal plastic surgery and mucosal augmentation – a narrative review. J Clin Periodontol. 2014;41(Suppl 15):S98–107.

Differential Diagnosis in Oral Lesions

Farnaz Hadaegh and Fargol Mashhadi Akbar Boojar

Premalignant Lesions

Leukoplakia

Any white oral mucosa lesion that cannot be rubbed off and diagnosed as any other white lesion (Fig. 39.1) [1].

Etiology is unknown. Tobacco, alcohol, and age above 40 years are contributing factors. A biopsy is a diagnostic tool since a clinical exam is not enough for diagnosis. The transformation of benign lesions to SCC is 5–15%. High-risk sites are the floor of the mouth and tongue.

Excision is the treatment of choice, but recurrence is not rare either [1].

Proliferative Verrucous Leukoplakia

It is a high-risk, recurrent, and multiple forms of leukoplakia. The lesion can start with a flat profile and progress to wart-like lesions. Etiology is unknown. Some cases are related to human papillomaviruses 16 and 18 [2]. Excision is the treatment of choice (Fig. 39.2) [3].

Erythroplakia

A high-risk red patch of the oral mucosa.

Etiology is unknown, but some are associated with tobacco and age between 50 and 70 years. High-risk sites are the floor of the mouth, tongue, and retromolar pad area. Erythroleucoplaki often gets secondarily infected with Candida Albicans, resulting in a red surface due to inflammation, dysplasia, or both (Fig. 39.3) [4]. Excision is the treatment of choice [4].

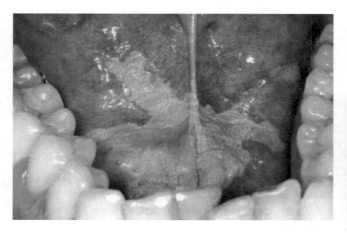

Fig. 39.1 Leukoplakia of the floor of the mouth. (Reproduced with permission from van der Waal [1])

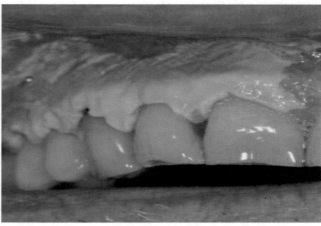

Fig. 39.2 Verrucous hyperkeratosis in the right maxillary gingiva at the first clinical examination. (Reproduced with permission from Bombeccari et al. [3])

F. Hadaegh (✉)
Department of Pediatric Dentistry, University of Pittsburgh, School of Dental Medicine, Pittsburgh, PA, USA
e-mail: fah30@pitt.edu

F. M. A. Boojar
School of Dentistry, Research committee of Golestan Medical University, Gorgan, Iran

© The Author(s), under exclusive license to Springer Nature Switzerland AG 2021
M. R. Stevens et al. (eds.), *Innovative Perspectives in Oral and Maxillofacial Surgery*,
https://doi.org/10.1007/978-3-030-75750-2_39

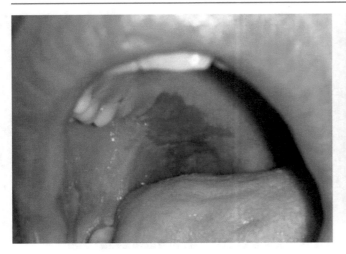

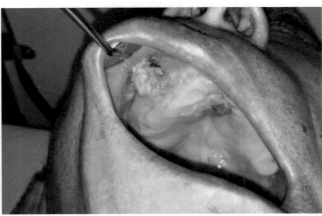

Fig. 39.4 Verrucous carcinoma. Clinical photograph showing papillary exophytic growths of the labial parts of the maxillary right anterior edentulous ridge and middle of the palate. (Reproduced with permission from Kang and Leem [9])

Fig. 39.3 Erythroleucoplakia. (Reproduced with Permission from Parasuraman et al. [4])

Oral Submucous Fibrosis (OSMF)

Overreaction to betel nut can make irreversible opaque changes in oral mucosa etiology of OSMF is multifactorial. Some risk factors are chewing of smokeless tobacco, high intake of chilies, toxic levels of copper in foodstuffs, vitamin deficiencies, and malnutrition resulting in low levels of serum proteins genetic predisposition. In one study in Malaysia, aside from anemia, recommended are the following clinical criteria for the diagnosis of OSF [5]:

1. Presence of palpable fibrous bands
2. Leathery mucosal texture
3. Blanching of the mucosa
4. Loss of tongue papillae
5. Burning sensation to spicy food
6. The rigidity of the tongue

These lesions can be transformed into SCC.

Treatment of choice will be a cessation of habit and temporary symptomatic relief [6].

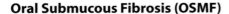

Mucosal Malignancies

Squamous Cell Carcinoma (SCC)

Squamous cell carcinoma presents as a chronic red or white patch or a nonhealing ulcer in high-risk areas such as the posterior lateral tongue and floor of the mouth. It affects males more than females.

Etiology can be related to genetic changes through tobacco, human papillomavirus (types 16 and 18). Also,

there is an increased risk in patients with Plummer-Vinson syndrome.

The treatment of choice is excision, or radiation surgery is the initial treatment of choice. Approximately 3% of cancer in men and 2% in women in the United States are SCC [7, 8].

Verrucous Carcinoma (Snuff Dipper's Cancer; Ackerman's Tumor)

Verrucous carcinoma is a broad-based verruciform of carcinoma that is well-differentiated and slow-growing.

Etiology can be related to tobacco and human papillomavirus (type 16 and 18) (Fig. 39.4) [9].

The treatment of choice is surgical excision [9].

Basal Cell Carcinoma (BCC)

Basal cell carcinoma is very rare in oral mucosa but usually seen in sun-damaged skin. It presents as a chronic nonhealing ulcer that rarely metastasis. The treatment of choice is surgery [10].

Oral Melanoma

It is the malignancy of melanocytes in high-risk areas such as the palate and gingiva. The 5-year survival rate is less than SCC. The treatment of choice is aggressive surgery [11].

Connective Tissue Tumors

Granular Cell Tumor

Most commonly seen in the tongue is a benign nonrecurring submucosal neoplasm of Schwann cell but microscopically copies carcinoma. This should not be confused with congenital epulis or congenital granular cell tumor, which is the infant counterpart of granular cell tumor.

The treatment of choice is surgery [12].

Neurofibroma

It is a solitary to multiple benign neoplasms of Schwann cells, mainly in the tongue and buccal mucosa. There is a type called neurofibromatosis syndrome, which appears as multiple neurofibromas, six or more café-au-lait macules, axillary freckling (Crowe's sign), and iris freckling (Lisch spots). There is not any known treatment for neurofibromatosis. Growth can be intervened by surgery or radiation therapy. Surgery may cause more injury to nerves and neurological problems [13].

Schwannoma

Schwannoma or neurilemmoma appears as a solitary, not syndrome-related benign neoplasm of Schwann cells in any site favorably in the tongue. Schwannoma is painless and slow-growing.

The treatment of choice is surgery [14, 15].

Mucosal Neuromas of Multiple Endocrine Neoplasia Syndrome Type III (MEN III)

It is a hereditary disease with an autosomal dominant pattern. It manifests as lingual hamartoma, thyroidal carcinoma, and adrenal pheochromocytoma. Treatment: Early diagnosis of MEN III syndrome is a prerequisite for a successful treatment. Dentists most likely can be the first health care providers to diagnose this potentially fatal syndrome. Also, patients with pheochromocytoma need surgical management [16].

Salivary Gland Tumors

Mucoepidermoid Carcinoma

It is the most common salivary malignancy of both minor and major glands. It mainly appears in the palate and is composed of epithelial cells and mucous. High-grade lesions

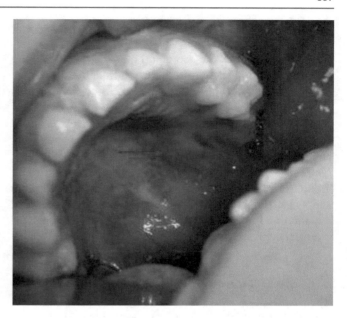

Fig. 39.5 Mucoepidermoid carcinoma of the left posterior hard palate appearing as a pale bluish-purple lump (arrow). A former incision scar is still visible. (Reproduced with permission from Baumgardt et al. [17])

metastasize, and the prognosis will be poor (Fig. 39.5) [17]. Treatment: Local surgical resection is the treatment of choice for low-grade tumors, while high-grade tumors are treated with surgical excision followed by postoperative radiotherapy [18].

Polymorphous Low-Grade Adenocarcinoma

It has a polymorphous microscopic pattern. Rarely, it may be seen in major salivary glands, but it is the second most common minor salivary gland malignancy that mainly manifests in the palate. And treatment of choice for the low-grade malignancy would be surgical excision [19].

Adenoid Cystic Carcinoma

It has a cribriform or "Swiss cheese" microscopic pattern that extends through perineural spaces. It is a high-grade salivary malignancy with a palate as the most common site. The treatment is surgery followed by radiation treatments [20].

Lymphoid Neoplasm

All lymphoid neoplasms that are malignant mostly appear in lymph nodes and occasionally in extranodal tissues such as mucosa-associated lymphoid tissue (MALT) as a mass or ulcerated mass [21].

Non-Hodgkin's Lymphoma

Epstein-Barr virus and chromosome translocations are important causative factors in some non-Hodgkin syndromes such as Burkitt's lymphoma. Most are B-cell types. It is microscopically classified as low-grade and high-grade. And the most common intraoral sites are the palate and tonsils. In Burkitt's lymphoma, bone involvement causes swelling, pain, tooth mobility, and lip paresthesia. Additionally, most lymph nodes or MALT appear in the head and neck. Treatment of choice varies depending on the classification and stage. Radiation, chemotherapy, and a combination of radiation and chemotherapy are used for localized, extensive, and aggressive types accordingly [22, 23].

Multiple Myeloma/Plasma Cell Myeloma

It appears as multiple lucencies in patients above 50 years old. Patients complain about pain, numbness, and swelling. Anemia, infection, fracture, and bleeding are seen in extensive punched-out bone involvement. The treatment of choice is chemotherapy. And the prognosis is poor. Approximately 10% of patients with multiple myeloma show a form of amyloidosis [24].

Leukemias

It is the neoplasm of bone marrow. Chromosome translocation and environmental agents such as virus, radiation, and benzene can be etiologic factors. It is classified based on the cell lineage (myeloid or lymphoid) and whether it is acute or chronic. Infection, fatigue, and bleeding are significant clinical signs of leukemia. Hemorrhagic and red gingiva are common oral manifestations of chronic monocytic leukemia. The treatment of choice for acute leukemia is chemotherapy, but chronic is not as successful as acute [25].

Odontogenic Cysts

Periapical Cyst

It is associated with nonvital teeth and the most common odontogenic cyst. Abscess forms when the cyst is acute. It becomes granuloma when the cyst is chronic. Treatment of choice is root canal filling, curettage, apicoectomy, or extraction [26, 27].

Dentigerous Cyst

It is a radiolucency around the crown of an impacted tooth. Canines and third molars are most affected. Tooth mobility or root resorption was maybe seen in DC.

The treatment of choice is enucleation and extraction of the involved tooth. The prognosis of the cyst is good, and recurrence is rare with regular follow-up.

In large cases, marsupialization will be done before enucleation to reduce the size of the bone defect [28, 29].

Lateral Periodontal Cyst

It is mostly found in the mandibular premolar area as unilocular radiolucency in the lateral PDL of a vital tooth. The multilocular radiolucency is called botryoid odontogenic cysts. Both should be removed surgically by conservative enucleation or excision, and usually, patients will be followed radiographically for recurrence years after surgery [30].

Gingival Cyst of the Newborn

It manifests as multiple small gingival nodules. It is called Bohn's nodules or Epstein's pearls when cysts appear in the palate of infants. There is no need for treatment. It goes away within a few weeks of the infant's birth [31].

Odontogenic Keratocyst

It is a rare and benign but locally aggressive developmental cyst. The posterior mandible is the most affected site that occurs in the third decade of life. It can appear in three forms; solitary, which has the lowest recurrence rate among the other two. Multiple cysts have a higher rate of recurrence comparing to solitary cysts. And the third form is syndrome-associated multiple cysts. In the last one besides multiple odontogenic keratocytes, the patient has numerous cutaneous basal cell carcinoma, skeletal abnormalities, and calcified falx.

Treatment of choice is a highly controversial protocol among oral and maxillofacial surgeons. Simple enucleation is for lesions smaller than 1 cm. Extensive resection is the choice of treatment in the case that the cyst extends into the skeletal base [32–34].

Calcifying Odontogenic Cyst

It is a rare condition with unpredictable behavior. It has the potential of recurrence (solitary ones). Keratinization of "ghost cells" is the characteristic of this cyst microscopically. Also, the cyst can be radiographically detected through the calcification of ghost cells that appear as radiolucency with opaque foci. The treatment of choice is enucleation and curettage [35, 36].

Glandular Odontogenic Cyst

It is a rare but locally aggressive odontogenic cyst with a recurrence potential that is called a sialo-odontogenic cyst. The name comes from gland-like spaces and mucous cells lining its epithelium. The treatment of choice for small unilocular lesions is enucleation. For large uni- or multilocular lesions, a biopsy is recommended. For large unilocular lesions, enucleation with peripheral ostectomy, and large multilocular cases, marginal resection or partial jaw resection is suggested. Marsupialization is an option for lesions approaching vital structures [37, 38] (Fig. 39.6) [39].

Odontogenic Tumors

Ameloblastoma

It is an aggressive benign tumor of the molar-ramus area in adults 40 years with a high recurrence rate. It can be unilocular or multilocular lucency. The cystic type does not show aggressive and recurrent nature as much. However, the malignant type, ameloblastic carcinoma, is very rare. Treatment of choice would be a range from excision to resection [40, 41].

Ameloblastic Fibroma and Ameloblastic Fibro-Odontoma

It affects children and teens in the molar-ramus area as benign and rare tumors. Ameloblastic fibroma and ameloblastic fibro-odontoma appear the same microscopically and radiographically (unilocular/multilocular or radiolucency with opacity or odontoma for the latter one). Enucleation or excision is the treatment of choice [42].

Adenomatoid Odontogenic Tumor

It is a rare and benign tumor that affects teens in the anterior of the jaws. It never recurs and appears as a radiolucency with opaque foci. The rule of thumb for this tumor is 2/3, over the crown of an impacted tooth in anterior of the maxilla of females. The treatment of choice would be enucleation [43, 44].

Odontogenic Myxoma

It affects both jaws of adults 30 years as a rare, aggressive benign tumor. The radiolucency follows a honeycomb pattern with small loculations. It can be treated with excision [45] (Fig. 39.7) [46].

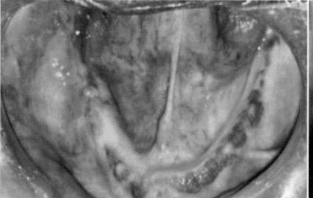
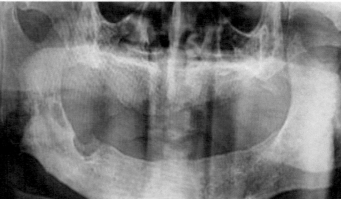

Fig. 39.6 Glandular odontogenic cyst. Left picture shows intraoral swelling over the right retromolar trigone (pre-op), right picture: OPG showing two radiolucencies in the retromolar area (preop). (Reproduced with permission from Gandra et al. [39])

Cementifying Fibroma

It appears as a radiolucency and sometimes with opaque foci in the mandible of young adults. It is considered identical to ossifying fibroma with well-circumscribed lucency. Treatment of choice is curettage or excision with rare recurrence [47, 48] (Fig. 39.8) [49].

Cementoblastoma

It is seen in patients under age 25 years as a well-circumscribed radio-opaque mass in the posterior of the mandible containing cementum replacing the involved tooth's root. The tooth should be removed with the lesion as the treatment of choice. There will not be a recurrence following excision [50].

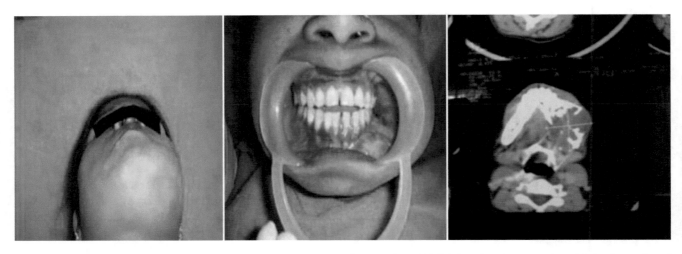

Fig. 39.7 Myxoma. (L) Preoperative showing expansion of lower border and buccal aspect of mandible middle (M). Preoperative intraoral view showing expansion and obliteration of buccal vestibule. (R) Preoperative axial CT view showing expansion with the destruction of the buccal and lingual cortical plate. (Reproduced with permission from Kumar et al. [46])

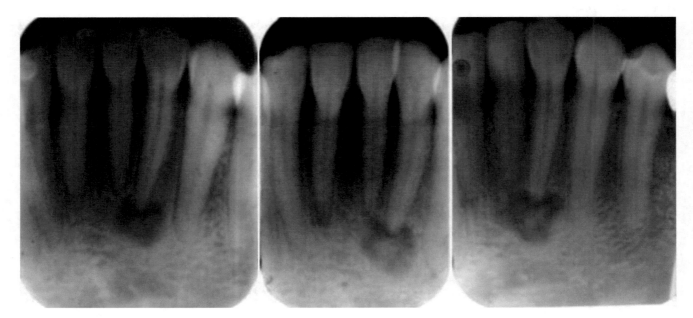

Fig. 39.8 Periapical osseous dysplasia. Serial radiographic of anterior mandible teeth how that the lesions "mature" over time, creating a mixed radiolucent and radiopaque appearance. (Reproduced with permission from El-Mofty [51])

Periapical Cemento-Osseous Dysplasia

It is a reactive process with an unknown cause that appears in middle-aged African-American women at apices of the mandible region's anterior teeth. Although the apices are involved, the teeth remain vital. This lesion starts as circumscribed lucency and then becomes opaque. Florid osseous dysplasia manifests as multi-quadrant radiopaque masses, an extreme type of periapical cemento-osseous dysplasia. It requires no treatment (Fig. 39.8) [51].

Odontoma

It is a benign tumor of dental hard tissue that appears as opaque lesions in children and teenagers. It includes two types of compound and complex. The first one more commonly manifests in the anterior of the maxilla and the latter in both jaws' posterior. The compound type contains small tooth-like masses, and the complex type is composed of a clustered opaque mass. Treatment of choice is curettage with no recurrence [52, 53] (Fig. 39.9).

Bone Lesions Fibro-Osseous Lesions

Ossifying Fibroma

It is seen in the body of the mandible of adults or younger adults. It is considered a relatively common fibro-osseous

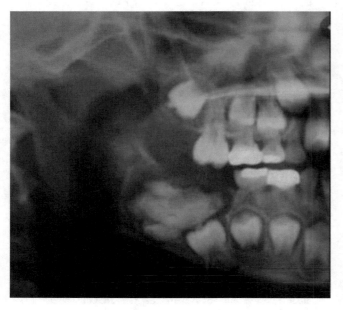

Fig. 39.9 Complex odontoma. Pano right mandible. (Reproduced with permission from Chi et al. [53], pp. 7–9)

benign tumor. It appears as a well-circumscribed radiolucency with opaque foci and identical to cementifying fibroma, but some might show significant size. Treatment of choice would be curettage or excision [54].

Fibrous Dysplasia

It affects more commonly half of the maxilla in children and stops growing at puberty. It is a relatively uncommon fibro-osseous lesion. Half of the patients experience pain. This lesion appears as a ground glass radiographically (diffuse opacity). It will be treated with surgical recontouring after puberty for cosmetic purposes. Also, this tumor can be associated with McCune-Albright syndrome that includes polyostotic fibrous dysplasia, café-au-lait macules, and endocrine abnormalities [55, 56].

Bone Lesions Giant Cell Lesions

Peripheral Giant Cell Granuloma

It is seen as red to purple (brown) gingival mass in the anterior and premolar area with occasional recurrence. Treatment of choice is excision extending to PDL [57, 58].

Central Giant Cell Granuloma

It is an unpredictable tumor. Some show an aggressive pattern with a high recurrence rate, but others might appear as mild in nature. It is usually seen as a radiolucency, more commonly anterior of the mandible in teenagers. It could be treated with excision. For larger lesions, calcitonin is an option [59, 60].

Aneurysmal Bone Cyst

It is a pseudocyst containing blood. It shows multilocular lucency in teenagers. It can be treated with excision, but occasional recurrence might happen [61].

Hyperparathyroidism

It is called Von Recklinghausen's disease of bone. It affects multiple bones due to excessive parathormone hormone. Patients might experience systemic signs such as osteoporosis, arrhythmias, neurologic problems, kidney stones, and metastatic calcification. It appears as multiple radiolucencies of multinucleated giant cells. Also, there is a loss of lamina dura around the involved teeth. Etiology can be attributed to a parathyroid tumor or parathyroid hyperplasia due to vitamin D deficiency, malabsorption, or renal failure [62].

Cherubism

It is an autosomal dominant disorder of the jaws in children. Radiographically, it appears as a soap bubble pattern bilaterally. It requires no treatment because it becomes stable after puberty [63].

Langerhans Cell Disease

It is also called idiopathic histiocytosis or Langerhans granulomatosis. It appears as a "punched out" lesion or "floating teeth" around the involved teeth. The treatment ranges from excision to radiation or chemotherapy. It has an excellent prognosis if the lesion is localized [64].

Paget's Disease

It is a metabolic disorder of multiple bones with unknown causes. It affects adults above 50 years old. Patients experience bone pain, headache, altered hearing, and vision. If it involves jaws, it will appear as diastema or hypercementosis. Some patients might complain of a tight denture or a tight ring. Jaw fracture and osteomyelitis are the late complications of the disease. However, in the early stages, bleeding makes the surgery hard due to the disease's highly vascular nature. Bisphosphonates and, to a lesser degree, calcitonin showed efficacy as a treatment [65].

Bone Malignancies

Osteosarcoma

It appears more commonly in the mandible of adults mean age of 35 years old. Etiology is unknown, but it might be contributed to specific genetic alterations. Swelling, pain, paresthesia, and widening of the PDL are the clinical features that can be seen. Treatment of choice will be resection and preoperative chemotherapy or postoperative chemotherapy. Prognosis is better for tumors in the mandible than the maxilla [66].

Chondrosarcoma

It is a rare sarcoma of jaws that tumor cells make cartilage. Clinical features and treatment of choice will be the same as osteosarcoma [67].

Ewing's Sarcoma

It is a malignant tumor of children with the onion skin radiolucency pattern. Treatment of choice includes aggressive multimodality therapy with a fair prognosis [68].

Conclusion

Premalignant and malignant entities of the head and neck area are mainly treated with excision, enucleation, marsupialization, chemotherapy, radiation, or partial resection of the involved jaw. Early diagnosis plays a significant role in the course of treatment of an aggressive lesion. This outline studies a list of entities that might need specific consideration.

References

1. van der Waal I. Oral leukoplakia: present views on diagnosis, management, communication with patients, and research. Curr Oral Health Rep. 2019;6(1):9–13.
2. Koh J, Kurago ZB. Expanded expression of toll-like receptor 2 in proliferative verrucous leukoplakia. Head Neck Pathol. 2019;13(4):635–42.
3. Bombeccari GP, Garagiola U, Candotto V, et al. Diode laser surgery in the treatment of oral proliferative verrucous leukoplakia associated with HPV-16 infection. Maxillofac Plast Reconstr Surg. 2018;40:16.
4. Parasuraman L, Bal M, Pai PS. Erythroplakia and erythroleucoplakia. In: Premalignant conditions of the oral cavity. Singapore: Springer; 2019. p. 87–95.
5. Warnakulasuriya S, Tilakaratne WM, Kerr A. Oral submucous fibrosis. In: Kuriakose M, editor. Contemporary oral oncology. Cham: Springer; 2017.
6. Rao NR, Villa A, More CB, Jayasinghe RD, Kerr AR, Johnson NW. Oral submucous fibrosis: a contemporary narrative review with a proposed inter-professional approach for early diagnosis and clinical management. J Otolaryngol Head Neck Surg. 2020;49(1):3.
7. Brocklehurst P, Kujan O, Glenny AM, Oliver R, Sloan P, Ogden G, Shepherd S. Screening programs for the early detection and prevention of oral cancer. Cochrane Database Syst Rev. 2010;11:CD004150.
8. Pérot P, Falguieres M, Arowas L, Laude H, Foy JP, Goudot P, Corre-Catelin N, Ungeheuer MN, Caro V, Heard I, Eloit M. Investigation of viral etiology in potentially malignant disorders and oral squamous cell carcinomas in non-smoking, non-drinking patients. PLoS One. 2020;15(4):e0232138.

9. Kang S, Leem DH. Verrucous carcinoma arising from a previous cystic lesion: a case report. Maxillofac Plast Reconstr Surg. 2018;40(1):31.

10. Varadarajan VV, Nasri E, Dziegielewski PT. Basal cell carcinoma of the oral cavity: a case report. Otolaryngol Case Rep. 2020;28:100159.

11. Bergman PJ. Melanoma. Clinical small animal internal medicine. Chichester: Wiley Blackwell; 2020. p. 1347–52.

12. Mobarki M, Dumollard JM, Dal Col P, Camy F, Peoc'h M, Karpathiou G. Granular cell tumor a study of 42 cases and systemic review of the literature. Pathol Res Pract. 2020;216(4):152865.

13. Ravindran DM, Ravi S, Muthukumar Santhanakrishnan BS. LASER assisted excision of solitary neurofibroma in the gingiva. Cureus. 2020;12(2):e7118.

14. Goldbrunner R, Weller M, Regis J, Lund-Johansen M, Stavrinou P, Reuss D, Evans DG, Lefranc F, Sallabanda K, Falini A, Axon P. EANO guideline on the diagnosis and treatment of vestibular schwannoma. Neuro-Oncology. 2020;22(1):31–45.

15. Lee E, Kim J, Seok H, et al. Schwannoma of the tongue: a case report with review of literature. Maxillofac Plast Reconstr Surg. 2017;39:17.

16. Abdullah B, Museedi O, Saif J, Basima A, Saja M. Multiple endocrine neoplasia type 2B: maxillofacial finding in one case. J Oral Maxillofac Surg Med Pathol. 2020;32(3):233–5.

17. Baumgardt C, Günther L, Sari-Rieger A, et al. Mucoepidermoid carcinoma of the palate in a 5-year-old girl: case report and literature review. Oral Maxillofac Surg. 2014;18:465–9.

18. Wang Y, Wang S, Zhang B. A population-based analysis of mucoepidermoid carcinoma of the oral cavity. Laryngoscope. 2020;131(3):E857–63.

19. Hong TU, Park SK, Kim DH, Choe S. Polymorphous low-grade adenocarcinoma in the nasopharynx: a case report and review of the literature. Korean J Otorhinolaryngol Head Neck Surg. 2020;64(2):119–23.

20. Högerle BA, Lasitschka F, Muley T, Bougatf N, Herfarth K, Adeberg S, Eichhorn M, Debus J, Winter H, Rieken S, Uhl M. Primary adenoid cystic carcinoma of the trachea: clinical outcome of 38 patients after interdisciplinary treatment in a single institution. Radiat Oncol. 2019;14(1):117.

21. Bhattacharyya S, Bains AP, Sykes DL, Iverson BR, Sibgatullah R, Kuklani RM. Lymphoid neoplasms of the oral cavity with plasmablastic morphology—a case series and review of the literature. Oral Surg Oral Med Oral Pathol Oral Radiol. 2019;128(6):651–9.

22. Kusuke N, Custódio M, de Sousa SC. Oral lesion as the primary diagnosis of non-Hodgkin's lymphoma: a 20-year experience from an oral pathology service and review of the literature. Eur Arch Otorhinolaryngol. 2019;276(10):2873–9.

23. Aggarwal A, Mittal A, Sasi A, Nischal N. Non-Hodgkin's lymphoma in AIDS. QJM Int J Med. 2020;113(5):362. –.

24. Abd BA, Mohammed MQ. Multiple myeloma, the plasma cell cancer: an overview. Med J Babylon. 2020;17(3):233.

25. Angst PD, Maier J, dos Santos NR, Manso IS, Tedesco TK. Oral health status of patients with leukemia: a systematic review with meta-analysis. Arch Oral Biol. 2020;120:104948.

26. Hasna AA, Carvalho CA. Endodontic treatment of a large periapical cyst with the aid of antimicrobial photodynamic therapy-case report. Braz Dent Sci. 2019;22(4):561–8.

27. Subramaniam K, Sethu G, Lochana P. Radicular cyst. Drug Invent Today. 2019;11(9):2143–46.

28. Saha SS, Gandhoke HK, Mahato B, Deb T. Dentigerous cyst with ameloblastomatous proliferation as well as calcifications: an unusual presentation. J Indian Acad Oral Med Radiol. 2020;32(3):297.

29. Alnofaie H, Alomran O, Ababtain R, Alomar A. Spontaneous eruption of a deeply impacted premolar after conservative treatment of an associated dentigerous cyst: a case report. Cureus. 2019;11(12):e6414.

30. Chrcanovic BR, Gomez RS. Gingival cyst of the adult, lateral periodontal cyst, and botryoid odontogenic cyst: an updated systematic review. Oral Dis. 2019;25(1):26–33.

31. Tavares TS, da Costa AA, Freire-Maia FB, Souza LN, Zarzar PM, Martins-Júnior PA, Aguiar MC, Mesquita RA, Caldeira PC. Unusual exophytic gingival lesion in a newborn treated with diode laser. Oral Surg Oral Med Oral Pathol Oral Radiol. 2020;130(3):e74–9.

32. Brannon RB. The odontogenic keratocyst: a clinicopathologic study of 312 cases. Part I. clinical features. Oral Surg Oral Med Oral Pathol. 1976;42(1):54–72.

33. Hsun-Tau C. Odontogenic keratocyst: a clinical experience in Singapore. Oral Surg Oral Med Oral Pathol Oral Radiol Endodontol. 1998;86(5):573–7.

34. Payne TF. An analysis of the clinical and histopathologic parameters of the odontogenic keratocyst. Oral Surg Oral Med Oral Pathol. 1972;33(4):538–46.

35. Freedman PD, Lumerman H, Gee JK. Calcifying odontogenic cyst: a review and analysis of seventy cases. Oral Surg Oral Med Oral Pathol. 1975;40(1):93–106.

36. Altini M, Farman AG. The calcifying odontogenic cyst: eight new cases and a review of the literature. Oral Surg Oral Med Oral Pathol. 1975;40(6):751–9.

37. Gardner DG, Kessler HP, Morency R, Schaffner DL. The glandular odontogenic cyst: an apparent entity. J Oral Pathol Med. 1988;17(8):359–66.

38. Van Heerden WF, Raubenheimer EJ, Turner ML. Glandular odontogenic cyst. Head Neck. 1992;14(4):316–20.

39. Gandra PK, Ali M, Goswami S, et al. Surgeons approach to glandular odontogenic cyst of mandible mimicking mucoepidermoid carcinoma. J. Maxillofac. Oral Surg. 2020; https://doi.org/10.1007/s12663-020-01406-y.

40. Neagu D, Escuder-de la Torre O, Vázquez-Mahía I, Carral-Roura N, Rubín-Roger G, Penedo-Vázquez Á, Luaces-Rey R, López-Cedrún JL. Surgical management of ameloblastoma. Review of literature. J Clin Exp Dent. 2019;11(1):e70.

41. McMillan MD, Smillie AC. Ameloblastomas associated with dentigerous cysts. Oral Surg Oral Med Oral Pathol Oral Radiol. 1981;51(5):489–96.

42. Tariq S, Chalkoo AF. Combined odontogenic tumor-odontogenic Keratocyst and Ameloblastic Fibroma: a case report. P Int J Maxillofac Imaging. 2020;6:24–628.

43. Chrcanovic BR, Gomez RS. Adenomatoid odontogenic tumor: an updated analysis of the cases reported in the literature. J Oral Pathol Med. 2019;48(1):10–6.

44. Sangalette B, Emídio T, Capelari M, Pastori C, Toledo G. Surgical therapy for removal of adenomatoid odontogenic tumor. Hum Pathol Case Rep. 2020;20:200366.

45. Zúñiga FI, Herrera LM, Díaz RA, Reppeto MA, Arratia AL. Surgical management of mandibular odontogenic myxoma: a case report. Oral Surg Oral Med Oral Pathol Oral Radiol. 2020;129(1):e30–1.

46. Kumar N, Kohli M, Pandey S, et al. Odontogenic myxoma. J Maxillofac Oral Surg. 2014;13:222–6.

47. Kaur T, Dhawan A, Bhullar RS, Gupta S. Cemento-ossifying fibroma in maxillofacial region: a series of 16 cases. J Maxillofac Oral Surg. 2021;20(2):240–45.

48. Silva F, Louro R, Cortezzi W, Torres M, Lima F, Sartoretto S, Correa R, Arantes E, Caetano D, Romanach M. Cemento-ossifying fibroma: prototype guided surgical approach for treatment of major lesions. Int J Oral Maxillofac Surg. 2019;48:242–3.

49. Trijolet JP, Parmentier J, Sury F, Goga D, Mejean N, Laure B. Cemento-ossifying fibroma of the mandible. Eur Ann Otorhinolaryngol Head Neck Dis. 2011;128(1):30–3.

50. D'Orto B, Busa A, Scavella G, Moreschi C, Capparè P, Vinci R. Treatment options in cementoblastoma. J Osseointegrat. 2020;12(2):172–6.
51. El-Mofty SK. Osseous dysplasia, periapical. In: Slootweg PJ, editor. Dental and oral pathology. Berlin; Heidelberg. Cham: Springer; 2016.
52. Patil S, Rahman F, Tipu SR, Kaswan S. Odontomas: review of literature and report of a case. Oral Maxillofac Pathol J. 2012;3(1):224–27.
53. Chi A. Odontoma, Complex. In: Slootweg PJ, editor. Dental and oral pathology. Berlin; Heidelberg. Cham: Springer; 2016.
54. Behl A, Ahmed J, Bali V, et al. Peripheral ossifying fibroma. J Stomat Occ Med. 2012;5:42–8.
55. DiCaprio MR, Enneking WF. Fibrous dysplasia: pathophysiology, evaluation, and treatment. JBJS. 2005;87(8):1848–64.
56. Couturier A, Aumaître O, Gilain L, Jean B, Mom T, André M. Craniofacial fibrous dysplasia: a 10-case series. Eur Ann Otorhinolaryngol Head Neck Dis. 2017;134(4):229–35.
57. Chrcanovic BR, Gomes CC, Gomez RS. Peripheral giant cell granuloma: an updated analysis of 2824 cases reported in the literature. J Oral Pathol Med. 2018;47(5):454–9.
58. Maheshwari S, Bhutada G, Baisane V, Palve D. Peripheral giant cell granuloma–a review and case report. Int J Healthc Biomed Res. 2017;5(02):53–8.
59. Alsufyani NA, Aldosary RM, Alrasheed RS, Alsaif RF. A systematic review of the clinical and radiographic features of hybrid central giant cell granuloma lesions of the jaws. Acta Odontol Scand. 2021;79(2):124–31.
60. Schreuder WH, van den Berg H, Westermann AM, Peacock ZS, de Lange J. Pharmacological and surgical therapy for the central giant cell granuloma: a long-term retrospective cohort study. J Cranio-Maxillofac Surg. 2017;45(2):232–43.
61. Grahneis F, Klein A, Baur-Melnyk A, Knösel T, Birkenmaier C, Jansson V, Dürr HR. Aneurysmal bone cyst: a review of 65 patients. J Bone Oncol. 2019;18:100255.
62. Palla B, Burian E, Fliefel R, Otto S. Systematic review of oral manifestations related to hyperparathyroidism. Clin Oral Investig. 2018;22(1):1–27.
63. Hamner JE, Ketcham AS. Cherubism: an analysis of treatment. Cancer. 1969;23(5):1133–43.
64. Madrigal-Martínez-Pereda C, Guerrero-Rodriguez V, Guisado-Moya B, Meniz-Garcia C. Langerhans cell histiocytosis: literature review and descriptive analysis of oral manifestations. Medicina Oral, Patologia Oral y Cirugia Bucal. 2009;14(5):E222.
65. Wollina U, Goldman A, Bieneck A, Abdel-Naser MB, Petersen S. Surgical treatment for extramammary Paget's disease. Curr Treat Options in Oncol. 2018;19(6):27.
66. Zhang Y, Yang J, Zhao N, Wang C, Kamar S, Zhou Y, He Z, Yang J, Sun B, Shi X, Han L. Progress in the chemotherapeutic treatment of osteosarcoma. Oncol Lett. 2018;16(5):6228–37.
67. Brimioulle M, Bowles PF, Pelser A. Maxillary chondrosarcoma mimicking torus palatinus. Case Rep. 2017;2017:bcr-2017.
68. Ahuja US, Puri N, Gupta D, Singh S, Kumar G. Ewing's sarcoma of mandible: a case report with review. Int J Clin Pediatr Dent. 2019;12(5):470.

Intraoral Biopsy Techniques

Mark R. Stevens and Alexander B. Faigen

A biopsy is done for a multitude of reasons; infection, inflammatory, and neoplastic cases all serve as viable indications to take a tissue sample for evaluation [1]. As an oral and maxillofacial surgeon, it is a primary responsibility to perform these diagnostic duties, to assist colleagues in the most appropriate management of oral lesions. When the surgeon is working to determine what the etiology of a lesion is, it is important to take into account its location when choosing the biopsy technique. Time, cost, and cosmesis are all factors in the decision and management for patients [2].

Before the procedure, it is imperative to obtain a thorough medical history along with dental history. Medications and allergies, systemic diseases, HPI, and risk factors all play a role in the pathologic evaluation of the specimen and patient as a whole. The patient exam includes an oral evaluation and exam of the head and neck. This exam will help to determine the types of radiographs and studies which the surgeon will order. Thorough examination gives the clinician what is needed to describe the lesion. Lesion location, tissue plane, size, color, associated symptoms, local tissue attachment, and tenderness all give a clinical picture which can begin to exclude unlikely differential diagnoses [1].

Surgical management by incisional and excisional biopsy is not the only means of identification when a biopsy is indicated. FNA or fine-needle aspiration and cytologic smear also can play a role in diagnosis. The factors that help to select the surgical technique are the size of the lesion itself, anatomic location, in soft tissues or osseous structures, and the surgeon's suspicion of malignancy [3].

Prior to Procedure

The initial diagnosis of a lesion begins with gathering information from the patient. This gathering of information includes obtaining a thorough medical history including medical comorbidities such as cardiovascular disease, pulmonary conditions, and endocrine disorders. These systemic illnesses could be a cause or a factor leading to certain lesions. In addition, it is vital to obtain a list of current medications, allergies, and previous surgical history. Documentation of risk factors such as smoking, alcohol consumption, use of illicit drugs, and unsafe sexual practices can also help in diagnosing a lesion.

Obtaining a thorough dental history is also required. For example, a lesion that presents after the placement of a polymethyl methacrylate temporary crown may represent a localized allergic reaction to the dental material. Another example could be a dark pigmented lesion present in the keratinized gingiva adjacent to a large amalgam restoration can represent an amalgam tattoo rather than something more sinister such as melanoma [4].

Pertinent information includes the duration of the lesion, whether the lesion is fast- or slow-growing, or if the lesion is symptomatic or asymptomatic. A final verdict of the lesion can be made at times with a clinical inspection; however, sometimes, further studies must be done to obtain conclusive diagnosis. It is vital to obtain an accurate medical and social history from the patient. Lesions that are symptomatic and of short duration may represent a reactive process, infection, or malignancy. Long-standing lesions that are asymptomatic can suggest a developmental or benign process. However, these are just generalizations that do not fit each and every case. Changes to a lesion can provide important insights into the diagnosis and must be thoroughly explored and documented.

After thoroughly reviewing the history of present illness from the patient, the practitioner can objectively collect data on the patient with a thorough clinical exam. Initially, the

M. R. Stevens (✉)
Department of Oral and Maxillofacial Surgery, Augusta University, Augusta, GA, USA
e-mail: MASTEVENS@augusta.edu

A. B. Faigen
Oral and Maxillofacial Surgery, Dental College of Georgia at Augusta University, Augusta, GA, USA
e-mail: afaigen@augusta.edu

practitioner should perform a comprehensive head and neck exam looking for external lesions, facial asymmetries, and/or lymphadenopathy. The head and neck exam should be performed with extensive scrutiny starting at the top of the scalp working down to the neck. This includes palpating lymph nodes in the postauricular and occipital regions and then working your way beneath the mandible and down along the sternocleidomastoid muscle. It is important to document any oddities and any differences noted from the right and left sides [5].

The clinician must be systematic in performing the comprehensive oral exam in order not to miss any minute details. This can include starting with soft tissues from right to left and top to bottom and then moving onto the hard tissue in a similar manner. The most important aspects of the lesion to document are location, size, color, surface texture, characteristics such as ulcerated, flat, or raised, borders, symptoms, and if the lesion is solitary in nature or found in multiples.

The location of the lesion can help differentiate one lesion from another. For example, recurrent herpetic lesions are only found on keratinized tissue within the oral cavity, while primary herpetic gingivostomatitis can occur on both keratinized and nonkeratinized tissue.

The size of the lesion also plays an important role in differentiation along with the duration of the lesion obtained from clinical exam or history provided by the patient. A rapidly growing lesion can indicate an aggressive neoplasm that should be biopsied immediately so that a definitive diagnosis can be made and treatment initiated as soon as possible. The surface texture of a lesion can also serve as a diagnostic marker. The different surface textures include papillary or granular, flat or raised, or smooth. Each of these different textures can hone into a specific diagnosis. For example, the papillary epithelial surface is often associated with squamous papilloma found with the human papillomavirus. After thorough and adequate documentation of the lesion is performed, a decision can be made in terms of which biopsy technique is best for that specific lesion. These techniques include surgical biopsy procedures such as incisional versus excisional biopsies, cytologic smears, and fine-needle aspiration. The factors that influence the selection of the surgical biopsy technique include the size of the lesion, the anatomic location whether it be in soft tissue or intraosseous, or if there is a suspicion of malignancy.

Excisional Biopsy

With excisional biopsies, a full-thickness excision of the entire lesion is taken. The lesions typically need to be less than 1 centimeter in diameter so that the whole lesion can be removed without leaving a significant defect in the soft tissue that will require healing by secondary intention. However, an excisional biopsy can be used with large, potentially malignant lesions as incisional biopsies may miss the malignant portion of the lesion. Disadvantages with the use of this technique include the removal of unnecessary tissue especially if the lesion is benign. This can ultimately lead to a higher chance of developing scarring. With excisional biopsies, it is possible that not all of the margins of the sample come back clear which will require additional treatment and removal of tissue [2].

The excisional biopsy is typically performed by making an elliptical incision that is three times the diameter of the lesion. The scalpel can then be used to excise the tissue from below the basement membrane into the deep dermal muscle layer as needed. This allows the pathologist an adequate sample of tissue to provide a definitive diagnosis. The purpose of the elliptical incision is to allow for primary closure of the tissue (Fig. 40.1).

In cases of vesiculobullous diseases, care must be taken in the selection of the transport media for the specimen. If direct immunofluorescence is a possible need, such as in pemphigoid, Michele's solution is the media of choice. Michele's solution preserves immunoglobulins, fibrin, and complement, along with maintaining an isotonic pH of 7.0–7.2 [7].

A punch biopsy is a variation that can allow excision for smaller lesions and incision of larger ones. This utilizes a circular blade with a handle to assist in positioning. Pressure applied at the blade will help decide depth, and then, a pickup can be used to provide traction of the tissues prior to using a 15 blade or scissor to amputate.

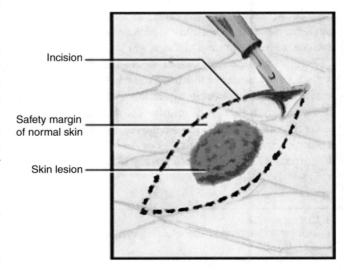

Fig. 40.1 Excisional margin in an elliptical fashion that is on healthy skin/tissues with lesion entirely within including at its depths [6]

Incisional Biopsy

An incisional biopsy refers to the excising of a portion of a lesion using full-thickness excision techniques, and this is typically reserved for lesions that measure greater than 1 cm in diameter, deeply invasive lesions, and suspicion of malignancy (Fig. 40.2). It is used to obtain large samples of a large lesion but not the entire lesion. If the entire lesion is obtained, a large defect would be created. When a lesion presents with multiple areas of erythema, leukoplakia, or ulcerations, then it might be necessary to take multiple incisional biopsies of each of these different areas. If ulcerations are present, then the clinician must take a sample of the ulcerated tissue along with adjacent healthy tissue if possible to allow the pathologist to visualize histologically the changes under a microscope. This ultimately allows the pathologist the best opportunity to provide a final diagnosis of the lesion [5].

Enucleation

Shelling out a lesion with its total cystic contents is termed enucleation. The fibrous connective tissue of a cyst gives the surgeon the ability to completely excavate the lesion without interruption of the surrounding tissue planes. Care should be taken to remove the cyst in its entirety with its contents; however, the unique variations sometimes don't allow this [8].

Enucleation is the method of choice for cystic jaw lesions that can be removed safely without compromising adjacent structures. Enucleation both allows the lesion to be removed entirely and for it to be examined by the pathologist. In the setting of a large lesion, a pathologic fracture of the jaw is possible if enucleation is improperly performed. Teeth could become devitalized, and impacted teeth in close proximity may be removed [2, 8].

Access the cyst through a window into the osseous structure (Fig. 40.3). Once visualized, use a curette which is the largest to fit the space and begin dividing the connective tissue associated with the cyst from the walls. Maintain the curette orientation so that the concave surface is facing the bone. Use of sinus curettes may be helpful to maneuver around roots and septae. Once the cyst has been removed, position and close tissues airtight [8].

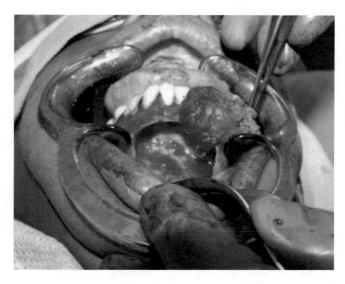

Fig. 40.3 The initial lesion with flap and tissue reflected. Osseous access gained with rongeur after tooth extraction, curette with a concave surface to bone used to remove contents in whole. Tight closure achieved [6]

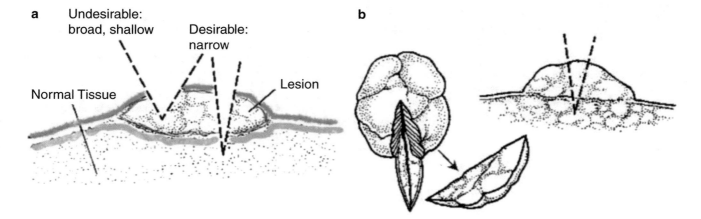

Fig. 40.2 Incisional biopsy including normal tissue and diseased tissues with depth to determine spread cross sectional view (**a**), inclusion of normal tissues (**b**) to get adequate specimen comparison [6]

Marsupialization

Creating a surgical window into a cystic lesion and removing its contents while maintaining its continuity with the oral cavity is called marsupialization (Fig. 40.4). Completing the removal of contents and maintaining egress will promote cavity shrinkage [8]. This will help to minimize the osseous defect left behind from enucleation. Marsupialization should be performed when the cystic lesion is closely associated with other vital structures like sinuses, nerve tissues, or healthy teeth. When the cyst is not easily removed in one piece and concerns for recurrence are present, it may be more advisable to marsupialize and come back secondarily. The advantages of this procedure are that it can be performed easily and preserve many closely associated vital structures; however, this comes with the price of leaving the pathology in the patient.

Once the aspiration of the lesion helps to indicate a cyst, you can then create a large window into the lesion. Removal of the contents precedes the suturing of the lining to the oral mucosa. In some cases, a nasal trumpet can be secured into the lesion to maintain a patent tract for decompression.

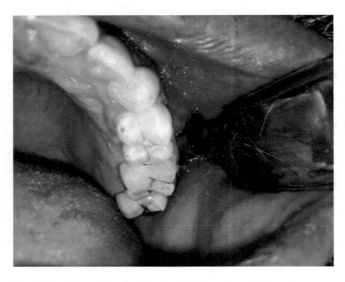

Fig. 40.4 Cyst within maxilla after incision through the oral mucosa and cystic wall into the center of cyst. Scissors are used to complete the excision of the window of mucosa and cystic wall. The oral mucosa and mucosa of the cystic wall sutured together around the periphery of the opening. Use of a nasal trumpet can help maintain patency [6]

Fine-Needle Aspiration (FNA)

This method is typically used for evaluating subcutaneous lesions in the most minimally invasive way possible. In the head and neck, it is typically used to obtain a final diagnosis for salivary gland and neck masses. FNA should be considered as the first-line diagnostic tool when appropriate cytologic assessment can be performed in a timely fashion. The armamentarium for FNA of the parotid gland and neck includes using a 22-gauge needle. The needle is inserted into the depth of the mass, and a small amount of fluid or tissue is aspirated. Normal salivary gland tissue obtained from FNA is composed of the ductal and acinar epithelium [2]. With a cancer-like mucoepidermoid carcinoma, a small number of cells are found with a predominance of mucin-containing cells with abundant foamy cytoplasm. These various cell types need a trained eye of a pathologist to differentiate. This type of biopsy, though minimally invasive, can provide a great deal of information in regard to what the mass may be whether a benign cyst or something more sinister such as cancer. An FNA biopsy is one of the simplest types of biopsies to perform, but it can sometimes miss a cancer if the needle does not go into the depth of the mass or if it does not remove enough cells for the pathologist to analyze. The minimally invasive nature of FNA, however, makes it a great first choice biopsy for salivary gland and neck masses as vital structures can be avoided.

References

1. Fornatura M. Biopsy of oral lesions. Academic presentation/lecture. 2014.
2. Pfenninger JL, Usatine R. Choosing the biopsy technique. J Fam Pract. 2014;63(1):1–3.
3. Pisharodi L, Guiter G, Layfield LJ. Fine-needle aspiration. In: Diagnostic surgical pathology of the head and neck; Academic presentation/lecture. 2009. p. 1069–130.
4. Usatine R. Punch biopsy. J Fam Pract. 2014;63(1):1–3.
5. McCoy JM. Biopsy techniques, Chapter 80. In: Atlas of oral and maxillofacial surgery. St. Louis: Elsevier; 2015. p. 840–7.
6. Oral and Maxillofacial Surgery, Dental College of Georgia at Augusta University, Augusta, Georgia, USA.
7. Fonseca RJ, Marciani RD, Turvey TA. Oral and maxillofacial surgery. St. Louis: Saunders/Elsevier. Chapter 31; 2009. p. 621.
8. Hupp JR, et al. Contemporary oral and maxillofacial surgery. 6th ed. St. Louis: Elsevier; 2013. p. 448–58.

Dental Anesthesiology

41

Saba Sefidabi and Mahmood Dashti

Introduction

The latest local anesthetic agents employed daily are presumed to be successful and secure in delivering an analgesic surgical domain. Usage of correct category of a local anesthetic and a complete medical history reduce the frequency of an unplanned allergic reaction. It is almost crucial regarding the anesthetic classification and to be careful about the infiltration procedure that is being administered. Overlooking the anatomic system and procedures, including the armamentarium's bad choice, can significantly increase the occurrence of serious allergic cases and complicated situations [1].

Dentists have access to multiple local anesthetics and numerous administration methods to avoid discomfort. The attributes that may affect the outcome comprise a rise in the challenge in anesthetizing teeth having inflammation, surgeries that are done on the tooth (e.g., it seems to be simpler to have favorable anesthesia for dental removal than for the root canal procedure), different sensitivities of other teeth to local anesthesia, and numerous remedies and procedures utilized to provide a local anesthetic.

Facing drug-related issues is quite common. Deciding on the right local anesthetic agent and employing a preoperative examination of the patient are essential. The numerous problems such as neuralgia or paresthesia, hypersensitivity, overdosing, allergy, hematoma, toxicity, and trismus, which can be noticed while administering an anesthetic agent.

Hence, the surgeon should be careful regarding the probable systems of handling and their complexities [1, 2].

Categorization and Chemical Composition of Local Anesthetics

Local anesthetics are grouped as per the rate of frequency, chemical composition, effectiveness, and the time they take to induce an effect. They are chemically known as amino amides or amino esters – esters: procaine and benzocaine, and amides: bupivacaine, prilocaine, mepivacaine, lidocaine, and articaine. Amides generate a more quick and significant anesthetic effect. Hence, they are administered more often compared to esters. Esters are not available as injections anymore. Ester local anesthetics are hydrolyzed in the plasma by pseudocholinesterase into para-aminobenzoic acid (PABA) and other derivatives, but the liver breaks down an amide-type local anesthetic. The speed of the hydrolysis influences the toxicity of a local anesthetic. The rates of biotransformation of mepivacaine, etidocaine, amide-group lidocaine, and bupivacaine are alike. Articaine, which consists of both ester and amide, is broken down in the blood and the liver. The class of esters (cenozoic acid esters) comprises tetracaine, procaine, cocaine, benzocaine, and chloroprocaine. The amide group comprises ropivacaine (Naropin), lidocaine, prilocaine (Citanest), dibucaine (nupercaine), bupivacaine (Marcaine), etidocaine (curanest), and mepivacaine (Carbocaine).

Ester local anesthetics are not accessible in dental cartridges mainly due to multiple factors like poor success rate, the benefits of amino amides, and the possibility of inducing allergies [3, 4]. Lidocaine is the high standard local anesthetic to be utilized in dentistry [5, 6]. Lidocaine is available as two dilutions of epinephrine – 1:80,000, 1:200,000, and 1:300,000 ratios in other nations and ratios of 1:50,000 and 1:100,000 in the United States and Canada. It is suggested (in North America) that epinephrine in a ratio of 1:100,000 be employed with lidocaine when there is a requirement to manage persisting discomforts [7].

S. Sefidabi · M. Dashti (✉)
Private Practice, Tehran, Iran
e-mail: dashti.mahmood72@gmail.com

© The Author(s), under exclusive license to Springer Nature Switzerland AG 2021
M. R. Stevens et al. (eds.), *Innovative Perspectives in Oral and Maxillofacial Surgery*,
https://doi.org/10.1007/978-3-030-75750-2_41

Injection Techniques

Infiltrative techniques Administer anesthesia to the maxillary teeth and canines, the mandibular incisors, and all teeth, comprising mandibular molars, in kids up to age five [7, 8].

1. *Posterior superior alveolar (PSA) infiltration:* This method is utilized to anesthetize the nearby buccal tender tissue, the maxillary molar, the PDL, periosteum, and the bone. The mesiobuccal section of the primary molar is not anesthetized efficiently by this procedure [9]. The insertion region of this injection is at an angle to the maxillary second premolar at the buccal vestibule level. The needle is entered at a depth of nearly 5 mm [10].
2. *Middle superior alveolar (MSA) infiltration:* MSA infiltration is utilized to anesthetize the mesiobuccal part of the primary molar, premolars, bone, PDL, periosteum, and the neighboring buccal tender tissue. The insertion region for this injection is at an angle to the maxillary second premolar at the level of the buccal vestibule. The needle is entered at a depth of nearly 5 mm, and on careful aspiration, the use of 1.0 ml anesthetic liquid ensues.
3. *Anterior superior alveolar (ASA) infiltration:* ASA infiltration anesthetizes teeth from the canine to the midline teeth and the adjacent PDL, buccal tender tissue, periosteum, and the bone. The insertion region is above the maxillary canine. After careful aspiration, a deposition of 1.0 ml of the liquid is administered [10].

Regional nerve blocks These blocks are utilized to give anesthesia across a wider region than the other surgical methods. Regional blocks are administered with others in the mandibular arch as infiltrative methods are not that successful because of bone density.

1. *Greater palatine foramen block:* This method anesthetizes the hard palate tissues at an angle till the midline and at the front end to the distal part of the canine [7, 10].
2. *Inferior alveolar nerve block:* This enables to anesthetize the mandibular teeth from the third molar up to the midline, buccal tender tissue at the front end of the premolars, the lower chin and lip, the periosteum, and the PDL. The canal is almost placed 1 cm higher than the mandibular occlusal surface, anterior to the pterygomandibular raphe. One must employ the thumb of the weaker arm to pull in the cheek. The tissue must be drawn in tight. The syringe should be gripped collateral to the mandibular occlusal plane, with the barrel lying on top of the premolars opposite the anesthetized area. It can be beneficial to bend the needle slightly. One must focus on the inferior alveolar canal. A common 27-gauge needle will be required to slide nearly 75% of its length, or 20–25 mm. The bone (mandibular ramus) must be accessed at that depth. Otherwise, the outcome is surely a debacle. Then aspiration is unavoidable [9].
3. *Maxillary nerve blocks:* The method applied to anesthetize half of the maxilla is to approve the different systems of surgical cure, which is to be done on the maxillary sinus and maxilla. Anesthesia could be effective if the High Tuberosity Anaesthesia Method or the Greater Palatine Nerve Block Method is adopted.
4. *Infraorbital nerve block:* It causes a prickle in the cheek, maxillary front teeth and gingiva, nostril, upper lip, and the lower eyelid. Anesthesia can be administered on the infraorbital nerve in three ways. The anesthetic drug's positioning into the buccal mucosa, opposite the upper second bicuspid tooth at 0.5 cm from the buccal plane, is the intraoral system. On the contrary, directing the drug into the tissues near the infraorbital foramen is the extraoral system [11].
5. *Gow-Gates nerve block:* The benefit of this method over the common inferior alveolar nerve block is its greater efficacy in creating anesthetic effects and the minimal danger of positive aspiration. This injection anesthetizes the buccal, inferior alveolar, lingual, mylohyoid, and auriculotemporal nerves.
6. *Nasopalatine nerve block:* This anesthetizes the palatal tissue of the premaxilla. The nasopalatine nerve passes via the incisive canal to the incisive papilla and generates a tingle to the anterior one-third of the palate. The access to the nasopalatine foramen is almost at the rear end of the maxillary incisors. This is mostly an agonizing injection [12].
7. *Mental nerve block:* This administers anesthesia to the chin's skin, buccal mucosa, and the lower lip [13]. One must palpate the mental foramen, situated close to the apices of the premolars. One must point the needle down when pulling in the lower lip and then direct 3–4 ml straight above the foramen [9, 14].

Intraseptal This procedure is beneficial when obtaining soft tissue, hemostasis, and osseous anesthesia for surgical flap operations, root planing, and scaling.

Intraosseous injections These are implemented when the usual block or the infiltration procedures do not work. They are utilized to anesthetize many teeth or a single tooth within a quadrant.

Intrapulpal When the traditional anesthetic methods are not successful, this procedure is mostly applied throughout the endodontic operations.

Complexities of Local Dental Anesthesia and Anatomical Factors

The complexities derived from many different aspects, the succeeding reasons can be classified as basically important side effects:

The local anesthetic and interaction with other medicinal products [15]; the patient's psychological stress level and overall well-being; the procedure implemented, and the anatomical condition [16].

There could be a threat of a considerable overdose of local anesthetic by an accidental intravascular injection due to the intimate anatomical link between the central nervous system's outcome and the selected spot for injection. It is hence essential to have an aspiration specimen when rotating the syringe before each injection [1, 7]. There could be distress if there is contact with the artery wall [16]. Lidocaine less than 200 µg is needed inside the internal cerebrovascular system to overcome the poisonous limit of the dosage. The circulatory path is sealed from inside by intravascular injection of a vasoconstrictor and a local anesthetic, thereby inhibiting the circulation to all the tissues and slowing down the metabolism. There are queries regarding why most positive blood aspirations and side effects happen during the block anesthesia at the mandibular foramen. The area that is selected for this injection method is the location over the mandibular foramen. In the direct procedure, the needle appears from the first premolar area of the opposite region and is then positioned between the anterior border of the mandibular ramus and the pterygomandibular raphe; the sliding then carries on to the mandibular foramen. The risk exists if the needle is driven into the inferior alveolar artery and also accidentally thrusting the needle tip and thereby releasing the local anesthetic into the maxillary artery as it is nearby.

If the injection pressure is high, it is rational to inject it in an opposite pathway of the bloodstream. The maxillary artery is placed at an angle to the lingual nerve and medial to the inferior alveolar nerve, or medial to the lingual nerve and at a particular angle to the inferior alveolar nerve.

Once the local anesthetic reaches the maxillary nerve, the bloodstream circulates it even more into sensitive cerebral areas. The ophthalmic artery originates from the frontal part of the medial meningeal artery above the anastomotic ramus that occurs in lower than 1% of the patients. The central retinal ramus derieved from ophthalmic artery, and inside the optic nerve, it progresses to the retina (Tillmann 1997). An extremely rare problem can occur if the local anesthetic circulates to the retina by this path and can cause short-term or long-lasting loss of vision [2].

Systemic Results Due to Local Anesthesia

Psychogenic Reactions

This psychogenic result is related to the patients' body neutralizing a stress-inducing condition or connected with their dental history [17]. Due to this, patients with high anxiety have a greater respiratory rate, heart rate, and blood pressure throughout and before employing local dental anesthesia than patients with no anxiety [16]. Patients usually have symptoms of blush or erythema, which resemble hyperventilation, allergic reactions, nausea, and puking [15]. It is critical to observe the patient and help them to de-stress. The patient should be calmed before giving local anesthetic injections to stop any more psychogenic episodes. Dental tensions can be successfully curbed by giving oral sedatives. The first dose should be based on the patient's age, weight, well-being, and operation period. For fit adult patients, for short-duration operations, antihistamines such as diphenhydramine (Benadryl) 50 mg should be given an hour before the surgery; for medium-duration surgeries (1–2 hours), benzodiazepines such as triazolam (Halcion) 0.125–0.5 mg should be administered an hour before the operation; and for longer-duration surgeries (2–4 hours), benzodiazepines such as lorazepam (Ativan) 1–4 mg can be injected 1–2 hours before the surgery or 30–60 minutes before the sublingual concentration can be advised and provided. Pharmacologically, mild and usually tensed dental patients can be handled by providing a sedative, or highly tensed patients can be managed with the help of general anesthesia [18, 19].

Systemic Toxicity

Local anesthetic systemic toxicity occurs due to an adequate (poisonous) amount of anesthetic drug observed in the blood that gets to the central nervous system and cardiovascular system. The early signs are denoted by the central nervous system like convulsions and excitation, succeeded by fainting and respiratory arrest. These reactions are usually followed by cardiovascular symptoms like tachycardia, hypertension, and premature ventricular contractions [1]. The critical indicators and reactions are mainly objective symptoms like twitching, talking fast, and shaking in the extremities [1, 5]. The influencing aspects are linked with weight, age, widespread vasoconstrictors, sex, different medications, genetics, the frequency of an ailment, concentration, vasoactivity, dosage, method of employing the drug, frequency of injection, and the vascularity of the injection area [4]. The patient should be examined to stop systemic toxicity. The dosage of the local anesthetic must be reduced; slim or young patients should not be operated on every four quadrants in one appointment by just utilizing a local anesthetic; the aspirating method, altering the dose by segregating the administration of the anesthetic, slow and precise injection procedure, implementing an aspiring examination, and using the least poisonous agents like levobupivacaine and ropivacaine are advised [20].

To avert a poisonous dose and its complexities, it should be recalled that for fit adults, the advised optimum safe dosage of 2% lignocaine in 1:80,000 adrenaline is (four-and-a-half) 2 or 2.2 ml cartridges (180–198 mg lignocaine); for 3% prilocaine and felypressin 0.03 IU/ml, the optimum safe dosage is 400 mg (6–2 ml cartridges). The other method to minimize toxicity is to utilize one-tenth cartridge per kilo as an estimated standard to the optimum dosage. Dentists should know that a very high dosage of topical anesthetics, though these agents are highly concentrated to simplify infiltration, can result in a poisonous reaction, especially in kids.

The dental clinic's treatment comprises supplying 100% oxygen, airway backup, supine placement, and safeguarding from wounds if seizures occur; treatment of convulsions (benzodiazepines or thiopental; propofol cannot be utilized in patients with an irregular heartbeat and blood pressure) [21]. If a serious hypotension arrhythmia takes place, a 1.5 ml/kg 20% lipid emulsion should be infused for more than around 60 seconds and then an extended dosage at 0.25 ml/kg/min = 1000 ml/h should be initiated. There have been cases as per research that documented a resuscitation outcome at a total dosage of ≤10 ml/kg; so the 12 ml/kg can be supplied as an assessment of the optimum dosage. The adrenaline dosage must be included in the resuscitation citation directions like the American Heart Association.

Allergy

Allergy is known as an abnormal hypersensivity reaction of the body to a previously introduced allergn; the repeated subjection to it can induce an increased potential to respond. The frequency of allergic reactions is unusual regarding the amide-type local anesthetics. Less than 1% of all problems are estimated due to an allergy. Many issues considered to be allergic, in reality, are reactions [22] generated by anxiety. Amide-type local anesthetics cause fewer allergies than ester-type local anesthetics, thereby making the amide-type anesthetics the frequently employed one, among which lidocaine is highly utilized for dental anesthesia for dental anesthesia involving epinephrine. Preservatives (e.g., methyl hydroxybenzoate), antiseptics (e.g., chlorhexidine), antioxi-

dants (e.g., bisulfate), vasoconstrictor (e.g., sulfites), and other antigens like latex and the local anesthetic drug itself can cause serious reactions. Mild allergic reactions like erythema, urticaria, and itching, also serious reactions such as angioedema and/or respiratory discomfort are commonly observed. The more serious anaphylactic responses that can be fatal comprise signs of hypotension, fainting, and apnea [22]. Skin prick examination is a highly recommended method to identify allergies. An intradermal examination must be employed for patients who have had an allergy in the past by using local anesthetics and should thus be made mandatory if the skin test outcomes turn out to be negative [22, 23]. The succeeding procedures should be utilized if a local anesthetic patient had tested negative for an allergy. The primary step should be the elimination of the causative agent for an allergic reaction in the clinic. Oral or intramuscular antihistamine such as diphenhydramine (Benadryl), 25 or 50 mg, should be authorized for handling less-severe symptoms. Hydrocortisone cream, too, can be advised to alleviate erythema or skin itching. In potentially fatal situations, intramuscular or subcutaneous epinephrine 0.3–0.5 mg, standard life support, and hospital care should be provided. Anaphylaxis is an acute, potentially fatal hypersensitivity reaction, and clinical signs are organ dependent. The dangerous signs of anaphylaxis are unmanageable co-existing asthma, distinct allergies like tree nut and peanut allergy, and mast cell defects. As per the directions of the Australasian Society of Clinical Immunology and Allergy regarding the critical handling of anaphylaxis in the clinic, the given procedures should be carried out: the patient should lie down flat, and in situations of breathlessness, the patient should be permitted to sit. Adrenaline at 1:1000 concentration (0.01 mg/kg up to 0.5 mg per dose) should be intramuscularly directed with 1 ml syringes and 21 gauge needles, and must be continued every 5 minutes as per requirement. Epinephrine is also suggested (0.3 mg) for kids and adults who are 30 kg and above, and the dosage is 0.15 mg for those weighing in the range 15–30 kg. Adrenaline auto-injector can also be given, which is usually used for overweight allergic patients. Patients themselves buy this for their use. Adrenaline should be given intravenously (IV) for anaphylaxis just in the case of extremely hypotensive patients or patients with cardiopulmonary arrest or those do not teatated with adrenaline due to the possible cardiovascular serious reactions of IV distribution of adrenaline. The examination of the proof-based pharmacologic cure of anaphylaxis was performed by Estelle and Simons. The primary procedure of using intramascular epinephrine was accepted as first step in the cure of anaphylaxis. There is a debate regarding the employment of glucocorticoids and antihistamines. The application of antihistamines is not successful, as presumed by a few writers, as they don't act on the lower or upper airway obstruction, shock, or hypotension. In contrast, others suggest that these drugs reduce the side effects of headache, flushing, urticaria, rhinorrhea, and hypotension. Glucocorticoids were introduced as the second most popular medications (following epinephrine) for anaphylaxis worldwide, despite the fact that glucocorticoids have no valid effect on anaphylaxis according to the research of the World Allergy Organization [18]. Therefore, the primary cure should be epinephrine followed by glucocorticoids, and antihistamines may be given to cure extreme systemic reactions.

Methemoglobinemia

Methemoglobinemia is a distinct dosage-reliant response when the iron in the hemoglobin remains unchanged in the ferric (Fe^{3+}) form that can't combine with oxygen, resulting in tissue hypoxia and cyanosis. Patients in such conditions are in danger of acquiring underlying health issues such as heart disease, pulmonary illness (chronic obstructive pulmonary disease, pneumonia), and liver cirrhosis, with underdeveloped hepatic and renal function. Local anesthetics, mainly prilocaine and benzocaine (90% of documented patients), and sometimes articaine and lidocaine, can also cause methemoglobinemia when given in high doses [20]. Cyanosis indicators will be noticed in mucous membranes and nail beds. Dizziness, headaches, dyspnea, extreme tiredness, and tachycardia are witnessed in dire situations. Pulse oximetry and in-hospital arterial blood examination are performed as a crucial part of dental clinic diagnosis [20]. The first stage of handling methemoglobinemia is promptly giving supplemental oxygen (100%). Hyperbaric oxygenation can also be utilized for extreme situations if it is accessible. Methylene blue should be used in 1–2 mg/kg doses, given as 1% solution (10 mg/ml) intravenously for more than 5–10 minutes per hour up to a maximum concentration of 7 mg/kg. Continuous dosage may be required within 30–60 minutes of the original dosage [21, 22]. Guay concluded 242 reports of methemoglobinemia issues related to dental local anesthetics like cocaine, bupivacaine, lidocaine, tetracaine, mepivacaine, and prilocaine in adults and kids. He declared to stop distributing benzocaine. Prilocaine should not be given to distinct classes of patients like toddlers younger than 6 months, patients having other oxidizing drugs, and pregnant women. The dosage is to be approved at 2.5 mg/kg [20].

Local Complications Associated with Local Anesthesia

Pain on Injection

Distress by injection can happen due to certain situations like the solution's temperature; rupturing of tender tissues, nerves, blood vessels, or the periosteum; velocity of injections; dull needles; needles with barbs; or rough positioning of the needle resulting in great distress and other problems. A burning sensation occurs due to the acidity of the solution and the volume of injection. A strong burning sensation is felt when lidocaine is injected locally. Patients can also sense an abrupt "electric" shock when the needle pierces a nerve, causing rapid head movements with a danger of self-inflicted injuries. To avoid any distress, warming the anesthetics to body temperature, implementing topical anesthetics, utilizing a tinier-gauge needle (27 gauge), changing over to a new needle when you have to inject numerous times at the identical wound or when you have many injection spots, and injecting slowly that too with minimal pressure to minimize distress are the various procedures being implemented. A measure of 30 seconds per milliliter of fluid is advised. An inappropriate injection region can cause an intraneural or intramuscular injection blunting of the needle; at the anatomic injection design (palate) position, it is unreasonable to experience pain when being injected [12, 23, 24].

Needle Fracture

Since the invention of the non-reusable, stainless steel dental local anesthetic needles, the complications arising due to the needle getting ruptured in the oral activity is very scarce. Usually, needle fractures occur with 30-gauge needles and through inferior alveolar nerve block due to a bad injection procedure, the assistant's or patient's unpredictable movement, or the wrong selection of hypodermic needle's dimension [25]. The injection needle must be inspected first to avert needle fractures. For inferior nerve block in kids or adults, a 30-gauge and smaller needles should be avoided. However, 25- to 27-gauge needles can be used. When sliding the needle into tender tissues, any bend should be averted [25, 26]. If there is a possibility of a traceable broken needle, it should be instantly eliminated with a hemostat. A computerized tomographic (CT) scan must be carried out if it is hard to locate the needle with the naked eye, and the patient must be operated on by general anesthesia. In reports regarding the elimination of the fragment, mainly the superficial mucosal opening – perpendicular to the needle's path succeeded by blunt supra-periosteal dissection to leave out the important structures – is suggested [27, 28]. Kim et al. in 2013 studied the complexities in the report regarding the needle fracture after dental local anesthesia in 36 publications and 59 needle rupturing incidents. According to them, three-dimensional visual procedures must be undertaken to observe the ruptured fragments and adjacent structures like the parotid gland and vessels. This is critical as 27 of the total 57 cannula fragments were seen in the pterygomandibular region. The method of eliminating the fragment by local or general anesthesia must be determined by the patient's systemic state [29].

Continuation of Anesthesia and Other Sensory Dysfunctions

Prolong anesthetic, neuralgia, or paresthesia can arise after dental local anesthesia blocks. This could be for a little while, and after some days, weeks, or months, the sensation could be restored, or it could be permanent [23]. This usually includes nervus mandibularis or [30]. The nerve may get ruptured through injection due to a first-hand wound, or the needle could cause physical injury to the medial pterygoid muscle causing trismus, or the needle could impair the intraneural blood supply, causing a hematoma. Neurotoxicity of the local anesthetic is a separate hypothesis for nerve dysfunction [31]. Lidocaine or bupivacaine is less harmful than tetracaine and procaine [24]. Neuralgia or paresthesia complication is usually temporary, but it can be long-lasting if the anesthetic agent is injected right into the nerve. Due to a feeling of immobility, the patient may endure side effects like drooling, lacking a sense of taste, tongue biting, and faltering of speech. Sullivan et al. implemented an unplanned, dual-blind, placebo-controlled study on 496 cases suffering from Bell's palsy they contiiued steroid therapy 3days after. the onset usually improves the possibility for a complete recovery by 3 or 9 months [32]. Piccinni et al. did a research of the documents and sent it to the FDA Adverse Event Reporting System; around 573 dysesthesia and paresthesia patients on taking local anesthetics during 2004 and 2011 were examined during these trials. They summarized that taking articaine or prilocaine or both drugs led to a greater threat of paresthesia [33]. If a nerve gets ruptured due to dental local anesthesia, the primary cure should be to handle the patient's discomfort. In order to decrease local anesthesia-dependent nerve injury, avoiding high concentration of anesthetic agent for inferior alveolar nerve blocks (use 2% lidocaine as standard), preventing iterative injections, and avoiding inferior alveolar nerve blocks are done by using high concentration agents (articaine) infiltrations only. The suggestion is to have a minimal regular dosage of multivitamin B to revive nerve health and function [34, 35].

Absence of Effect

A wrong procedure or method of operation and resolution, anatomical variants, and psychological and pathological aspects are contributed to anasthetic failure [23]. Anatomical attributes include a change in the placement of foramen, accessory nerve supply, bone density, and atypical formation of the nerves (bifid mandibular canals) [36, 37]. Any past surgery or bruises, infections, inflammation, and trismus are the pathological factors of the ineffectiveness of anesthesia. The inflammatory ailments changing the pharmacodynamics and pharmacokinetics of the local anesthetics result in alleviation of a reaction and a rise in bad outcomes [38]. Local anesthetic deficiency or the challenge to gain moderate analgesic usually happens in conditions of inflammation like apical periodontitis pulpitis, pericoronitis, or acute periodontal abscess [39]. The ineffectiveness of local anesthetics is also a result of psychological factors like anxiety and worry [36]. The non-success of an inapproptiate procedure is a result of poor access to mandibular anesthesia. The terminal branches of the facial nerve in the parotid gland's deep lobe can get damaged if the needle is placed inward and moves very deep and very dorsally. Anesthesia in the facial nerve (first hand) can cause a quick onset when the anesthetic agent is injected; facial nerve palsy is the result of reflex vasospasms of the external carotid artery, causing ischemia of the facial nerve. As a result, the patient cannot raise their eyebrows, form wrinkles on the forehead, pull in the commissure of the lips to smile, shut the upper eyelid, and turn down the lower lip at the dysfunctional portion. The elimination of the contact lenses and shutting of the eye on the damaged part in Bell's palsy avert drying or corneal abrasion. In a majority of the patients, on injecting the mandibular anesthesia, the result is instant paralysis, and delayed paralysis is also observed on a few occasions. Cakarer et al. reported a case study for delayed paralysis. In a patient, they removed simple teeth with no issues, and the patient came back with troubles after a day of feeling frail on the left facial muscles. On observation, they deduced Bell's palsy symptoms on the left region and unilateral blankness, without any pathologic symptom in the bruise or any herpetic lesions. They discussed with the patient and with the Department of Physical Therapy, Rehabilitation, and Department of Ophthalmology. They prescribed tobramycin ophthalmic solution (4 × 1), lanolin eye ointment (at night), and lubricant eye drops (4 × 1); eye patches were utilized. Galvanic stimulation of the damaged regions of the facial nerve was carried out for 4 weeks by advocating mime therapy. All the symptoms vanished in a fortnight [25]. The auriculotemporal nerve will be damaged if the needle is slid in very deep and high. There has been a case of immediate deafness on one side after administering inferior dental nerve anesthesia.

Trismus

Trismus is a discomforting situation where one can't open their mouth in general. Many trismus-like circumstances result in numerous injections in quick time in the identical region, an inferior type of infection, intramuscular injections in the muscle or injury to the muscles (either the temporal muscle or the lateral pterygoid muscle) can result in the development of hematoma and fibrosis, incorrect placement of the needle when administering the inferior nerve block or posterior maxillary injections or the inflammation of the masseter and various masticatory muscles, needle fracture of the muscles by sliding it during the styloid procedure, and high concentration of local anesthetic solutions collected within a confined area which lead to the tissue enlargement. Discomfort due to hemorrhage causes muscle contraction and restricted movement in the acute stage. A few conditions can be cured naturally once trismus occurs. The development of trismus to fibrous ankylosis and chronic hypomobility can be averted by the non-delayed procedure of good care comprising a simple diet, heat treatment, advising analgesics, antibiotics, anti-inflammatory drugs, physiotherapy, or muscle relaxants. Antibiotics are given to cure trismus due to an infection. Trismus is mostly cured in 6 weeks or within 4–20 weeks. Understanding of the anatomical regions and muscles: palpation of bony anterior ramus for temporalis muscle, the right angulation of the needle and touching of bone before injecting, and the pterygomandibular fold for pterygoid muscle are effective techniques to prevent trismus by local anesthesia. by applying intraoral Vazirani-Akinosi procedures, the extraoral procedures, or the closed-mouth mandibular sealing system, can be administered anesthesia to patients suffering from trismus [40–42].

Infection

Complications arising due to infections are rare due to the application of glass cartridges and throwaway needles. Insertion of a needle via an infected tissue can result in the spreading of infection, as the needle can be infected before surgery or by the poor composition of local anesthetic solutions. On the contrary, lateral viral contamination can reoc-

cur because of the surgery's trauma, which can cause neural sheath inflammation. The spot to be inserted should be sterilized with a topical antiseptic before sliding in the needle. Chlorhexidine gluconate – one of the antiseptic mouthwashes – should be used for every regional procedure. Local anesthesia should not be injected via the contaminated region. Due to high infection risk, it is critical to inject the local anesthesia to improve the PH level of the anesthetic agent to improve its success rate as the infected tissue is more acidic. This method is defined as anesthetic buffering and results in the patient feeling at ease through the injection, a quicker onset of anesthesia, and negligible post-injection tissue abrasions. Prescribed method to cure the contamination is by giving antibiotics (penicillin V 500 mg every 6 hours for 7–10 days), physiotherapy, [2, 23, 43].

Edema

Tissue swelling may occur due to an injection, injection of reaction-inducing solutions, allergy, infection, and hemorrhage [24]. Management of the edema is determined by its origin. Allergy-induced edema can be cured by administering intramuscular epinephrine, communicating with an allergist to ascertain the edema's exact origin, and supplying corticosteroid and antihistamine. Edema due to trauma should be treated as a hematoma. Antibiotics should be authorized to cure edema caused by contamination.

Hematoma

One of the complications of local anesthesia is hematoma due to arterial or venous tearing. If there is a high pressure during an injection, it could be a sign of inserting the needle against the bloodstream. Aspiration can be implemented to avert hematoma before injecting the anesthetic solution by utilizing a tiny needle and by minimizing the number of needle insertions into the tissues. The density of the damaged tissue ascertains the magnitude of the hematoma. The varying outcomes on the nerve can induce hematoma on distinct areas like the superior anterior alveolar (infraorbital) nerve block at the bottom of the lower eyelid, posterior superior alveolar nerve block extraoral in the lower buccal area of the mandible, intraoral distal to maxillary tuberosity, buccal nerve block or any palatal injection inside the mouth, and incisive (mental) nerve block at the chin region [16, 25]. A localized pressure should be administered within 2 minutes at least if the swelling occurs right after the injection to avert the hemorrhage. The patch and swelling mostly wane off within 10–15 days. Ice packs must be placed on the first day after surgery, after which hot moist packs at random can be utilized and massage treatment with heparin cream is advised. Antibiotics should be prescribed if the hematoma is serious to stopping the spread of a contaminated gash [25].

Gingival Lesions

Gingival bruises constitute repeated aphthous stomatitis and the onset of herpes simplex following a local anesthetic injection or succeeded by a trauma to the intraoral tissues. The precise technique is inconclusive. There is no need for any supervision till the onset of extreme discomfort [26]. Topical anesthetic solutions (e.g., viscid lidocaine) can be administered to the concerned regions to alleviate agony. Syrup of magnesia and diphenhydramine should be properly rinsed in the mouth to successfully spreads over the ulceration and alleviate the ache. Triamcinolone acetonide of corticosteroid can resolve the suffering [27].

Soft Tissue Injury

Complications documented due to local anesthesia is the chewing or biting wounds of the lip and tongue, especially in disabled patients or kids, after injecting local anesthesia [28]. Local anesthetics such as plain mepivacaine must be used for temporary results, and following instructions should be given to the patients or guardian regarding drinking hot fluids, eating, and biting on the lips or tongue for any anesthesia assessment; to stop chewing, cotton rolls can be positioned between the tender tissues and the teeth. To speed up the recuperation for any feeling, injection of phentolamine mesylate (OraVerse) and alpha-adrenergic receptor can be administered. The advised dose for adults is 1–2 cartridges of phentolamine mesylate (a dose of 0.4–0.8 mg), and for kids, the directed dose is 0.5–1 cartridge (0.2–0.4 mg) [7, 29]. Swelling may subside after 2–3 days. The injury will recover in the following 10–14 days. Analgesics can be authorized for any issues with discomfort, and topical local anesthetic gel may be spread over the affected region.

Conclusion

Application of local anesthesia can be related to serious problems. The patient's medical history should be examined periodically in depth, and a productive anxiety-management technique should be implemented to avert any local anes-

thetic complexities. The dosage relating to local anesthetics should be examined thoroughly every time as per body weight, and the optimum suggested doses should be reviewed. The injection must not be agonizing while giving anesthesia so as to prevent intramuscular or intravascular or first-hand trauma to the nerve. Modern advancements should be implemented by the surgeons to minimize any probable complications linked with local anesthesia.

References

1. Yalcin B. Complications associated with local anesthesia in oral and maxillofacial surgery. 2019.
2. Meyer F-U. Complications of local dental anesthesia and anatomical causes. Ann Anat. 1999;181(1):105–6.
3. Giovannitti J, Rosenberg M, Phero J. Pharmacology of local anesthetics used in oral surgery. Oral Maxillofac Surg Clin North Am. 2013;25:453.
4. Becker DE, Reed KL. Essentials of local anesthetic pharmacology. Anesth Prog. 2006;53(3):98–108; quiz 9–10.
5. Sekimoto K, Tobe M, Saito S. Local anesthetic toxicity: acute and chronic management. Acute Med Surg. 2017;4(2):152–60.
6. Jung RM, Rybak M, Milner P, Lewkowicz N. Local anesthetics and advances in their administration – an overview. J Pre-Clin Clin Res. 2017;11(1):94–101.
7. Malamed SF. Handbook of local anesthesia. Elsevier Health Sciences; USA. 2004.
8. Rusu M, Matei M, Bucur A. Local anaesthetics used in dentistry. 2009.
9. Moskovitz JB, Sabatino F. Regional nerve blocks of the face. Emerg Med Clin North Am. 2013;31(2):517–27.
10. Reed KL, Malamed SF, Fonner AM. Local anesthesia part 2: technical considerations. Anesth Prog. 2012;59(3):127–36; quiz 37.
11. Nardi NM, Alvarado AC, Schaefer TJ. Infraorbital nerve block. StatPearls. Treasure Island (FL): StatPearls Publishing. Copyright © 2020, StatPearls Publishing LLC; 2020.
12. Fitzpatrick TH, Downs BW. Anatomy, head and neck, nasopalatine nerve. StatPearls. Treasure Island (FL): StatPearls Publishing. Copyright © 2020, StatPearls Publishing LLC; 2020.
13. Whitworth JM, Kanaa MD, Corbett IP, Meechan JG. Influence of injection speed on the effectiveness of incisive/mental nerve block: a randomized, controlled, double-blind study in adult volunteers. J Endod. 2007;33(10):1149–54.
14. Zide BM, Swift R. How to block and tackle the face. Plast Reconstr Surg. 1998;101(3):840–51.
15. Haas DA. An update on local anesthetics in dentistry. J Can Dent Assoc. 2002;68(9):546–51.
16. Brand H, Bekker W, Baart JA. Complications of local anaesthesia. An observational study. Int J Dent Hyg. 2009;7:270–2.
17. Sharma A, Pant R, Priyadarshi S, Agarwal N, Tripathi S, Chaudhary M. Cardiovascular changes due to dental anxiety during local anesthesia injection for extraction. J Maxillofac Oral Surg. 2019;18(1):80–7.
18. Donaldson M, Gizzarelli G, Chanpong B. Oral sedation: a primer on anxiolysis for the adult patient. Anesth Prog. 2007;54(3):118–28; quiz 29.
19. Appukuttan DP. Strategies to manage patients with dental anxiety and dental phobia: literature review. Clin Cosmet Investig Dent. 2016;8:35–50.

20. Safety Committee of Japanese Society of Anesthesiologists. Practical guide for the management of systemic toxicity caused by local anesthetics. J Anesth. 2019;33(1):1–8.
21. Bosack RC, Lieblich S. Anesthesia complications in the dental office; 2015. p. 1–346.
22. Batinac T, Sotošek Tokmadžić V, Peharda V, Brajac I. Adverse reactions and alleged allergy to local anesthetics: analysis of 331 patients. J Dermatol. Wiley-Black: USA. 2013;40:522.
23. Lee J, Lee JY, Kim HJ, Seo KS. Dental anesthesia for patients with allergic reactions to lidocaine: two case reports. J Dent Anesth Pain Med. 2016;16(3):209–12.
24. Presman B, Vindigni V, Tocco-Tussardi I. Immediate reaction to lidocaine with periorbital edema during upper blepharoplasty. Int J Surg Case Rep. 2016;20:24–6.
25. Biočić J, Brajdić D, Perić B, Đanić P, Salarić I, Macan D. A large cheek hematoma as a complication of local anesthesia: case report. Acta Stomatol Croat. 2018;52(2):156–9.
26. Phore S, Panchal R. Traumatic oral lesions: pictorial essay. Med J Dr DY Patil Vidyapeeth. 2018;11(2):94–8.
27. Rawal S, Claman L, Kalmar J, Tatakis D. Traumatic lesions of the gingiva: a case series. J Periodontol. 2004;75:762–9.
28. Bagattoni S, D'Alessandro G, Gatto MR, Piana G. Self-induced soft-tissue injuries following dental anesthesia in children with and without intellectual disability. A prospective study. Eur Arch Paediatr Dent. 2020;21(5):617–22.
29. Bendgude V, Akkareddy B, Jawale BA, Chaudhary S. An unusual pattern of self-inflicted injury after dental local anesthesia: a report of 2 cases. J Contemp Dent Pract. 2011;12(5):404–7.
30. Schatz M. Skin testing and incremental challenge in the evaluation of adverse reactions to local anesthetics. The Journal of allergy and clinical immunology. 1984;74(4 Pt 2):606–16.
31. Macy E. Local anesthetic adverse reaction evaluations: the role of the allergist. Annals of allergy, asthma & immunology : official publication of the American College of Allergy, Asthma, & Immunology. 2003;91(4):319–20.
32. Troise C, Voltolini S, Minale P, Modena P, Negrini AC. Management of patients at risk for adverse reactions to local anesthetics: analysis of 386 cases. Journal of investigational allergology & clinical immunology. 1998;8(3):172–5.
33. Tomoyasu Y, Mukae K, Suda M, Hayashi T, Ishii M, Sakaguchi M, et al. Allergic reactions to local anesthetics in dental patients: analysis of intracutaneous and challenge tests. The open dentistry journal. 2011;5:146–9.
34. Olson ML, McEvoy GK. Methemoglobinemia induced by local anesthetics. American journal of hospital pharmacy. 1981;38(1):89–93.
35. Taleb M, Ashraf Z, Valavoor S, Tinkel J. Evaluation and Management of Acquired Methemoglobinemia Associated with Topical Benzocaine Use. American Journal of Cardiovascular Drugs. 2013;13(5):325–30.
36. Dahshan A, Donovan GK. Severe methemoglobinemia complicating topical benzocaine use during endoscopy in a toddler: a case report and review of the literature. Pediatrics. 2006;117(4):e806–9.
37. Udeh C, Bittikofer J, Sum-Ping STJ. Severe methemoglobinemia on reexposure to benzocaine. Journal of Clinical Anesthesia. 2001;13(2):128–30.
38. Guay J. Methemoglobinemia related to local anesthetics: a summary of 242 episodes. Anesthesia and analgesia. 2009;108(3):837–45.
39. Mansuri S, Bhayat A, Omar E, Jarab F, Ahmed MS. A Randomized Controlled Trail Comparing the Efficacy of 0.5% Centbucridine to 2% Lignocaine as Local Anesthetics in Dental Extractions. International Journal of Dentistry. 2011;2011:795047.
40. You JS, Kim SG, Oh JS, Choi HI, Jih MK. Removal of a fractured needle during inferior alveolar nerve block: two case reports. Journal of dental anesthesia and pain medicine. 2017;17(3):225–9.
41. Kim JH, Moon SY. Removal of a broken needle using three-dimensional computed tomography: a case report. Journal of the Korean Association of Oral and Maxillofacial Surgeons. 2013;39(5):251–3.
42. Stone J, Kaban LB. Trismus after injection of local anesthetic. Oral surgery, oral medicine, and oral pathology. 1979;48(1):29–32.
43. Brooke RI. Postinjection trismus due to formation of fibrous band. Oral surgery, oral medicine, and oral pathology. 1979;47(5):424–6.

Systemic Diseases with Oral Manifestations

42

Mohammad Hosein Amirzade-Iranaq
and Fargol Mashhadi Akbar Boojar

Introduction

Oral manifestations of systemic conditions and diseases are an excellent assistant for dental and maxillofacial surgeons in predicting outcomes and improving the prognosis of surgical interventions. Due to the wide range of systemic condition and diseases that upset the maxillofacial and oral area, clinicians should be aware of the signs of these conditions. This chapter will briefly discuss the distinguishing features and main manifestations of the most common systemic conditions. The aim is to classify these manifestations and treatment options, and consideration of each systemic disease is not the subject of the current review due to the wide range and expansion of the subject.

Gastrointestinal Diseases

Because the oral cavity is where the gastrointestinal (GI) tract begins, oral lesions may be the first evidence of GI disease, even before abdominal signs and symptoms appear. These oral symptoms might appear during the course of the disease or even after the gut infection has cleared up. Oral symptoms such as oral ulcerations, widespread mucosal edoema, cobblestone mucosa, and localised mucogingivitis, for example, may be the earliest indicator of GI disease in inflammatory bowel disorders (IBDs), Crohn's disease (CD), and ulcerative colitis (UC). Due to tooth enamel exposure to acidic stomach content, GERD, bulimia, or anorexia can result in irreparable dental erosion [1, 2].

M. H. Amirzade-Iranaq (✉)
Universal Network of Interdisciplinary Research in Oral and Maxillofacial Surgery (UNIROMS), Universal Scientific Education and Research Network (USERN), Tehran, Iran
e-mail: h.amirzade@gmail.com

F. M. A. Boojar
School of Dentistry, Research committee of Golestan Medical University, Gorgan, Iran

Gastroesophageal Reflux Disease

The rise of acidic and nonacidic stomach contents over the gastroesophageal junction causes GERD. GERD affects both men and women equally and affects people of all ages, albeit it is more common in middle-aged and older people [3, 4]. GERD is caused by a number of factors. Obesity, hiatal hernia, delayed stomach emptying, diabetes, asthma, pregnancy, smoking, and dry mouth are all risk factors for GERD. Also, GERD can be caused by particular foods and beverages, including as chocolate, peppermint, fried or fatty foods, coffee, alcoholic beverages, and connective tissue illnesses such progressive systemic sclerosis (scleroderma) [2, 5–7].

Heartburn, regurgitation, dysphagia, and retrosternal pain are all common GERD symptoms. Furthermore, coughing, sleep disturbances, laryngitis, hoarseness, asthma, chronic obstructive pulmonary disease, angina, unexplained chest discomfort, halitosis, sinusitis, otalgia, dental erosion, and other dental indications can all be caused by aberrant reflux [8–10].

Periodic increases in salivation, xerostomia (dry mouth), burning sensation, tongue sensitivity, halitosis, palatal erythema, oral ulcers, dysgeusia (bad taste), gingivitis, periodontitis, dental thermal sensitivity (pulpitis), and dental erosion are all common oral symptoms in people with GERD. The severity of GERD dental erosion is linked to the reflux's severity, frequency, and pH. Saliva quantity and quality are also important considerations [2–4, 10].

The occlusal surfaces of the posterior mandibular teeth and the palatal surfaces of the anterior maxillary teeth are affected by erosion in GERD patients. Affected teeth have worn enamel that is smooth, silky glazed, or shiny. As the underlying dentin is exposed, they may appear yellow and become sensitive to temperature fluctuations. Advanced phases of dental erosion reveal changes in tooth morphology, resulting in an enamel concavity with a width greater than its depth. Occlusal erosion progresses to the point where the cusps round and, in severe cases, the entire occlusal morphology vanishes, exposing the pulp may occur [2, 10, 11].

Ulcerative Colitis

Remissions and exacerbations characterize by UC, an inflammatory reaction that can harm the large intestine. The mucosa may seem grainy under the microscope in mild illness. Stripping of the mucosa, with areas of sloughing, ulceration, and bleeding, is a symptom of advanced illness. Dehydration is a common problem among patients. Due to water and electrolyte malabsorption, UC patients may experience exhaustion, weight loss, and fever. Oral alterations are non-specific and infrequent in UC cases, with a prevalence of roughly 8%. On a clinical evaluation of a patient with UC, oral health care specialists can find them [2, 12].

Multiple small white or yellow pustules on an erythematous and edematous mucosal backdrop characterise Pyostomatitis Vegetans (PV) oral lesions, which are not premalignant. The pustules can rupture, merge, and appear scattered, clumped, or like a snail's track [13]. Pustules can affect practically any area of the mouth. The buccal gingiva, labial, and buccal mucosa are the most usually affected areas, whereas the tongue and floor of the mouth are the least impacted [14]. PV lesions can be harmless or cause significant oral irritation, and they have nothing to do with the clinical activity of UC. With a male/female ratio of roughly 3:1, there is a preference for men. PV can strike at any age, but it is most common between the ages of 20 and 59, with an average age of 34 [2].

Another oral manifestation of UV is pyoderma gangrenosum, which causes deep sores, occasionally through the tonsillar pillar. Aphthous stomatitis, hairy leukoplakia, and halitosis are other oral symptoms of UC [2, 15].

Due to vitamin K-dependent liver factors, UC is linked to persistent bleeding. Before dental operations, a blood test for haemoglobin, hematocrit, platelet count, and red blood cell count should be performed to rule out anaemia (macrocytic and microcytic) and bleeding proclivity [2, 16].

Vitamin K, vitamin B12, and folic acid malabsorption may occur in patients who have had significant intestinal operations. They should be checked for bleeding disorders caused by vitamin K deficiency (fibrin clot formation). A partial thromboplastin time (PT) and a prothrombin time (PT) or an international normalised ratio (INR) will reveal the patient's ability to produce clots.

Crohn's Disease

CD is a chronic inflammatory illness of the gastrointestinal system that affects either the small or large intestine. The segmental distribution of intestinal ulcers is punctuated by normal-appearing mucosa in this condition. This pattern has been labelled as skip lesions. Granulomas are found in around half of all patients. CD is most common in women between the ages of 20 and 39 who live in cities [2, 17].

CD lesions are less susceptible to surgery than UC lesions because to the skip lesion distribution. Oral lesions affect anywhere from 0.5 percent to 20% of CD patients. The majority of CD oral symptoms occur in patients who have active intestinal disease, and their existence is often linked to disease activity. Oral symptoms appear 60 percent of the time before intestinal signs. The most prevalent oral sign of CD is recurrent aphthous ulcers [17].

Oral manifestations of CD can be characterised as specific or non-specific lesions based on the granulomatous alterations seen on histology. PV, cobblestone mucosal architecture, and minor salivary gland duct disease all show granulomatous alterations, which are a characteristic of CD. Inflammatory hyperplasia of the oral mucosa with a cobblestone pattern, indurated polypoid tag-like lesions in the vestibule and retromolar pad area, and chronic deep linear ulcers with hyperplastic edges are all symptoms of CD. Pallor, angular cheilitis, glossitis, candidiasis, perioral dermatitis, lichenoid responses, and an increased risk of dental caries are some clinical findings in CD [18, 19].

Liver Disease

In the body, the liver is the principal organ for protein synthesis, catabolic processes, and detoxification. The liver is involved in the immunological response as well as the excretion of heme pigments. Gluconeogenesis is controlled by the liver. Lipids are converted to cholesterol and triglycerides in the liver. The liver synthesises and stores proteins, albumin, and coagulation factors (factors I, II, V, VII, IX, and X).

Coagulopathy can result from hepatocyte dysfunction and vitamin K deficiency since various clotting factors (e.g., II, VII, IX, and X) are vitamin K dependent. The cytochrome P-450 microsomal enzyme system in the hepatocyte is primarily responsible for drug metabolism. The liver metabolises local anaesthetics, analgesics, sedatives, antibiotics, and antifungals. As a result, when a person has liver failure, it is critical to utilise these medicines with caution. Insulin, aldosterone, antidiuretic hormone, estrogens, and androgens are all inactivated or metabolised by the liver. Obviously, liver dysfunction can manifest itself in a variety of ways. The most common symptom of liver illness is jaundice, and the disease can progress to liver failure and death [2, 20, 21].

The etiologically of oral symptoms of liver disease is linked to primary liver functioning. Immunotherapy given after a liver transplant to prevent organ rejection can develop oral candidiasis, also known as angular cheilitis. Other significant oral symptoms of liver illness include atrophic glossitis, petechiae, lichen planus, and oral metastases of hepatocellular carcinoma, which primarily present as hemorrhagic growing masses in the premolar and mandibular ramus area [20, 21].

Hematologic Diseases

Lymphoma

B and T lymphocytes, as well as monocytes, are involved in Lymphomas, which are solid tumor malignancies. The lymph nodes are the most prevalent site for these tumors, with extra-nodal sites being less common. The cause is unknown; however immunodeficiency, viral infections, and chemical exposures have all been cited as risk factors [22, 23].

Hodgkin lymphoma (HL) is distinguished from non-Hodgkin lymphoma (NHL) by one categorization system (NHL). HL primarily affects teens and young adults, with a middle-aged peak in frequency. HL used to be a condition that was always fatal, but improved diagnostic and treatment methods have given a newly diagnosed patient a 90% chance of survival. NHL most commonly affects people in their forties and fifties. Men are more likely to develop HL and NHL [24, 25].

Lymphoma can present with a variety of symptoms, including painless lymphadenopathy, hepatosplenomegaly, and secondary infections. Fever, night sweats, weight loss, and pruritus (all B-cell lymphoma symptoms), as well as itching, indicate advanced disease and a bad prognosis. Histologic and immunohistochemical findings in sick tissues are used to make the diagnosis [22].

In NHL, especially Burkitt's lymphoma and AIDS-associated lymphoma, oral signs and symptoms are significantly more common. The lymphoid tissues of Waldeyer's ring, as well as the vestibule and gingivae, are preferentially affected by oral involvement in NHL. Soft masses that are painless and involve the palate and buccal mucosa, with or without acute ulceration, are also possible. Slow-growing,

painless, bluish soft masses have been characterised as palatal lesions, which have been mistaken for tiny salivary gland cancers. Loose teeth and facial paresthesia may be connected with intraosseous lesions. A major swelling of the salivary glands could also be a symptom of NHL [25–27].

Burkitt's lymphoma is a type of aggressive lymphoma that often has oral symptoms in children. The Epstein-Barr virus has been linked to the disease's development. Burkitt's lymphoma appears as a fast growing mass that destroys bone and soft tissue around the teeth, causing painful loosening. It affects the maxilla more than the mandible [22, 26].

Patients with cutaneous T-cell lymphoma have also been reported to have oral lesions (mycosis fungoides). These lesions are defined as ulcerated tumors or indurated plaques having a red or white surface. The tongue is the most common location of involvement, and it usually occurs after skin lesions [28].

Multiple Myeloma

Multiple myeloma (MM) is a malignant plasma cell dyscrasia in which immunoglobulin light chains are produced in excess. It's a plasma cell malignancy with a multicentric genesis in the bone that's quite uncommon. MM is more common in middle-aged and older people, with a male predisposition and a higher frequency among African-Americans [29, 30]. Bone pain induced by osteolytic lesions or pathologic fractures due to bone loss is the most prevalent presenting symptom in MM. There may also be anaemia and petechial haemorrhages. In individuals with MM, haemorrhage and infection are major problems. Thrombocytopenia, poor platelet function, and aberrant coagulation are all possible causes of bleeding [30, 31]. Hypercalcemia, proteinuria, renal failure, and thrombocytopenia are all possible symptoms. Multiple "punched-out" well-defined or ragged radiolucencies on radiography are highly diagnostic of advanced MM. These may be particularly noticeable on skull films. Renal failure may be the first symptom of immunoglobulin buildup in the kidneys caused by tumours. In 30–50% of patients, light chains (Bence Jones protein) can be identified in the urine [30, 32].

MM has been linked to a number of oral symptoms. Swelling, discomfort, paresthesias, and tooth loss can occur in up to 30% of individuals with mandibular involvement. If thrombocytopenia is caused by malignant plasma cells infiltrating the bone marrow, you may see gingival bleeding or oral petechiae. Extramedullary plasmacytomas are a rare side effect of MM. These lesions appear as dome-shaped lumps that have a tendency to ulcerate when discovered in the oral cavity, most typically on the gingivae or hard palate [22, 30].

Leukemia

Leukemia is a cancer that affects the bone marrow's white blood cells. This neoplastic process causes a significant increase in circulating immature or defective white blood cells, suppressing normal hematopoiesis and resulting in secondary anemias, thrombocytopenia, and a lack of normal functioning leukocytes [33].

The clinical course of leukemia (acute or chronic) or the progenitor cell lineage are used to classify it (lymphoid or myeloid). There are two types of acute leukemias: acute lymphocytic leukaemia (ALL) and acute myelogenous leukaemia (AML) (AML). ALL is more common in youngsters, whereas AML is more common in adults. Chronic myelocytic leukaemia (CML) and chronic lymphocytic leukaemia (CLL) are the two most common kinds of chronic leukaemia in adults [34, 35].

Lymphadenopathy, recurrent infection, and bone and stomach discomfort can all be symptoms of impaired leucocyte activity. Leukemia cutis is an infiltration of leukemic cells into the skin that manifests as stiff and rubbery papules, plaques, and nodules and can be a precursor to systemic leukaemia. Blisters and ulcers are less common. Dermal nodules having a green colour can be caused by myelogenous leukemias, chloromas, or granulocytic sarcomas [36, 37].

Acute (rather than chronic) and myeloid (rather than lymphoid) leukemias have more oral symptoms. Gingival hypertrophy, petechiae, ecchymosis, ulcers, and haemorrhage, primarily spontaneous gingival bleeding, are all common findings. Immunosuppression frequently leads to viral, fungal, and bacterial oral infections. Chemotherapeutic medicines' direct action on the oral mucosa can cause ulcers, which must be distinguished from herpes simplex virus (HSV) or cytomegalovirus (CMV). A rare presenting ailment is mental nerve neuropathy, sometimes known as "numb chin syndrome." AML and acute promyelocytic leukaemia are the most common causes of gingival hyperplasia. Edematous, erythematous, and friable gingiva are seen. Chemotherapy helps to improve gingival hyperplasia. Lichinoid or keratotic papules and plaques, desquamative gingivitis, atrophy, and ulcerations are all consequences of hematopoietic stem cell transplantation (HSCT) [33, 36–38].

Neutropenia

Neutropenia is a condition in which the number of circulating neutrophils in the blood drops below 1500/mm3.

Neutropenia can strike anyone at any age, with congenital neutropenia affecting children and acquired neutropenia affecting adults. Increased susceptibility to bacterial infections, which most usually affect the oral cavity, ear, and perirectal areas, is linked to neutropenia. Neutropenic ulcers are most commonly found on the gingiva. Premature exfoliation of deciduous teeth has been described, which has resulted in attachment loss and periodontal damage [22].

Iron-Deficiency Anemia

The most frequent cause of anaemia in the world is iron deficiency anaemia. The most vulnerable are women of reproductive age, as both menstruation and pregnancy increase the risk of iron deficiency. Athletes, obese patients who have undergone bariatric surgery and young children are among the other groups at risk [39].

Mucosal pallor, particularly pallor of the gingivae and vermilion border of the lips, angular cheilitis, and atrophic glossitis due to loss of filiform and fungiform papillae of the tongue, leading the tongue to look smooth and red, are all oral manifestations of iron deficiency anaemia. Pain, a burning feeling, or dysphagia may precede atrophic glossitis. Oral candidiasis is made more likely by iron deficient anaemia [30, 40, 41].

Pernicious Anemia

Pernicious anemia (PA) is a multi-system illness that affects the blood, immune system, and gastrointestinal tract. Alterations in the IF-mediated vitamin B12 absorption due to loss of parietal cells, small intestine disorders, genetic mutations, and gastric surgery account for many cases of PA [42, 43]. The presence of a painful or burning, atrophic or "bald" tongue is a characteristic oral finding in PA. Atrophy of the oral mucosa occurs when both the filiform and fungiform papillae are lost, resulting in erythema and glossitis. In addition to changes in taste sense, angular cheilitis can occur (dysgeusia) [44, 45].

Sickle Cell Anemia (SCA)

Sickle cell anemia is a kind of hemolytic anaemia that is caused by a point mutation in the b-globin gene, which causes an aberrant haemoglobin S chain. The haemoglobin S chain is prone to aggregation and polymerization, which results in red blood cell distortion and final lysis. This type of hemolytic anaemia can manifest itself in a variety of ways. Major clinical signs of sickle cell crises include pain, ischemia, and infarction, which most typically affect the long bones, lungs, liver, brain, and spleen. Another symptom that requires immediate attention is increased susceptibility to infection and cerebrovascular accident. SCA oral symptoms include non-specific intraoral alterations such as diminished trabecular bone pattern in the mandible, hair-on-end appearance on skull radiographs, and higher frequency of osteomyelitis [22].

Thalassemia

Thalassemias are inherited disorders that result in inadequate erythropoiesis and consequent hemolysis due to genetic abnormalities in haemoglobin synthesis. Males and females are both affected, with the majority of those infected hailing from Africa, the Mediterranean, and Southeast Asia. The bones of the face and skull may show "hair on end" striations due to vertical trabeculation subsequent to hematopoiesis growth, in addition to the mucosa's pallor and yellowing due to jaundice. The outer plate is thinned, while the diploic space is expanded. The involvement of the facial bones, which results in frontal growth of the head, extension of the maxillary bones, and dental malalignment, is far less prevalent (hemolytic facies) [46, 47].

Langerhans Cell Histiocytosis

Langerhans cell histiocytosis (LCH), formerly known as histiocytosis X, is a rare disorder characterised by damaging tissue infiltration by aberrant histiocytes mixed with lymphocytes and eosinophils of uncertain aetiology and pathophysiology. Depending on the location and level of organ involvement, LCH has a wide range of clinical symptoms. The widespread type, previously known as Letterer-Siwe disease, and the confined variant, Hand-Schüller-Christian disease, are the two most prevalent forms of LCH, while the third form, eosinophilic granuloma, is the most common. LCH is a rare condition that primarily affects infants and children, with adults being affected only rarely [48–50].

LCH typically affects bone, with 10–20 percent of patients experiencing symptoms similar to an odontogenic infection or periodontal disease in the maxilla or mandible. Irregular ulcerations of the hard palate, which may be the disease's initial presentation, are one of the oral signs. Edema and ulceration of the overlaying mucosa can occur as a result of osteolytic lesions. Gingival inflammation, necrosis, recession, increased tooth mobility, and early tooth loss can all be caused by lesions in the alveolar bone. The teeth show a characteristic floating look inside the radiographic lucency caused by osteolytic degradation [51–53].

Thrombocytopenia

Thrombocytopenia is a low platelet count caused by a reduction in platelet generation, survival, or splenic sequestration. Petechial haemorrhages, spontaneous gingival haemorrhage, and minor trauma bleeding are examples of oral symptoms that can be the first indicator of disease [22, 30].

Hereditary Hemorrhagic Telangiectasia (Osler-Weber-Rendu Disease)

Hereditary hemorrhagic telangiectasia (HHT) is a genetic disorder that causes blood vessel structural abnormalities. HHT has been divided into two subtypes. HHT type 1 is characterised by arteriovenous malformations (AVMs) in the lungs and brain, whereas HHT type 2 is characterised by hepatic involvement. HHT is characterised by telangiectasias, which are tiny "1-mm to 2-mm" vascular lesions that blanch with pressure and affect the skin and mucous membranes. The vermilion, tongue, and buccal mucosa are frequently affected. Other clinical indications of this systemic illness include epistaxis and arteriovenous malformations (AVMs) of the lung, brain, or liver [22, 30].

Hemophilia

Hemophilia is a bleeding disorder caused by a quantitative deficiency in a certain clotting factor. Hemophilia A is caused by a factor VIII deficiency, while haemophilia B is caused by a factor IX deficiency. Prolonged bleeding due to a clotting delay is the clinical characteristic. Uncontrolled or delayed bleeding after surgical treatments, extractions, and periodontal procedures, easy bruising and spontaneous haemorrhage in places prone to stress, and bleeding into joints (hemarthrosis), resulting in deformity impairment are some of the symptoms [22, 30].

Endocrine Diseases

The endocrine system is made up of glands that produce and release hormones directly into the bloodstream. Metabolism, tissue growth, homeostasis, sexual development, reproduction, immunological control, cognitive function, and emotional stabilisation are just a few of the processes that these hormones regulate. The neurological system and the delicate bio-feedback mechanism that maintains well-balanced hormones throughout the body have a strong grip on the endocrine glands. Any change in this balance can disrupt physiological function and cause sickness, which can have a severe influence on an individual's health and well-being [33, 54].

Pituitary Gland Disorders

The pituitary gland is known as the "master gland" since it is involved in the functions of multiple organs. It is located in the sella turcica, a bony compartment of the sphenoid bone, and is stimulated by the hypothalamus directly. The intermediate and posterior lobes of the pituitary have limited storage and secretion functions for melanocyte-stimulating hormone and antidiuretic hormone, respectively. The anterior pituitary lobe, on the other hand, is in charge of producing and secreting hormones like growth hormone (GH), puberty hormones (gonadotropins), thyroid-stimulating hormone, Prolactin, and adrenocorticotrophic hormone (ACTH) [33, 54].

Hypopituitarism

Pituitary hormone insufficiency can be caused by a variety of circumstances. In terms of this gland's multifunctional activity, hypopituitarism can impair people's growth, puberty, thyroid, and adrenal functioning. GH and gonadotropins are the pituitary hormones with the highest sensitivity to shortage, with the former being connected to head and neck signs. Pituitary dwarfism is the result of GH insufficiency in childhood. The illness is characterised by a slow rate of growth, short stature, and a wide range of clinical symptoms. Adult GH shortage, on the other hand, has been linked to reduced effect and non-specific clinical characteristics [33, 54].

Hypopituitarism causes a hypognathic maxilla and mandible in childhood, resulting in reduced facial features. Dental crowding and malocclusion are also caused by the smaller jaws and normal-sized teeth. Furthermore, the deciduous dentition's exfoliation pattern is delayed, resulting in a delay in the eruption of permanent teeth. Clinical signs in adulthood include fixed expression, thin lips, sparse brows, and eyelash loss, with no specific oral manifestations recorded [33, 54].

Hyperpituitarism

The most common form of hyperpituitarism is excessive GH production. If the illness arises in adulthood (about the age of 40), it is known as acromegaly, whereas gigantism is a childhood disorder equivalent. Generalized enlargement of bodily parts while maintaining symmetry and proportionality is referred to as gigantism. Acromegaly, on the other hand, is marked by deformity of the face and extremities that develops over time [33, 54].

Frontal bossing, mandibular prognathism, interdental spacing, and root hypercementosis are some of the maxillofacial signs of gigantism. Glabellar protrusion and face height increase, mandibular prognathism, Interdental spac-

ing, open bite, enlarged pulp chambers (taurodontism), roots hypercementosis, facial skin and lips thickening, macroglossia, and mucosal hypertrophy of the oropharyngeal tissues are some of the maxillofacial manifestations of acromegaly [33, 54].

Hypothyroidism

Hypothyroidism is characterised by a lack of thyroid hormones, which can be inherited or acquired. If the illness appears in early childhood, it is referred to as cretinism, whereas severe hypothyroidism acquired in maturity is referred to as myxedema [24–27].

Severe congenital hypothyroidism can progress to cretinism, which is characterised by physical and mental impairment. Bradycardia, dyspnea, and decreased activity are all symptoms of the disease. A huge head, short neck, broad nose, lack of facial expressions, hypertelorism, and thick, dry, and wrinkled skin are all characteristics of the head and neck region.

Adult-onset hypothyroidism is related with decreased metabolic activity, which appear as obesity, a slower respiratory rate, bradycardia, and widespread edoema (myxedema). The majority of oral and maxillofacial signs of myxedema include face swelling, thickened dry skin, brittle scalp, sparse eyebrows, hoarseness, delayed tooth eruption, enamel hypoplasia, micrognathia, open bite, macroglossia, glossitis, and dysgeusia [33, 54].

Hyperthyroidism

Thyroid hormone production is excessive in Hyperthyroidism (thyrotoxicosis). Graves disease, toxic thyroid adenoma, toxic multinodular or diffuse goitre, ectopic thyroid tissue (e.g., lingual thyroid), and subacute thyroiditis are the most prevalent etiologic reasons for thyroid problems in women [23, 27].

Weight loss despite an increased appetite, warm-sweaty skin, brittle hair and nails, tachycardia, irritability, and heat sensitivity are all indications of hyperthyroidism. Oral and head and neck signs of this illness include exophthalmos, enlarged thyroid, extra-glandular thyroid tissue, maxillomandibular osteoporosis, burning mouth syndrome, periodontitis, and increased susceptibility to dental caries [33, 54].

Hyperparathyroidism

PTH hypersecretion is classified as Hyperparathyroidism. The most frequent hyperparathyroidism symptoms include bone loss, kidney stones, stomach pain, proximal myopathy, and depression. Enamel and dentin hypoplasia, hypocalcification shortened roots, widening of pulp chambers, pulpal calcifications, hypodontia, dental growth delay, maxillomandibular tori, orofacial paresthesia, facial muscles aching, and susceptibility to oral candidiasis are all symptoms of hyperparathyroidism in the head and neck [33, 54].

Hypoparathyroidism

Hypoparathyroidism is the lack or deficiency of PTH, resulting in hypocalcemia and hypophosphatemia. Tetany, paresthesia, and seizures are all symptoms of hypocalcemia. 33 Ectodermal tissues in the head and neck region might be damaged, and baldness and skin scaling are common symptoms. 33 Loss of jawbone density, brittle teeth, expanded pulp chambers, loss of lamina dura, malocclusions, Brown tumour of hyperparathyroidism, and soft-tissue calcifications are further head and neck signs [33, 54].

Hypoadrenocorticism (Addison's Disease)

Primary adrenocortical insufficiency, often known as Addison's disease, is characterised by a lack of glucocorticoid and mineralocorticoid hormones. Muscle weakness, hypoglycemia, hypotension, anorexia, nausea, weight loss, and anxiety are all symptoms of corticosteroid shortage. The elbows, creases of the palms, and areolas of the breasts are all prone to hyperpigmentation. This hyperpigmentation is caused by an increase in ACTH levels, which stimulates the synthesis of melanocyte-stimulating hormone. Black-bluish plaques are particularly common in the perioral and intraoral tissues [35].

Hyperadrenocorticism (Cushing Syndrome)

Cushing syndrome is a state of hyperadrenocorticism caused by an excess of endogenous glucocorticoids produced by the adrenal cortex or by long-term use of exogenous corticosteroids (iatrogenic Cushing syndrome) [37]. Obesity, humpback, hypertension, hyperglycemia, osteoporosis, thinner skin, muscle atrophy, immunosuppression, emotional disturbance, and cognitive failure are all symptoms of Cushing syndrome [38, 39]. Moon face, acne breakouts, and hirsutism are symptoms of the condition in the head and neck region. In addition, people with hyperadrenocorticism are more prone to mouth infections and bone fractures [33, 54].

Diabetes Mellitus

According to the American Diabetes Association, diabetes is categorised as follows:
- Type I DM is commonly found in the pediatric population. The etiology is autoimmune, in which insulin-producing beta islets are majorly destroyed.
- Type II DM is highlighted by cellular resistance to insulin. The etiology is unknown but has been strongly linked to genetic predisposition. The risk of the disease increases with age.
- Gestational DM is the onset of hyperglycemia during pregnancy that normalizes after delivery.
- Others are relatively uncommon and include genetic, infectious, traumatic, or iatrogenic factors affecting beta islets.

The hallmark symptoms of DM include polyuria, polydipsia, polyphagia, and weight loss. Vasculopathy, retinopathy, nephropathy, and neuropathy may become substantial and negatively impact the patient's quality of life if the condition is left untreated or inadequately controlled. Gingivitis and periodontitis are the most common oral problems in diabetic people. Salivary gland dysfunction, sialadenosis, fungal infections, oral burning sensation and taste dysfunction, dental caries, oral ulceration, and irritant fibroma are further orofacial consequences of diabetes [33, 54].

Pregnancy

Increased oestrogen, progesterone, and human chorionic gonadotropin cause many physical and physiologic changes during pregnancy, which have a substantial impact on several body organs, including the mouth cavity. During various phases of pregnancy, certain oral symptoms can be noticed [33, 54]:
- Pregnancy gingivitis due to increased estrogen and progesterone levels, as well as a change in the host-immune response.
- Periodontitis and tooth mobility as a result of a continuous hormone-mediated inflammatory response and gingivitis progression.
- Gingival hyperplasia and pyogenic granuloma (pregnancy tumor) develop near the end of the first trimester, with most instances resolving on their own following birth.
- Dental erosion, especially during the first trimester, due to frequent vomiting.
- Gastroesophageal reflux becomes more common in the third trimester as the fetus grows larger and the stomach sphincter weakens owing to elevated estrogen levels.

- Chloasma, also known as pregnancy mask, is a condition in which estrogen and progesterone stimulate melanocytes in the face, trunk, and extremities.
- Salivary flow disturbance and changes in oral pH.
- Increased susceptibility to dental caries.

Immunological Diseases

Pemphigus Vulgaris

Pemphigus is an autoimmune blistering illness that is rare and possibly fatal. The disease is most common among Jews, especially those of Ashkenazi descent, in Eastern countries like Malaysia, China, and Japan, with a minor female predisposition. PV nearly always starts with numerous mucosal site involvement in the clinic. Oral involvement can occur up to a year before cutaneous involvement. Lesions start out as flaccid vesicles or bullae that swiftly rupture, producing painful shallow ulcerations that heal without scarring [55].

Mucous Membrane Pemphigoid

Pemphigoid illness is a blistering condition that affects the subepithelia or sub-epidermis of the skin or mucosa. Mucous membrane pemphigoid is a condition that mostly affects the mucous membranes of the mouth. Other mucosal surfaces, such as the conjunctiva of the eyes, nasopharynx, anogenital, larynx, and oesophagus, are less usually affected. Vesicles or bullae, in contrast to PV, may be more visible in the oral cavity. Scarring is a common occurrence when an ulcer heals. Adhesions (symblepharons), eyelid inversions (entropion), and corneal abrasion from eyelashes can all be caused by scarring of the conjunctiva (trichiasis). In severe cases, laryngeal involvement could result in voice changes and breathing restrictions [1, 56].

Systemic Lupus Erythematosus

Systemic lupus erythematosus (SLE) is a multiorgan autoimmune disease that is complicated and systemic. Oral ulceration, erythematous erosions, and lichenoid lesions were the most prevalent lesions identified. The buccal mucosa and lip are the most typical sites for lesions.

Sjögren Syndrome

Sjogren syndrome is a chronic inflammatory immune-mediated disease that is becoming more common. The moisture-producing glands, most often the lacrimal and salivary glands, are destroyed and dysfunctional in Sjogren syndrome, resulting in dry eyes and xerostomia. Patients' ability to eat certain foods or lack of desire to eat, difficulty chewing and swallowing certain foods, burning mouth complaints, mucosal irritation and associated mouth pain, and dietary changes related to sensitivity to spicy, hot, or acidic foods may all be affected by a lack of saliva or thickened saliva. Swallowing and speech issues, as well as a difficulty to create an appropriate seal under full dentures, may arise depending on the level of salivary gland damage. Caries, salivary gland infections, and candidiasis are all frequent oral infections [57, 58].

Rheumatoid Arthritis

Rheumatoid arthritis (RA) is a common systemic autoimmune disease that primarily affects the joints, but can also present as rheumatoid nodules, lung involvement, or vasculitis. Tempromandibular joint (TMJ) erosions with concomitant temporomandibular myofacial discomfort may be present in this syndrome, despite the absence of particular mouth lesions. Patients with advanced joint degeneration may develop malocclusion. Patients with RA nearly usually have adequate mouth opening, which allows them to keep their joints mobile. However, when the malocclusion worsens, patients may acquire a clinically visible anterior open bite [57, 58].

Sarcoidosis

Sarcoidosis is a systemic disease characterized by noncaseating granulomatous inflammation in multiple organ systems, especially the lungs, heart, brain, eyes, and skin. Salivary gland involvement is the most prevalent symptom in the head and neck, however intraoral soft tissue lesions are also seen sometimes. Symptoms include exhaustion and sadness, "asthma symptoms" (wheezing, chronic cough), arthritis, and muscle discomfort or weakness, among others. Patients with lymphadenopathy, erythema nodosum, and localised skin or ocular lesions may appear clinically. Single or many nodules or ulcerations of the tongue, lips, palate, or gingiva; asymptomatic enlargement of the affected mucosa; or teeth mobility due to fast alveolar bone loss are all symptoms of oral sarcoidosis. Involvement of the face nerve (cranial nerve VII) manifests clinically as facial nerve palsy [55, 58].

Recurrent Aphthous Stomatitis

Recurrent aphthous stomatitis (RAS) is a painful, self-limited, recurrent oral ulcer with unclear aetiology.

Various triggers have been described, including stress, hormonal impacts, dietary allergies, trauma, and quitting smoking. The use of systemic medicines, such as nonsteroidal anti-inflammatory drugs, beta-blockers, and nicorandil, can also activate RAS. RAS manifests itself in three clinical forms: minor, major, and herpetiform, all of which affect nonkeratinized mucosa. Aphthous ulcers are painful and have a whitish-grey pseudomembrane with an erythematous halo in all forms [55, 58].

Behçet Disease

Behçet disease (BD) is an uncommon systemic vasculitis with recurring oral, ocular, and vaginal involvement that is more common in nations along the "silk route," such as Turkey, Japan, and the eastern Mediterranean countries. Oral ulcers are the disease's first symptom, and practically every patient will experience them at some point during their illness. The disease's initial signs are recurrent, aphthous-like ulcerations (small, severe, or herpetiform), which are the main criteria for diagnosis. Common cutaneous signs include erythema nodosum, pseudofolliculitis, and acneiform nodules on the back, face, and neck, particularly around the hairline [58].

Erythema Multiforme

Erythema multiforme (EM) is a self-limiting disorder that affects the skin and mucous membranes and causes erythema, erosions, vesicles, and ulcers. Acute onset with flu-like symptoms such as low-grade fever, malaise, headache, and sore throat that occur over a few days. Asymmetric targetoid lesions of the hands and feet are common skin lesions. The presence of hemorrhagic crusting on the lips is a prominent symptom [59].

Oral Lichen Planus

Oral lichen planus (OLP) is a common mucosal inflammatory disorder that causes discomfort and burning in the mouth as a result of erosions and shallow ulcerations, which is aggravated by spicy or acidic foods. The most prevalent type of OLP is reticular OLP, which is asymptomatic most of the time. The buccal mucosa, buccal vestibule, tongue, and gingiva are the most common sites of involvement in lesions. Purplish, pruritic, polygonal papules, most usually on the arms and legs, are the four Ps that characterize skin lesions. Desquamative gingivitis is a sign of gingival involvement [22, 55] .

Oral Lichenoid Lesions

Oral mucosa lesions can have a similar clinical appearance to lichen planus, such as white reticular patches, plaques, papules, erosions, or ulcerations, but they are caused by a different source or underlying disease. These are known as oral lichenoid lesions, and they're treated by either removing the cause or treating the underlying condition. Contact reaction to dental materials, mucosal reactivity to systemic drugs, chronic graft versus host disease (GVHD), and discoid or systemic lupus erythematosus oral lesions are the four types of oral lichenoid lesions [22, 56, 58].

Viral, Bacterial, and Fungal Infections

Primary Oral Herpes

Primary herpetic gingivostomatitis (PHGS) develops when a nonimmune individual is exposed to HSV-1 for the first time. The majority of cases involve youngsters aged one to five years old and are generally asymptomatic. Patients with lymphadenopathy, fever, sore throat, and vesiculo-ulcerative lesions in the oral and perioral regions are symptomatic. The oral mucosa, both movable and non-movable, might be impacted, and an acute start of global gingival inflammation and pain is a common symptom [60].

Secondary Oral Herpes

In the trigeminal ganglion, HSV 1 induces life-long latency. Stress, exhaustion, fever, menstruation, immunosuppression, and exposure to heat, cold, or sunshine are all potential triggers for viral reactivation. The mucocutaneous junction of the lips or keratinized intraoral tissues may be affected by recrudescence. There are no systemic signs with recrudescence, unlike PHGS. However, a local prodrome of tingling, burning, or itching often precedes the beginning of HSL. Recrudescent intraoral herpes (RIH) is less prevalent than herpes simplex labialis (HSL), and it affects keratinized tissues including the gingiva and palate in immunocompetent hosts [60, 61].

Varicella Zoster (Chickenpox)

Varicella-zoster virus (VZV) is a human herpesvirus that can cause both primary and secondary infections. A nonimmunized person who is exposed to VZV for the first time develops chickenpox, an acute disease. The onset of a widespread, pruritic skin rash that spreads centripetally may be preceded by a prodrome. Fever and malaise are also possible symptoms. Macular lesions evolve through papular, vesicular, pustular, and crusty stages. Despite the fact that the mouth and oropharynx are impacted, intraoral lesions are rarely symptomatic [60, 61].

Herpes Zoster (Shingles)

Reactivation of VZV dormant in a sensory nerve ganglion can cause herpes zoster (HZ) or shingles. A prodrome of mild fever, malaise, and pain, burning, itching, or paresthesia in the afflicted area characterises herpes zoster. Regional lymphadenopathy and a unilateral vesicular rash in the dermatome of a sensory nerve follow this disease. Bilateral or multiple dermatome involvement is unusual and should raise suspicions of immunosuppression. HZ instances may affect the trigeminal nerve's mucocutaneous distribution, with a preference for the ophthalmic division. The latter can cause serious eye consequences such corneal ulcers and blindness, requiring immediate medical intervention. Ipsilateral vesicular eruptions in the midface and mucous membranes of the nose, nasopharynx, palate, and tonsils occur when the maxillary division of CN5 is involved. Ipsilateral lesions of the side of the head, ear, lower lip, and matching oral mucosa result from HZ impacting the mandibular nerve. Only the oral mucosa and the spare cutaneous dermatome may be affected by lesions. Exfoliation of teeth, root resorption, and osteonecrosis are all possible oral consequences of HZ [60, 61].

A serious HZ consequence is postherpetic neuralgia (PHN), which is characterised by persistent, refractory pain following the clearance of lesions. It is particularly common in the trigeminal nerve's ophthalmic division. Ramsey Hunt syndrome is caused by the reactivation of latent VZV in the geniculate ganglion, which is characterised by cranial nerve seven and occasionally cranial nerve eight dysfunctions. A vesicular rash affecting the ear and pharynx, as well as ipsilateral facial paralysis, earache, taste abnormalities, vertigo, tinnitus, and hearing loss, may be experienced by those who are affected [60, 61].

Coxsackievirus Infections

Coxsackieviruses are divided into two groups, group A and group B, each with multiple serotypes. Group A coxsackieviruses have a predilection for mucocutaneous tissues and cause herpangina or hand-foot-mouth disease (HFMD). In contrast, group B coxsackieviruses often infect visceral organs. Most coxsackievirus infections are subclinical or manifest with a non-specific rash or febrile illnesses. Complications are more likely in neonates and immunocompromised [62, 63].

Fever, malaise, and symptomatic oral lesions are the most common symptoms of herpangina in young children. Before widespread erythema and punctate erosions emerge in the posterior oral cavity, developing in to clusters and advance through macular, popular, and vesicular stages. Sore throat, odynophagia, dysphagia, and throat exudates are all symptoms of lesions that affect the soft palate, uvula, posterior pharyngeal wall, and tonsils. There may also be headaches, vomiting, and abdominal pain [62, 63].

HFMD is a highly transmissible disease that mostly affects youngsters. Patients develop a low-grade fever and vesicular lesions, which eventually condense into symptomatic oral erosions. The tongue, palate, and buccal mucosa are common sites [62–64].

Human Papillomavirus

Human papillomavirus (HPV) is spread throughout the world and is most commonly transmitted through intimate vaginal, anal, or oral contact. HPV infection is more likely in people who have had multiple sexual encounters and are immunocompromised. Mucocutaneous warts, respiratory papillomatosis, mucocutaneous epithelial dysplasia, and different epithelial malignancies are all symptoms of HPV. Respiratory papillomatosis and oral warts are two oral symptoms of HPV infection. The presence of high-risk HPV 16 in the posterior oral cavity raises the risk of oropharyngeal malignancies, which affect the base of the tongue, the posterior throat, and the tonsillar tissues. Consistent sore throat or hoarseness, a neck lump, bloody sputum on coughing, and lingual paresthesia or ear pain are all signs and symptoms of HPV positive oropharyngeal malignancies [62–64].

Tuberculosis

Tuberculosis (TB) is a systemic bacterial infection that seldom involves the oral cavity. Globally, TB is the second most common death-causing infectious disease after human immunodeficiency virus (HIV). TB is known to affect men more than women, mostly adults. Lungs are typically the primary infection site, but other sites may be affected, including skin, central nervous system, lymphatic system, kidneys, and gastrointestinal tract [65].

The majority of TB oral symptoms are caused by the original pulmonary infection. Primary oral TB, on the other hand, can be caused by direct injection of organisms into the mouth mucosa, with younger individuals being the most afflicted [3, 5]. The most typically afflicted areas are the tongue, buccal mucosa, lip, palate, and gingiva. Single chronic ulcerations with uneven edges are the most common lesions. Multiple ulcers, swelling, nodular masses, and mandibular osteomyelitis, on the other hand, have been recorded [65, 66].

Bacterial Salivary Gland Infection

Sialadenitis is an inflammation of salivary glands caused by a variety of causes, including infectious pathogens (bacterial and viral). Hyposalivation may help bacteria cause sialadenitis. When massaging the infected gland, a quick onset of sensitive swelling of the auricular area with intermittent pus discharge is a clinical sign of acute bacterial infection. Recurrent episodes of severe enlargement of the salivary glands and chronic purulent discharge characterise the chronic bacterial infection. Both the parotid and submandibular glands are susceptible to infection [1, 65].

Syphilis

Syphilis is a sexually transmitted infectious disease that, if left untreated, can lead to serious problems. Syphilis is classified as acquired or congenital depending on the mode of transmission. Primary Syphilis oral symptoms include a solitary ulcer on the upper lip in males and lower lip in females, a deep ulcerative region with a red or brown base and irregular elevated borders, and a solitary ulcer on the upper lip in males and lower lip in females. Macular syphilides, papular syphilides, mucous patches, snail track ulcers, Lues maligna (ulceronodular illness), Gumma, hard plate perforation, oronasal communication, and interstitial glossitis are secondary and tertiary Syphilis oral symptoms [65].

Actinomycosis

Actinomycosis is a chronic infectious disease caused by a group of bacteria belonging to Actinomyces species. At the initial infection site, an acute local infection may develop (injured mucosa). If the pathogen is not treated, it steadily invades the underlying tissue and causes a chronic granulomatous infection. Single or several masses with peripheral fibrotic boundaries (wooden region) and central necrotic tissues intermixed with bacterial colonies that may exude yellowish material known as sulphur granules are seen in the clinic. Actinomycosis usually manifests itself clinically as a painless indurated swelling or, in more advanced cases, a mass that drains through the skin. The most commonly impacted area is the mandibular angle (lumpy jaw). Also affected are the salivary glands, cheeks, and jawbone. With a history of recurrent sinus tract, periapical actinomycosis is linked to non-resolving periapical lesions [65].

Cat-Scratch Disease

Cat-scratch disease is a bacterial infection that occurs following a scratch or a bite by infected cats. Some recent reports have shown that the disease may also be transmitted to humans via other infected mammals hosts such as dogs. Three to ten days after being scratched by an infected cat, a red papule develops at the wound site, and a few days later, it becomes vesiculated and crusted. Regional lymphadenopathy, proximal to the infected site, occurs 1–2 weeks after the papule eruption. Axillary lymph nodes are frequently affected. Patients mostly complain of fever, malaise, and nausea, and a few may develop severe complications involving the nervous system, heart, lung, liver, and bone. Submandibular lymph nodes are the most commonly affected, followed by preauricular and submental lymph nodes. Cervical lymph nodes and parotid tail lymphadenopathy have been reported. Overlying skin shows erythematous discoloration in most cases with tenderness on palpation [65].

Other Bacterial Infections

Erysipelas is a superficial skin infection that is common in infants, young children, and older adults. Lower extremities are the most commonly affected sites, followed by the face. Skin lesions are well-demarcated, erythematous, swollen, raised with red margins; facial erysipelas affect mostly the butterfly area (cheeks and nose bridge); and advanced lesions can cause swelling of the eyes. Fever, chills, and toxicity are reported [65].

Impetigo is also a superficial skin infection in which the face and lower extremities are commonly affected. This infection starts as skin papules that enlarge, gradually forming vesicles and finally forming a thick crust. Regional lymphadenitis may occur [65].

Scarlet fever manifestation is a diffuse skin red-bluish rash that appears on the second day of clinical illness. Sandpaper skin texture caused by blocked sweat glands, petechiae, and skin desquamation may occur later. Oral manifestations of scarlet fever are exudative pharyngitis and tonsillitis, petechiae on the palate, tongue coverage with the white coating with red papillae (white strawberry tongue), which later, the tongue becomes red (red strawberry tongue) [65, 67].

Oral Candidiasis

Oral candidiasis is the most common opportunistic infection of the oral mucosa (primary candidiasis). Pseudomembranous candidiasis is a creamy white plaque (cottage cheese appearance) consisting of debris, desquamative epithelium, and fungal organisms and can be wiped off, leaving an inflamed area. This type of candidiasis can also be acute (with antibiotics and immunosuppressive therapy) or chronic (with impaired immunity). Erythematous candidiasis is a diffuse erythematous macule (no wipeable white plaque) that might be accompanied by a burning sensation. Median rhomboid glossitis, palatal erythema (kissing lesions), angular cheilitis, and denture stomatitis are different types of this infection. Chronic hyperplastic candidiasis (candida leukoplakia) is an uncommon form of candida infection characterized by a white patch that cannot be wiped off. Mucocutaneous candidiasis is an immunologic disorder associated with candida infections of nails, skin, and mucosal surfaces that affect young children. Oral lesions present as non-removable white patches (hyperplastic candidiasis) [68–71].

Other Fungal Infections

Histoplasmosis oral manifestation is most commonly detected in HIV-infected patients, which begins as erythematous macule and then forms a painful ulcerative lesion indistinguishable from malignancy [65].

Mucormycosis is an opportunistic infection found in the nose, throat, and mouth of a healthy individual. Rhinocerebral mucormycosis may be associated with nasal obstruction, epistaxis, facial pain, and visual disturbance. Also, maxillary sinus involvement can present as intraoral swelling of the maxillary ridge or palate. If left untreated, palatal destruction and necrosis may occur [65].

Aspergillosis is the most prevalent opportunistic infection after candida. The oral manifestation of this infection is allergic fungal sinusitis or aspergilloma. In immunosuppressed patients, the pathogen may spread and invade the oral mucosa forming a yellow-black necrotic area commonly in the palate and tongue [72, 73].

Conclusion

Oral cavity exhibits manifestations of systematic disease and serves as an indicator in oral health. As reviewed in this chapter, numerous systematic conditions, including gastrointestinal, hematologic, endocrine, immunological, and infections, cause pathologic manifestation in the oral cavity. Clinicians and dental practitioners play a crucial role in preventive medicine to identify and enhance their treatments' prognosis considering these conditions regarding related oral manifestations.

References

1. Chi AC, Neville BW, Krayer JW, Gonsalves WC. Oral manifestations of systemic disease. Am Fam Physician. 2010;82(11):1381–8.
2. Mejia LM. Oral manifestations of gastrointestinal disorders. Atlas Oral Maxillofac Surg Clin North Am. 2017;25(2):93–104.
3. Vakil N, Van Zanten SV, Kahrilas P, Dent J, Jones R. The Montreal definition and classification of gastroesophageal reflux disease: a global evidence-based consensus. Am J Gastroenterol. 2006;101(8):1900–20.
4. Roesch-Ramos L, Roesch-Dietlen F, Remes-Troche JM, Romero-Sierra G, Mata-Tovar Cde J, Azamar-Jácome AA, et al. Dental erosion, an extraesophageal manifestation of gastroesophageal reflux disease. The experience of a center for digestive physiology in Southeastern Mexico. Rev Esp Enferm Dig. 2014;106(2):92–7.
5. El-Serag HB, Petersen NJ, Carter J, Graham DY, Richardson P, Genta RM, et al. Gastroesophageal reflux among different racial groups in the United States. Gastroenterology. 2004;126(7):1692–9.
6. Herbella FA, Sweet MP, Tedesco P, Nipomnick I, Patti MG. Gastroesophageal reflux disease and obesity. Pathophysiology and implications for treatment. J Gastrointest Surg. 2007;11(3):286–90.
7. Di Fede O, Di Liberto C, Occhipinti G, Vigneri S, Lo Russo L, Fedele S, et al. Oral manifestations in patients with gastro-oesophageal reflux disease: a single-center case–control study. J Oral Pathol Med. 2008;37(6):336–40.
8. Malfertheiner P, Hallerbäck B. Clinical manifestations and complications of gastroesophageal reflux disease (GERD). Int J Clin Pract. 2005;59(3):346–55.
9. Ranjitkar S, Smales RJ, Kaidonis JA. Oral manifestations of gastroesophageal reflux disease. J Gastroenterol Hepatol. 2012;27(1):21–7.
10. Farrokhi F, Vaezi M. Extra-esophageal manifestations of gastroesophageal reflux. Oral Dis. 2007;13(4):349–59.
11. Preetha A, Sujatha D, Patil BA, Hegde S. Oral manifestations in gastroesophageal reflux disease. Gen Dent. 2015;63(3):e27–31.
12. Baumgart DC. The diagnosis and treatment of Crohn's disease and ulcerative colitis. Dtsch Arztebl Int. 2009;106(8):123.
13. Baumgart DC, Sandborn WJ. Crohn's disease. Lancet. 2012;380(9853):1590–605.
14. Tan C, Brand H, de Boer N, Forouzanfar T. Gastrointestinal diseases and their oro-dental manifestations: part 1: Crohn's disease. Br Dent J. 2016;221(12):794–9.
15. Femiano F, Lanza A, Buonaiuto C, Perillo L, Dell'Ermo A, Cirillo N. Pyostomatitis vegetans: a review of the literature. Med Oral Patol Oral Cir Bucal. 2009;14(3):E114–7.
16. Nico MM, Hussein TP, Aoki V, Lourenco SV. Pyostomatitis vegetans and its relation to inflammatory bowel disease, pyoderma gangrenosum, pyodermatitis vegetans, and pemphigus. J Oral Pathol Med. 2012;41(8):584–8.
17. Antunes H, Patraquim C, Baptista V, Silva-Monteiro L. Oral manifestations of Crohn's disease. BMJ Case Rep. 2015;2015:bcr2015212300.
18. Lankarani KB, Sivandzadeh GR, Hassanpour S. Oral manifestation in inflammatory bowel disease: a review. World J Gastroenterol: WJG. 2013;19(46):8571.
19. Vasovic M, Gajovic N, Brajkovic D, Jovanovic M, Zdravkovaic N, Kanjevac T. The relationship between the immune system and oral manifestations of inflammatory bowel disease: a review. Cent Eur J Immunol. 2016;41(3):302.
20. Guggenheimer J, Close J, Eghtesad B, Shay C. Characteristics of oral abnormalities in liver transplant candidates. Int J Organ Transplant Med. 2010;1(3):107.
21. Hong C, Scobey M, Napenas J, Brennan M, Lockhart P. Dental postoperative bleeding complications in patients with suspected and documented liver disease. Oral Dis. 2012;18(7):661–6.
22. McCord C, Johnson L. Oral manifestations of hematologic. Oral Manifestations of Systemic Diseases, An Issue of Atlas of the Oral & Maxillofacial Surgery Clinics, E-Book. 2017;25(2):149.
23. Word ZH, Matasar MJ. Advances in the diagnosis and management of lymphoma. Blood and Lymphatic Cancer. 2012;2:29.
24. Campo E, Swerdlow SH, Harris NL, Pileri S, Stein H, Jaffe ES. The 2008 WHO classification of lymphoid neoplasms and

beyond: evolving concepts and practical applications. Blood. 2011;117(19):5019–32.

25. Townsend W, Linch D. Hodgkin's lymphoma in adults. Lancet. 2012;380(9844):836–47.

26. Molyneux EM, Rochford R, Griffin B, Newton R, Jackson G, Menon G, et al. Burkitt's lymphoma. Lancet. 2012;379(9822):1234–44.

27. Bower M. Acquired immunodeficiency syndrome-related systemic non-Hodgkin's lymphoma. Br J Haematol. 2001;112(4): 863–73.

28. Kolokotronis A, Konstantinou N, Christakis I, Papadimitriou P, Matiakis A, Zaraboukas T, et al. Localized B-cell non-Hodgkin's lymphoma of oral cavity and maxillofacial region: a clinical study. Oral Surg Oral Med Oral Pathol Oral Radiol Endod. 2005;99(3):303–10.

29. Merlini G, Bellotti V. Molecular mechanisms of amyloidosis. N Engl J Med. 2003;349(6):583–96.

30. Messadi DV, Mirowski GW. Oral signs of hematologic disease. In: Oral signs of systemic disease. Basel: Springer International Publishing; 2019. p. 25–43.

31. Biewend ML, Menke DM, Calamia KT. The spectrum of localized amyloidosis: a case series of 20 patients and review of the literature. Amyloid. 2006;13(3):135–42.

32. Stoopler ET, Sollecito TP, Chen S-Y. Amyloid deposition in the oral cavity: a retrospective study and review of the literature. Oral Surg Oral Med Oral Pathol Oral Radiol Endod. 2003;95(6):674–80.

33. Glick M. Burket's oral medicine: PMPH USA; 2015.

34. Swerdlow S, Campo E, Harris N. WHO classification of tumours of haematopoietic and lymphoid tissues. Revised 4th ed. Lyon: International Agency for Research on Cancer; 2017. World Health Organization Classification of Tumours. 2.

35. Hou GL, Huang JS, Tsai CC. Analysis of oral manifestations of leukemia: a retrospective study. Oral Dis. 1997;3(1):31–8.

36. Weckx L, Hidal L, Marcucci G. Oral manifestations of leukemia. Ear Nose Throat J. 1990;69(5):341–2, 5–6.

37. Wu J, Fantasia JE, Kaplan R. Oral manifestations of acute myelomonocytic leukemia: a case report and review of the classification of leukemias. J Periodontol. 2002;73(6):664–8.

38. Francisconi CF, Caldas RJ, Oliveira Martins LJ, Fischer Rubira CM, da Silva Santos PS. Leukemic oral manifestations and their management. Asian Pac J Cancer Prev. 2016;17(3):911–5.

39. Kassebaum NJ, Jasrasaria R, Naghavi M, Wulf SK, Johns N, Lozano R, et al. A systematic analysis of global anemia burden from 1990 to 2010. Blood. 2014;123(5):615–24.

40. Love AL, Billett HH. Obesity, bariatric surgery, and iron deficiency: true, true, true and related. Am J Hematol. 2008;83(5):403–9.

41. Eisen D, Lynch DP. The mouth: diagnosis and treatment. St. Louis: Mosby Incorporated; 1998.

42. Stover PJ. Vitamin B12 and older adults. Curr Opin Clin Nutr Metab Care. 2010;13(1):24.

43. Bizzaro N, Antico A. Diagnosis and classification of pernicious anemia. Autoimmun Rev. 2014;13(4–5):565–8.

44. Stabler SP. Vitamin B12 deficiency. N Engl J Med. 2013;368(2):149–60.

45. Macleod R, Hamilton P, Soames J. Quantitative exfoliative oral cytology in iron-deficiency and megaloblastic anemia. Anal Quant Cytol Histol. 1988;10(3):176–80.

46. Vogiatzi MG, Macklin EA, Fung EB, Cheung AM, Vichinsky E, Olivieri N, et al. Bone disease in thalassemia: a frequent and still unresolved problem. J Bone Miner Res. 2009;24(3):543–57.

47. Azam M, Bhatti N. Hair-on-end appearance. Arch Dis Child. 2006;91(9):735.

48. Willman CL, Busque L, Griffith BB, Favara BE, McClain KL, Duncan MH, et al. Langerhans'-cell histiocytosis (histiocytosis X) – a clonal proliferative disease. N Engl J Med. 1994;331(3):154–60.

49. Howarth DM, Gilchrist GS, Mullan BP, Wiseman GA, Edmonson JH, Schomberg PJ. Langerhans cell histiocytosis: diagnosis, natural history, management, and outcome. Cancer. 1999;85(10):2278–90.

50. Adeyemo TA, Adeyemo WL, Adediran A, Akinbami AJ, Akanmu AS. Orofacial manifestation of hematological disorders: hemato-oncologic and immuno-deficiency disorders. Indian J Dent Res. 2011;22(5):688–97.

51. Caldemeyer KS, Parks ET, Mirowski GW. Langerhans cell histiocytosis. J Am Acad Dermatol. 2001;44(3):509–11.

52. Milián MA, Bagán JV, Jiménez Y, Pérez A, Scully C, Antoniades D. Langerhans' cell histiocytosis restricted to the oral mucosa. Oral Surg Oral Med Oral Pathol Oral Radiol Endod. 2001;91(1):76–9.

53. Hicks J, Flaitz CM. Langerhans cell histiocytosis: current insights in a molecular age with emphasis on clinical oral and maxillofacial pathology practice. Oral Surg Oral Med Oral Pathol Oral Radiol Endod. 2005;100(2):S42–66.

54. Farag AM. Head and neck manifestations of endocrine disorders. Atlas Oral Maxillofac Surg Clin North Am. 2017;25(2):197–207.

55. Heath KR, Fazel N. Oral signs of connective tissue disease. In: Oral signs of systemic disease. Basel: Springer International Publishing; 2019. p. 91–112.

56. Johnson L, Perschbacher K, Leong I, Bradley G. Oral manifestations of immunologically mediated diseases. Atlas Oral Maxillofac Surg Clin North Am. 2017;25(2):171–85.

57. dos Santos PR, Franca TT, Ribeiro CMB, Leao JC, De Souza IPR, Castro GF. Oral manifestations in human immunodeficiency virus infected children in highly active antiretroviral therapy era. J Oral Pathol Med. 2009;38(8):613–22.

58. Sankar V, Noujeim M. Oral manifestations of autoimmune and connective tissue disorders. Atlas Oral Maxillofac Surg Clin North Am. 2017;25(2):113.

59. Ayangco L, Rogers RS 3rd. Oral manifestations of erythema multiforme. Dermatol Clin. 2003;21(1):195–205.

60. Birek C. Herpesvirus-induced diseases: oral manifestations and current treatment options. J Calif Dent Assoc. 2000;28(12):911–21.

61. Betz SJ. HPV-related papillary lesions of the oral mucosa: a review. Head Neck Pathol. 2019;13(1):80–90.

62. Lynch DP. Oral manifestations of viral diseases. In: Mucosal immunology and virology. Cham: Springer; 2006. p. 99–156.

63. Fatahzadeh M. Oral manifestations of viral infections. Atlas Oral Maxillofac Surg Clin North Am. 2017;25(2):163–70.

64. Van Heerden WFP. Oral manifestations of viral infections. S Afr Fam Pract. 2006;48(8):20–4.

65. Amr Bugshan B, Farag AM, Desai B. Oral complications of systemic bacterial and fungal infections. Oral Manifestations of Systemic Diseases, an Issue of Atlas of the Oral & Maxillofacial Surgery Clinics, E-Book. 2017;25(2):209.

66. Betz SJ, Padilla RJ. Oral cavity. In: Practical head and neck pathology. Basel: Springer International Publishing; 2019. p. 1–38.

67. Perschbacher K. Mucocutaneous diseases of the oral cavity. Diagn Histopathol. 2018;24(5):166–71.

68. Langlais RP, Miller CS, Gehrig JS. Color atlas of common oral diseases. Burlington: Jones & Bartlett Learning; 2020.

69. Millsop JW, Fazel N. Oral candidiasis. Clin Dermatol. 2016;34(4):487–94.

70. Akpan A, Morgan R. Oral candidiasis. Postgrad Med J. 2002;78(922):455–9.

71. Singh A, Verma R, Murari A, Agrawal A. Oral candidiasis: an overview. J Oral Maxillofac Pathol. 2014;18(Suppl 1):S81.

72. Ashack KA. Dermatologic manifestations in the oral mucosa dermatologic manifestations in the oral mucosa.

73. Schubert M. Oral manifestations of viral infections in immunocompromised patients. Curr Opin Dent. 1991;1(4):384.

Principles in Exodontia

43

Mahmood Dashti and Setareh Zareh

Introduction

Exodontia is the process of removing teeth from the dental alveolus within the alveolar bone. It is one of the common dental procedures, and it is a fundamental skill of all dentists. However, it could become a challenging procedure. Dentists may decide to extract teeth due to many reasons, such as carious lesions, impacted teeth, periodontal treatments, orthodontic treatments, or trauma [1]. This chapter reviews and highlights simple and complex exodontia, techniques, complications, and tips on how to prevent any complication caused by the surgeon during the procedure.

When Is Extraction the Only Solution?

Teeth may be evaluated for removal at the level of individual teeth, full mouth, or for the overall health of the patient. At the level of individual teeth, the decision of extraction is very simple; if there is a presence of gross dental decay, advanced periodontal disease, or trauma, dentist will decide to remove the tooth in question. Teeth may also be subject to extraction either when they have a hopeless prognosis or when an orthodontist requests the extraction(s) to open more space to bring back the rest of the dentition into an alignment within the jaw [1].

Unfortunately, inexperienced dentists have extracted the wrong tooth over the years because the patient presented with a chief complaint of having severe toothache and insisted on the extraction of the tooth, when the tooth was clinically and radiographically fully intact [1]. This error can be prevented if proper history and examination are considered when assessing a patient.

Exodontia requires a full diagnostic process, including discussion with the patient regarding his or her chief complaint, clinical examination, dental and medical history, radiographic analysis, and special tests. Prior radiographic analysis of the dentition will not only confirm the diagnosis but will also indicate the presence of any potential difficulties the dentist might encounter [1].

Instruments

The most frequently used instruments when extracting a tooth are elevators and forceps.

Elevators

Elevators are used primarily for luxation of teeth. In Fig. 43.1, the basic components of an elevator are shown. This instru-

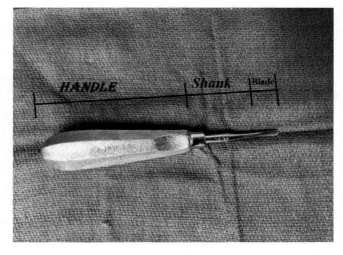

Fig. 43.1 Basic component of an elevator

M. Dashti
Private Practice, Tehran, Iran
e-mail: dashti.mahmood72@gmail.com

S. Zareh (✉)
Stony Brook University, School of Dental Medicine, Stony Brook, NY, USA
e-mail: Setareh.Zareh@stonybrookmedicine.edu

© The Author(s), under exclusive license to Springer Nature Switzerland AG 2021
M. R. Stevens et al. (eds.), *Innovative Perspectives in Oral and Maxillofacial Surgery*,
https://doi.org/10.1007/978-3-030-75750-2_43

ment helps with cleaving the periodontal ligament, which is the connection between the tooth particles along the surface area of the tooth roots to the surrounding alveolar bone [2–4]. By luxating the tooth, the space between the tooth roots and the alveolar bone can be expanded. This pocket expansion allows for a more degree of freedom of tooth movement within the pocket. Complications that can arise are the potential of fracturing the alveolar bone, which can be due to excessive luxation forces, or necrosis of the bone cells lining the socket, which can be caused by pressure-induced or compression-induced necrosis [5–7]. To minimize forces on the alveolar bone when luxating a tooth, tooth particles should be sectioned in such manner that the individual tooth particles impart fewer forces on the alveolar bone when performing the technique [8].

The elevator should be placed so that the tip of the instrument's ventral surface contacts the hardpoint(s) on the tooth being extracted, and the instrument's dorsal surface touches a hard intra-oral point(s). This technique prevents the loss of anchorage of the elevator position in a way that when a force with a specific direction and magnitude is applied to the tooth at the ventral contact point (at the tip of the elevator), the tooth will move gradually, yet the force applied will not damage the dorsal or ventral contact points. "Purchase point" is a commonly used term to describe the dental elevator position, yet this term is imprecise due to the fact that the tip of the dental elevator should concurrently contact at least two points (a dorsal and a ventral point) in order for the elevator to leverage a tooth. Then again, an elevator's position can be depicted as a blend of two luxation factors; the ventral and dorsal contact focuses on the tip of the elevator and the direction and extent of the power applied at the tip [9]. To "create a purchase point" for the tip of the elevator, teeth and bone can be sectioned and removed, respectively [3, 4]; however, the more accurately sectioned teeth and removed bone will lead to more positioning of the elevator tip. Thus, different combinations of hard ventral and dorsal tip contact points are more readily available for luxation.

Elevators are categories based on the differences between the shape and size of their blade. There are three basic elevators:

(a) The straight type: most commonly used to luxate teeth.
(b) The triangle or pennant-shape type: most useful when a broken root remains in the tooth socket and the adjacent socket is empty.
(c) The pick type: used to remove roots. (The heavy version of the pick is the Crane pick.)

Forceps

Extraction forceps are instruments utilized for removing teeth from the alveolar bone. Preferably, forceps are used to

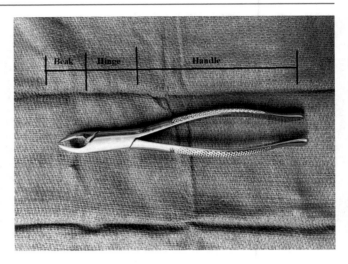

Fig. 43.2 Basic component of extraction forceps

elevate the luxated teeth from the socket instead of pulling them out. Conventional extraction is accomplished by cutting the periodontal ligament, luxation with elevators, and removal with forceps. In cases where the elevator fails to disconnect the socket's tooth, the forceps will carry out the process with intermittent lateral and apical forces [10, 11]. When properly used, forceps can help expand the bone. In Fig. 43.2, the basic component of an extraction forceps is shown.

Maxillary forces are grasped with the palm located underneath the forceps, such that the beak is pointed in an upward direction. However, the mandibular forceps are held such that the palm is located on top of the forceps, so the beak is directed down toward the teeth.

The biggest variation among extraction forceps is the beak, which is designed to modify the tooth root close to the root and crown junction. One important note to remember is that the beak of the forceps is designed to alter the root of the tooth, not the crown. Thus, there are different beaks developed for single-rooted teeth, two-rooted teeth, and three-rooted teeth.

Extraction technique for each tooth, including which instrument to use, where to put instruments on the tooth, the movement required, and pathway of extraction

1. *Maxilla*
   (a) *Incisor, Canine, Premolar (Single Rooted)*
       Single-rooted maxillary teeth are commonly removed with maxillary universal forceps (No.150) after performing proper elevation techniques. No. 150 forceps are straight when observed from the above and moderately S-shaped when viewed from the side. The beaks of the forceps curve and meet at the tip. This slight curve allows the surgeon to access the incisors and the premolars easily. The No. 150A forceps have some slight modifications from the No.

150 forceps. No.150A is used for maxillary premolars. If No.150A forceps are used for incisors, it will lead to fewer alterations to the incisors' roots. Straight forceps are another type of forceps available for the extraction of single-rooted teeth. No.1 forceps can be used for maxillary incisors and canines and are much simpler to use than the No. 150 for upper incisors [3].

Extraction steps for single-rooted teeth are as follows:

Rotation with No. 1 forceps or No. 150 maxillary universal forceps. The forceps should be positioned against the tooth and forced apically. Continue applying apical pressure and begin buccal luxation and subsequently palatal luxation. Upon observing some mobility, the conical root for the upper anterior dentition will allow rotational forces. The tooth should be rotated distally and later mesially. Continue this process until the tooth is removed from the socket. This extraction method can be used for both maxillary lateral incisor and canine; yet, the canine might require a tremendous effort and force to be removed from the socket [12].

With respect to maxillary premolar extraction, the steps are as follows:

Due to the maxillary premolars having two delicate and thin roots, they are easily fractured if proper techniques are not used. The No. 1 and No. 150 are the commonly used forceps for the upper premolar extractions. First, place the forceps and push apically, start buccal luxation to start expanding the alveolar, and then push palatally. This should be repeated in a conscious manner, and eventually, the beaks can be used to push the tooth out of the socket [12].

(b) *First Molar*

Maxillary molars have three roots, comprising a buccal bifurcation and a single palatal root. Forceps for maxillary molars are designed to have beaks that are pointed to fit within the buccal bifurcation and a smooth, concave surface for the palatal root. For this reason, maxillary molar forceps come in pairs of left and right. For the surgeon to reach the posterior part of the mouth and remain in the correct position, forceps should be balanced. Forceps No. 53 right and left are the most commonly used molar forceps. These forceps are designed so that the pointed buccal beak fits into the buccal bifurcation and sits anatomically around the palatal. For good positioning for the surgeon, the beak is offset. The No. 88 right and left forceps have a different design, such that they have long pointed beaks formation. They are commonly used for maxillary molars with severely carious crowns. The sharp pointed beak can extend deep past the trifurcation into sound dentin. However, one dis-

advantage of this design is the fact that it will crush the crestal alveolar bone, and if it is used without caution on intact teeth, it can fracture a large amount of buccal alveolar bone [3].

Extraction steps for maxillary first molar are as follows:

Due to maxillary molars commonly being in close contact with the maxillary sinus, careful radiographic analysis can help prevent possible antral involvement. Maxillary molars can be removed using No. 150, No. 210s, No. 53, or No. 88 forceps. Although it might be a simple extraction, their three roots can lead to a more complex extraction due to root dilacerations. First, position the forceps and apply apical force; then apply careful and slow forces in the palatal and buccal directions to allow for the socket's primary expansion. Due to maxillary bone not being too compacted, great initial forceps can lead to buccal plate fractures and, subsequently, tuberosity fractures. Substantial forces and movements follow the buccal and palatal direction, which allows for a greater expansion of the alveolar bone. The tooth is deliberately removed from the socket buccally. In the gingiva tear, stop the extraction and free the gingiva from the fractured buccal plate to prevent extra tearing of the gingiva [12].

(c) *Second and Third Molars*

At times, maxillary molars and erupted third molars have a single conical root, and during extraction, the No. 201S forceps offset from the handle with a wide, smooth beak are used. No. 65 forceps, also known as root-tip forceps, are another type of forceps with alteration of beak (narrower). They are primarily used to remove fractured maxillary molar roots and remove narrow premolars and mandibular incisors [3].

These traditional techniques have complication such as fracturing of the maxillary tuberosity, luxation of the adjacent tooth when used as a support, and post-operative complications such as infection, alveolitis sicca, and radix in antro highmori [12–16]. The use of No. 217 lower cowhorn forceps can lower the risk of these complications during a conventional extraction of the maxillary third molar [17].

2. *Mandible*

(a) *Incisor, Canine*

The lower universal forceps or the No.151 is the most commonly used instrument to extract single-rooted teeth. Their handle shape resembles the No.150 forceps, yet the beaks on the No.151 are pointed more inferiorly for the mandibular dentition and are smooth and narrow and have the beaks meet at the tip. This design allows the beaks to anchor at the cervical line of the tooth and hold the root [3].

The extraction technique is the same as the maxillary incisors [12].

(b) *Premolars*

The forceps used for mandibular premolars are the modified No. 151A forceps. The form of this instrument prevents it from fully adapt to the tooth roots, which is why these forceps should not be used for other mandibular teeth besides the premolars [3].

Extraction steps for mandibular premolars are as follows:

The No. 151 or the English/Asch forceps are the ideal forceps for extracting mandibular premolars. All mandibular anterior can be removed using this technique. Forceps are positioned apically, followed by a small luxation to push the tooth in buccal and lingual movements. Due to the roots being single or conical in shape, rotational movements can be used as well. Due to the mental foramen being in close contact with the roots, a thorough radiographic analysis must be done prior to the procedure to prevent compressing the nerve [12].

(c) *Molars*

Mandibular molars are two-rooted teeth with a bifurcation which allows the use of forceps that anatomically fits the tooth. Due to the bifurcation being located on both buccal and lingual sides, single molar forceps can be used for both sides, unlike the maxillary molar forceps, which required right and left forceps. No.17 forceps are the most commonly used lower molar forceps; they have a straight handle and beaks that are designed obliquely downward, with centrally pointed tips to fit into the bifurcation of the mandibular molars. The rest of the beak adjusts to the sides of the furcation. Due to the molar teeth' fused conical roots, the No. 17 forceps can't be used because of the pointed tips. No. 151 is mainly used for molar teeth. No. 87 (cowhorn) forceps are the modified lower molar forceps, which are designed to have two heavy pointed beaks that enter the bifurcation. Once the forceps are placed in the correct position, gently start pumping the handles up and down; this will elevate the tooth when squeezing the handles together tightly. When squeezing the beaks into the bifurcation, the buccal and lingual cortical plates should be used as a fulcrum to allow squeezing the tooth out of the socket [3].

Extraction steps for mandibular molars are as follows:

Substantial pressure should be applied apically. When using cowhorn forceps, place the tips of the beak in furcation of the tooth and gently rock the beak back and forth in position while squeezing the instrument handles. As the beaks are closely situated around the crown, heavy luxation should be performed in a buccal and lingual direction. When the tooth is sufficiently mobile, it can be removed from the socket with a wiggling motion [12].

In cases where simple extractions cannot be accomplished, surgical extraction can be used to remove the teeth in question. Below is a list of possible indications of using surgical extraction techniques [12]:

- Accidental fracture of the crown during simple extraction leaves the root buried in the socket
- Retained roots
- Severely carious teeth that will fracture with forceps extraction
- Endodontically treated teeth
- Teeth with internal resorption
- Teeth with divergent roots
- Teeth with dilacerated or greatly curved roots
- Ectopic teeth in positions where forceps cannot be used
- Teeth that are positioned close to vital anatomic structures
- Unerupted teeth other than third molars
- Hypercementosis
- Ankylosed teeth
- Mandibular third molar in the proximal segment of a fracture of the mandibular angle region
- Multirooted teeth located in areas of the jaw where bone preservation is critical for implant placement.
- Tooth that will be used for autotransplant

Surgery for Impacted and Ankylosed Teeth

Impacted teeth must be considered for extraction. They can often result in pathological findings. The most commonly observed pathology is periodontal bone loss and root resorption, cysts and tumors, and tooth decay [18]. Partially impacted teeth that are unable to erupt into a functional occlusal position should be considered for extraction due to not having enough space, intrusion of adjacent teeth, or other reasons [3]. The most commonly impacted teeth are the maxillary and mandibular third molars.

Steps for Surgical Removal of Impacted Tooth

1. *Reflecting Adequate Flaps for Accessibility*

The preferred technique is the envelope flap technique, which is easily sutured and takes less time to heal than the three-cornered flap that is an envelope flap with a releasing incision. The surgeon should consider using a three-cornered flap when requiring greater accessibility to the more apical side of the tooth, which may result in the stretching or tearing of the envelope flap. An enveloped incision is the preferred incision for the extraction of impacted mandibular third molars. This incision extends from the mandibular first molar's mesial papilla, surrounding the tooth; it further extends to the mandibular second molar's distobuccal line angle, laterally up and posteriorly to the mandible's ramus's anterior border. The enveloped incision is also the preferred method for the incision of the maxillary third molar. This incision will allow for an extension from the second molar's distal (posteriorly above the tuberosity) to the mesial aspect of the first molar (anteriorly). When greater accessibility is needed (i.e., in deeply embedded impactions), a release incision can be used, expanding from the second molar's mesial aspect [3].

2. *Removal of Overlying Bone*

Initially, the bone on the occlusal, buccal, and distal aspects below the impacted tooth's cervical line should be extracted. The volume of bone that should be removed varies depending on the morphology of the roots, the tooth's angulation, and the depth of impaction. Due to the risk of damaging the lingual nerve, the bone should not be extracted from the lingual aspect if not necessary. The usage of burs when removing bone from above the impacted tooth is dependent on the surgeon's preference. For mandibular third molar impaction, bone is initially removed from the tooth's occlusal aspect to expose the crown. Subsequently, the cortical bone located on the buccal aspect down to the cervical line should be removed. The bur can further remove bone from the cancellous area of bone located between the tooth and the cortical bone with a ditching technique. This will allow greater access for the elevators to achieve purchase points and a pathway to remove the tooth. To protect the lingual nerve from injury, the extraction of bone occurs from the lingual aspect. Bone removal is not necessary for maxillary teeth; yet when it is, bone is predominantly extracted from the buccal aspect down to the cervical like to expose the whole crown. Bone removal is typically accomplished by using a periosteal elevator. For the elevator to have sufficient purchase area to remove the tooth, the bone must be extracted on the tooth's mesial aspect [3].

3. *Sectioning the Tooth*

The direction in which the impacted tooth should be divided varies based on the impacted tooth's angulation and any root curvature. Although it is necessary to modify teeth with divergent roots or deeply impacted teeth, the most critical factor is the tooth's angulation. The tooth is sectioned three-fourths of its length in the lingual aspect with a bur. Due to the risk of damaging the lingual nerve, the bur should not be used to section the tooth completely in the lingual aspect. To split the tooth, insert a straight elevator in the point made with the bur and rotate.

The mesioangular mandibular impaction is usually one of the least complicated impacts to remove concern-

ing the four basic angulation types. After an adequate amount of bone is extracted, the crown's distal half is separated at the buccal groove to just underneath the cervical line on the distal aspect and removed. The remaining tooth particle is removed with a No. 301 elevator positioned at the cervical line's mesial side. A mesioangular impaction can also be extracted by developing a purchase point in the tooth with the drill. A crane pick elevator can then be used to elevate the tooth from the alveolus.

Horizontal impactions are one of the most challenging impactions to extract. Following the removal of adequate bone from below the cervical line to expose the distal root from the superior aspect and most of the crown's buccal surface, the tooth is divided at the cervical line to separate the crown from the roots. Once the crown is removed, the roots can be dislodged with a Cryer elevator into space formerly employed by the crown. If the impacted third molar has divergent roots, they should be divided into two separate portions and removed individually.

Vertical impaction is also a very complex impaction to extract. The technique for bone removal and sectioning closely resembles the mesioangular impaction techniques, in which the buccal, distal, and occlusal bones are removed. After the distal portion of the crown has been divided and extracted, the tooth can be elevated by applying an elevator to the cervical line at the tooth's mesial aspect. As the accessibility surrounding the mandibular second molar is difficult to obtain and requires the extraction of significantly more bone on the distal and buccal sides, this technique is more complicated than the mesioangular removal. Teeth with distoangular impaction are the most difficult to extract. The crown is sectioned above the cervical line after an adequate amount of bone is removed from the distal and the tooth's bucco-occlusal sides. The crown is obliterated to prevent interference with the visibility and accessibility of the root structure. Due to the roots being fused, straight or Cryer elevators can be used to elevate the tooth in the space formerly resided by the crown. Divergent roots should be sectioned into two pieces and removed separately. Removal of this impaction is very complicated because a remarkable amount of distal bone must be removed, and teeth tend to rotate distally upon elevation and impact the mandibular ramus.

As the bone overlying the maxillary teeth is thin and elastic, impacted maxillary teeth are rarely split. In cases where the patient is older (loss of bone elasticity) or has a thicker bone, the tooth is removed by bone removal [3].

4. *Delivery of the Sectioned Tooth with Elevator*

After sufficient bone is extracted to expose the tooth and the tooth is divided appropriately, the tooth is extracted with elevators from the alveolus. The most commonly used elevators for the mandible are the straight elevators, the paired Cryer elevators, and the Crane pick [3].

5. *Preparing for Wound Closure*

A bone file is mainly used to smooth any sharp and rough edges on the bone, especially where the elevator came in contact with the bone. The surgeon should remove all particulate bone chips and debris left from the wound, which can be achieved with full irrigation with sterile saline.

Surgeons begin to administer an antibiotic like tetracycline into mandibular third molars' sockets to prevent osteitis sicca, also known as dry socket. Primary closure is used for closing the incision made for the impacted third molar. During the surgical procedure, a well-designed and none-traumatized flap will fit into its original location. Place the initial suture through the attached tissue located on the posterior aspect of the second molar. Additional sutures can be placed posteriorly from the same position and anteriorly past the papilla on the second molar's mesial side. Usually, no more than three sutures are needed to close an envelope incision. If used, a releasing incision must also be closed. If the maxillary third molar flap sits passively in position, post-operatively suturing will not be needed [3].

Complications

Complications are unexpected outcomes of a surgical procedure. Management and prevention of a surgical complication are best achieved by a thorough preoperative assessment (clinical examination, radiographic analysis, complete medical and dental history) and a comprehensive treatment plan, and precise execution of the surgical procedure [19].

Although complications are rare, they can lead to prolonged treatment and inconvenience to both the patient and dentist. There are a variety of complications that can occur. The most common complication is alveolar osteitis, also known as dry socket. This condition is associated with fibrinolysis of the blood clots and exposure to the socket's bony walls. This is a painful and self-limiting condition that resolves in 2–3 weeks with the incidence of 3–5% of extractions with risk factors being traumatic extraction, smoking, posterior teeth, and the extraction of mandibular dentition more than maxillary can increase the incidence of alveolar osteitis, yet they are unpredictable [1].

This post-operative condition is associated with pain around and inside the extraction site. The severity of the pain can increase between the first- and third-day post-extraction, along with partial or total disintegration of the blood clots. Dry socket can also be associated with halitosis. If the patient's signs and symptoms exceed that of the alveolus, then the diagnosis should be reviewed for a possible spread of infection due to remnant pieces of tooth or bone. A thorough review of the case history, radiographs, and past medical/dental history can help reduce these complications. Other complications that can arise post-extraction are listed below [1].

Post-extraction Complications

- Fractured tooth (including crown and/or root fracture)
- Laceration
- Soft tissue injury
- Luxation of adjacent tooth/teeth
- Fracture of cortical plates (both buccal (labial) and lingual (palatal) plates)
- Fracture of maxillary tuberosity
- Fracture mandible
- Hemorrhage (only primary hemorrhage)
- Displacement of tooth/root in the maxillary antrum
- Displacement of tooth/root into adjacent tissue space
- Dry socket
- Trismus
- Post-operative pain
- Infection
- Wound dehiscence

A complication of posterior maxillary teeth extractions is penetration into or loss of tooth roots into the maxillary sinus, which is a complication that must always be considered. It is crucial to check that all the pieces of the teeth are complete post-extraction carefully. A method of examining for the presence of an oro-antral communication is to hold the patient's nose and having them blow and listen for any passage of bubbles or air. If the communication is small and the tooth is intact, compress the socket and suture the communication close. Advise the patient not to blow their nose or create any negative pressure; discuss thoroughly with the patient the reason for this distressing complication. However, if the communication is extensive and more than 4 mm of a piece of the tooth is missing, refer the patient to an oral and maxillofacial surgeon (OMFS), after you have placed a two-layer mucoperiosteal flap with a buccal fat pad [20].

Another complication that the patient should be promptly referred to an OMFS is the displacement of tooth or root beyond the alveolus into the soft tissue, which is usually a sign of excessive or misdirected force. Do not ignore this because the probability of infection is high. A short course of antibiotics should be prescribed if the patient has a delay in being seen by the OMFS [20].

A series of prevention tips are listed corresponding to their complications, respectively, in Table 43.1 [18].

Table 43.1 A series of prevention tips corresponding to the complications that might rise during a surgical extraction procedure [18]

Prevention of soft tissue injury	1. Pay close attention to soft tissue injury 2. Develop adequate-sized flaps 3. When retracting soft tissue, use minimal force
Prevention of root and displacement fracture	1. Plan for root fraction (always!) 2. If high possibility of a fracture exists, use a surgical extraction 3. In case of broken root, do not use strong apical force
Prevention of injury to adjacent teeth	1. Note the potential fracture to large restoration 2. Inform the patient pre-operatively 3. Use elevators accordingly 4. Have the assistant inform the surgeon when pressure is put on adjacent teeth
Prevention of extraction of wrong teeth	1. Check the patient's chart, records, and radiographs to confirm the correct tooth 2. Check with the assistant and the patient to ensure that the correct tooth is being extracted 3. Pay close attention during the surgical procedure
Prevention of fracture of alveolar process	1. Do not use excessive force 2. Use surgical extraction techniques to reduce force needed for extraction 3. Perform a thorough preoperative clinical exam and radiographs
Prevention of nerve injury	1. Be sure to have the knowledge of the correct nerve anatomy in the surgical site 2. Avoid excising and affecting the periosteum in the nerve area
Prevention of injury to the temporomandibular joint	1. Do not open the mouth too widely 2. Support the mandible during the surgical procedure
Prevention of oroantral communications	1. Perform a thorough preoperative clinical exam and radiograph analysis 2. Avoid extreme apical pressure
Prevention of post-operative bleeding	1. Perform a complete medical and dental history to obtain information about history of bleeding problems 2. Atraumatic surgical technique should be used 3. Have good hemostasis during surgery 4. Provide the best post-operative instructions to the patient
Prevention of wound dehiscence	1. Implement aseptic technique 2. Perform atraumatic surgery 3. Be sure to close the incision over the intact bone 4. Suture the surgical site without applying tension

Post-extraction Patient Instructions

Bleeding

Place a gauze on the area and have the patient bite down firmly for 30 minutes. If the gauze is spotted red or pink through and through, no additional gauze is necessary. However, if the gauze is soaked red, have the patient bite down more firmly on a new clean gauze for another 30 minutes. Make sure to tell your patient to contact you if the bleeding does not stop after several gauze pads. Advise the patient to not spit or drink through a straw for 24 hours; explain to them that this can result in a clot becoming dislodged [21].

Swelling

An ice pack should be used for 24 hours to help reduce the swelling. Explain to the patient that post-operative swelling is normal to develop within 24 hours; however, if the swelling does not subside after 48 hours or a large swelling develops, the patient should seek care. Advise the patient not to lie flat down for 24 hours. Sitting in a comfortable chair or using pillows to keep the head elevated in bed should be advised to the patient for the first 24 hours. The patient should be advised to call the doctor or seek care if the swelling continues to increase after 48 hours [21].

Discomfort

When counseling the patient regarding post-operative discomfort, be sure to explain that some discomfort is expected during the first day, yet it should subside to soreness with some occasional throbbing the next day. However, if the discomfort becomes severe or persists after 48 hours, the patient should call the doctor. The patient should be advised to take over-the-counter (OTC) analgesics immediately after the procedure. Two Advil® tablets every 4 hours are best (unless the patient is allergic to aspirin or other NSAIDs or told by their physician to avoid these medications). If the patient's pain and discomfort do not taper down with OTC medication, the doctor should prescribe analgesics [21].

Home Care

Patients should be told to avoid chewing any food, eating, or drinking anything hot until the local anesthetic has worn off completely. Cold beverages, ice cream, ices, pudding, and yogurt can help wear off the local anesthetic. The patient should avoid brushing the surgical site for 24 hours, and after 24 hours gentle tooth brushing of the surgical site is permitted. Advise the patient to rinse with warm saltwater after 24 hours. Advise the patient to refrain from smoking during the post-surgical period. Patients should contact the doctor if they experience fever above 100.5 °F, difficulty swallowing, difficulty breathing, severe discomfort, significant swelling, and persistent bleeding [21].

References

1. Sambrook PJ, Goss AN. Contemporary exodontia. Aust Dent J. 2018;63 Suppl 1:S11–8. https://doi.org/10.1111/adj.12586. Erratum in: Aust Dent J. 2018;63(2):266.
2. Fragiskos FD. Oral surgery. Berlin, Heidelberg, New York: Springer; 2007.
3. Hupp JR, Ellis E, Tucker MR. Contemporary oral and maxillofacial surgery. 6th ed. St. Louis: Mosby-Elsevier; 2018.
4. Koerner KR, Tilt LV, Johnson KR. Color atlas of minor oral surgery. London: Mosby-Wolfe; 1994.
5. Goga Y, Chiba M, Shimizu Y, Mitani H. Compressive force induces osteoblast apoptosis via caspase-8. J Dent Res. 2006;85:240–4.
6. Matsui H, Fukuno N, Kanda Y, Kantoh Y, Chida T, Nagaura Y, et al. The expression of Fn14 via mechanical stress-activated JNK contributes to apoptosis induction in osteoblasts. J Biol Chem. 2014;289:6438–50.
7. Nettelhoff L, Grimm S, Jacobs C, Walter C, Pabst AM, Goldschmitt J, et al. Influence of mechanical compression on human periodontal ligament fibroblasts and osteoblasts. Clin Oral Investig. 2016;20:621–9.
8. Mamoun J. Use of elevator instruments when luxating and extracting teeth in dentistry: clinical techniques. J Korean Assoc Oral Maxillofac Surg. 2017;43(3):204–11. https://doi.org/10.5125/jkaoms.2017.43.3.204. Epub 2017 Jun 28. PMID: 28770164; PMCID: PMC5529197.
9. Kaminishi RM, Davis WH, Nelson NE. Surgical removal of impacted mandibular third molars. Dent Clin N Am. 1979;23:413–25.
10. Peterson LJ, Ellis E, Hupp JR, Tucker MR. Contemporary oral and maxillofacial surgery. St Louis: CV Mosby; 1988. p. 265–83.
11. Waite DE. Textbook of practical oral and maxillofacial surgery. Philadelphia: Lea & Febiger; 1987. p. 120–34.
12. Oluseye SB. Exodontia: a retrospective study of the reasons, methods and complications of tooth extraction in oral and maxillofacial surgery clinic, Lagos University Teaching Hospital. NPMC dissertation. National postgraduate medical college of Nigeria. 1993.
13. Heasman PA, Jacobs DJ. A clinical investigation into the incidence of dry alveolus. Br J Oral Maxillofac Surg. 1984;22:115–22.
14. Wagaiyu EG, Kaimenyi JT. Frequency of alveolar osteitis (dry alveolus) at Kenyatta National Hospital Dental outpatient Clinic—a retrospective study. East Afr Med J. 1989;66:658–62.
15. Simon E, Matee M. Post-extraction complications seen at a referral dental clinic in Dar es Salaam, Tanzania. Int Dent J. 2001;51:273–6.
16. Belinfante LS, Marlow CD, Meyers W, et al. Incidence of dry socket: complications in third molar removal. J Oral Surg. 1973;3(1):106–9.
17. Edward J, Aziz MA, Madhu Usha A, Narayanan JK. Comparing the efficiency of two different extraction techniques in removal of maxillary third molars: a randomized controlled trial. J Maxillofac Oral Surg. 2017;16(4):424–9. https://doi.org/10.1007/s12663-016-0935-1. Epub 2016 Jul 13. Erratum in: J Maxillofac Oral Surg. 2017;16(4):430. PMID: 29038624; PMCID: PMC5628062.
18. Courtesy of Stony Brook dental school, Postoperative Patient Home Care Instructions.
19. Tarakji B, Saleh LA, Hanouneh S. Systematic review of dry socket: aetiology, treatment and prevention. J Clin Diagn Res. 2015;9:ZE10–3.
20. Asanami S, Kasazaki Y. Expert third molar extractions. Tokyo: Quintessence Publishing; 1990.
21. Hupp JR, et al. Contemporary oral and maxillofacial surgery. 5th ed. Mosby Elsevier; 2008.

Trauma and Management in Oral Surgery

44

Nima Dehghani [iD], Xaniar Mahmoudi,
Mohadeseh Azarsina, and Amir Reza Sharifnia

Introduction

Trauma to the oral cavity is a common occurrence and requires medical attention. The growing population of patients with traumatic dentoalveolar injuries and the exiting challenges in managing such injuries has led to an increase in suggested diagnostic and therapeutic strategies. The frequency of traumatic injuries to the face is higher in children than adults; nonetheless, a smaller percentage of children experience fractures in the maxillofacial region. The diagnosis and treatment of traumatic facial injuries are highly important, particularly in children, since such injuries can lead to eventual malocclusion and facial asymmetry if not adequately managed. Moreover, such patients are at high risk of aspiration, infection, and bleeding. Depending on the type of dentition, preoperative assessments and the final management may vary in different patients. Prompt diagnosis and correct management greatly impact jaw function, quality of life, and life satisfaction of patients. In this chapter, the common causes of trauma, preoperative assessments, classification of traumatic injuries, and the existing treatment modalities for managing dentoalveolar traumatic injuries are discussed.

Etiology

The causes of trauma may vary in different age groups. Children have the lowest rate of facial trauma, probably due to the fact that adults mostly supervise them. Maxillofacial fractures in children mainly occur due to regular daily activities such as playing, cycling, and falls. When adolescents become more independent, they start to drive and participate in team sports. Trauma in adults is often due to motor vehicle accidents, fights, sports accidents, and occupational accidents [1]. Also, the teeth may be unintentionally injured in the process of intraoral surgical procedures or endotracheal intubation [2]. The severity of injury often increases with age and is greater in males than females. The prevalence of dentoalveolar injuries is 30% in children during the primary dentition period and 5–20% during the mixed dentition period. Trauma due to sports activities has a prevalence of 36% in adults [3]. Some medical conditions such as radiation-induced osteonecrosis of the jaw, osteoporosis, vitamin D deficiency, oral cancer, and odontogenic infections can also cause dentoalveolar injuries. Child abuse is another cause of dentoalveolar trauma. The abovementioned causes account for 7% of oral injuries [4]. Moreover, seizure attacks can cause dentoalveolar injuries due to severe clenching of teeth [5].

Pre-incident Preparation

Management of dentoalveolar trauma requires pre-planning in order to be able to provide the patients with the best treatment possible. Such accidents occur with no prior notice and cannot be predicted. Thus, having the necessary equipment and instruments and assisting the clinician in such cases is imperative and should be planned ahead. The International Association of Dental Trauma has offered a suitable guideline in this respect, which can be of great help at the time of such incidents. The required instruments and materials that

N. Dehghani (✉)
Department of Oral and Maxillofacial Surgery, Tehran University of Medical Sciences, Tehran, Iran
e-mail: nimadt2002@gmail.com

X. Mahmoudi
Dental School, Tehran University of Medical Sciences, Tehran, Iran
e-mail: xaniarmahmoudi@yahoo.com

M. Azarsina · A. R. Sharifnia
Private Practice, Tehran, Iran
e-mail: azarsina2012@yahoo.com; amir.shar.19.80.1@gmail.com

© The Author(s), under exclusive license to Springer Nature Switzerland AG 2021
M. R. Stevens et al. (eds.), *Innovative Perspectives in Oral and Maxillofacial Surgery*,
https://doi.org/10.1007/978-3-030-75750-2_44

need to be available in medical centers include restorative materials, endodontic instruments, necessary instruments for tooth splinting, and surgical equipment such as sutures and surgical instruments.

Patient Assessment

Accurate patient assessment is imperative for prompt and correct intervention. Taking a medical history is particularly important and should be precisely performed. Each child presenting with facial trauma should be stabilized first. The patients should be assessed according to the Advanced Trauma Life Support protocol. Life-threatening injuries should be detected and managed at the earliest time possible. Several differences exist in the assessment of traumatic injuries in children, compared with adults, which should be taken into account. These include airway maintenance in children due to their lower respiratory capacity, larger and looser oral and pharyngeal soft tissue, a more cephalic larynx, and a narrower epiglottis. These differences make intubation and ventilation of children more difficult [6]. Children who have suffered trauma are at higher risk due to higher surface-to-volume ratio, metabolism rate, oxygen demand, and cardiac output. The low blood volume in children also makes them more susceptible, particularly to hemodynamic instability. All these factors increase children's susceptibility to post-traumatic hypotension, hypoxia, and hypothermia [7, 8]. Dental and skeletal injuries can lead to aspiration of the broken segment and compromise the airway. After ensuring airway patency, the hemorrhagic wounds should be sutured to enhance visibility and access to the oral cavity. Since the prognosis of dentoalveolar injuries depends on the diagnosis and correct intervention, precise timing is of critical importance. Nonetheless, in case of the presence of life-threatening emergencies, treatment of dentoalveolar injuries must be postponed. In case of severe trauma, the nervous system, vertebral column, skull, temporomandibular joints, and head and neck soft tissue should be carefully examined [9]. Moreover, we should search for any sign/symptom of child abuse when examining pediatric patients. These signs/symptoms may include multiple injuries in various locations, a prolonged lag time between the occurrence of injury and time of seeking medical attention, misleading answers provided by the parents, and suspicious conditions [10].

Medical History of the Patient

Taking the patient's medical history is an integral part of clinical examination and helps the clinician become familiar with the patient. Taking a medical history is particularly important in emergencies. Patient's allergy history to medications, history of hemorrhagic disorders, the need for antibiotic prophylaxis, history of seizure, recent medication intake, cardiovascular conditions, and respiratory diseases should be particularly questioned [11].

Dental History of the Patient

In taking the dental history of the patient, previous dental treatments, current ongoing dental treatments, and history of dentoalveolar trauma should be asked. History of previous dental treatments can help in the diagnosis and management of the recent traumatic injury. Next, the patient or his/her companions should be questioned about the history of current trauma. The time interval between the incident and seeking treatment can help the clinician in determining the treatment prognosis. The nature of trauma is also important in determining the mechanism of injury and the injured tissues. The extent of trauma can also be determined to some extent as such. The location where the incident happened can also provide some information about the severity of injury and the degree of tissue contamination and determine the need for antibiotics prescription.

Radiographic Examination

Radiographic examination is imperative to obtain additional information about root injuries such as root fracture, PDL widening, bone fracture, and bone density. The commonly requested radiographic modalities for this purpose often include periapical radiography, occlusal radiography, and panoramic radiography. Intraoral periapical radiography is often the first radiographic modality requested for patients with dental trauma. If a periapical radiograph is obtained at a correct position, it can reveal the injured tooth's slightest details. In cases suspected of a concussion, periapical radiography can reveal the size of the PDL space. Repeated radiographs at regular intervals are often prescribed for the follow-up and monitoring of the change in the size of the pulp chamber and tooth root. Occlusal radiography is beneficial for the assessment of root fractures, the palate, tongue, cheeks, and lips. It is easy to obtain and does not apply pressure to the oral cavity. Panoramic radiography is the most beneficial modality in such cases since it provides a comprehensive view of the teeth, alveolar ridge, and supporting bone. Radiography should be necessarily used in children with traumatic dentoalveolar injuries to assess root development, root canal size, and the permanent successor of the traumatized primary tooth [12].

Classification of Dentoalveolar Injuries

In dentoalveolar traumas, using a classification system can help a more enhanced diagnosis and treatment planning. Several classification systems have been introduced for the classification of dental traumas and injury to the surrounding tissues (Table 44.1). These systems have been designed based on the anatomical location of traumatic injury, etiology of injury, emergency management, pathology, and treatment. Andreasen's classification system is a combination of the World Health Organization classification system and other classifications introduced in the literature. This classification system includes details of injuries and trauma to the dentition, alveolar bone, supporting tissues, gingiva, and oral mucosa, as well as anatomical and therapeutic considerations and prognosis [13]. This classification can be used for both primary and permanent dentitions. Table 44.1 presents Andreasen's classification.

Management and treatment of Dentoalveolar Injuries

The type of injury can be determined according to Andreasen's classification, and an efficient treatment plan can be designed based on the patient's requirements. Factors that should be considered in treatment planning include age and level of patient cooperation, type of injury to the primary, mixed, or permanent dentition, the extent of the injury, associated injuries, and patient's medical condition. The main treatment goal in such cases includes resuming the teeth' function and optimal esthetics, gingiva, and the surrounding bone. Deciding to retain or extract a particular tooth can be difficult, depending on the condition. Although preservation of teeth and the supporting structures is of utmost importance, we may need to extract a tooth that would play no role in the final treatment plan. In some cases, despite the poor prognosis of the avulsed tooth, we may have no choice other than to replant the avulsed tooth to preserve the contour and volume of the broken alveolar ridge to enhance healing.

Traumatic Dental Injuries

Traumatic dental injuries commonly occur, and dental clinicians need to learn the correct management of such injuries. In-time and correct management can stop the bleeding, prevent infection and aspiration, and preserve the injured tissues' viability and enhance achieving a better treatment outcome. Herein, we will briefly review and discuss traumatic dental injuries.

Table 44.1 Andreasen's classification for dentoalveolar injuries

Dental hard tissue injury	Alveolar bone injuries	Periodontal injuries	Gingival injuries
Enamel infraction	Intrusion of teeth into alveolar socket wall	Concussion	Contusion
Enamel fracture	Alveolar socket wall fracture	Subluxation	Abrasion
Enamel dentin fracture	Alveolar wall fracture	Extrusive luxation	Laceration
Uncomplicated crown fracture		Lateral luxation	Degloving
Complicated crown root fracture		Intrusive luxation	
Root fracture		Avulsion	

Crown Fracture

Crown fracture is common and may be associated with the loss of tooth structure. The crown fracture may involve the enamel alone, both the enamel and dentin, or even the pulp chamber. Fractures not causing pulpal involvement are referred to as simple fractures, while those involving the pulp are referred to as complex fractures. In complex fractures, the tooth may become sensitive to thermal alterations and require treatment. Exposure to dentinal tubules can enhance the leakage of bacteria into the pulp chamber and lead to pulpitis. In simple fractures, restoring the broken area with restorative materials prevents tooth hypersensitivity and inhibits pulpal inflammation progression. Pulp therapy may be indicated in complex fractures. Direct pulp capping is a type of pulp therapy that involves applying a layer of calcium hydroxide over the exposed pulp. In case of noticing further changes in the pulp tissue, partial or complete pulpotomy may be indicated.

Crown-Root Fracture

Crown-root fractures often occur following direct trauma to the anterior teeth and indirect trauma to the posterior teeth. Enamel, dentin, cementum, and dental pulp may be involved in this type of fracture (Fig. 44.1). Determining the extension (depth) of fracture below the gingival margin or alveolar bone is essential in determining the treatment prognosis. The traumatic force causes oblique fracture starting from the middle third to beneath the alveolar bone crest. Since such fractures involve cementum, the biologic width should be evaluated for correct treatment planning [14]. In case of the absence of adequate space to observe the biologic width in the restoration of a tooth, orthodontic treatment or a surgical procedure may be required prior to tooth restoration. Younger patients are better candidates for orthodontic extraction. If appropriate conditions are not met for the abovementioned treatments, the tooth needs to be extracted and replaced with a dental implant.

Root Fracture

A root fracture is uncommon and, in case of occurrence, involves the cementum, dentin, and dental pulp. A root fracture is often classified based on fracture line location in the apical third, middle third, or coronal third of the root. The location of the fracture line determines the treatment plan and prognosis. The majority of fractures in the middle third and apical third can have a fair/good prognosis in correct management [15]. The majority of root fractures can be observed on periapical radiographs. Computed tomography scans can more accurately determine fracture line location and direction since they provide a 3D image of the area. Fractures in the coronal third of the root often have the poorest prognosis, and such teeth often need to be extracted (in adults). Fractures of the middle third and apical third of the root can be managed by shortening the tooth's coronal portion and its subsequent splinting. Splinting with rigid and semirigid wires is recommended for 4 weeks to 4 months.

Periodontal Tissue Injury

In this section, injury to the tooth-supporting structures, particularly the periodontal tissue, is discussed. Luxation injuries often occur in the anterior maxillary teeth, particularly central incisors. Such injuries can irreversibly damage the PDL and dental pulp. We will review each type of injury in detail.

Concussion

A concussion is the mildest trauma applied to the PDL in which the tooth position does not change. The tooth is sensitive to palpation, percussion, and mastication due to edema and pos-

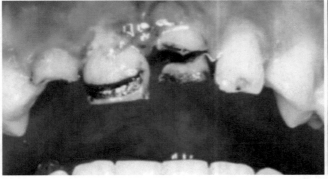
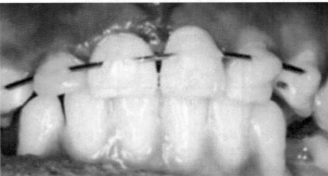

Fig. 44.1 A patient with a crown-root fracture of maxillary central incisors. After root canal treatment, the broken pieces were reattached using dental restorative materials. (Reproduced with permission from Roettger et al. [21])

sible bleeding in the PDL. No specific treatment is required, and healing often occurs without requiring treatment.

Subluxation

Subluxation is a mild injury to the PDL, which increases the tooth mobility without displacement. Clinical examination reveals bleeding around the gingival margin. The tooth is mobile and sensitive to palpation, percussion, and mastication. Radiography is indicated to rule out more severe injuries. No treatment is required. If the patient complains of unbearable pain, the opposing tooth can be slightly adjusted to be out of occlusion or the tooth can be splinted with a nonrigid wire for 2 weeks. A small number of teeth may undergo pulp necrosis following subluxation. Pulp vitality tests should be performed.

Extrusion

The tooth is displaced from its original location. Tooth mobility and bleeding are evident on clinical examination. The percussion test produces a dull sound. In most cases, pulp necrosis occurs, and the tooth requires root canal ther-

apy. The tooth should be repositioned into its original position as soon as possible and splinted (Fig. 44.2). To ensure the return of the tooth to its original position, periapical radiography can be performed. Teeth with closed (mature) apices have a low chance of revascularization, and such teeth need to undergo root canal treatment after removing the splint wire.

Lateral Luxation

The tooth is displaced but is still in its socket. Lateral luxation often occurs in the anterior maxillary teeth and is usually associated with an alveolar bone fracture. Unlike other types of injuries, the tooth is not mobile and is locked in its place. On percussion, a high bony sound is heard. The load applied to the tooth crown causes palatal displacement of the crown and labial displacement of the root apex. This movement applies labial force to the alveolar bone and increases the risk of bone fracture and locking of the tooth in this position. The supplying vasculature is also injured with minimal possibility of healing. For treatment, after anesthetic injection, the pressure is applied to the apex of the locked tooth, allowing its return to its original position. The tooth is subsequently splinted for 4 weeks.

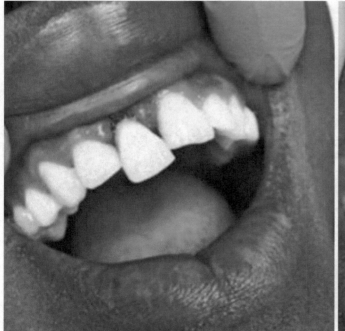 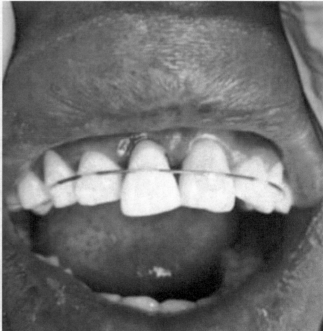

Fig. 44.2 Extrusion of maxillary right central incisor due to trauma. After repositioning the tooth in its socket, it is splinted to the adjacent teeth using wire and composite resin. (Reproduced with permission from Roettger et al. [21])

Intrusion

Intrusion refers to a type of trauma that causes apical movement of the tooth and damage to the PDL, alveolar bone, and dental pulp vasculature. Following intrusion trauma, the tooth appears shorter than the adjacent teeth and is not often mobile. Percussion produces a metal sound. If the tooth has an open apex, it is expected to extrude spontaneously. If pulp necrosis occurs during the follow-up period, the tooth must undergo endodontic treatment. Mature teeth should be extruded either surgically or by orthodontic treatment. After extrusion of the tooth in its original position, it should undergo endodontic therapy within 2 weeks to prevent pulpitis and subsequent complications. The need for splinting of the tooth should also be considered.

Avulsion

Avulsion refers to a relatively uncommon injury-causing displacement of a tooth from its socket. It more commonly occurs in the maxillary central incisors (Fig. 44.3). Sports accidents and fights are the most common causes of avulsion. There is a theory stating that if an avulsed tooth is replanted within 60 minutes, the tooth-supporting structures may reinstatement. According to most of the available literature, fibroblasts can survive and remain viable on the root surface for up to 60 minutes after an avulsion and can reform a complete PDL and prevent ankylosis if the tooth is replanted within this time period [16–18]. If the avulsed tooth is stored in a storage medium with optimal osmolarity (milk, saliva, Hank's balanced salt solution), the final treatment prognosis would be more favorable [19]. Prompt treatment is required for avulsed teeth. The likelihood of optimal healing and prognosis of treatment increase if the avulsed tooth is placed back in the socket or stored in a storage medium with optimal osmolarity within the first 5 minutes after avulsion [20]. Replantation of the tooth back into its socket and its subsequent splinting is the best-suggested treatment strategy. In some cases, however, the patient may suffer severe trauma, and quick replantation of the tooth may not be possible due to alveolar fracture. In such cases, the tooth should be monitored after splinting, and endodontic treatment should be considered in the follow-up period for mature teeth. Revascularization and healing may occur in open-apex teeth. The patient is at risk of tetanus when the tooth falls on the soil. In such cases, the patient's tetanus vaccination status should be evaluated. Antibiotics are often prescribed for such patients for 7–10 days.

Alveolar Bone Injury

Alveolar bone injury is uncommon. An alveolar bone fracture can be easily detected by clinical examination. If the mucosa is intact, irregularity or mobility of bone can be easily detected by palpation of the area. Trauma causing alveolar bone fracture can also cause jaw fracture. Complementary examinations are imperative to ensure no fracture of the maxilla and mandible. Fracture of the alveolar process often occurs at the site of incisors and premolars. Treatment includes the reduction of bone and stabilization of the fracture site. The reduction can be performed by the open or closed methods. In closed reduction, the adjacent structures' injury would be minimal, and the area is fixed by rigid splinting for 4 weeks [3]. Open reduction is performed for cases with complex fractures when closed reduction is not indicated. After surgical access to the area, resorbable or non-

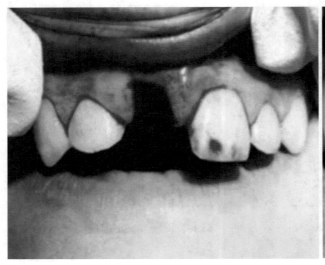
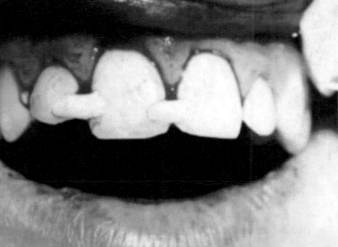

Fig. 44.3 Avulsed tooth splinted to the adjacent teeth after replantation. (Reproduced with permission from Roettger et al. [21])

resorbable plates are used to splint the fracture segments in open reduction. A suitable splint must be able to fix the fracture segments in place, not interfere with the patient's occlusion, and provide optimal fixation throughout treatment.

References

1. Grunwaldt L, Smith DM, Zuckerbraun NS, et al. Pediatric facial fractures: demographics, injury patterns, and associated injuries in 772 consecutive patients. Plast Reconstr Surg. 2011;128(6):1263–71.
2. Ozcelik O, Haytac C, Akkaya M. Iatrogenic trauma to oral tissues. J Periodontol. 2005;76:1793–7.
3. Leathers R, Gowans R. Offce-based management of dental alveolar trauma. Atlas Oral Maxillofac Surg Clin North Am. 2013;21:185–97.
4. Cairns AM, Mok JY, Welbury RR. Injuries to the head, face, mouth and neck in physically abused children in a community setting. Int J Paediatr Dent. 2005;15:310–8.
5. Lagunju I, Oyinlade A, Babatunde O. Seizure-related injuries in children and adolescents with epilepsy. Epilepsy Behav. 2016;54:131–4.
6. Vyas RM, Dickinson BP, Wasson KL, Roostaeian J, Bradley JP. Pediatric facial fractures: current national incidence, distribution, and health care resource use. J Craniofac Surg. 2008;19(2):339–49; discussion 350.
7. Holland AJA, Broome C, Steinberg A, Cass DT. Facial fractures in children. Pediatr Emerg Care. 2001;17(3):157–60.
8. Siy RW, Brown RH, Koshy JC, Stal S, Hollier LH Jr. General management considerations in pediatric facial fractures. J Craniofac Surg. 2011;22(4):1190–5.
9. Criden MR, Ellis FJ. Linear nondisplaced orbital fractures with muscle entrapment. J AAPOS. 2007;11(2):142–7.
10. Ryan ML, Thorson CM, Otero CA, et al. Pediatric facial trauma: a review of guidelines for assessment, evaluation, and management in the emergency department. J Craniofac Surg. 2011;22(4):1183–9.
11. Bickley LS. Bates guide to physical examination and history taking. 11th ed. Philadelphia: Lippencott Williams & Wilkins; 2013.
12. Woodward T. Interpretation of dental radiographs. Top Companion Anim Med. 2009;24:37–43. Zero D, Zandona A, Vail M, Spolnik K. Dental caries and pulpal disease. Dent Clin North Am. 2011;55:29–46.
13. Andreasen JO. Periodontal healing after replantation and autotransplantation of incisors in monkeys. Int J Oral Surg. 1981;10:54–61.
14. Tsukiboshi M. Treatment planning for traumatized teeth. 2nd ed. Quintessence: Hanover Park; 2012.
15. Cvek M, Tsilingardis G, Andreasen JO. Survival of 534 incisors after intra-alveolar root fracture in patients aged 7-17 years. Dent Traumatol. 2008;24:379–08.
16. AAE, American Association of Endodontists. The recommended guidelines of the American Association of Endodontists for the treatment of traumatic dental injuries. AAE; 2013.
17. IADT. Guidelines for the management of traumatic dental injuries: 2. Avulsion of permanent teeth. Dent Traumatol. 2012;28:88–96.
18. Krasner P, Rankow H. New philosophy fr the treatment of avulsed teeth. Oral Surg Oral Med Oral Pathol. 1995;79:616.
19. Blomlof L. Milk and saliva as possible storage media for traumatically exarticulated teeth prior to replantation. Swed Dent J Suppl. 1981;8:1–26.
20. Lin DG, Kenny DJ, Barrett EJ, Leckic P, McCullough CAG. Storage conditions of avulsed teeth affect the phenotype of cultured human periodontal ligament cells. J Periodontal Res. 2000;35:42–50.
21. Roettger M, Greaves M, Ahmad M, Leon-Salazaar V. Sports-related oral and dentoalveolar trauma: pathophysiology, diagnosis, and emergent care. In: Roettger M, editor. Modern sports dentistry. Textbooks in contemporary dentistry. Cham: Springer; 2018. https://doi.org/10.1007/978-3-319-44416-1_3.

Reconstructive Surgery in Oral and Maxillofacial Region

45

Reza Tabrizi and Parsa Behnia

The reconstruction of oral and maxillofacial defects can be both challenging and satisfying. The orofacial defects most often result from trauma or pathologic lesions surgery and congenital problems. The aims of reconstructing orofacial defects consist of the restoration of complex functional, anatomic, and aesthetic characteristics. The decision-making in reconstruction surgery depends on patients and defects status, which should be considered case by case. This chapter discusses the significant options in soft tissue and bone reconstruction.

Evaluation of Patients with Orofacial Defects

The first step in a comprehensive patient evaluation is taking a history. The time and etiology of defects are essential. If the patient's health condition permits, the reconstruction should be done as soon as possible. Also, there are few exceptions in immediate reconstruction: (1) acute infection and (2) uncertainty in safe margin following cancer resection.

The etiology of defects can affect treatment planning. In traumatic patients, primary care is the treatment priority. For example, immediate reconstruction in gunshot patients is advocated if the patients' condition is stable [1]. Immediate reconstruction is necessary for through-and-through defects, covering vital anatomical structures and facial defects that affect patients' appearance.

Treatment planning can be modified according to the patient's health condition. A simple reconstruction option with a short operation duration is desirable for patients in American

Society of Anesthesiologists (ASA) III or IV. In particular, the use of reconstruction plate or pre-fabricated titanium mandible in compromised patients following segmental mandibular resection without continuity is recommended.

Radiographic Assessment

In hard tissue defects, a CT scan is beneficial. A three-dimensional CT scan can help estimate the size of defects and make 3D models. Studies showed that 3D models and the use of patient-specific pre-bent plates significantly decrease operation time and provide precise surgery [2, 3]. Furthermore, CT models can help surgeons determine any vital anatomical structure in proximity to defects.

Soft Tissue Defects in the Oral and Maxillofacial Region

Accurate preoperative planning, including flap design, is important than the technique of harvest flap harvesting. The "right" flap selection is essential, as otherwise, if an incorrect flap is chosen, the entire reconstructive attempt is downfallen to failure, despite how meticulously the surgical technique is done.

Regional Soft Tissue Flaps

Generally, regional flaps are the most common techniques used for the reconstruction of oral and maxillofacial defects. These techniques have the advantage of the donor site proximity to the recipient site and mostly depend on an "arc of rotation" as a limiting factor for regional flaps. Other benefits of such flaps are easy harvesting, reliability, short operation time, and requirement of no special instruments. The main

R. Tabrizi (✉)
Department of Oral and Maxillofacial Surgery, Dental School, Shahid Beheshti University of Medical Sciences, Tehran, Iran
e-mail: rtabrizi@sbmu.ac.ir

P. Behnia
Department of Oral and Maxillofacial Surgery, Shahid Beheshti University of Medical Sciences, Tehran, Iran
e-mail: Parsabehnia1@sbmu.ac.ir

disadvantages of local flaps are limited application due to the arc of rotation and a limited soft tissue for reconstruction. To overwhelm these limitations, free flap transportation should be considered as an alternative treatment option. A local flap is preferable when it is available to avoid the risks of a free tissue transfer.

Forehead and Scalp

The forehead and scalp defects have familiar characters: an inherent resistance to tissue distension, cosmetically noticeable areas such as the brows and hairline, and the potential involvement of neurovascular structures [4]. Defects can be of various sizes, from a small skin defect to a full-thickness defect.

The scalp defects may be large that the reconstruction is challenging due to relative scalp immobility. Tissue quality and coverage aims can differ in patients based on previous surgery, radiation, or other comorbidities. Surgical planning should provide function and aesthetics related to adjacent tissues to prevent overlooking. The knowledge of the scalp and forehead anatomy is essential to reach an acceptable outcome.

Secondary Intention Healing

A secondary intention is a nonsurgical technique that can be suitable for selected patients. In the absence of intrinsic wound-healing problems, particularly heavy smoking or a history of local radiation, the granulation tissue will form and secondary healing occurs. It is a good option for non-hair-bearing areas of the scalp (the temple or vertex) when defects consist of a partial-thickness wound. Patients who cannot tolerate a surgical procedure or are medically compromised are candidates for secondary intention healing. However, it is associated with significant scar formation and is not advocated for visible aesthetic zoon, such as the frontal. Smaller defects (less than 2 cm) with a vascularized bed wounds heal in a few weeks, whereas more extensive wounds may last a few months to completely close. Although secondary intention healing is associated with contraction (up to 60%), it should be noted that it can distort adjacent tissues [5].

Primary Wound Closure

Subcutaneous undermining around defects can decrease wound tension. Primary closure is useful for small defects less than 1–2 cm. It should be cautioned that the use of primary closure does not distort anatomic landmarks (Fig. 45.1a, b). For temple defects with size 3 cm or less, reconstruction with a distensible tissue is recommended. The surface anatomy relationships of the forehead, the hairline, and brow should be considered [6].

Tissue Expansion

Tissue expansion is a preferred approach for large defects in the scalp and frontal. Gradual tissue expansion depends on the phenomenon of biologic creep, which leads to permanent

Fig. 45.1 (**a**) Traumatic injuries in the left eyebrow, frontal, and the perioral area, which were repaired by primary closure; (**b**) the patient's view 6 months after repair

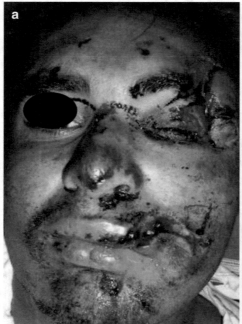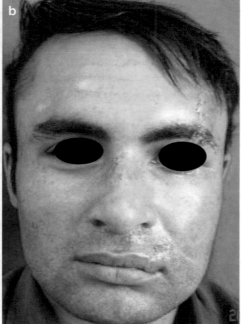

elongation of tissues due to tan external force. The biological effect concept in tissue expansion includes the adjacent skin movement, enhanced mitotic activity, cell proliferation, and endorsed angiogenesis [7]. The complications of tissue expansion consist of infection, implant or port exposure, hematoma, seroma implant leak, skin necrosis, and neurosensory disturbance overlying the implant. These complications can be prevented by correct placement of the implant, antibiotic prophylaxis for 2–3 weeks, and post-operative drain.

Skin Grafting

The skin has a dual role as a graft and recipient in reconstruction. It was used for resurfacing superficial defects in the scalp and frontal. Full-thickness skin grafts are useful in patients with tight skin and large defects that adjacent tissue transfer is difficult or result in distortion surface anatomy. Skin grafts often reduce the need for additional facial skin incisions; however, they are vulnerable to the formation of a "patch-like" appearance because of a mismatch of color, contour, or texture if not meticulously planned. Skin grafts should be used with caution. The skin graft is recommended in cases that cannot be reconstructed with local flaps or significant distortion [8].

Local Flaps

When primary closure is not possible, the local soft tissue flap is the workhorse for forehead and scalp reconstruction. Local flaps are not only advocated for small or medium defects, but they may also reconstruct select large defects. In general, local flaps can be characterized as advancement, transposition, or rotation flaps. The forehead region is cosmetically essential, and any alteration of the adjacent anterior hairline or brow position can lead to aesthetic disharmony and patient dissatisfaction. Furthermore, critical neurovascular structures cross the forehead and temporal regions and should not be injured to make reconstruction more convenient [9]. The unilateral or bilateral advancement flaps can reconstruct small (less than 3 cm) forehead defects. These flaps rely on random blood supply in the dermal and subdermal plexus. Advancement flaps should be designed with a length-to-width ratio of at least 4:1 [10].

Nose Reconstruction

The nasal pyramid locates in the middle face. Nasal prominence and central location are often associated with behavior and personal identity [11]. The local and regional flap reconstruction has advantages over skin grafts or free flaps in certain situations.

The restoration of the nasal mucosal lining is challenging. The ideal donor site should be similar to the nasal lining in vascularity and pliability. Skin grafts, free mucosal grafts, and local mucoperichondrial flaps are applied for restoration of the nasal lining.

Bone and cartilage graft replacement prevent soft tissue from collapsing under the forces of scar contracture. Moreover, they maintain airway patency during inspiration. Any reconstruction without restoration of cartilage and bony components results in scar contracture or soft tissue collapse and nasal deformity. Three donor sites are recommended for cartilage replacements: auricular cartilage, costal cartilage, and nasal septum. Cartilage grafts depend on the vascularity of the recipient site and the overlying flap. It is advocated that grafts should be placed in the early reconstruction stage before scar formation, which compromises the final aesthetic outcome. Reconstruction of the bony nasal pyramid or dorsum needs autogenous bone grafts. Different donor sites have been used for nasal bone reconstruction: calvaria graft, rib, iliac crest, the lateral ramus.

Skin coverage is the final stage of nasal reconstruction and is essential to achieve a desired aesthetic result. Local and distant flaps are used to restore soft tissue in nasal defects. The flap selection primarily depends on anatomic location, defect size, defect location, and the adjacent skin's quality. If soft tissue defects are in an area with thin and smooth and mobile skin, particularly the nasal dorsum, primary closure may be possible. In larger defects, a skin graft may be suitable. The skin and cartilage composite grafts may be used in a one-stage reconstructive for the alar rim defects. A sandwich graft of skin and cartilage from the root of the auricular helix is commonly used to restore full-thickness defects. The paramedian forehead flap is a gold standard for the reconstruction of extensive defects of the nose (Fig. 45.2a–d). It is an axial flap that relies on the supratrochlear artery [11].

Periorbital Reconstruction

Reconstruction aims in the periorbital region consist of providing ocular surface lubricity with an internal layer in the smooth mucus membrane structure to prevent corneal irritation. Forming tars that restore the lid's shape and hardness with fixed lid edges are essential for lashing out corneal contact. Restoration of eyelid defects with thin skin are necessary to allow lid movement and enough levator movement to permit the upper lid lifting. The periorbital aesthetic is another crucial issue that should be considered in treatment planning [12]. The defect zone, size, and type of defect (the full or partial layer thickness) are the significant factors that should be considered in treatment planning (Fig. 45.3a–c).

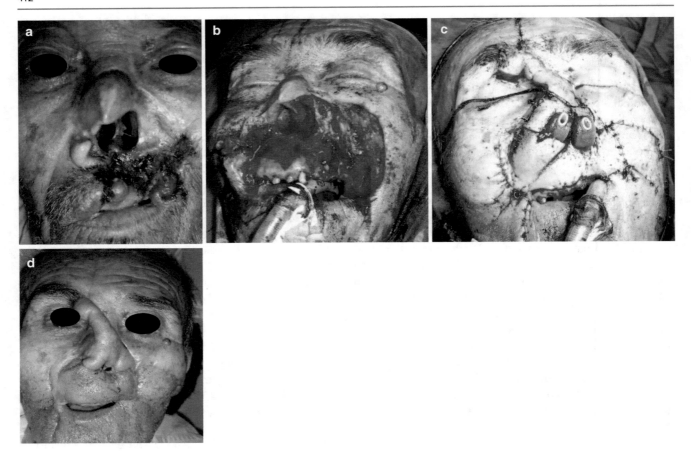

Fig. 45.2 (**a**) A patient with a massive basal cell carcinoma in the nasal and upper lip. (**b**) The nasal and perioral area's defect due to the tumor resection (**c**). A paramedian forehead flap for nose reconstruction and Kazanjian flap for closing the upper lip flap. (**d**) The patient 4 weeks after reconstruction

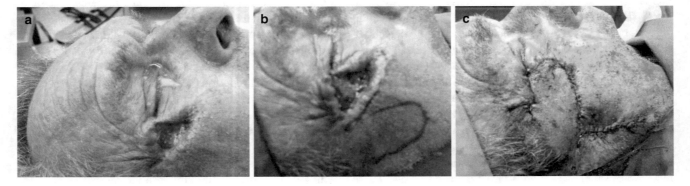

Fig. 45.3 (**a**) Ulcerative lesion (basal cell carcinoma) in the lateral of the left orbit. (**b**) The design of rotational flap for closure of the defect. (**c**) Reconstruction of the defect

The standard methods used in the reconstruction of periorbital defects include the split-thickness skin grafting, lid switch flap, Tenzel rotational flap, Cutler-Beard flap, forehead flap, Tripier flap, transconjunctival advancement (Hughes), and Mustarde's lid switch flap.

Lip Reconstruction

Lips are one of the essential components in a facial structure which maintains oral competence. Furthermore, lips have a role in mastication, communication, facial expression, and also beauty. Phonation of various sounds needs the advanced function of the lips and surrounding musculature. Defects of the lips are most often acquired, which are secondary to traumatic injuries or oncologic excision. The vermilion superficial defects usually heal by secondary intention. Minimal distortion occurs in this way. However, contraction should be expected in all wound healing.

Lip vermilion is a particular tissue that is different from any other soft tissue in the body. Furthermore, lip vermilion covers the orbicularis muscles, important to maintaining a proper sphincteric function of the lip. If vermillion defects are small, lateral, and superficial, the secondary intention healing may have an acceptable outcome. If such defects locate medially, primary closure is suitable. Anatomic landmarks, mainly the vermilion border and the white roll, should be marked and aligned with sutures. Three-layer closure of the buccal mucosa, orbicularis oris, and skin must be done. Mucosal closure should be performed using a fast absorbable suture, while the muscle layer is approximated with a slowly absorbable suture. Precise re-approximation of the orbicularis oris muscle prevents lips incompetency. The skin defects that include less than 50% of the philtrum can often be closed primarily when the philtrum is wide enough. This technique is mainly useful for the small skin defects of the lower philtrum that permits a wedge excision and local advancement. In partial-thickness defects in this area, preauricular full-thickness skin grafts have good clinical results [13].

Large defects of the vermilion need more advanced procedures such as vermilion switch flaps or vermilion advancement flaps. Vermilion advancement flaps are advocated in repairing midline vermilion defects. These flaps rely on the labial artery.

Larger defects in the central area of lips can also be closed primarily in men that can grow facial hair and conceal otherwise unappealing scars and asymmetry. In defects more significant than 50% of the philtrum that involves both skin and vermilion, an Abbe flap is the best choice [14].

Cheek Reconstruction

The cheek consists of four anatomic subunits: medial, lateral, buccal, and zygomatic. Inferiorly and laterally, the cheek abuts the mandible's inferior border, the preauricular crease, and the temporal hairline. The central subunits form the superior and medial borders: the lower eyelid, nasal sidewall and ala, the lip and oral commissure, and nasolabial fold. The size, shape, and subunit location of the defect are important factors in cheek reconstruction [15]. Small defects, particularly in concave areas, can heal by secondary intention. On convex regions such as the central expanse of the cheek, secondary healing is not suitable. The exception is the preauricular area that large defects can be left to granulate with acceptable aesthetic results. The nasofacial groove is also a desirable location in which to hide scars due to secondary intention. The secondary intention healing should be avoided in juxtaposition to the lower eyelid because scar contracture can lead to ectropion.

As significant elasticity and laxity inherent in the cheek skin with extensive subcutaneous fatty tissue lead in primary closure of relatively large wounds of the cheek. It is preferred that the closure be placed in peripheral subunit borders of the cheek or Relaxed skin tension lines (RSTLs). Medially, repairs should be paralleled to the nasofacial sulcus or nasolabial fold. Laterally, the closure should follow RSTLs. Long, linear closures of the cheek from the superomedial to inferolateral should be located parallel to both the nasolabial fold and RSTLs. Several regional and distant flaps can be used to restore extensive and composite defects in the cheek area, such as nasolabial flap, submental flap, and pectoralis major flap (Figs. 45.4 and 45.5).

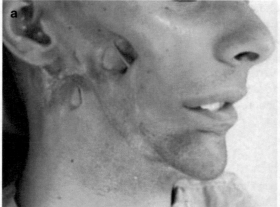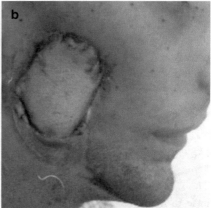

Fig. 45.4 (**a**) A buccal defect due to tumor resection and post-op radiotherapy. (**b**) The use of pectoralis major flap for reconstruction of the defect

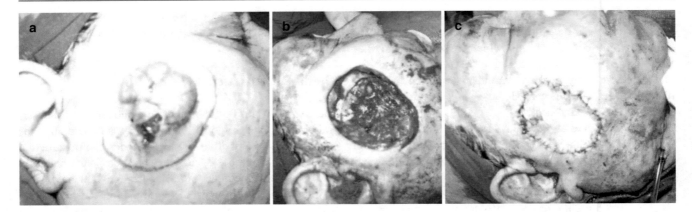

Fig. 45.5 (**a**) A tumoral lesion (basal cell carcinoma) in the malar area. (**b**) The defect of the malar area after tumor resection. (**c**) The reconstruction of the defect using a submental flap

Bone Defects in Maxillofacial Reconstruction

Frontal Defects

Reconstruction of the frontal bone defects aims to restore the normal contour and aesthetics. Various reconstruction options are available for frontal reconstruction. An ideal reconstruction material should be biocompatible, malleable, stable, and cost-effective. Alloplastic materials do not need a donor site and can be individually customized according to defects' size and shape. Furthermore, the use of alloplastic materials can reduce operation time and is associated with acceptable clinical results. Foreign body reaction and infection are the main disadvantages of alloplastic material applications. Autogenous sources such as calvaria grafts and iliac bone grafts can be used to restore the frontal defects. The second surgery in the donor site, unpredictable bone resorption, and difficulty forming grafts are disadvantages of using autogenous grafts [16].

Zygomatic Defects

The defects of zygoma can be due to traumatic injuries or oncologic surgeries. Zygomatic defects can compromise the patient's aesthetic. The use of customized alloplastic prosthesis is advocated for extensive zygomatic defects. The evidence advocates overall acceptable survival rates for the use of zygomatic implants [17]. Autogenous bone is another treatment option for zygomatic reconstruction.

Maxillary Defects

The maxilla is an anatomical structure connecting the skull base to the occlusal plane, anchors the maxillary dentition, resists the forces of mastication, separates the oral and nasal cavities, and is a prominent part of the orbit floor supporting the facial musculature [18]. The midface and maxillary defects may range from an oroantral fistula to a large defect from the skull base to the oral cavity.

The maxillary reconstruction aims include the restoration of the bone defect to provide a recipient site for dental implants, separation of the oral and nasal cavities, support of the orbital contents, and retorsion of facial contours.

Brawn and Shaw have classified the maxillary and midface defect as follows [19] – Vertical type: I. maxillectomy does not lead to an oronasal fistula; II. no orbital involvement; III. the orbital adnexae are involved with orbital retention; IV. maxillectomy with orbital enucleation or exenteration; V. orbitomaxillary defect; VI. nasomaxillary defect; Horizontal classification: (a) Palatal defect only, not involving the dental alveolus; (b) less than or equal to 1/2 unilateral; (c) less than or equal to 1/2 bilateral or transverse anterior; (d) greater than 1/2 maxillectomy.

Several techniques are available to reconstruct maxillary defects according to the patient's health condition, defect size, and location (Fig. 45.6). Historically, maxillary defects were reconstructed with a skin graft to provide a mucosal barrier and followed by an obturator [20]. Nowadays, free flaps are extensively used in the reconstructive field, and free flaps have successfully restored restoration function, quality of life, and improved cosmetics [21]. Limited maxillectomy defects that include a palatal defect without the orbital floor, cranial base, cheek involvement can be applied as an obturator. Obturators have many advantages: the treatment cost is cheaper than complex reconstruction procedures, a simple procedure without any operation, which is preferred in patients with a compromised health condition.

In using an obturator, surgeons should consider the size and location of the defect and may perform adjuvant procedures such as (1) removing the inferior turbinate to permit a sufficient space to accommodate the prosthesis, (2) coronoidectomy to prevent the obturator from getting dislodged in mandibular movement, or (3) skin grafting inside the

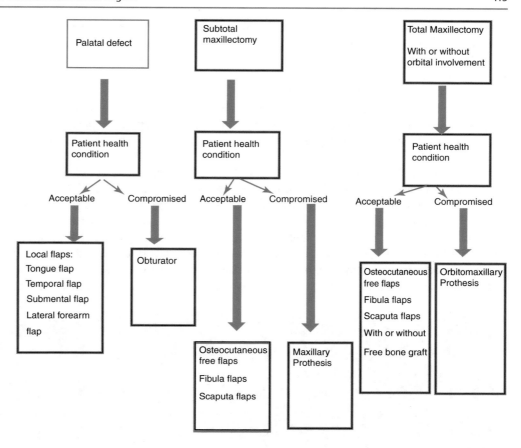

Fig. 45.6 The algorithm of reconstruction in the maxillary defects

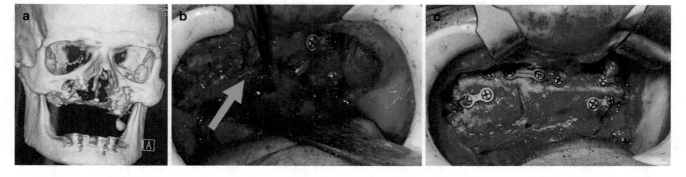

Fig. 45.7 (**a**) A maxillary defect due to a previous tumor surgery. (**b**) A pedicle of vascular fibula graft. (**c**) Reconstruction of the maxillary defect using a vascular fibular graft

defect to provide a scar band to aid in retention. Many free flaps have been used in the reconstruction of hard and soft tissues in the maxillary region. The radial forearm free flap is a workhorse in head and neck reconstructions; it could be relatively easily harvested, has a reliable and long pedicle, can be harvested simultaneously with maxillofacial cancer ablation, and often provides acceptable skin color match for maxillofacial reconstruction. The disadvantages of radial forearm flap include donor site morbidity, the risk of tendon exposure, and requirement of a split-thickness skin graft by the donor site for closure [22]. Osteocutaneous free flaps are

used to restore soft tissue components and bone defects simultaneously (Fig. 45.7a–c). The common free osteocutaneous flaps include the fibular free flap, scapular flap, radial forearm, and iliac crest free flap.

Mandibular Defects

Defects of the mandible following ablative surgery or traumatic injuries can be disfiguring and disabling. There are several reconstructive techniques for the reconstruction of mandibular continuity as well as oro-mandibular function. Soft tissue reconstruction should be considered before hard tissue reconstruction. Perioral soft tissue defects are challenging because of functional and aesthetic concerns (Fig. 45.8a–c). Early attempts for mandibular reconstruction relied on using non-vascularized, autogenous bone grafts (Fig. 45.9a–c). The risk of graft infection and soft tissue dehiscence was high due to salivary contamination and adjuvant radiation, leading to bone loss or bone resorption. It is advocated for mandibular defects whose sizes are more than 5 cm; pedicled osteomyocutaneous flaps should be used [23]. Today, osteocutaneous free tissue transfer is the gold standard for mandibular reconstruction (Fig. 45.10a–c).

A simple classification of mandibular defects includes total mandibular defects, subtotal hemimandibular defects, mandibular defects with continuity and without continuity, and concomitant soft tissue (buccal or lingual) defects.

The mandibular reconstruction goals are to restore the lower third of the face and reestablish the patient's function (mastication, speech).

The tongue defect due to cancer resection affects the patient's prognosis for recovery of oral function. If patients have tongue defects with mandibular defects, the reconstruction approach should start by addressing the tongue. In most cases, restoration of tongue bulk and improvement of mobility are more important in the post-operative functional recovery than simple management of the bony defect. Loss of oral mucosa in the mouth floor is critical in evaluating whether to reconstruct it with non-native tissue. Restoration of tongue bulk and preservation of mobility permit palatoglossal contact, which is essential for improving articulation during speech and manipulating bolus during swallowing. Dentition and occlusion are two crucial factors in treatment planning for mandibular reconstruc-

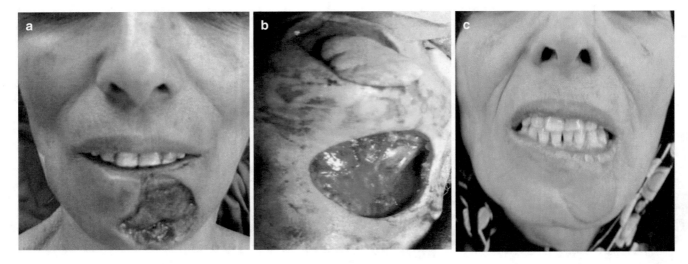

Fig. 45.8 (a) The defect of the lower lip and submental area due to human bite. (b) The reconstruction of the defect using a submental flap. (c) The patient 2 months after reconstruction

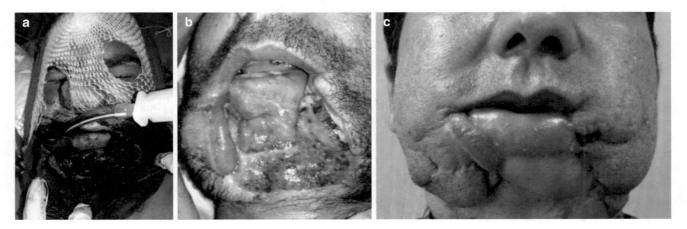

Fig. 45.9 (a) The soft tissue and hard tissue defects of the mandible and lower lip. (b) The defect after debridement. (c) The reconstruction of the mandible and lower lip using an osteocutaneous fibula graft

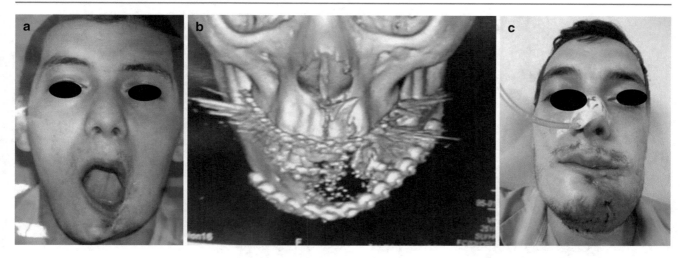

Fig. 45.10 (**a**) A mandibular and soft tissue defect due to a gunshot injury. (**b**) The primary reconstruction with a reconstruction plate before referring to our department. (**c**) The defects were restored with an osteocutaneous fibula graft

tion. The final aim of mandibular reconstruction is the restoration of oral function and dentition.

A free bone graft is advocated for small bone defects (<5 cm) with sufficient soft tissue coverage. It can be used in mandibular defects with or without continuity. Rigid fixation with a reconstruction plate is essential for achieving good clinical results. In mandibular defects with continuity, miniplates can be applied for rigid fixation.

It is essential to preserve mandibular symmetry by using the mirror technique and individually customized plates. Simultaneously, tumor resection and reconstruction, construction of a three-dimensional mandibular model, and mirror technique help receive a desirable result. The placement reconstruction plate before resection can prevent the condylar segment (proximal segment) displacement.

In extensive bone defects (>5 cm) or small bone defects with concomitant soft tissue defects, osteocutaneous free flaps are the gold standard. Free osteocutaneous fibula graft is the right choice for such defects, which restore hard and soft tissues. The vascular pedicle supplying the fibula flap is relatively long, and 20–26 cm of bone may be harvested in adults, sufficient for total mandibular defects. The fibula flap's pedicle can reach vessels in the inferior and the contralateral neck in mandibular reconstruction. The fibular bone quality is ideal for mandibular reconstruction, and dental implants can be placed with reliable results. The major drawback of using the fibula graft in mandibular reconstruction is the restoration of mandibular height. The alveolar height of a normal dentate mandible is more than the diameter of the fibular bone. For restoring the alveolar height, the double-barrel technique is recommended [24] (Fig. 45.11a–e).

The iliac crest flap is another flap for mandibular reconstruction. It has advantages such as sufficient bone volume,

good shape, and height, making it an optimal choice for plate fixation and implant placement for dental restoration [25]. The harvested bone is mainly cancellous. The iliac bone can be contoured to restore segmental mandibular defects. The hemimandible defect can be reconstructed from the ipsilateral ilium. The internal oblique muscle can be harvested and intraoral mucosal defect can be repaired by including the deep circumflex iliac artery's ascending branch. The internal oblique muscle is pliable, thin, and can be manipulated independent of the bone and more reliably than the overlying skin flap.

Custom-Made Titanium Prosthesis for Mandibular Reconstruction

The gold standard in the restoration of large mandibular defects is free bone flaps. In a few conditions, free flaps are contraindicated, such as stenosis or a lack of good-quality cervical vessels, lupus anticoagulants, stenosis of the fibula flap pedicle, patient's health condition is not suitable for an extended surgery. The use of custom-made titanium prosthesis through 3D designing helps to restore the mentioned situations. The 3D design restores the anatomy of the mandible, and the operation is simplified with the use of the cutting guides and pre-drilling. There is no donor site morbidity. Long-term tolerance with use of custom-made titanium is not yet well known [26]. Custom-made titanium prosthesis can be used as a titanium mesh in combination with autogenous particle bone grafts. It allows placing dental implants after bone healing (Fig. 45.12a–c). The use of custom-made prostheses is advocated in older patients who cannot tolerate an extended operation for microvascular reconstruction. In the same condition, reconstruction with autografts (free or vascular) is prioritized on the use of alloplastic devices.

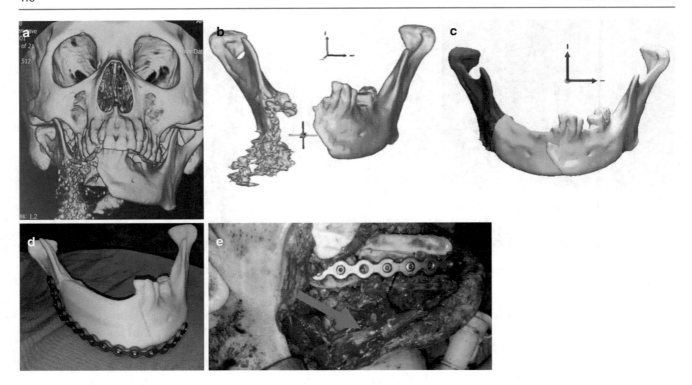

Fig. 45.11 (**a**) A mandibular defect due to a gunshot injury. (**b**) Three-dimensional models of the mandible show a collapse of mandibular segments. (**c**) The displaced segments were aligned in a computer model to demonstrate the actual size of the defect. (**d**) The mandibular model was reconstructed based on the computer model, and a reconstruction plate was bent on the model. (**e**) A double-barrel vascular fibula graft was used to reconstruct the mandible

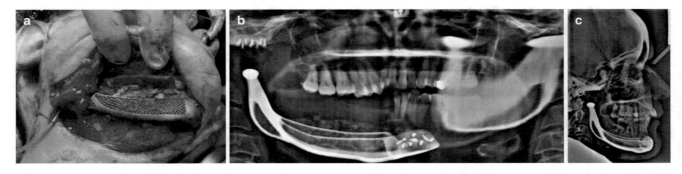

Fig. 45.12 (**a**) A custom-made titanium mesh, combined with autogenous particles from the iliac, was used to reconstruct the hemimandibular defect. (**b**) OPG view after reconstruction. (**c**) The lateral cephalometric view after reconstruction. (Courtesy of Hamed Kermani, DMD)

References

1. Jose A, Arya S, Nagori S. High-velocity ballistic injuries inflicted to the maxillofacial region. J Craniofac Surg. 2019;30(6):e511–e4.
2. Naros A, Weise H, Tilsen F, Hoefert S, Naros G, Krimmel M, et al. Three-dimensional accuracy of mandibular reconstruction by patient-specific pre-bent reconstruction plates using an "in-house" 3D-printer. J Craniomaxillofac Surg. 2018;46(9):1645–51.
3. Liang Y, Jiang C, Wu L, Wang W, Liu Y, Jian X. Application of combined osteotomy and reconstruction pre-bent plate position (CORPPP) technology to assist in the precise reconstruction of segmental mandibular defects. J Oral Maxillofac Surg. 2017;75(9):2026.e1–e10.
4. Bradford BD, Lee JW. Reconstruction of the forehead and scalp. Facial Plast Surg Clin North Am. 2019;27(1):85–94.
5. Leedy JE, Janis JE, Rohrich RJ. Reconstruction of acquired scalp defects: an algorithmic approach. Plast Reconstr Surg. 2005;116(4):54e–72e.
6. Olson MD, Hamilton GS 3rd. Scalp and forehead defects in the post-Mohs surgery patient. Facial Plast Surg Clin North Am. 2017;25(3):365.
7. Han Y, Zhao J, Tao R, Guo L, Yang H, Zeng W, et al. Repair of craniomaxillofacial traumatic soft tissue defects with tissue expansion in the early stage. J Craniofac Surg. 2017;28(6):1477–80.
8. Brenner MJ, Moyer JS. Skin and composite grafting techniques in facial reconstruction for skin cancer. Facial Plast Surg Clin North Am. 2017;25(3):347–63.

9. Desai SC, Sand JP, Sharon JD, Branham G, Nussenbaum BJ. Scalp reconstruction: an algorithmic approach and systematic review. JAMA Facial Plast Surg. 2015;17(1):56–66.

10. Lee S, Rafii AA, Sykes J. Advances in scalp reconstruction. Curr Opin Otolaryngol Head Neck Surg. 2006;14(4):249–53.

11. Skaria AM. The median forehead flap reviewed: a histologic study on vascular anatomy. Eur Arch Otorhinolaryngol. 2015;272(5):1231–7.

12. Yüce S, Demir Z, Selçuk CT, Çelebioğlu S. Reconstruction of periorbital region defects: a retrospective study. Ann Maxillofac Surg. 2014;4(1):45.

13. Salibian AA, Zide BM. Elegance in upper lip reconstruction. Plast Reconstr Surg. 2019;143(2):572–82.

14. Shipkov H, Stefanova P, Djambazov K, Uchikov A. Upper lip reconstruction. Plast Reconstr Surg. 2018;142(1):102e–3e.

15. Cass ND, Terella AM. Reconstruction of the cheek. Facial Plast Surg Clin North Am. 2019;27(1):55–66.

16. Dova S, Karkos PD, Constantinidis J. Reconstruction of frontal defects with calvarial grafts. Rhinology. 2018;56(3):297–302.

17. Hackett S, El-Wazani B, Butterworth C. Zygomatic implant-based rehabilitation for patients with maxillary and mid-facial oncology defects: a review. Oral Dis. 2020;27(1):27–41.

18. O'Connell DA, Futran ND. Reconstruction of the midface and maxilla. Curr Opin Otolaryngol Head Neck Sur. 2010;18(4):304–10.

19. Brown JS, Shaw RJ. Reconstruction of the maxilla and midface: introducing a new classification. Lancet Oncol. 2010;11(10):1001–8.

20. Costa H, Zenha H, Sequeira H, Coelho G, Gomes N, Pinto C, et al. Microsurgical reconstruction of the maxilla: algorithm and concepts. J Plast Reconstr Aesthet Surg. 2015;68(5):e89–e104.

21. Vincent A, Burkes J, Williams F, Ducic Y. Free flap reconstruction of the maxilla. Semin Plast Surg. 2019;33(1):30–7.

22. Lyons AJ. Perforator flaps in head and neck surgery. Int J Oral Maxillofac Surg. 2006;35(3):199–207.

23. Bak M, Jacobson AS, Buchbinder D, Urken ML. Contemporary reconstruction of the mandible. Oral Oncol. 2010;46(2):71–6.

24. Likhterov I, Roche AM, Urken ML. Contemporary osseous reconstruction of the mandible and the maxilla. Oral Maxillofac Surg Clin North Am. 2019;31(1):101–16.

25. Zheng L, Lv X, Zhang J, Zhang J, Zhang Y, Cai Z, et al. Deep circumflex iliac artery perforator flap with iliac crest for oromandibular reconstruction. J Craniomaxillofac Surg. 2018;46(8):1263–7.

26. Qassemyar Q, Assouly N, Temam S, Kolb F. Use of a three-dimensional custom-made porous titanium prosthesis for mandibular body reconstruction. Int J Oral Maxillofac Surg. 2017;46(10):1248–51.

Cleft Lip and Palate Diagnosis and Surgical Intervention

Reihaneh Heidari and Behrooz Amirzargar

Epidemiology

Cleft lip and palate are congenital deformities seen in newborns and need special considerations to prevent aesthetic deformity or functional problems. The prevalence of cleft lip is about 1 in every 2800 newborns and the prevalence of cleft palate is approximately 1 in every 1700 newborns in the United States [1]. However, it has been reported that the overall and worldwide incidence of cleft lip or palate is 1 in every 700 births. The incidence of cleft lip with or without cleft palate is highest among Native Americans and lowest among blacks, but the incidence of cleft palate does not vary between ethnic groups. Cleft lip with or without cleft palate is two times more common in males, but cleft palate alone is two times more common in females. Unilateral clefts are more common than bilateral clefts, and left clefts are also more common than right clefts [2, 3].

Etiology

The etiology of cleft lip and palate is multifactorial. Genetic and environmental factors both play a role in developing these deformities. It has been shown that many genes contribute to the cleft lip and palate etiology. Environmental factors such as several teratogens have been associated with the development of the cleft lip and palate. They include smoking, alcohol consumption, phenytoin, valproic acid, thalidomide, dioxins, and retinoic acid [4–7].

Embryologic Development

Knowing the normal development of the lip and palate is critical to understand the clefts and associated anatomical anomalies. As shown in Fig. 46.1, normal facial development occurs during the 4th to 10th embryonic week from frontonasal prominence, maxillary prominence, mandibular prominence, lateral and medial nasal prominence. The fusion of the medial nasal prominences (nasomedial processes) and maxillary prominences at each side forms the upper lip.

Normal development of the palate occurs during the 5th to 12th embryonic week. Fusion of the deeper surface of the two medial nasal prominences forms the primary palate which is the anterior part of the palate and located anterior to the incisive foramen. After the development of the primary palate, the secondary palate develops which is the posterior part of the palate and located posterior to the incisive foramen. Bilateral ingrowth of the maxillary prominences forms the palatine shelves which fuse in the midline and form the secondary palate (Fig. 46.2).

Associated Anomalies

In patients with cleft lip and cleft palate deformities, special consideration should be given to the nose. Because the development of these structures depends on each other, defects in the development of the lip or nose can cause deformity of the nose, especially in the floor of the nose. Furthermore, other facial, dental, and alveolar deformities may be seen in these patients. Also, associated genetic disorders should be considered in these patients.

R. Heidari (✉) · B. Amirzargar
Otorhinolaryngology Research Center,
Department of Otorhinolaryngology-Head and Neck Surgery,
Imam Khomeini Hospital Complex, Tehran University of Medical Sciences, Tehran, Iran
e-mail: rheidari@sina.tums.ac.ir; amirzargarb@sina.tums.ac.ir

© The Author(s), under exclusive license to Springer Nature Switzerland AG 2021
M. R. Stevens et al. (eds.), *Innovative Perspectives in Oral and Maxillofacial Surgery*,
https://doi.org/10.1007/978-3-030-75750-2_46

Fig. 46.1 Development of facial structures

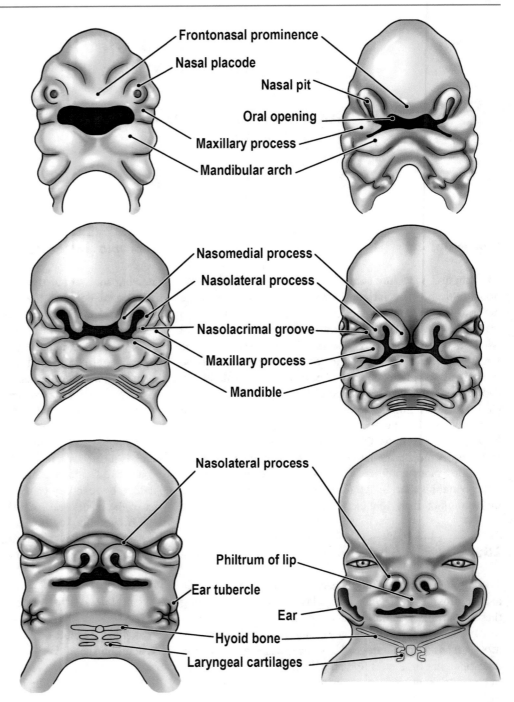

Diagnosis

Diagnosis of cleft lip is easily made in the newborn because of an unusual form of the upper lip, but the diagnosis of cleft palate may be done during infancy or even during childhood as a result of recurrent regurgitation or aspiration.

Prenatal diagnosis of the cleft lip and palate can be made using prenatal ultrasonography and more accurately using three-dimensional ultrasonography. However, the diagnosis of cleft palate is more difficult and requires special consideration. The accuracy of diagnosis improves with age and can be made as early as 18 weeks of the embryo.

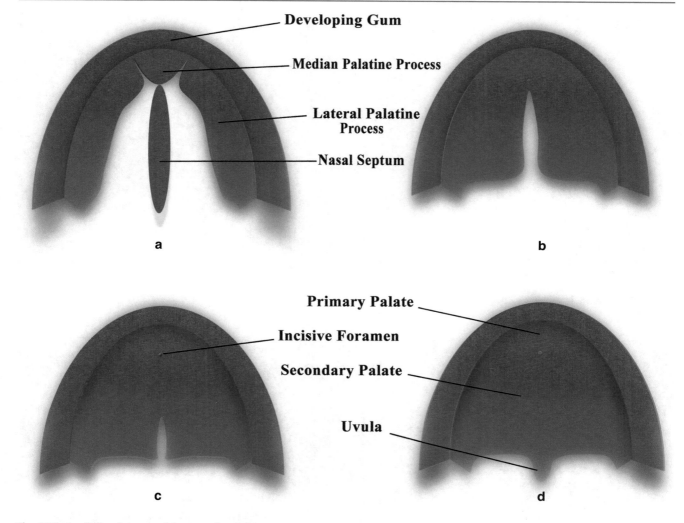

Fig. 46.2 (a–d) Development of the secondary palate

Cleft Lip

The normal upper lip consists of the skin, orbicularis oris muscle, and the mucous membrane. The junction between the skin and the upper lip's mucous membrane is called the vermilion border, which is a key structure during cleft lip repair. The orbicularis oris muscle is a sphincter of the mouth and creates a muscular sling around the oral cavity. In patients with cleft lip, the orbicularis oris muscle has an abnormal direction and insertion and, therefore, an abnormal function.

Classification

Cleft lip deformity can be classified as unilateral or bilateral, and each category consists of incomplete or complete types (Figs. 46.3 and 46.4). Sometimes there is a complete cleft of

the upper lip on one side and an incomplete cleft on the other side (Fig. 46.4a). In patients with incomplete cleft lip deformity, a notch in the upper lip appears, and the cleft does not completely involve the vertical height of the upper lip. In these patients, a variety of skin and muscular structures may be present in this segment. But in the complete cleft lip deformity, all the vertical height of the upper lip is involved. It is usually associated with the cleft of the alveolar process and the nasal floor.

In patients with an incomplete cleft lip, the orbicularis oris muscle's lower fiber abnormally inserts into the tissue at the cleft margins. Still, upper muscle fibers have a horizontal direction and form a partial oral sphincter. In patients with complete unilateral cleft lip, the muscle fibers have a vertical direction along the cleft's margin and insert into the nasal alae in the lateral part and into the columella medially. In patients with complete bilateral cleft lip, the muscle fibers at

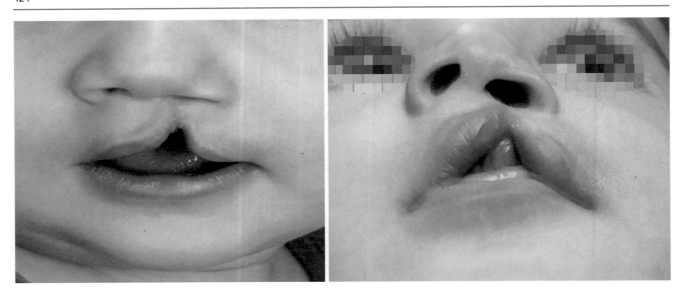

Fig. 46.3 Unilateral incomplete cleft lip

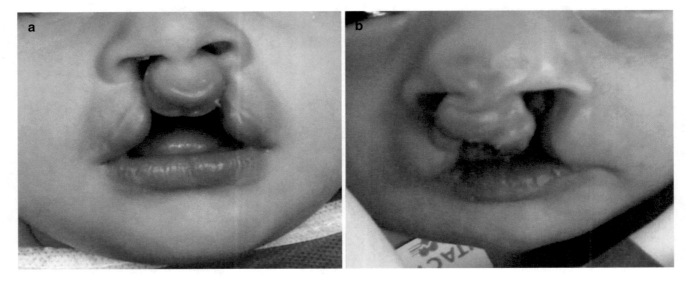

Fig. 46.4 (**a**) Bilateral cleft lip (complete at the right side and incomplete at the left side). (**b**) Bilateral complete cleft lip

the lateral segments insert into the nasal alae laterally, but the prolabial segment lacks muscle fiber. Also, these patients have varying degrees of premaxillary protrusion and short columella.

Nasal deformities in patients with unilateral cleft lip include deviation of the columella toward the normal side, short columella and lack of tip projection on the cleft side, short medial crus and long lateral crus on the cleft side, displacement of the alar base on the cleft side to the lateral, caudal, and posterior, wide or absent nasal floor on the cleft side, horizontally oriented nostril on the cleft side, and deviation of the septum to the normal side. Furthermore, the maxillary bone is underdeveloped on the affected side.

Nasal deformities in patients with bilateral cleft lip include a broad and flat tip, varying degrees of short columella or even absent columellar skin on surface inspection, short caudal septum, short lower lateral cartilage, laterally displaced alae, horizontally oriented nostrils, and bilaterally wide or absent nasal floor. Also, the entire premaxilla is underdeveloped in these patients.

Cleft Lip Repair

Initial management of patients with cleft lip depends on the width of the cleft. Incomplete clefts usually require fewer tensions on the lip closure site during surgery. There is no need for initial management but wide unilateral or bilateral clefts may need orthodontic or molding techniques to narrow the cleft gap's width. One of the simplest and easiest ways to narrow the gap is lip taping across the cleft several weeks before the surgery. Another technique used to narrow the wide gap is nasoalveolar molding (NAM). It is a presurgical treatment modality that Grayson first described in the 1990 [8]. NAM is an orthodontic technique that is used to reduce the severity of both hard and soft tissue deformities. These maneuvers help narrow the gap and help retract the protruded premaxilla, especially in patients with bilateral cleft lip, thereby leading to improved cosmetic results [8–10].

The timing of surgical repair depends on the infant's prematurity, general condition, application of molding, and preference of the surgeon. It is usually performed during the second to third months of the infant's life.

There are many described techniques for cleft lip repair. We only discussed the most common technique in this chapter. Millard technique or rotation advancement technique is the most common technique used for surgical repair of cleft lip. Unilateral left lip is repaired by lateral rotation of the medial segment of the cleft lip in conjunction with the cleft's lateral segment's medical advancement. First of all, before the injection of the solution of 1/200,000 epinephrine and lidocaine 2%, skin marking should be done. It can be done using a marker pen and a 27-gauge needle is inserted into methylene blue dye to mark the basic points (Fig. 46.5). These points are from 1 to 12 and 6 points on each side. The first one is a point at the exact low point of Cupid's bow at the mucocutaneous junction, which marks the upper lip's central point. Second point is made at the peak of the Cupid's bow on the noncleft side. Then the distance between points 1 and 2 is measured and used to locate point 3, which is the peak of the Cupid's bow on the cleft side. Alar base and the columella base at the noncleft side mark as points 4 and 5, respectively. Point 5 is the superior-most extent of the vertical portion of the rotation flap. Also, there is an extra back-cut point at the noncleft side which represents X in Fig. 46.3, which depends on the difference in the vertical height of the lip between the two sides, and it should not cross the philtral ridge of the noncleft side. Oral commissures on the noncleft and cleft side mark as points 6 and 7, respectively. The distance between points 2 and 6 is measured and used to locate the peak of the Cupid's bow on the cleft side, which is at an equal distance from point 7, and it marks as point 8. Point 9 is the medial-most point of the advancement flap. The distance between points 8 and 9 is equal to the distance between point 3 and point 5 + X. Points 10 and 11 are marked at the alar base and along the alar-facial crease at the cleft side. The estimated lateral-most aspect of the advancement flap also marks as point 12 [11].

The procedure starts with a sharp blade to make the incisions according to the skin markings. The rotation and the advancement flap are made, starting with through and through incisions and the mucosa at the edge of the cleft should be removed. A triangular skin flap then remains between the rotation flap and the edge of the cleft, sutured to point 12. To help the mobility of the flap and decrease tension on the closure site, usually, gingivobuccal sulcus mucosa is released from the face of the maxilla.

The release of the lower lateral cartilage at the cleft side is done through the alar base and columellar incisions. It

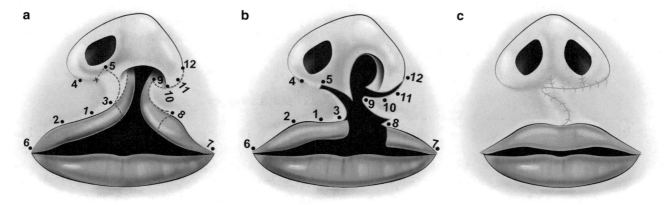

Fig. 46.5 (**a–c**) Millard technique for unilateral left lip repair

will help to reposition the lower lateral cartilage during primary rhinoplasty. Usually, one or two suspension sutures are placed from the lower lateral cartilage to the upper lateral cartilage to suspend the lower lateral cartilage on the cleft side in the superior-medial direction. It will help to reposition the lower lateral cartilage and alar base medially, increase tip projection, and also create greater symmetry.

For the closure of the cleft, the oral mucosa's closure should be done first using 4-0 Vicryl or Monocryl. Then the muscle layer should be sutured using 4-0 nylon or prolene. The first stitch attaches the muscle at the tip of the advancement flap to the muscle at point X. The next important stitch attaches the muscles at the level of the vermilion border. This is a key stitch for the alignment of the vermilion border. After that, these two stitches retract in the opposite direction, and two or three additional stitches are used to complete the muscle layer closure. Finally, skin closure can be done using a 6-0 nylon without any tension. Undermining along the edge of the flap incisions will help to evert the skin edge during wound closure. Attention should be done during skin closure, especially at the vermilion border, to achieve a straight and non-broken line of the vermilion border.

The most preferred method for the repair of the bilateral cleft lip is the Millard technique. Repair of bilateral cleft lip follows the same rules. Orthodontic devices are also used to retract the protruded premaxilla and reduce the gap before the surgery. Marking for the repair of the bilateral cleft lip is shown in Fig. 46.6. Points 1 and 2 are placed 2 mm lateral to the midpoint at the columellar-labial junction, which creates the philtral flap base. Point 5 is at the low point of Cupid's bow at the mucocutaneous junction, which marks the upper lip's central point. Points 3 and 4 are at the same distance (3 mm) from point 5, which is the peak of the Cupid's bow on both sides. There are c and d skin flaps with two forked flaps and use to place in the nasal sills. The central part's mucosa may be used as an e flap to reinforce the lip tubercle from behind. The markings of the lateral segments are the same as the lateral segments of the unilateral cleft lip. Incisions and elevation of the flaps and also suturing of the flaps are shown in Fig. 46.6.

Complications

One of the most common complications of cleft lip repair is partial wound dehiscence or separation. Placement of the tension-free sutures can prevent this complication. Other possible complications of cleft lip repair are vermilion notching, lip asymmetry, hypertrophic or keloid scar formation, stitch abscess, stitch marks formation, wound infection, bleeding, hematoma, feeding problems, airway obstruction, and rarely complete wound breakdown.

Cleft Palate

The normal palate consists of an anterior bony compartment (hard palate) and a soft tissue posterior component (soft palate). Soft palate consist of six paired muscles which work together, including levator veli palatine (the major muscle of soft palate, that orient transversally and work as a sling of the soft palate for speech and swallowing function, [12] musculus uvulae (help for velopharyngeal sufficiency and speech) [13], tensor veli palatine (major function for Eustachian tube dilation) [14], palatopharyngeus muscle, palatoglossus muscle, and superior constrictor.

In all forms of cleft palate, the orientation of the muscles is abnormal, and also the muscle and mucosa that overlay it are deficient [15], except for the submucosal cleft palate in which the integrity of mucosa is normal.

Classification of Cleft Palate

The incisive foramen is the landmark for classification. The defects anterior and posterior to this foramen named primary cleft palate (which includes primary palate, prolabium, premaxilla, anterior septum) and secondary cleft palate, respectively, also depend on the severity. They are classified as complete or incomplete and unilateral or bilateral cleft palate (Fig. 46.7).

In the submucosal cleft palate, the soft palate muscles are abnormally oriented, and the junction of levator veli palatine in the midline is dehiscence, but the mucosa is normal. Therefore, the cleft cannot be seen during the physical examination, but a translucent zone in the midline, notch in the posterior hard palate, or bifid uvulae can be detected [16].

Cleft Palate Surgery

Palatoplasty is a challenging surgery because the palate has very important functions such as swallowing, speech, the barrier of the nose to prevent regurgitation of saliva and food, preserve stable airway pathway. Therefore, in this surgery, all of these functions need to be considered. Also, the development of the palate has an important impact on facial growth. Hence, it will be affected by the type and severity of

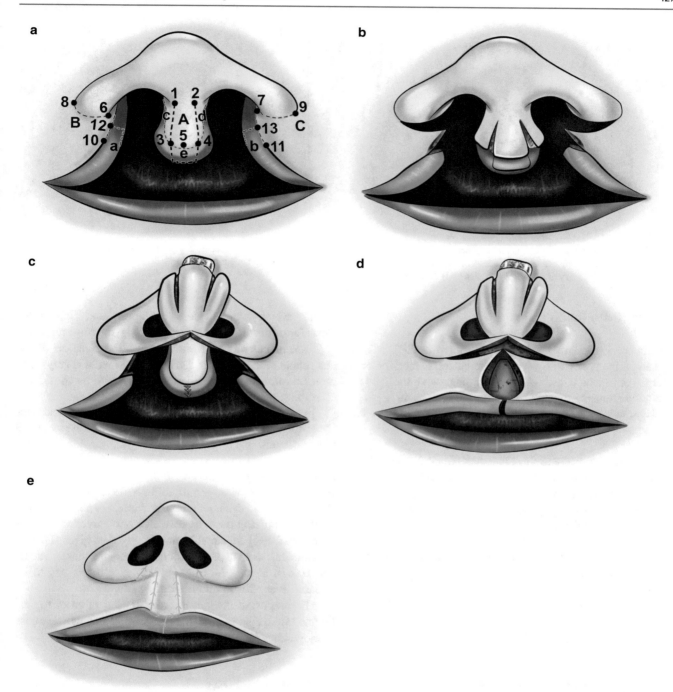

Fig. 46.6 (**a–e**) Bilateral left lip repair

the cleft. The timing of surgery is critical, too, because immediate reconstruction of this malformation will help maximize the coordination of the neuromuscular system and help result in better outcome of speech function [17, 18]. On the other hand, some studies demonstrated that manipulating hard palate mucoperiosteum during early infancy may have advers effect on facial growth if this surgery done in early-stage [19–21], thus recommend surgery in two stages [22, 23] and some studies are against that and emphasize the advantages of earlier surgery [17, 18].

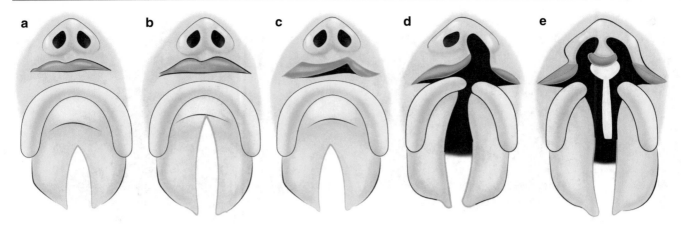

Fig. 46.7 Classification of cleft palate: (**a**) incomplete cleft of the secondary palate, (**b**) complete cleft of the secondary palate, (**c**) incomplete cleft of the primary and secondary palate, (**d**) unilateral complete cleft of the primary and secondary palates, (**e**) bilateral complete cleft of the primary and secondary palates

Palatoplasty Techniques

There are several methods for repairing the cleft palate. Based on the type and severity of the palatal defect, the best technique can be chosen. Therefore, diagnosing the type of cleft and choosing the best technique are important.

Here are some of the most common techniques used for the repair of cleft palate:

– Primary veloplasty (Schweckendiek palatoplasty)
– Bipedicle flap palatoplasty (Von Langenbeck)
– V-Y pushback palatoplasty
– Double-opposing Z-plasty (Furlow palatoplasty)
– Sommerlad palatoplasty

The best outcomes of all of these techniques are based on three primary rules:

1. Discrimination and preservation of these three soft palate layers: oral mucosa layer, the palatal muscle layer, and the nasal mucosa layer during dissection
2. Preservation of neurovascular bundle at the greater palatine foramen
3. Reorientation of palatal muscle in the best situation

Surgical Intervention

Preoperative Consideration

Patients with cleft palate may have other problems due to impaired embryologic development, and also it may be accompanied by syndromic problems like Pierre Robin sequence that can compromise the anesthesia and surgical process because these patients have micrognathia and retrognathia which complicate ventilation and intubation. Therefore, consult with an anesthesiologist before surgery.

Also, in patients with cleft palate, the function of the eustachian tube is disturbed. Thus, otitis media is very common, and insertion of ventilation tube should be considered after the surgical repair of the cleft palate.

As with the other surgeries, past medical history and family history, especially coagulopathy and heart disease, need to be checked.

Intraoperative Attention

Injection of perioperative antibiotics for decreasing infection after surgery and dexamethasone sodium phosphate 0.25 mg/kg for minimizing postoperative airway obstruction are recommended [24]. A suitable mouth gag that gives the best exposure has to be used, and for decreasing the tongue edema and risk of airway obstruction after surgery, it has to be released every 30–45 minutes during surgery.

After exposing the surgical site, the injection of topical lidocaine and epinephrine to the dissection area will decrease intraoperative hemorrhage.

Surgical Techniques

Two Flap Palatoplasty

This technique for repairing the cleft palate is one of the most used procedures and includes incisions that extend from the incisive foramen to the alveolar part of the cleft. In this technique, four flaps are designed to repair a cleft palate and two flaps are elevated from both sides of the vomer and transposed laterally for attaching to the medial edge of the nasal floor mucosa to repair the nasal side. Two mucoperiosteal flaps are then rotated in the middle to close the gap

a   b

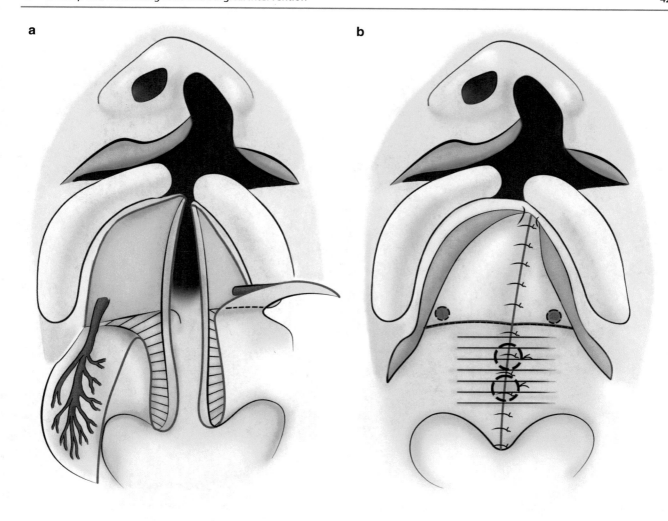

Fig. 46.8 (**a**) The red line presents the incision location for providing the flap. (**b**) Closure of the oral layer after suturing the vomer and nasal side mucosa

(Fig. 46.8). This method has limitations, like the alveolar cleft will not be closed with this technique, and it also can't help if a longer palate is needed [11].

Furlow Palatoplasty: Double-Opposing Z-Plasty

Double-opposing Z-plasty was first described by Furlow in 1986 [25]. If lengthening of the soft palate and repair of the palate muscle function are needed, this technique can be helpful. Moreover, this method often is used to repair the complete primary and secondary cleft palates. It also repairs the submucosal cleft palate.

It is not only a useful but also a hard technique because it requires dissection of mucosa and muscle from each other on each side of the cleft and moves the muscle layers backward and the mucosal layer forward.

The advantage of this method is preservation of the mucosa and muscle layers and reconstruction of muscle function. Therefore, speech outcome of this technique is superior compared to two-flap palatoplasty [26, 27].

Surgical Procedure

Surgical procedure for a left side cleft (for a right-handed surgeon) is as follows:

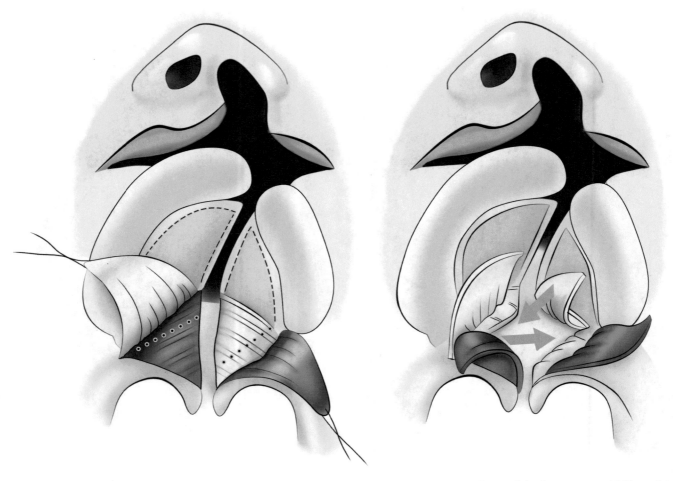

Fig. 46.9 Left: Dotted lines show the incisions to design the flap. Areas with red color show the muscle-containing layers, areas with blue color show submucosa-only layer. Right: The muscle-containing layers transpose posteriorly and the mucosa-only layer transposes anteriorly

1. Oral and nasal mucosa are separated by a sharp incision to the medial border of the left cleft.
2. The incision is made parallel to the posterior border of the hard palate, starting 3 mm posterior of the hard palate and soft palate junction and continuing to the posterior border of hamulus.
3. Dissection of oral mucosa and soft palate muscle from nasal mucosa starts from the incisions and continues to the lateral pharyngeal wall, in which the superior border is the hamulus and the inferior border is the top of the tonsillar fossa.

Surgical procedure for the right side of the cleft is as follows:

1. Oral and nasal mucosa are separated by a sharp incision to the medial border of the right cleft.
2. The incision is made parallel to the incision of left cleft but starts from the posterior border of right hamulus to the posterior endpoint of right cleft (base of uvula).
3. Dissection of oral mucosa and submucosa from the muscle layer is made (Fig. 46.9).

Mucosal and muscle layer flaps from the right and left sides transpose posteriorly. The mucosa-only flaps transpose anteriorly (Fig. 46.9). An absorbable stitch can do the sutures.

Helpful Points

- Careful dissection is needed to prevent damage to the tooth buds and large neurovascular stems.
- Nasal mucosa needs to be dissected without any tearing.
- Preserve 2–3 mm of mucosal and muscle flap near the hard palate to give the space for suturing.
- Use of a small and high degree of curvature needle will help with suturing the flap layers, especially near the hard palate.
- If the cleft involves a hard palate, two-flap palatoplasty is performed to repair this area.

Complications

Airway obstruction after cleft palate surgery because of mouth gag pressure can occur and lead to prolonged intubation.

The most common and significant complications of this surgery are fistula formation and velopharyngeal insufficiency. Risk factors for such complications are severity and type of cleft, and the method of surgery.

Some studies have shown that Furlow palatoplasty is associated with a statistically significant reduction in fistula rates and velopharyngeal insufficiency compared to both the VY pushback and the von Langenbeck repair techniques [28, 29].

It is important to know that after cleft surgery, patients remain at increased risk for middle ear disease, velopharyngeal dysfunction, and malocclusion. Therefore long-time follow-up with a multidisciplinary team is essential for a good result [30].

References

1. Mai CT, Isenburg JL, Canfield MA, Meyer RE, Correa A, Alverson CJ, et al. National population-based estimates for major birth defects, 2010-2014. Birth Defects Res. 2019;111(18):1420–35. https://doi.org/10.1002/bdr2.1589.
2. Bender PL. Genetics of cleft lip and palate. J Pediatr Nurs. 2000;15(4):242–9. https://doi.org/10.1053/jpdn.2000.8148.
3. Bernheim N, Georges M, Malevez C, De Mey A, Mansbach A. Embryology and epidemiology of cleft lip and palate. B-ENT. 2006;2(Suppl 4):11–9.
4. Bosi G, Evangelisti R, Valeno V, Carinci F, Pezzetti F, Calastrini C, et al. Diphenylhydantoin affects glycosaminoglycans and collagen production by human fibroblasts from cleft palate patients. J Dent Res. 1998;77(8):1613–21. https://doi.org/10.1177/00220345980770080901.
5. Lammer EJ, Chen DT, Hoar RM, Agnish ND, Benke PJ, Braun JT, et al. Retinoic acid embryopathy. N Engl J Med. 1985;313(14):837–41. https://doi.org/10.1056/NEJM198510033131401.
6. Shaw GM, Lammer EJ. Maternal periconceptional alcohol consumption and risk for orofacial clefts. J Pediatr. 1999;134(3):298–303. https://doi.org/10.1016/s0022-3476(99)70453-1.
7. Wyszynski DF, Duffy DL, Beaty TH. Maternal cigarette smoking and oral clefts: a meta-analysis. Cleft Palate Craniofac J. 1997;34(3):206–10. https://doi.org/10.1597/1545-1569_1997_034_0206_mcsaoc_2.3.co_2.
8. Grayson BH, Santiago PE, Brecht LE, Cutting CB. Presurgical nasoalveolar molding in infants with cleft lip and palate. Cleft Palate Craniofac J. 1999;36(6):486–98. https://doi.org/10.1597/1545-1569_1999_036_0486_pnmiiw_2.3.co_2.
9. Garfinkle JS, King TW, Grayson BH, Brecht LE, Cutting CB. A 12-year anthropometric evaluation of the nose in bilateral cleft lip-cleft palate patients following nasoalveolar molding and cutting bilateral cleft lip and nose reconstruction. Plast Reconstr Surg. 2011;127(4):1659–67. https://doi.org/10.1097/PRS.0b013e31820a64d7.
10. Rau A, Ritschl LM, Mucke T, Wolff KD, Loeffelbein DJ. Nasoalveolar molding in cleft care--experience in 40 patients from a single centre in Germany. PLoS One. 2015;10(3):e0118103. https://doi.org/10.1371/journal.pone.0118103.
11. Flint PW, Haughey BH, Lund VJ, Robbins KT, Thomas JR, Lesperance MM, et al. Cummings otolaryngology-head and neck surgery. 7th ed. Philadelphia: Elsevier; 2020.
12. Huang MH, Lee ST, Rajendran K. Anatomic basis of cleft palate and velopharyngeal surgery: implications from a fresh cadaveric study. Plast Reconstr Surg. 1998;101(3):613–27.; ; discussion 28-9. https://doi.org/10.1097/00006534-199803000-00007.
13. Huang MH, Lee ST, Rajendran K. Structure of the musculus uvulae: functional and surgical implications of an anatomic study. Cleft Palate Craniofac J. 1997;34(6):466–74. https://doi.org/10.1597/1545-1569_1997_034_0466_sotmuf_2.3.co_2.
14. Bailey BJ, Johnson JT, Newlands SD. Head & neck surgery--otolaryngology. 4th ed. Philadelphia: Lippincott Williams & Wilkins; 2006.
15. Stal S, Hicks MJ. Classic and occult submucous cleft palates: a histopathologic analysis. Cleft Palate Craniofac J. 1998;35(4):351–8. https://doi.org/10.1597/1545-1569_1998_035_0351_caoscp_2.3.co_2.
16. Seagle MB, Patti CS, Williams WN, Wood VD. Submucous cleft palate: a 10-year series. Ann Plast Surg. 1999;42(2):142–8. https://doi.org/10.1097/00000637-199902000-00006.
17. Dorf DS, Curtin JW. Early cleft palate repair and speech outcome. Plast Reconstr Surg. 1982;70(1):74–81. https://doi.org/10.1097/00006534-198207000-00015.
18. Haapanen ML, Rantala SL. Correlation between the age at repair and speech outcome in patients with isolated cleft palate. Scand J Plast Reconstr Surg Hand Surg. 1992;26(1):71–8. https://doi.org/10.3109/02844319209035186.
19. Kremenak CR Jr, Huffman WC, Olin WH. Maxillary growth inhibition by mucoperiosteal denudation of palatal shelf bone in non-cleft beagles. Cleft Palate J. 1970;7:817–25.
20. Landheer JA, Breugem CC, van der Molen AB. Fistula incidence and predictors of fistula occurrence after cleft palate repair: two-stage closure versus one-stage closure. Cleft Palate Craniofac J. 2010;47(6):623–30. https://doi.org/10.1597/09-069.
21. Willadsen E. Influence of timing of hard palate repair in a two-stage procedure on early speech development in Danish children with cleft palate. Cleft Palate Craniofac J. 2012;49(5):574–95. https://doi.org/10.1597/09-120.
22. Friede H, Priede D, Moller M, Maulina I, Lilja J, Barkane B. Comparisons of facial growth in patients with unilateral cleft lip and palate treated by different regimens for two-stage palatal repair. Scand J Plast Reconstr Surg Hand Surg. 1999;33(1):73–81. https://doi.org/10.1080/02844319950159659.
23. Rohrich RJ, Love EJ, Byrd HS, Johns DF. Optimal timing of cleft palate closure. Plast Reconstr Surg. 2000;106(2):413–21; discussion 23–5. https://doi.org/10.1097/00006534-200008000-00026.
24. Senders CW, Di Mauro SM, Brodie HA, Emery BE, Sykes JM. The efficacy of perioperative steroid therapy in pediatric primary palatoplasty. Cleft Palate Craniofac J. 1999;36(4):340–4. https://doi.org/10.1597/1545-1569_1999_036_0340_teopst_2.3.co_2.
25. Furlow LT Jr. Cleft palate repair by double opposing Z-plasty. Plast Reconstr Surg. 1986;78(6):724–38. https://doi.org/10.1097/00006534-198678060-00002.
26. Kirschner RE, Wang P, Jawad AF, Duran M, Cohen M, Solot C, et al. Cleft-palate repair by modified Furlow double-opposing Z-plasty: the Children's Hospital of Philadelphia experience. Plast Reconstr Surg. 1999;104(7):1998–2010.; ; discussion 1–4. https://doi.org/10.1097/00006534-199912000-00009.
27. Spauwen PH, Goorhuis-Brouwer SM, Schutte HK. Cleft palate repair: Furlow versus von Langenbeck. J Craniomaxillofac Surg. 1992;20(1):18–20. https://doi.org/10.1016/s1010-5182(05)80190-8.
28. Cohen SR, Kalinowski J, LaRossa D, Randall P. Cleft palate fistulas: a multivariate statistical analysis of prevalence, etiology, and surgical management. Plast Reconstr Surg. 1991;87(6):1041–7.
29. Stein MJ, Zhang Z, Fell M, Mercer N, Malic C. Determining post-operative outcomes after cleft palate repair: a systematic review and meta-analysis. J Plast Reconstr Aesthet Surg. 2019;72(1):85–91. https://doi.org/10.1016/j.bjps.2018.08.019.
30. Worley ML, Patel KG, Kilpatrick LA. Cleft lip and palate. Clin Perinatol. 2018;45(4):661–78. https://doi.org/10.1016/j.clp.2018.07.006.

Innovations in Orthognathic Surgery

47

Ali Heidari and Shohreh Ghasemi

Introduction

Oral and maxillofacial surgery improves the health, beauty, function, and mental state of human society.

This field has gone through many ups and downs since the first paper of Simon Hullihen on the correction of maxillary malformations was published in 1849 [1].

It is impossible to name the countless number of scientists whose efforts to develop oral and maxillofacial surgery have resulted in an escalating growth in this science field.

This chapter intends to give readers a preliminary introduction to the latest achievements in orthognathic surgery in recent decades by taking a brief look at new topics in this field. More complete and detailed information on each topic can be found in the relevant references.

In recent decades, the development of this science to reduce the surgery time, complications, and costs and to increase the accuracy of the surgery and patients' satisfaction is rapidly increasing and is still moving forward.

Computer-Aided Surgical Simulation for Orthognathic Surgery

In recent years, there has been a significant development in various treatments using virtual 3D modeling in medicine and dentistry. This has also been considered in the field of oral and maxillofacial surgery. The use of software for 3D

reconstruction of craniofacial defects and anomalies has grown significantly in the last decade [2, 3].

Improvement of new imaging technologies and exploitation of computed tomography (CT) and cone-beam CT (CBCT) have led clinicians to produce high-precision 3D models of the facial skeleton [4, 5].

Three-dimensional computer-assisted virtual planning has highly increased the success rate of treatment of cranio-maxillofacial anomalies and orthosurgery. This technique is gaining its place in the maxillofacial treatments and will become one of the most widely used and practical treatment methods in the near future [6–8].

In traditional orthodontic treatment models, the maxillary arch and temporomandibular joint (TMJ) relationship is transferred to a semi-adjustable articulator using a face-bow. A new relationship is reconstructed using plaster models and, finally, one or more occlusal splints are designed and constructed to be used during surgery.

Traditional treatment models are associated with at least two of the following errors: first, the condyle may be designed in an incorrect position in the joint cavity and, second, the maxilla may be in a false position relative to the skull base in all three dimensions [9, 10].

These errors may arise from the fact that in the traditional method, the plaster casts are displaced in a linear direction (two dimensional), relying on the therapist's visual skills. Still, in the virtual reconstruction method, in addition to linear movement, angular changes in the degree scale are also reconstructed.

These limitations in the traditional method have led to the increasing use of computer-aided designed and computer-aided manufactured (CAD/CAM) methods.

Computer-based methods should regenerate all the cranio-maxillofacial region tissues, including hard tissues (teeth and bones), soft tissue, and TMJ joint. In addition, they should be able to mark specific reference points for

A. Heidari (✉)
Department of Oral and Maxillofacial Surgery, Hamadan University of Medical Sciences, Hamadan, Iran
e-mail: dr.heidari68@umsha.ac.ir

S. Ghasemi
Department of Oral and Maxillofacial Surgery, Augusta University, Augusta, GA, USA
e-mail: sghasemi@augusta.edu

© The Author(s), under exclusive license to Springer Nature Switzerland AG 2021
M. R. Stevens et al. (eds.), *Innovative Perspectives in Oral and Maxillofacial Surgery*,
https://doi.org/10.1007/978-3-030-75750-2_47

repetition of movements and reconstruction and imitation of jaw relationships. The most important requirement of this tool is the ability to make repeatable changes in all three dimensions in the form of linear and angular movements.

These methods are first initiated with a CT and CBCT image of the skull up to the mandible's lower border, providing the clinician with a 3D craniofacial view.

These images are adjusted using the virtual references plan in all three planes of horizontal, sagittal, and coronal so that the head is adjusted in its natural position and the symmetry of the images is achieved (Fig. 47.1).

Then the face planes are designed virtually (virtual face plane).

The Frankfurt plane can be used to adjust the images because it is less affected by jaw anomalies.

Since CT images of the teeth may not be accurate enough due to distortion, some clinicians prefer to use a scanner to scan plaster casts or use an intraoral scanner to scan the dental arch [11] directly.

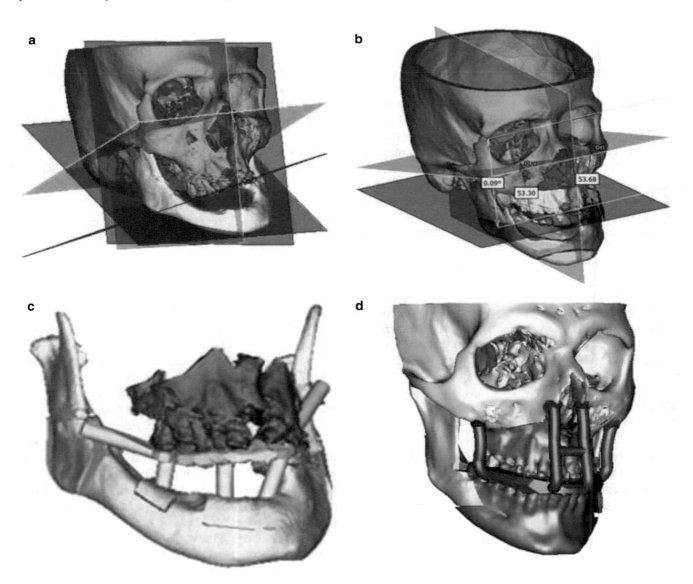

Fig. 47.1 (**a**) Preoperative screen capture of severe facial asymmetry and partially edentulous mandible, including the constructed facial coordinates. (**b**) Virtual bimaxillary osteotomy and genioplasty according to ideal facial symmetry. (**c**) The final computer-aided designed and computer-aided manufactured splint repositions the mandible in the final position after the sagittal split. (**d**) Experimental computer-aided designed and computer-aided manufactured splint, which uses the anatomic landmarks (zygomatic buttress and nasal aperture). This initial idea was rejected because of massive soft tissue exposure. (Adapted from Zinser et al. [3])

In this case, the CT or CBCT images must be matched and merged with the scanned images to provide an accurate 3D model of the bone and tooth complex.

A bite-recording jig also is used to match these images accurately. This device is designed and manufactured to contain fixed and unchangeable reference points so that they can be used to merge the scanner images to the CT images in an entirely correct position [12, 13].

These reference points can be intraoral or extraoral. The intraoral reference points beyond the osteotomy lines can adapt different splints in a fixed point (so that they do not change during osteotomy).

An initial splint is constructed, which records the dental arch's details and at least 4 points of bone above the osteot-omy line. This splint is mounted in the first stage of surgery before osteotomy, and holes are drilled at the fixed points. In the later stages of surgery, these indices will help position the next splints correctly (Fig. 47.2).

In the next step, the maxilla is moved in software. At this stage, the maxillary dental midline should be aligned in the midsagittal line so that the maxilla's left and right sides become symmetric and no roll or yaw movement is seen in the maxilla. After applying the necessary movements to the maxilla, a second splint is designed and constructed. This splint will determine the location of the maxilla during surgery and after maxillary osteotomy, and it will keep the maxilla in place during fixation time. Finally, the necessary movements are performed in software to correct the mandi-

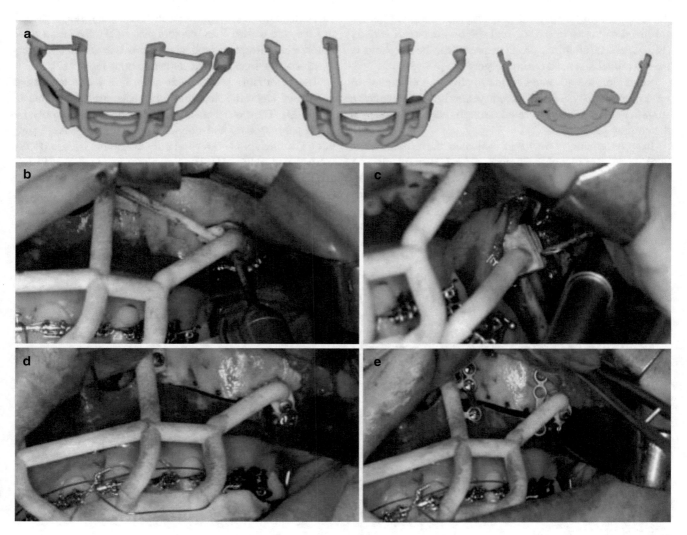

Fig. 47.2 (**a**) Computer-aided designed and computer-aided manufactured splints 1, 2, and 3 in vivo. Splint 1 indicates landmarks to the (**b**) maxilla and the (**c**) condyles. (**d**) Splint 2 positions the maxilla accord-ing to the virtual planning using temporary miniscrews. (**e**) Then, osteosynthesis can be performed using microplates. (Adapted from Zinser et al. [3])

ble, and a third splint will be made relying on the fixed reference points, which will stabilize the final occlusion position during surgery and after the mandibular osteotomy.

In another method, some clinicians use the surgical navigation system without providing a surgical wafer along with the image-guided visualization display system [13, 14]. First, the maxilla's new position is determined through virtual design and surgery. Then, the osteotomized maxilla is moved during the surgery to match the image of the maxilla in a new position.

Simpler virtual surgical methods can be used in simpler surgeries such as genioplasty. In this method, after preparing the 3D model, the genioplasty treatment plan is performed virtually, and the location of the osteotomy lines and the location of the hole needed for placing the fixing screws are determined using a surgical guide so that these splints are sterilized and used in the surgical site on the day of surgery (Fig. 47.3). In addition, pre-bent plates can be prepared in the 3D model and used during surgery [15].

Regarding the advances in the quality and efficiency of virtual surgical systems in recent years, most orthognathic surgeries seem to be performed through these techniques in the coming years.

In a systematic review that evaluated the accuracy and benefits of orthognathic surgery virtual systems, it was shown that maxillary surgeries performed through this method have an error of <1.2 mm in the vertical plane and <1.5° in the rotational movement.

In the mandible, this error was <1.1 mm in the sagittal plane and <1.8° in the mandible rotational movements [16].

Bioactive/Bioresorbable Plate Systems

Lack of access to tools and equipment to create a proper fixation will lead to the failure of surgical procedures and osteotomies in the jaw and face area [17]. Titanium screws and plates have been the main tool of surgeons to achieve this fixation for many years. However, these metal plates and screws have disadvantages, such as disruption of the facial skeletal growth, their palpability over time, mutagenic effects, production of corrosive products, and interference with imaging techniques [18, 19], which may eventually necessitate their removal from the surgical site.

The use of resorbable materials can solve many of these problems due to the lack of corrosive products, no need to their removal, and their radiolucency [20]. However, their mechanical strength has always been debated, and it is widely believed that they are weaker than titanium plates [21]. Besides, sometimes, their absorption products can provoke an inflammatory reaction to the foreign body, impairing bone repair [22].

The resorbable plates made of poly-L-lactic acid have been used since the first study on these animals' plates in 1966 [23]. They were mainly made of polymers of poly-L-lactic acid (PLLA) and poly-D-lactic acid (PDLA). Later, poly-glycolic acid (PGA) and polydioxanone sulfate (PDS) were also used [21, 24]. The first plates were made of PLLA and PDLA. In the second generation, PGA was added to the composition to improve its biomechanical properties. PGA increases the resorption rate of the plates and reduces the side effects of their long life. Different percentages of each of these polymers result in products with different proper-

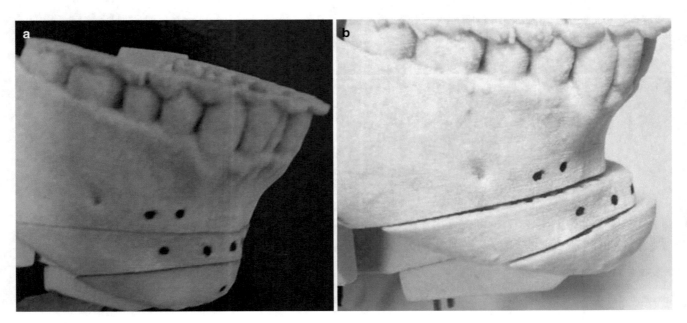

Fig. 47.3 (**a**) 3D rapid-prototyping multi-position model, initial position. (**b**) Final position corresponding to virtual planning. (Adapted from Olszewski et al. [15])

ties. These products are decomposed through hydrolysis of the ester bond and the final products are exhaled from the lungs in the form of water and carbon dioxide [21, 25]. These two generations of fixing devices have been used successfully in orthognathic surgery and had acceptable results [26, 27].

Recently, in the third generation of resorbable plates and screws, the most attention has been paid to bioactive constituents to stimulate the formation of new bone. To this end, hydroxyapatite (HA) was added to the structural composition of the new-generation products to improve the treatment results using its osteoconductivity [22, 24, 28].

It is expected that the addition of HA to the structural composition of the plates and screws stimulates ossification in the area and results in a complete replacement of the plates and screws by new bone tissue [29].

In maxillofacial surgeries, these new products have higher bonding strength than traditional PLLA products, which reach even the cortical bone's bonding strength up to 25 weeks after surgery [30].

Many clinicians in orthodontic surgery prefer titanium plates because they do not require a second operation to remove them [31, 32].

The resorbable plates are used similarly to titanium plates. In the maxillary fixation technique, two plates are placed in the piriforms and two plates in the zygomatic buttress. In the bilateral sagittal split osteotomy (BSSO) fixation, three screws or two plates or resorbable meshes can be used at the top and bottom of the mandibular nerve canal (Fig. 47.4).

The effectiveness of resorbable plates and screws in fixing LeFort osteotomy, in BSSO, and in maxillary and mandibular surgery has been reported [33].

Minimally Invasive Orthognathic Surgery

With the advancement of surgical techniques, minimally invasive methods are currently more preferred by surgeons and patients. These methods are associated with a minimal incision size and surgical manipulation, reduced need for hospitalization, reduced surgical complications, and better results.

Endoscopic surgery is a method that minimizes the invasive nature of surgeries. This technique has been used in various surgery fields and has recently been considered by oral and maxillofacial surgeons.

In the field of orthognathic surgery, endoscopy has been used for intraoral vertical ramus osteotomy (IVRO) [34]. First, the area of surgery is determined and marked on the skin. The mandible's lower border, the ramus's anterior and posterior borders, and the coronoid notch are also marked. A small incision (<2 cm) is made in the jaw area, 2 cm apart from the lower border of the mandible. A sharp incision separates the pterygomasseteric sling, and the procedure continues under the sub-periosteum. A periosteum elevator, suction, light source, and retractors designed for this purpose are inserted through the tunnel and provide access to the entire condyle and ramus complex. Then osteotomy is performed using a Stryker saw and treatment continues. This surgical procedure has advantages such as small incision of soft tissue and reduced dissection, pain, and postoperative swelling, which ultimately lead to a reduction in the recovery period and length of hospital stay [35, 36].

Endoscopy enables the fixation of osteotomy pieces in IVRO method [36]. Three screws with divergent angles or two plates can be used for this operation (depending on the amount of overlap of the parts).

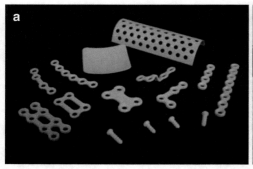
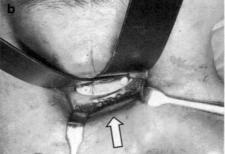
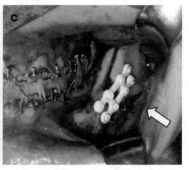

Fig. 47.4 Maxillofacial osteosynthesis systems using third-generation bioactive/bioresorbable materials. (**a**) The SuperFIXORB-MX® (OsteotransMS®) system. (**b**) Bioresorbable sheet and tack fixation for right orbital reconstruction in a case with naso-orbitoethmoidal (midfacial) fractures using the SuperFIXORB-MX® (OsteotransMS®) system, with use of the RapidSorb® system for infraorbital rim fixation. (**c**) Three-dimensional bioresorbable plate osteosynthesis of advancement mandibular bilaterally sagital split ramus osteotomy (BSSRO) using the SuperFIXORB-MX® (OsteotransMS®) system in orthognathic surgery. (Adapted from Kanno et al. [22])

Endoscopy has shown good capability and efficiency in mandibular osteotomies, although certain complications such as marginal mandibular nerve dysfunction have been reported [36].

Surgically Assisted Orthodontic Treatment

The length of treatment has always been a great challenge for orthodontists and people undergoing orthodontic treatment. Surgically (corticotomy)-assisted orthodontic treatment has been proposed in recent decades as a treatment modality to increase orthodontic treatment speed [37]. This method has tried to reduce the duration of orthodontic treatment with the help of surgical methods. This method can be performed for people who want to reduce the length of orthodontic treatment and can pay extra costs for surgery [38].

The process of bone remodeling is a permanent physiological process resulting from bone formation by osteoblasts and bone removal by osteoclasts. This process is responsible for maintaining, regenerating, and health of the skeleton.

Regarding the mechanism of tooth movement under the influence of orthodontic forces, the destruction and necrosis process begins in the periodontal ligament (PDL), and the regional bone at the tooth surface where the force enters adjacent tissues is pressed. After the local tissues are necrotized, osteoclasts and macrophages infiltrate and remove necrotic tissue remnants, moving the tooth toward the tissue removal site. On the opposite side, new bone and PDL are formed due to the resulting tension force [38]. The destruction and necrosis process and the necrotic tissue removal by osteoclasts take about a month, which is considered the *lag phase* [38, 39].

Surgery and bone removal result in temporary osteopenia and reduce the amount of bone regenerated by osteoblasts by stimulating the process of acute inflammation at the surgical site [38]. Compared to the normal bone in the same area, the osteopenic bone is more prone to orthodontic dental movements [39].

Selective corticotomy of the bone at the surgery site creates transient osteopenia and results in the completion of healing process due to osteoblastic activity and increased ossification [40].

The healing process sequence accelerates orthodontic movements and reduces the treatment period [41]. The bone remodeling process is completed up to 6 months after surgery, orthodontic treatment and dental movements should be done during this period. The movement of teeth will be limited [42, 43]. Therefore, orthodontic force should be applied during the first 2 weeks after surgery and reactivated at 2-week interval.

In this procedure, the flap is first removed with the full thickness of the sub-periosteum on both buccal and lingual sides, and then the cortical bone is removed on both sides at the interdental spaces. The area is then filled with bone grafts, and the flaps are returned to their place and sutured (Fig. 47.5). The graft material is placed to increase the bone volume in the area where the tooth will later move. This prevents problems such as fenestration, dehiscence, and gingival resorption in later stages [35, 44, 45].

Recently, 3D modeling and CBCT have enabled the designing and building of the surgical guide in advance. This increases the accuracy of the surgery and the speed of the surgeon. The utilization of piezoelectric instruments for surgery can also help reduce surgery complications [46, 47].

Some clinicians do not elevate the flap completely; instead, they create a narrow tunnel through a small longitudinal incision through which the corticotomy is performed at the buccal level. Corticotomy is performed by piezosurgery and its thin tip, and the graft material is placed through the tunnel [48].

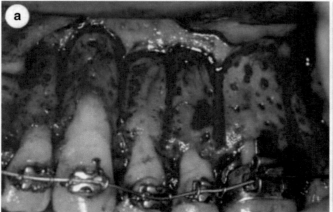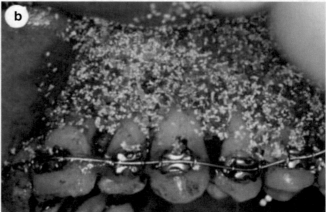

Fig. 47.5 Corticotomy-facilitated orthodontics. (**a**) Interdental buccal corticotomy. (**b**) Augmentation with bone allograft. (Adapted from Wilcko et al. [37])

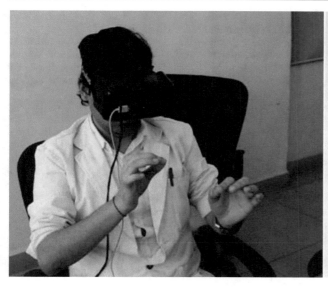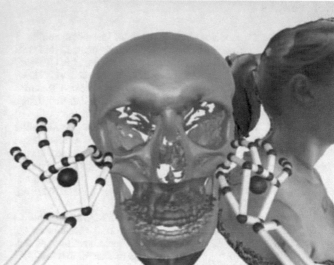

Fig. 47.6 3D interaction with the patient's CBCT data. (Adapted from Pulijala et al. [52])

A more conservative technique may be used, in which a micro-osteoperforation (MOP) is created in the cortical bone without making an incision or elevation of the flap. These perforations stimulate the bone remodeling process, reducing the complications of the methods mentioned above [49, 50].

In a study on the effectiveness of MOP, it was shown that in addition to the acceleration of orthodontic movements as much as the usual corticotomy, this method could increase the number of osteoclasts at the surgical site [51].

Virtual Reality Training Tool for Orthognathic Surgery

In recent years, we have witnessed an increasing growth in the methods and tools for teaching and promoting the practice of medicine and dentistry [52]. Training of various surgical procedures requires high levels of practice, repetition, and care [53]. Virtual reality is a new method of practical training for oral and maxillofacial residents in the field of orthognathic surgery. This technology helps improve residents' knowledge and skills before initiating patients' treatment in simulated and almost real conditions of surgery.

The following conditions are required to provide virtual orthognathic surgery training:

1. Providing a highly accurate 3D image of the workplace and the operating field
2. The possibility of comprehensive intervention in the 360-degree space of the surgery site

3. Creating an appropriate and almost real sense of touch for learners in all surgical movements

In recent years, significant progress has been made in producing and presenting accurate 3D space of the surgery site and the operating field. The possibility of comprehensive intervention in the operating room and performing activities related to surgery is well provided; however, more measures are still needed to create a real and appropriate sense of touch for learners (Fig. 47.6).

In a study using the Oculus Rift Development Kit 2 (DK2) virtual reality, the LeFort surgery was reconstructed in 3D for learners [52], and the efficiency and face validity of this method were approved, and it was recommended as a suitable tool as part of the training program for oral and maxillofacial residents. However, this method has some limitations, such as the inability to give surgeons a proper sense of touch.

Conclusion

Knowledge and practical activities in the field of oral and maxillofacial surgery are changing and renewing rapidly like any other field of science. Therefore, maxillofacial surgeons should improve their skills by getting acquainted, learning, and using these methods and should try to work at the first level of modern science. Given the unfamiliarity of some aspects of these technologies, they are recommended to be used with caution based on each case's conditions, in addition, accurate follow-ups.

References

1. Hullihen SP. Case of elongation of the under jaw and distortion of the face and neck, caused by a burn, successfully treated. Am J Dent Sci. 1849;9(2):157–65. PMID: 30749486; PMCID: PMC6059554.

2. Macchi A, Carrafiello G, Cacciafesta V, Norcini A. Three-dimensional digital modeling and setup. Am J Orthod Dentofac Orthop. 2006;129(5):605–10. https://doi.org/10.1016/j.ajodo.2006.01.010. PMID: 16679200.

3. Zinser MJ, Sailer HF, Ritter L, Braumann B, Maegele M, Zöller JE. A paradigm shift in orthognathic surgery? A comparison of navigation, computer-aided designed/computer-aided manufactured splints, and "classic" intermaxillary splints to surgical transfer of virtual orthognathic planning. J Oral Maxillofac Surg. 2013;71(12):2151.e1–21. https://doi.org/10.1016/j.joms.2013.07.007. PMID: 24237776.

4. Cevidanes LH, Bailey LJ, Tucker GR Jr, Styner MA, Mol A, Phillips CL, Proffit WR, Turvey T. Superimposition of 3D cone-beam CT models of orthognathic surgery patients. Dentomaxillofac Radiol. 2005;34(6):369–75. https://doi.org/10.1259/dmfr/17102411. PMID: 16227481; PMCID: PMC3552302.

5. Hsu SS, Gateno J, Bell RB, Hirsch DL, Markiewicz MR, Teichgraeber JF, Zhou X, Xia JJ. Accuracy of a computer-aided surgical simulation protocol for orthognathic surgery: a prospective multicenter study. J Oral Maxillofac Surg. 2013;71(1):128–42. https://doi.org/10.1016/j.joms.2012.03.027. Epub 2012 Jun 12. PMID: 22695016; PMCID: PMC3443525.

6. Gateno J, Teichgraeber JF, Xia JJ. Three-dimensional surgical planning for maxillary and midface distraction osteogenesis. J Craniofac Surg. 2003;14(6):833–9. https://doi.org/10.1097/00001665-200311000-00004. PMID: 14600624.

7. Gateño J, Teichgraeber JF, Aguilar E. Computer planning for distraction osteogenesis. Plast Reconstr Surg. 2000;105(3):873–82. https://doi.org/10.1097/00006534-200003000-00008. PMID: 10724245.

8. Gateno J, Allen ME, Teichgraeber JF, Messersmith ML. An in vitro study of the accuracy of a new protocol for planning distraction osteogenesis of the mandible. J Oral Maxillofac Surg. 2000;58(9):985–90; discussion 990–1. https://doi.org/10.1053/joms.2000.8740. PMID: 10981978.

9. Ellis E 3rd. Accuracy of model surgery: evaluation of an old technique and introduction of a new one. J Oral Maxillofac Surg. 1990;48(11):1161–7. https://doi.org/10.1016/0278-2391(90)90532-7. PMID: 1698956.

10. Marmulla R, Mühling J. Computer-assisted condyle positioning in orthognathic surgery. J Oral Maxillofac Surg. 2007;65(10):1963–8. https://doi.org/10.1016/j.joms.2006.11.024. PMID: 17884523.

11. Santler G. 3-D COSMOS: a new 3-D model based computerised operation simulation and navigation system. J Craniomaxillofac Surg. 2000;28(5):287–93. https://doi.org/10.1054/jcms.2000.0156. PMID: 11467392.

12. Chapuis J, Schramm A, Pappas I, Hallermann W, Schwenzer-Zimmerer K, Langlotz F, Caversaccio M. A new system for computer-aided preoperative planning and intraoperative navigation during corrective jaw surgery. IEEE Trans Inf Technol Biomed. 2007;11(3):274–87. https://doi.org/10.1109/titb.2006.884372. PMID: 17521077.

13. Zinser MJ, Mischkowski RA, Dreiseidler T, et al. Computer-assisted orthognathic surgery: waferless maxillary positioning, versatility, and accuracy of an image-guided visualisation display. Br J Oral Maxillofac Surg. 2013;51(8):827–33. https://doi.org/10.1016/j.bjoms.2013.06.014.

14. Mischkowski RA, Zinser MJ, Kübler AC, Krug B, Seifert U, Zöller JE. Application of an augmented reality tool for maxillary positioning in orthognathic surgery - a feasibility study. J Craniomaxillofac Surg. 2006;34(8):478–83. https://doi.org/10.1016/j.jcms.2006.07.862. Epub 2006 Dec 8. PMID: 17157519.

15. Olszewski R, Tranduy K, Reychler H. Innovative procedure for computer-assisted genioplasty: three-dimensional cephalometry, rapid-prototyping model and surgical splint. Int J Oral Maxillofac Surg. 2010;39(7):721–4. https://doi.org/10.1016/j.ijom.2010.03.018. Epub 2010 Apr 22. PMID: 20417056.

16. Haas Jr OL, Becker OE, de Oliveira RB. Computer-aided planning in orthognathic surgery-systematic review. Int J Oral Maxillofac Surg. 2014. pii: S0901–5027(14)00430-5. https://doi.org/10.1016/j.ijom.2014.10.025.

17. Buijs GJ, van Bakelen NB, Jansma J, de Visscher JG, Hoppenreijs TJ, Bergsma JE, Stegenga B, Bos RR. A randomized clinical trial of biodegradable and titanium fixation systems in maxillofacial surgery. J Dent Res. 2012;91(3):299–304. https://doi.org/10.1177/0022034511434353. Epub 2012 Jan 23. PMID: 22269272.

18. Schumann P, Lindhorst D, Wagner ME, Schramm A, Gellrich NC, Rücker M. Perspectives on resorbable osteosynthesis materials in craniomaxillofacial surgery. Pathobiology. 2013;80(4):211–7. https://doi.org/10.1159/000348328. Epub 2013 May 6. PMID: 23652285.

19. Yang L, Xu M, Jin X, Xu J, Lu J, Zhang C, Tian T, Teng L. Complications of absorbable fixation in maxillofacial surgery: a meta-analysis. PLoS One. 2013;8(6):e67449. https://doi.org/10.1371/journal.pone.0067449. PMID: 23840705; PMCID: PMC3696084.

20. Sukegawa S, Kanno T, Katase N, Shibata A, Takahashi Y, Furuki Y. Clinical evaluation of an unsintered hydroxyapatite/poly-L-lactide osteoconductive composite device for the internal fixation of maxillofacial fractures. J Craniofac Surg. 2016;27(6):1391–7. https://doi.org/10.1097/SCS.0000000000002828. PMID: 27428913; PMCID: PMC5023762.

21. Pina S, Ferreira JMF. Bioresorbable plates and screws for clinical applications: a review. J Healthcare Eng. 2012;3:846435, 18 pages. https://doi.org/10.1260/2040-2295.3.2.243.

22. Kanno T, Sukegawa S, Furuki Y, Nariai Y, Sekine J. Overview of innovative advances in bioresorbable plate systems for oral and maxillofacial surgery. Jpn Dent Sci Rev. 2018;54(3):127–38. https://doi.org/10.1016/j.jdsr.2018.03.003. Epub 2018 Apr 5. PMID: 30128060; PMCID: PMC6094489.

23. Sukegawa S, Kanno T, Nagano D, Shibata A, Sukegawa-Takahashi Y, Furuki Y. The clinical feasibility of newly developed thin flat-type bioresorbable osteosynthesis devices for the internal fixation of zygomatic fractures: is there a difference in healing between bioresorbable materials and titanium osteosynthesis? J Craniofac Surg. 2016;27(8):2124–9. https://doi.org/10.1097/SCS.0000000000003147. PMID: 28005767; PMCID: PMC5110331.

24. Park YW. Bioabsorbable osteofixation for orthognathic surgery. Maxillofac Plast Reconstr Surg. 2015;37(1):6. https://doi.org/10.1186/s40902-015-0003-7. PMID: 25722967; PMCID: PMC4333128.

25. Suuronen R, Kallela I, Lindqvist C. Bioabsorbable plates and screws: current state of the art in facial fracture repair. J Craniomaxillofac Trauma. 2000 Spring;6(1):19–27; discussion 28–30. PMID: 11373737.

26. Mohamed-Hashem IK, Mitchell DA. Resorbable implants (plates and screws) in orthognathic surgery. J Orthod. 2000;27(2):198–9. https://doi.org/10.1093/ortho/27.2.198. PMID: 10867078.

27. Turvey TA, Bell RB, Tejera TJ, Proffit WR. The use of self-reinforced biodegradable bone plates and screws in orthognathic surgery. J Oral Maxillofac Surg. 2002;60(1):59–65. https://doi.org/10.1053/joms.2002.28274. PMID: 11757010.

28. Shikinami Y, Matsusue Y, Nakamura T. The complete process of bioresorption and bone replacement using devices made of

forged composites of raw hydroxyapatite particles/poly l-lactide (F-u-HA/PLLA). Biomaterials. 2005;26(27):5542–51. https://doi.org/10.1016/j.biomaterials.2005.02.016. PMID: 15860210.

29. Sukegawa S, Kanno T, Kawai H, Shibata A, Sukegawa-Takahashi Y, Nagatsuka H, et al. Long-term bioresorption of bone fixation devices made from composites of unsintered hydroxyapatite particles and poly-L-lactide. J Hard Tissue Biol. 2015;24:219–24. https://doi.org/10.2485/jhtb.24.219.

30. Kanno T, Tatsumi H, Karino M, Koike T, Ide T, Sekine J. The applicability of an unsintered hydroxyapatite particles/poly-L-lactide composite sheet with tack fixation for orbital fracture reconstruction. J Hard Tissue Biol. 2016;25:329–34.

31. Gareb B, van Bakelen NB, Buijs GJ, Jansma J, de Visscher JGAM, Hoppenreijs TJM, et al. Comparison of the long-term clinical performance of a biodegradable and a titanium fixation system in maxillofacial surgery: a multicenter randomized controlled trial. PLoS One. 2017;11:e0177152.

32. van Bakelen NB, Boermans BD, Buijs GJ, Jansma J, Pruim GJ, Hoppenreijs TJ, et al. Comparison of the long-term skeletal stability between a biodegradable and a titanium fixation system following BSSO advancement——a cohort study based on a multicenter randomised controlled trial. Br J Oral Maxillofac Surg. 2014;52:721–8.

33. Sukegawa S, Kanno T, Matsumoto K, Sukegawa-Takahashi Y, Masui M, Furuki Y. Complications of a poly-L-lactic acid and polyglycolic acid osteosynthesis device for internal fixation in maxillofacial surgery. Odontology. 2018;106(4):360–8. https://doi.org/10.1007/s10266-018-0345-6. Epub 2018 Feb 7. PMID: 29417376.

34. Troulis MJ, Kaban LB. Endoscopic approach to the ramus/condyle unit: clinical applications. J Oral Maxillofac Surg. 2001;59(5):503–9. https://doi.org/10.1053/joms.2001.22706. PMID: 11326371.

35. Papadaki ME, Kaban LB, Troulis MJ. Endoscopic vertical ramus osteotomy: a long-term prospective study. Int J Oral Maxillofac Surg. 2014;43(3):305–10. https://doi.org/10.1016/j.ijom.2013.09.012. Epub 2013 Nov 15. PMID: 24246948.

36. Troulis MJ, Kaban LB. Endoscopic vertical ramus osteotomy: early clinical results. J Oral Maxillofac Surg. 2004;62(7):824–8. https://doi.org/10.1016/j.joms.2003.12.021. PMID: 15218560.

37. Wilcko MT, Wilcko WM, Pulver JJ, Bissada NF, Bouquot JE. Accelerated osteogenic orthodontics technique: a 1-stage surgically facilitated rapid orthodontic technique with alveolar augmentation. J Oral Maxillofac Surg. 2009;67(10):2149–59. https://doi.org/10.1016/j.joms.2009.04.095. PMID: 19761908.

38. Feller L, Khammissa RAG, Siebold A, Hugo A, Lemmer J. Biological events related to corticotomy-facilitated orthodontics. J Int Med Res. 2019;47(7):2856–64. https://doi.org/10.1177/0300060519856456. Epub 2019 Jun 24. PMID: 31234667; PMCID: PMC6683901.

39. Feller L, Khammissa RAG, Schechter I, Moodley A, Thomadakis G, Lemmer J. Periodontal biological events associated with orthodontic tooth movement: the biomechanics of the cytoskeleton and the extracellular matrix. Scientific World Journal. 2015;2015:894123, 7 pages. https://doi.org/10.1155/2015/894123.

40. Pfeilschifter J, Wüster C, Vogel M, Enderes B, Ziegler R, Minne HW. Inflammation-mediated osteopenia (IMO) during acute inflammation in rats is due to a transient inhibition of bone formation. Calcif Tissue Int. 1987;41(6):321–5. https://doi.org/10.1007/BF02556670. PMID: 3124941.

41. Kim SJ, Park YG, Kang SG. Effects of Corticision on paradental remodeling in orthodontic tooth movement. Angle Orthod.

2009;79(2):284–91. https://doi.org/10.2319/020308-60.1. PMID: 19216591.

42. Amit G, Jps K, Pankaj B, Suchinder S, Parul B. Periodontally accelerated osteogenic orthodontics (PAOO) - a review. J Clin Exp Dent. 2012;4(5):e292–6. https://doi.org/10.4317/jced.50822. PMID: 24455038; PMCID: PMC3892210.

43. Kaipatur N, Major P, Stevenson T, Pehowich D, Adeeb S, Doschak M. Impact of selective alveolar decortication on bisphosphonate burdened alveolar bone during orthodontic tooth movement. Arch Oral Biol. 2015;60(11):1681–9. https://doi.org/10.1016/j.archoralbio.2015.08.008. Epub 2015 Aug 25. PMID: 26355528.

44. Wilcko W, Wilcko MT. Accelerating tooth movement: the case for corticotomy-induced orthodontics. Am J Orthod Dentofac Orthop. 2013;144(1):4–12. https://doi.org/10.1016/j.ajodo.2013.04.009. PMID: 23810038.

45. Bhattacharya P, Bhattacharya H, Anjum A, Bhandari R, Agarwal DK, Gupta A, Ansar J. Assessment of corticotomy facilitated tooth movement and changes in alveolar bone thickness - A CT scan study. J Clin Diagn Res. 2014;8(10):ZC26–30. https://doi.org/10.7860/JCDR/2014/9448.4954. Epub 2014 Oct 20. PMID: 25478442; PMCID: PMC4253260.

46. Cassetta M, Giansanti M, Di Mambro A, Calasso S, Barbato E. Minimally invasive corticotomy in orthodontics using a three-dimensional printed CAD/CAM surgical guide. Int J Oral Maxillofac Surg. 2016;45(9):1059–64. https://doi.org/10.1016/j.ijom.2016.04.017. Epub 2016 May 10. PMID: 27178968.

47. Milano F, Dibart S, Montesani L, Guerra L. Computer-guided surgery using the piezocision technique. Int J Periodontics Restorative Dent. 2014;34(4):523–9. https://doi.org/10.11607/prd.1741. PMID: 25006769.

48. Caruso S, Darvizeh A, Zema S, Gatto R, Nota A. Management of a facilitated aesthetic orthodontic treatment with clear aligners and minimally invasive corticotomy. Dent J (Basel). 2020;8(1):19. https://doi.org/10.3390/dj8010019. PMID: 32075255; PMCID: PMC7148540.

49. Cheung T, Park J, Lee D, Kim C, Olson J, Javadi S, Lawson G, McCabe J, Moon W, Ting K, Hong C. Ability of mini-implant-facilitated micro-osteoperforations to accelerate tooth movement in rats. Am J Orthod Dentofacial Orthop. 2016;150(6):958–67. https://doi.org/10.1016/j.ajodo.2016.04.030. PMID: 27894545; PMCID: PMC5131371.

50. Alikhani M, Raptis M, Zoldan B, Sangsuwon C, Lee YB, Alyami B, Corpodian C, Barrera LM, Alansari S, Khoo E, Teixeira C. Effect of micro-osteoperforations on the rate of tooth movement. Am J Orthod Dentofac Orthop. 2013;144(5):639–48. https://doi.org/10.1016/j.ajodo.2013.06.017. PMID: 24182579.

51. Kim J, Kook YA, Bayome M, Park JH, Lee W, Choi H, Abbas NH. Comparison of tooth movement and biological response in corticotomy and micro-osteoperforation in rabbits. Korean J Orthod. 2019;49(4):205–13. https://doi.org/10.4041/kjod.2019.49.4.205. Epub 2019 Jul 22. PMID: 31367575; PMCID: PMC6658902.

52. Pulijala Y, Ma M, Pears M, Peebles D, Ayoub A. An innovative virtual reality training tool for orthognathic surgery. Int J Oral Maxillofac Surg. 2018;47(9):1199–205. https://doi.org/10.1016/j.ijom.2018.01.005. Epub 2018 Feb 15. PMID: 29398172.

53. Elsey EJ, Griffiths G, Humes DJ, West J. Meta-analysis of operative experiences of general surgery trainees during training. Br J Surg. 2017;104(1):22–33. https://doi.org/10.1002/bjs.10396. PMID: 28000937.

Vahid Akheshteh

Ameloblastoma

Ameloblastoma usually occurs in the posterior jaw and has distinct cortical boundaries [1]. Its lesions can be seen as either unilocular or multilocular. The multilocular types usually have curved and rough septa, and terms like "soap bubble" or "honeycomb" are used to describe them depending on the size and number of loculus they have [2–4].

In radiographic images, root resorption and tooth displacement are common sightings. Although the use of advanced imaging is recommended for many lesions today, in the case of ameloblastoma, due to the tendency of this lesion to expand and the possibility of perforation of bone cortices, the use of imaging modality techniques, such as soft tissue CT scans and MRI, are highly recommended (Fig. 48.1).

Dentigerous Cysts

They usually occur behind the mandible or maxilla surrounding tooth number eight, in the anterior maxilla surrounding tooth number 3, or around the extra mesiodens teeth in the anterior maxilla [1, 5, 6].

Like most cysts, their shape is curved or round and their borders are clear and corticated. Like ameloblastoma, these cysts have the ability to resorb and move adjacent teeth, but the important and fundamental point is that in dentigerous cysts, dental displacement is usually very significant.

It is possible to diagnose dentigerous cysts by their attachment to the CEJ (cementoenamel junction), which can also be seen on many conventional radiographs. Considering all these points, it is sometimes impossible to differentiate dentigerous cysts from cases such as ameloblastic fibroma [1, 5, 6] (Figs. 48.2, 48.3, and 48.4).

V. Akheshteh (✉)
Oral and Maxillofacial Radiology Department, Alborz Medical Science University, Karaj, Iran
e-mail: V.Akheshteh@gmail.com

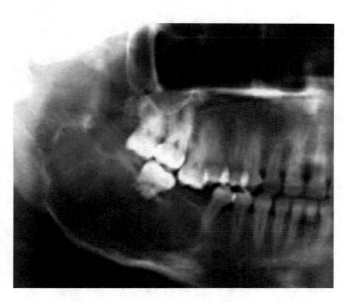

Fig. 48.1 Cropped panoramic view shows ameloblastoma in the posterior region of the right mandible. The lesion developed from the tooth's periapical of the second premolar to the mid ramus. Note the lesion's expansile nature, root resorption, and the displacement of the tooth second molar, a typical feature of ameloblastoma

Keratocystic Odontogenic Tumors

This lesion usually occurs behind the mandible and unlike ameloblastoma, which is characterized by its bony expansion, the keratocystic odontogenic tumor tends to expand less and spread more extensively [1, 7]. The external boundaries of this lesion are also clear, corticated, and can also be scallop-like.

In multicellular cases such as ameloblastoma, curved and rough septa are seen. Root resorption and tooth displacement occur in both ameloblastoma and dentigerous cysts, although to a lesser extent [1, 7].

An important point about keratocystic odontogenic tumor is that it can be peri-coronal like a dentigerous cyst, even

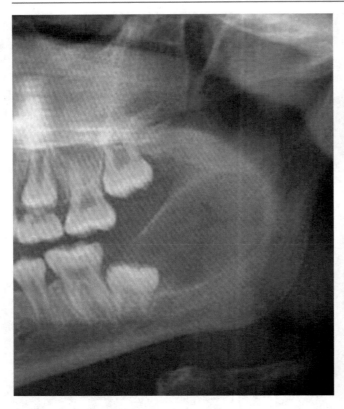

Fig. 48.2 Cropped panoramic view shows a dentigerous cyst on the left side of the mandible. Attached to the CEJ, both radiographically and surgically, is a prominent feature of dentigerous cysts

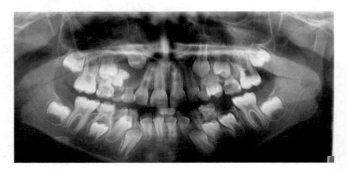

Fig. 48.3 A common area for dentigerous cyst is the maxillary canine tooth. A lesion is seen on the right side of the anterior maxilla and canine area in the panoramic image. The superior displacement of the canine tooth is seen

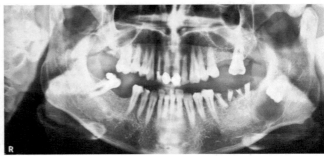

Fig. 48.4 In the panoramic image on the left side of the mandible, a dentigerous cyst is seen

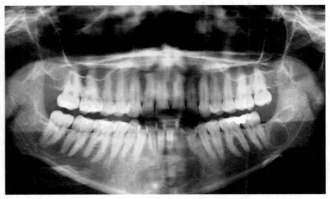

Fig. 48.5 An odontogenic keratocyst tumor is seen in the panoramic view on the left side of the mandible and third molar. This lesion is bilocular. The internal structure is radiolucent with well-defined corticate border. Unlike ameloblastoma, it usually does not tend to expand

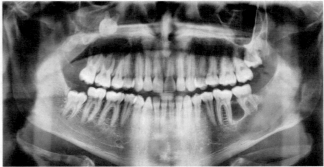

Fig. 48.6 In the panoramic view, the odontogenic keratocyst tumors are seen (one lesion on the left side of the mandible and one lesion on the maxilla's right side). These lesions can be unifocal or multifocal with the syndrome

though it is less expansive than a dentigerous cyst (Figs. 48.5, 48.6, and 48.7).

Odontoma

Odontoma is either complex or compound. The compound type occurs mostly in the anterior maxilla, and the complex type occurs more often behind the mandible. The internal structure of the odontoma is opaque and consists of a lucent rim (soft tissue capsule) next to a corticated border [1, 8].

Concerning their shape, compound odontomas are tooth-like structures, while complex odontomas are irregular and shapeless [9, 10] (Figs. 48.8 and 48.9).

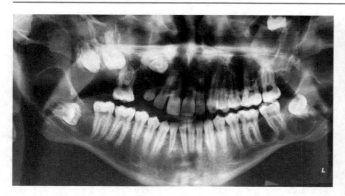

Fig. 48.7 Another example is the multiple KOT found in all four quadrants

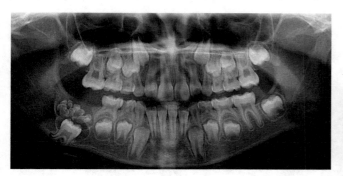

Fig. 48.8 To the right of the mandible can be seen a complex odontoma lesion in the panoramic view. Unlike compound odontoma, the masses are irregular in shape and cause displacement of the first molar

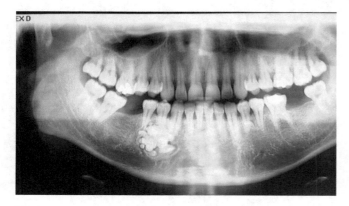

Fig. 48.9 In the panoramic view, a compound odontoma lesion can be seen to the right of the mandible

Radicular Cysts

Radicular cysts are the most common maxillary cysts and usually occur when there is a necrotic tooth. Therefore, the presence of deep caries or deep repairs is an important indicator for the diagnosis of this cyst. This cyst has a completely radiolucent internal structure with definite corticated borders [1, 11].

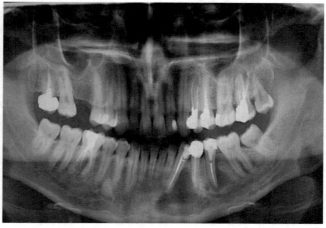

Fig. 48.10 In the panoramic view on the left side of the mandible, radicular cyst lesions related to teeth 3, 4, and 5 can be seen. In addition to the displacement of the teeth, these lesions can also cause root resorption of adjacent teeth

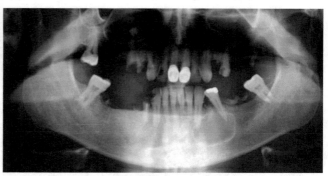

Fig. 48.11 In the panoramic view, a radicular cyst associated with the first premolar is seen on the mandible's left side. This lesion has well-defined corticated borders

Their shape, like other cysts, is like a balloon or a water-filled balloon and hydraulics. However, in the long run, the internal structure could lose its radiolucency and may contain small calcified particles (dystrophic calcification). Furthermore, like radicular ameloblastomic cysts, they can cause root resorption and displacement of adjacent teeth [12, 13] (Figs. 48.10, 48.11 and 48.12).

Fibrous Dysplasia

Fibrous dysplasia usually occurs unilaterally and generally in the maxilla. A major difference with previous lesions is its obscure limits. Its internal structure compared to normal bones can be more radiolucent or radiopaque or a combination of both. Needless to say, in more mature lesions, the internal pattern is opaquer. Various sources have suggested different names for the pattern of radiopacity resulting from fibrous dysplasia, referring to them as "orange peel-like" or "frosted glass" [1, 14, 15].

Fibrosis dysplasia usually causes spindle-shaped expansion of bone along the longitudinal axis while maintaining the cortex of bone. Moreover, a unique feature is the reduction of air-filled space of sinuses while maintaining a normal shape [1] (Figs. 48.13 and 48.14).

Florid-Osseous Dysplasia

It is similar to periapical osseous dysplasia in many ways, and a major difference that distinguishes the two is the occurrence of florid-osseous dysplasia in multiple quadrants of the jaw. Usually, the internal structure of these lesions is a radiolucent-radiopaque mixture, and in older lesions, it may be completely radiopaque [1].

The borders of these lesions are usually clear and can also have soft tissue capsules, although it may not be possible to see them in very mature radiopaque lesions [16, 17].

A differential diagnosis of fibrous dysplasia is that here the inferior alveolar canal moves upward, while as it moves downward in osseous florid [18] (Figs. 48.15 and 48.16).

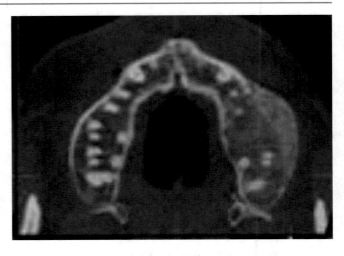

Fig. 48.14 In the axial view of the CBC images, there is a fusiform expansion to the left of the maxilla

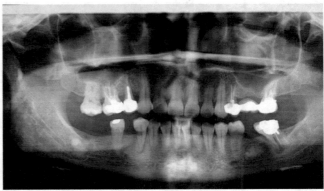

Fig. 48.15 Florid cemento-osseous dysplasia in a panoramic view seen in several quadrants. In this view, a lesion can be seen on both sides of the mandible

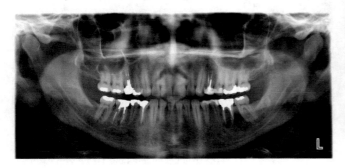

Fig. 48.12 Infected radicular cysts are seen on the left side of the mandible. These infected cysts can be sclerotic or ill-defined

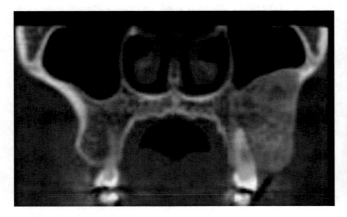

Fig. 48.13 Coronal view of CBCT image: on the maxilla's left side, there is an increase in bone density due to a fibrous dysplasia lesion. In this case, the superior displacement of the sinus floor is seen

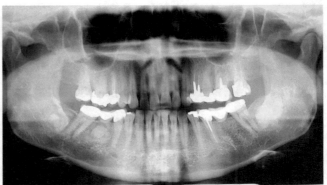

Fig. 48.16 Another example of Florid Osseous Dysplasia (FOD) in different quadrants

Osteosarcoma

Osteosarcoma is a malignant lesion that usually occurs in the mandible, and due to its malignant nature, its boundaries are unclear, and its internal structure can vary from a range of completely radiolucent to completely radiopaque. One of the hallmarks of this lesion is the resemblance of bone spicules to the sunbeams [1, 19].

It can have a variety of effects on surrounding structures due to its malignant nature. For example, it can dilate the periodontal membrane, which is not specific to osteosarcoma. The destruction of bone structures, such as the walls of the corticated sinuses and canal, is another effect of this lesion on the surrounding structures [1, 20].

References

1. White SC, Pharoah MJ. Oral radiology: principles and interpretation. Elsevier Health Sciences; 2019.
2. Yuan M, Ya-Ning Z, Ya-Qiong Z. Three-dimensional radiographic features of ameloblastoma and cystic lesions in the maxilla. Dentomaxillofac Radiol. 2019;48(6):20190066.
3. Bruno AM, Bruno A, Michelle A. Radiographic estimation of the growth rate of initially underdiagnosed ameloblastomas. Med Oral Patol Oral Cir Bucal. 2019;24(4):e468–72.
4. Petrovic ID, Migliacci J, Ganly I. Ameloblastomas of the mandible and maxilla. Ear Nose Throat J. 2018;97(7):E26–32.
5. Cheranjeevi J, Anila B, Nikunj P. A case of impacted central incisor due to dentigerous cyst associated with impacted compound odontome. BMJ Case Rep. 2014;2014:bcr2013202447.
6. Masahiko T, Satoshi A, Junya K. An analysis of dentigerous cysts developed around a mandibular third molar by panoramic radiographs. Dent J (Basel). 2019;7(1):13.
7. Andrea B, Cosimo N, Caterina G. Odontogenic keratocyst: imaging features of a benign lesion with an aggressive behavior. Insights Imaging. 2018;9(5):883–97.
8. Bhavana A, Harshkant G, Preeti N. Infected complex odontoma: an unusual presentation. BMJ Case Rep. 2012;2012:bcr2012006493.
9. Pillai A, Moghe S, Gupta MK, Pathak A. A complex odontoma of the anterior maxilla associated with an erupting canine. BMJ Case Rep. 2013: bcr2013200684. https://doi.org/10.1136/bcr-2013-200684. PMID: 24225732; PMCID: PMC3830212.
10. de Cintia V, Luégya A, Maria C. Impacted permanent incisors associated with compound odontoma. BMJ Case Rep. 2015;2015:bcr2014208201.
11. Peeyush S, Ankur S, Naqoosh H. Multilocular radicular cyst – A common pathology with uncommon radiological appearance. J Clin Diagn Res. 2016;10(3):ZD13–5.
12. Shibani S, Punnya V, Angadi K. Radicular cyst in deciduous maxillary molars: a rarity. Head Neck Pathol. 2010;4(1):27–30.
13. De J, Ratika S. Giant radicular cyst of the maxilla. BMJ Case Rep. 2014;2014:bcr2014203678.
14. Andrea B, Michael TC, Alison MB. Fibrous dysplasia of bone: craniofacial and dental implications. Oral Dis J. 2018.
15. Deepak G, Preeti G, Amit M. Computed tomography in craniofacial fibrous dysplasia: a case series with review of literature and classification update. Open Dent J. 2017;11:384–403.
16. McCarthy EF. Fibro-osseous lesions of the maxillofacial bones. Head Neck Pathol. 2013;7(1):5–10.
17. Brenda L, Billy J. Benign fibro-osseous lesions of the head and neck. Head Neck Pathol. 2019;13(3):466–75.
18. Victor D, Anne-Laure E, Charles G. Differentiating early stage florid osseous dysplasia from periapical endodontic lesions: a radiological-based diagnostic algorithm. BMC Oral Health. 2017;17(1):161.
19. Tadahide N, Yasushi S, Naruo O. A modified preauricular and transmandibular approach for surgical management of osteosarcoma of the mandibular condyle within the masticator space and infratemporal fossa: a case report. J Med Case Rep. 2019;13(1):58.
20. Guo Dong W, Yun Fu Z, , Yuan L.Periosteal osteosarcoma of the mandible: case report and review of the literature. J Oral Maxillofac Surg 2011 ; 69(6): 1831–1835.

Skull Reconstruction for Craniosynostosis

Moosa Mahmoudi and Sara Samiei

Craniosynostosis is a congenital defect defined as a premature fusion of one or more sutures in craniosynostosis [1]. According to a recent prevalence survey, this condition affects about 1 in 2000–2500 births worldwide [2–4]. Craniosynostosis usually occurs as an isolated event (non-symptomatologic craniosynostosis), but it can also be associated with a particular syndrome (symptomatologic craniosynostosis).

Morphological abnormalities linked with craniosynostosis include atypical skull vaults and facial asymmetry. According to Virchow's law, calvaria's growth occurs in a plane parallel to the fused suture's growth, but the growth in the vertical plane is interrupted [5]. As a result, the calvaria deformity provides information about which sutures are fused. Therefore, craniosynostosis is divided into coronary (frontal cranial), sagittal (scapula), lambdoid (occipital), and metopic (pyramid head) in terms of the affected sutures and the resulting malformations [6]. These morphological abnormalities can also have functional consequences, such as impaired brain growth and increased intracranial pressure [7].

Although significant improvements have been made in craniosynostosis management, surgical management is the preferred treatment in most cases. Minimally invasive techniques have been proposed [8], but these approaches are usually reserved for patients <6 months of age with mild malformations with only one suture [9]. The most commonly accepted treatment is modifying an open skull vault to normalize the bald shape to increase intracranial volume and reduce the risk of increased intracranial pressure. Surgery consists of three stages: (1) removal of affected bone, (2) bone remodeling in the most suitable form for the patient, and (3) remodeled bone placement and fixation [10]. The

consensus is to operate on patients 1 year before birth to maximize reoxidation by taking advantage of this childhood bone malleability [11].

Today, the diagnosis and surgical correction of craniosynostosis are based primarily on the surgeon's subjective judgment, the degree of deformation, and the modification of the affected bone to best restore the skull's standard shape. Decide on an approach. This approach usually lengthens the duration of surgery and relies heavily on the surgeon's experience. Computer-assisted surgical plans have been proposed to improve these surgical procedures' accuracy and efficiency [12, 13]. Therefore, an osteotomy can be designed preoperatively, and the bone can be virtually constructed to achieve the desired shape and features. For a more objective plan, the normative skull model can be used as a reference when remodeling the virtual skull taking into account the patient's age and gender [14–16]. In addition, realistic 3D-printed skull models can simulate surgery before surgery to improve the quality of treatment and medical education [17–19].

Syndromic Craniosynostosis

Pfeiffer, Crouzon, Saether-Chotzen, Apert, and Muenke syndromes are the five most common forms of syndromic craniosynostosis. Even though each has a different genetic basis and associated abnormalities, their hallmark is turribrachycephaly, which is most often associated with craniosynostosis.

Early local or partial cranial resection may be urgently indicated in multistore cases with signs of increased intracranial pressure. Others can be well managed with posterior vault distraction, central vault dilation, or anterior orbital advancement. Some authors advocate early monobloc advances for patients in need of acute airway intervention and globe protection, but the risks of these procedures are high.

Many patients require central facial advancement by joining, monoblock, or bisected facial relocation in addi-

M. Mahmoudi (✉)
Department of OMFS, Kerman University of Medical Sciences, Kerman, Iran
e-mail: mahmoodimusa@gmail.com

S. Samiei
Kerman University of Medical sciences, Kerman, Iran
e-mail: sarah.Samiei89@gmail.com

M. R. Stevens et al. (eds.), *Innovative Perspectives in Oral and Maxillofacial Surgery*,
https://doi.org/10.1007/978-3-030-75750-2_49

tion to Le Fort III and Le Fort II. This step in the treatment algorithm provides the greatest functional and aesthetic benefits and the potential for maximum morbidity, thus providing indications, risks, and benefits for each central facial procedure. It is not uncommon for patients to require traditional orthopedic surgery and other bone and soft tissue modeling procedures during peak facial growth. Finally, understanding the psychological aspects of craniofacial differences in both the affected individual and their families is essential to the success of holistic approach (*Plast. Reconstr. Surg.* 140: 82e).

Main goals in syndromic craniosynostosis cases include (1) to optimize cerebral blood flow, increase cranial volume to prevent sequelae of intracranial pressure, and (2) to the skull, orbit, and maxilla. These goals are to improve abnormal morphology [20]. Multiple operations are often required to achieve these goals, but careful response times and methods play an essential role in minimizing operations and providing the best results. There is evidence of psychological sequel in syndromic craniosynostosis cases in contrast with cases whom underwent surgery in the first year of life [21, 22]. This is especially true for apert syndrome and Crouzon and Pfeiffer syndromes, but not Muenke syndrome [21]. Mathijssen and Arnaud provided evidence to privilege the first surgery within the first year of life. More current data from Utria narrowed the window to 6–9 months of age [23] (Table 49.1).

The timing of surgery for symptomatological craniosynostosis is controversial, and more prospective comparative studies are needed to address this critical issue adequately.

Types of Surgery

Early case series from several prominent international centers report evidence of early success with frontal dilatation of syndromic craniosynostosis [24–27]. Some have begun to report high reoperation rates for both intracranial pressure and morphological problems [28]. Non-invasive methods such as local cranial resection, occipital flap release, and remodeling through the cranial fornix ensure that the fountain increases the skull's volume in very young people [29].

In a direct volume comparison between anterior orbital advancement and posterior fornix extension, we found that the posterior fornix extension allows nearly twice the volume increase at similar perioperative morbidity.

Surgical Techniques and Approaches

Bicoronal Synostosis

Early closure can occur unilaterally or bilaterally. Bicoronal craniosynostosis, known as turribrachycephaly, is most commonly related to symptomatological craniosynostosis. Cranial deformities look like barium with shorter anterior-posterior dimensions and flatter and higher vertical dimensions. This is due to stunts in a plane perpendicular to the fused suture. Both trajectories are also affected by the vertical elongation of the bone and the flat top surface.

In monocoronary fusion, barium and orbital restrictions progress along with a typical pattern with orbital harlequin deformity and procerus deviation to the affected side due to flattening and growth limitation of the frontal and parietal bones. Opposite anterior and posterior protrusions are often seen.

Facial skeletal distraction for cases with previous intervention may help to improve facial asymmetry. However, each intervention should be weighed against the tolerance of complex postoperative care, the underlying function, and the psychosocial impact of multiple surgeries (Table 49.2).

Innovative surgical approaches to correct severe obstructive sleep apnea and facial growth limitation include monoblock advancement, Le Fort III, combined Le Fort III and Le Fort I Ostectomy, Le Fort III, and zygomatic bone splitting [30–32].

The author's preferred approaches are a combination of Le Fort III and Le Fort I, a split sagittal bilateral osteotomy if the facial deformities, including occlusal inconsistencies, can be completely corrected. Monoblock progress is an important tool. However, if a well-performed frontal orbital advance has already been made, this can overcorrect or displace the upper third of the face and nose. An important subdivision of Le Fort III's progress is the use of different advances in the central face

Table 49.1 Surgical time for syndromic craniosynostosis

<3 month	Strip craniectomy if evidence of elevated ICP, multi suture synostosis
6–8 month	Posterior vault distraction
10–18 month	Fronto-orbital advancement
5–9 year	Le Fort III, Le Fort I DO (early mixed dentition)
9–12 year	Le Fort III/monobloc advancement (late mixed dentition)
15–20 year	Orthognathic surgery to set occlusion, facial balance

Table 49.2 Surgical rehabilitation options for midface dysmorphism

Findings	Surgical goals	Surgical approach
Exorbitism	Increase volume	Le Fort III
Exposure keratopathy	Orbital protection	Monobloc
Airway obstruction	Nasal and pharyngeal airway	Component surgical
Tracheostomy	Decannulate	Combination of Le Fort III, Le Fort I, DO
Short radix tip	Normalize nasal length	
Anterior crossbite	Positive overjet	

through the cheekbones, which may allow for better correction in the presence of significant asymmetry [32].

Focusing on delaying frontal surgery, some patients eliminated anterior orbital advancement and switched directly to monoblock surgery at about 5 years of age. It was recently announced that the use of early posterior cranial fornix extension would reduce the number of major craniofacial surgeries experienced by patients with apartment syndrome in the first 5 years of life, thereby reducing exposure to general anesthesia and its consequences of perioperative blood loss [33].

Figure 49.1 shows an algorithm for treating syndromic craniosynostosis with the posterior fornix's early extension. Data from previous case studies based in Netherlands further support this algorithm, based on the large occipital peri-frontal dilation and low incidence of posterior tonsillar hernia in the occipital region as early surgery for Apert and Crouzon-Pfeiffer syndromes. Dilation is preferred for follow-up surgery and reduced incidence of papilledema [34].

Apert, Crouzon, and Pfeiffer syndromes are associated with varying degrees of maxillary hypoplasia, disturbance, and hypertelorism [35]. It is important to emphasize that hypoplasia exists in the vertical, sagittal, and lateral planes and makes an accurate anatomical diagnosis of which plane

is involved. Both degrees help guide surgical choices to correct physical and functional deformities [35]. Orthodontic indications include acute or chronic visual impairment, obstructive sleep apnea, inferior obstruction, and appearance problems [34]. The surgery timing is tailored to functional needs, preferably delaying surgery at age 5–8, at which point the trajectory is essentially physically mature [36].

An important principle of mid-face surgery is an excessive sagittal correction, especially if performed early. If the patient is not overcorrected to the point where he appears to be "sniffing," he may need to move his central face further forward in later years. If there is anterior bar retraction, then after repeated anterior cranial dilations, one should choose between central facial advancement and single-block osteotomy with or without facial halving.

Proponents of Separating

Cranial dilatation from central facial advance generally points to a relatively high prevalence of the combination of the two [37]. Proponents of monoblocks, with or without facial dichotomy, highlight the inherent benefits of surgical

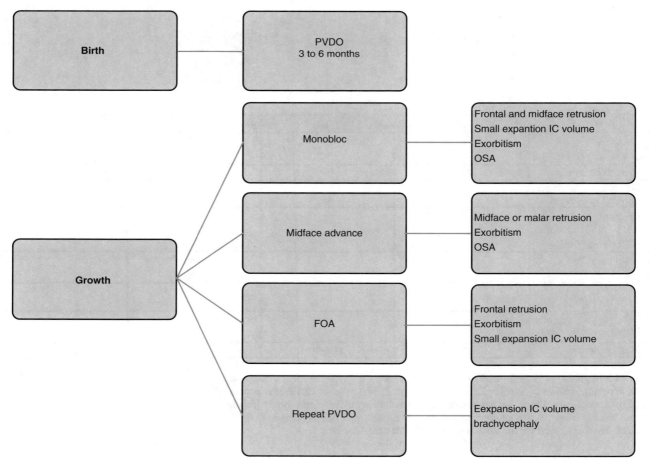

Fig. 49.1 Management algorithm for children with syndromic craniosynostosis. PVDO posterior vault distraction osteogenesis, FOA fronto-orbital advancement, OSA Obstructive sleep apnea

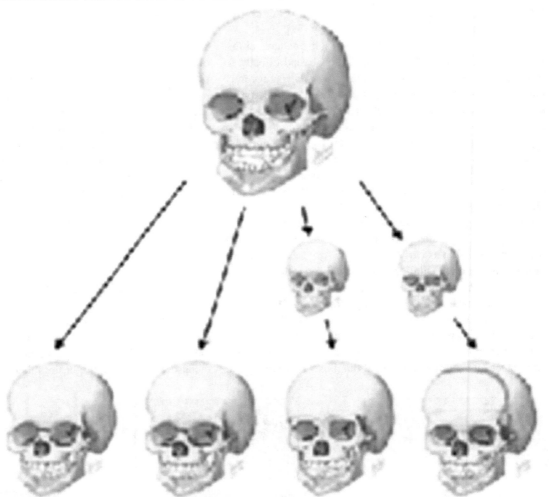

	Lefort III	Lefort II + ZR	Facial Bipartition	Monobloc
Levels palpebral fissure	–	++	++	–
Expands cranium	No	No	Yes	Yes
Nastal Lengthening	–	++	–	–
Lengthens midface	–	++	++	–
Differential advancement: central vs peripheral	–	++	++	–
Close anterior open bite	–	++ (level)	++ (V-shaped)	–
Correct hypertelorism	–	–	++	–
Decrease bi-zygomatic width	–	–	++	–
Morbidity profile	Lower	Lower	Higher	Higher

Fig. 49.2 Options for central facial osteotomy in children with syndromic craniosynostosis, including Le Fort III, Le Fort II with zygomatic relocation, monoblock, and monoblock with the dichotomy of the face. The table below the line art provides a comparative assessment of the risk-to-benefit ratios for the various options. The extension of Le Fort II's central face with zygomatic relocation is accompanied by a different relocation of the lateral orbital junction complex from the central face, which tends to be more hypoplastic in patients with Apert syndrome [39]

load reduction with an acceptable morbidity profile, especially when performing distractions [38] (Fig. 49.2).

Monobloc Distraction with Facial Bipartition

A competing surgical choice in some Pfeiffer patients with Apert and biconcave facial dysmorphism is a monobloc with a bisected facial procedure. Popularized by Craig et al. and Ponniah et al., combined monobloc facial bipartition with distraction (MFBD) put facial halves to "open" or "relax" the face, improve hyperm, teloriscorrect disturbances, close anterior (V-shaped) open bites, improve central one-third canthal tilt, and reduce face width [40, 41] (Figs. 49.3 and 49.4). It allows for more significant advancement of the central midline than the sides, similar to the Le Fort II central surface's distraction with zygomatic relocation, but without lengthening the ventral midline [42].

Non-syndromic Craniosynostosis

Craniosynostosis occurs more often in men than in women. Single-sutured non-syndromic symmetric bone union (metopic, sagittal) is more common in boys, and asymmetric (single crown or lambdoid) fusion is more common in girls [43].

Hydrocephalus

Hydrocephalus rarely occurs in both syndromic and non-syndromic craniosynostosis but is much more common in the earlier group.

Visually Impaired

Elevated intracranial pressure can cause papilledema and optic nerve atrophy. Once more, these findings are more common in multi-sutured craniosynostosis and symptomatic craniosynostosis than in single-sutured non-syndromic craniosynostosis because of the potential for higher intracranial pressure in the previous.

Timing of Surgery

The optimal timing and type of surgical correction for non-syndromic craniosynostosis with a single suture remain controversial (see form and function below). Most surgeons agree that such procedures are ideally performed within 6–9 months for vault remodeling procedures such as anterior orbital advancement and posterior vault remodeling.

The general purpose of vault modifications is to correct the deformation with some overcorrection. Stabilization of relocated bone segments is achieved by using intervening bone grafts, sutures, and resorbable plates and screws. The goal is to create a stable structure but not to limit brain growth and subsequent skull expansion. Titanium or metal plates are not used for infants undergoing cranial remodeling due to the risk of transcranial migration and growth limitation [44–46].

Limited incision and endoscopic techniques for suture resection use smaller incisions in different locations, not fixation. Blood loss is generally the most crucial consideration during skull surgery [47]. Blood loss should be closely tracked and resurrected according to the patient's hemodynamics.

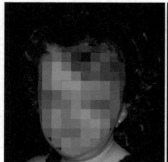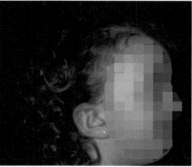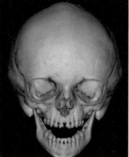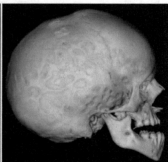

Fig. 49.3 (Left) Anteroposterior photograph of a 2-year-old girl with Crouzon syndrome. (Second from left) Lateral photograph of a 2-year-old girl with Crouzon syndrome. (Second from right) Anteroposterior view of a three-dimensional computed tomographic scan. (Right) Lateral view of a three-dimensional computed tomographic scan

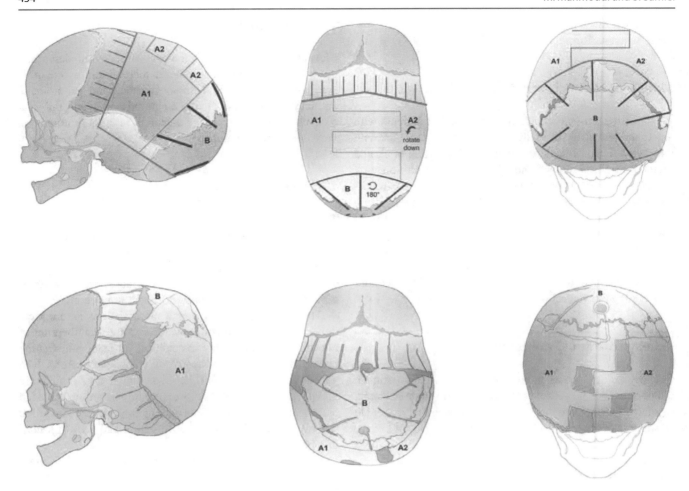

Fig. 49.4 Schematic representation of a posterior vault reconstruction for correction of sagittal synostosis. Note the transposition of the parietal segments (A1 and A2) to the occiput to facilitate shortening and expansion using a tongue-and-groove osteotomy pattern. The bulleted occiput (B) is flattened using radial osteotomies and transposed to the vertex

A significant portion of total blood loss occurs during skin incisions and exposures. Options for limiting blood loss at these stages include peri-incision ("blocking") hemostatic sutures, runny clips, electrocautery of Colorado tips, and swollen solutions containing adrenaline [48]. Other causes of routine blood loss are transosseous perforators and osteotomy.

Specific Features and Treatment Modalities

Sagittal Presentation

Sagittal fusion causes the scalp (a characteristic "boat-shaped" head) secondary to limiting lateral bitemporal growth and promoting anterior-posterior dilation. This is the most common form of non-syndromic single suture osteo-synthesis (about 60% of cases). The 70 cranial index, the ratio of bilateral parietal diameter to frontal-occipital distance, is the most common measure used to assess the scapular skull. The index of the head is between 76 and 82, usually less than 76 in sagittal fusion. On investigation, the sagittal suture can be palpated at the top of scalp, and one or both fontanels can be closed.

Treatment

The treatment of sagittal fusion has undergone a steady evolution over the last two decades. There remains considerable disagreement about the best way to correct these patients [49] surgically. Traditional treatments include open vault remodeling or skull resection, and endoscopic techniques (strip skull resection) have evolved as less invasive alternatives since they were reported in the literature of 1998 [50].

Traditional ball remodeling is still considered the standard treatment for sagittal fusion, especially in patients treated at an older age (6 months or older). Some surgeons advocate a one-step complete vault reconstruction [51], while others suggest posterior vault reconstruction (Fig. 49.3) or anterior, depending on the deformity's location and severity.

Metopic Presentation

Metopic synostosis, also known as the triangular skull, results in a characteristic "keel"-shaped forehead and triangular head shape. This is the second most common form of skull fusion, with about 30% in new cases. Unlike other cranial sutures, forehead sutures usually fuse within 8 months. Therefore, mild head shape abnormalities are detected in late childhood and do not necessarily require aggressive diagnosis and/or surgery [52]. Upper orbital advancements may be needed to be performed [53, 54].

Division of the anterior orbital bar at the midline and enlargement with intervening bone grafts allows for increased occlusion and interorbital distance. The new structure shows a dull intracranial angle, evidenced by the lateral boundary and temporal region's advancement and enlargement. This fascia corresponds to the junctional frontal and nasal frontal regions and is temporarily held in place by suturing with an absorbent plate. Advanced fascial recurrence (or limited growth of fused sutures) ensures overcorrection for better long-term results [54].

Unicoronal Presentation

Single coronary fusion, also known as the anterior-cranial, shows ipsilateral forehead growth limitation, resulting in a flattened forehead and supraorbital border and in a temporal defect. On the contrary, a compensatory uplift occurs on the forehead. The ipsilateral orbit is higher and narrower, raising the eyebrows and keeping the eyes "more open," instead of the normal opposite side. Radiologically, this appears as a peak on the orbital bone's superior lateral surface and is called a "harlequin deformity."

In addition, the base of the nose is also directed to the affected ipsilateral, and the ipsilateral ear is usually displaced above and/or anterior to the unaffected side. In rare cases, a shift of the jaw to the unaffected side may be present following a change in the glenoid fossa position [55]. Single coronary bone union accounts for about 10% of all non-symptomatologic single suture bone union [56].

Treatment

Monocoronal fusion's primary surgical treatment involves reconstructing the anterior forehead with anterior advancement of the ipsilateral forehead and supraorbital border. This can be reliably done using variations of frontal orbit advanced technology. Depending on the deformity's severity, bilateral or unilateral advancement of the bandeau and frontal bone may occur [57]. This approach allows correction of ipsilateral orbital deformity and remodeling of the ipsilateral and contralateral foreheads. Supraorbital bands are usually split and enlarged with intervening bone grafts to accommodate differences in orbital width.

Overcorrection is needed in anticipation of the loss of facial growth potential and continued skull growth. Depending on the deformity's required correction and severity, various techniques and modifications of the typical frontal orbitofrontal cortex are used for monocoronal fusion [58]. As the ipsilateral orbit and forehead advance, the orbit can be lowered (bone graft or downward repositioning), and the contralateral forehead can be submerged or shaped to reduce protrusions. Occasionally, the frontal segment is ectopically replaced with or without rotation.

Once the fascia is positioned, an intraoperative evaluation is needed to define the optimal fit before taking the bone graft (to avoid defects in the forehead's visible part). If desired, canthopexy can be performed on the affected lateral canthus. Distraction bone formation has also been proposed to treat monocoronary osteosynthesis, with early data showing promising results [59]. Endoscopic suture resection followed by helmet therapy has also been reported and is used in several institutions [8].

Lambdoid Presentation

Unilateral craniosynostosis is very rare and is the least common among non-symptomatological craniosynostosis (<1%) [56, 60]. Patients affected show ipsilateral occipital flattening, ipsilateral occipital displacement, and milky swelling. Mastoid swelling was demonstrated by Ploplys et al. [61] as an essential feature in the pre-imaging diagnosis of lambdoid osteosynthesis. Secondary protrusions on the opposite side of the forehead are often observed, forming a trapezoidal head [61]. It is important to distinguish between patients with unilateral lambdoid osteoarthritis (usually a trapezoidal head shape) and patients with a deformed positional cranial head (parallelogram head shape). Ear position remains a clinically unreliable function. However, computed tomography has shown that the affected ear is closer to the anterior nasal spine [61].

Treatment

Surgical treatment of lambdoid bone fusion depends on the severity of the deformity. In mild to moderate cases, open suture resection with a fracture of the barrel stave and ipsilateral occipital bone has been proposed. Due to the baby's supine position after sleep surgery, the correction is likely to recur. Infants and children with more severe deformities require treatment by remodeling the cranial fornix.

Some authors used switch cranioplasty with occipital bar advance with resorbable fixation to maintain correction [62, 63]. This technique involves half of the posterior fornix bone flap. Then, each half is transposed to the other side and rotated 90–180 degrees for an optimal fit. Discarding the conventional supraorbital fascia for a simplified single-segment anterior reconstruction requires long-term evaluation but may improve the forehead's aesthetics.

Patients and Methods

Surgical Technique

To change the shape of the frontal bone in a single segment, first measure the area under the skin on the forehead that does not support the weight to determine the donor's bone flap's approximate size. A scalp-shaped coronal incision (modified from the zigzag pattern above) provides access to the skull, and the scalp flap is lifted above the humeral surface [64]. A peri-bone incision is made in parallel, just behind the suture. The pericranial flaps based on the coronary arteries and anterior and posterior are elevated. The temporalis muscle rises continuously with the anterior flap, and the dissection advances anteriorly to the supraorbital margin level. No intraorbital incision is required. The donor site's specific location is then determined by visual perception of the entire posterior skull, selecting the ideal curvature for reconstructing the forehead as a single unit.

In most cases, the second half of the lateral bone appears to provide the best overall shape. This piece of bone is

removed by a neurosurgeon, usually after mapping a suitable size of about 20 × 6 cm. For several reasons, the recommended timing for this procedure is 11 months or older. When making previous repairs, special care must be taken to ensure that the two wall bones do not separate along the more active and unentangled sagittal suture. After the removal of the frontal bone, the lower part of the supraorbital region is removed to the floor of the anterior orbit to facilitate anterior and lateral dilation of the anterior orbit. The removed bilateral parietal bones, frontal bone, and supraorbital bone are posterior tables to collect enough bone for reconstructing the posterior donor site and all other defects left by the expected skull enlargement and divided above.

Forehead reconstruction proceeds with proper placement of both parietal flaps. During treatment of the triangular skull, this flap is fixed to the midline, a U-shaped resorbable suture passes through two holes in the glabellar bone, and the outer surface of this flap advances on both sides. In unilateral correction of coronary fusion, this flap is properly advanced to overcorrect the concave side. This one-piece reconstruction replaces both the fascia and the frontal bone, with the lower end of this segment on the new orbit. You can create a subtle contour at this bottom edge to create a normal arched look at the top track edge. You can also use the bone bender to change the lateral curvature if desired.

Therefore, this single bone flap's underside is repositioned in the same way as the fascia repositioning to reconstruct the supraorbital region. Placing a new frontal bone allows you to mark the bone removal areas on both sides of the temporal area underneath this new bone flap. This bone removal allows precise end-to-end insertion of the new frontal bone's posterolateral surface, similar to the insertion of traditional fascia secured with resorbable sutures [65].

If the new bone flap's curvature appears to fill the temporal fossa too much, a cut can be made in the bone beneath the temporalis muscle (Fig. 49.5) to mitigate this transition. The posterior parietal donor site is then rebuilt using the previous supraorbital and frontal bones enlarged by the split calvaria

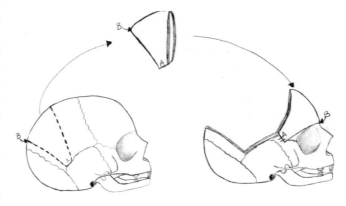

Fig. 49.5 Bone flap's curvature

graft. Large grafts are secured with absorbent sutures, and small grafts are secured with Surgicel (Ethicon, Inc., Somerville, N.J.). Single-segment reconstruction eliminates the supraorbital/frontal joint. This can become more apparent later if not fitted correctly and reduce the likelihood of local overgrowth that can occur in discontinuous bone segments.

The use of single-segment frontal reconstruction offers theoretical benefits. Still, the need to harvest additional bone from areas of the skull that traditionally remain intact raises questions about the effects of supplemental skull incisions.

Conclusion

Surgery for craniosynostosis consists of three steps:

1. Removal of the affected bones
2. Remodeling of the bones into the most appropriate shape for the patient
3. Placement and fixation of remodeled bones

Timing of surgery for both syndromic and non-syndromic craniosynostosis is controversial, and further research is needed to address this critical question adequately. Options for midface osteotomy in children with syndromic craniosynostosis include Le Fort III, Le Fort II with zygomatic repositioning monobloc, and monobloc with facial bipartition.

An essential part of midface surgery is a sagittal overcorrection, especially when performed early. Treatment for non-syndromic craniosynostosis is dependent on the involved suture (metopic, sagittal, unicoronal, or lambdoid) and indicate suturectomy with vault reconstructions. Endoscopic suturectomy with helmet therapy has also been reported and is used in some centers.

References

1. Sharma R. Craniosynostosis. Indian J Plast Surg. 2013;46:18.
2. Lajeunie E, Le Merrer M, Bonaiti-Pellie C, Marchac D, Renier D. Genetic study of nonsyndromic coronal craniosynostosis. Am J Med Genet. 1995;55:500–4.
3. Boulet SL, Rasmussen SA, Honein MA. A population-based study of craniosynostosis in metropolitan Atlanta, 1989-2003. Am J Med Genet Part A. 2008;146:984–91.
4. Kweldam CF, Van Der Vlugt JJ, Van Der Meulen JJNM. The incidence of craniosynostosis in the Netherlands, 1997-2007. J Plast Reconstr Aesthetic Surg. 2011;64:583–8.
5. Virchow R. Uber den cretinismus, namentilich in franken, und uber pathologische schadelformen. Verh Phys Med Ges Wurzbg. 1851;2:230–56.
6. Kirmi O, Lo SJ, Johnson D, Anslow P, BChir M. Craniosynostosis: a radiological and surgical perspective. 2009; https://doi.org/10.1053/j.sult.2009.08.002.
7. Cohen SR, Frank RC, Meltzer HS, Levy ML. Craniosynostosis. Handb Craniomaxillofacial Surg. 2014:343–68. https://doi.org/10.1142/9789814295109_0013.
8. Jimenez DF, Barone CM. Early treatment of anterior calvarial craniosynostosis using endoscopic-assisted minimally invasive techniques. 2007:1411–9. https://doi.org/10.1007/s00381-007-0467-6.
9. Cohen SR, Holmes RE, Meltzer HS, Nakaji P. Immediate cranial vault reconstruction with bioresorbable plates following endoscopically assisted sagittal synostectomy. J Craniofac Surg. 2002;13:578–82.
10. Persing JA. MOC-PS(SM) CME article: management considerations in the treatment of craniosynostosis. Plast Reconstr Surg. 2008;121:1–11.
11. Slater BJ, et al. Cranial sutures: a brief review. Plast Reconstr Surg. 2008;121:170–8.
12. Steinbacher DM. Three-dimensional analysis and surgical planning in craniomaxillofacial surgery. J Oral Maxillofac Surg. 2015;73:S40–56.
13. Seruya M, et al. Computer-aided design and manufacturing in craniosynostosis surgery. J Craniofac Surg. 2013;24:1100–5.
14. Saber NR, et al. Generation of normative pediatric skull models for use in cranial vault remodeling procedures. Childs Nerv Syst. 2012;28:405–10.
15. Mendoza CS, et al. Personalized assessment of craniosynostosis via statistical shape modeling. Med Image Anal. 2014;18:635–46.
16. Soleman J, Thieringer F, Beinemann J, Kunz C, Guzman R. Computer-assisted virtual planning and surgical template fabrication for frontoorbital advancement. Neurosurg Focus. 2015;38:1–8.
17. Ghizoni E, et al. 3D-printed craniosynostosis model: a new simulation surgical tool. World Neurosurg. 2017;109:356–61.
18. Eastwood KW, et al. Development of synthetic simulators for endoscope-assisted repair of metopic and sagittal craniosynostosis. J Neurosurg Pediatr. 2018;22:128–36.
19. Jiménez Ormabera B, et al. Impresin 3 D en neurocirugía: modelo específico para pacientes con craneosinostosis. Neurocirugia. 2017;28:260–5.
20. Taylor JA, Derderian CA, Bartlett SP, Fiadjoe JE, Sussman EM, Stricker PA. Perioperative morbidity in posterior cranial vault expansion: distraction osteogenesis versus conventionalosteotomy. Plast Reconstr Surg. 2012;129:674e–80e.
21. Renier D, Lajeunie E, Arnaud E, Marchac D. Management of craniosynostoses. Childs Nerv Syst. 2000;16:645–58.
22. Arnaud E, Meneses P, Lajeunie E, Thorne JA, Marchac D, Renier D. Postoperative mental and morphological outcome for nonsyndromic brachycephaly. Plast Reconstr Surg. 2002;110:6–12; discussion 13
23. Mathijssen IM, Arnaud E. Benchmarking for craniosynostosis. J Craniofac Surg. 2007;18:436–42.
24. Thompson D, Jones B, Hayward R, Harkness W. Assessment and treatment of craniosynostosis. Br J Hosp Med. 1994;52:17–24.
25. Marchac D, Renier D, Broumand S. Timing of treatment for craniosynostosis and facio-craniosynostosis: a 20-year experience. Br J Plast Surg. 1994;47:211–22.
26. McCarthy JG, Glasberg SB, Cutting CB, et al. Twenty-year experience with early surgery for craniosynostosis: II. The craniofacial synostosis syndromes and pansynostosis—results and unsolved problems. Plast Reconstr Surg. 1995;96:284–95; discussion 296–298
27. Posnick JC. The craniofacial dysostosis syndromes: staging of reconstruction and management of secondary deformities. Clin Plast Surg. 1997;24:429–46.
28. Honnebier MB, Cabiling DS, Hetlinger M, McDonald-McGinn DM, Zackai EH, Bartlett SP. The natural history of patients treated for FGFR3-associated (Muenke-type) craniosynostosis. Plast Reconstr Surg. 2008;121:919–31.

29. Nowinski D, Di Rocco F, Renier D, SainteRose C, Leikola J, Arnaud E. Posterior cranial vault expansion in the treatment of craniosynostosis: comparison of current techniques. Childs Nerv Syst. 2012;28:1537–44.

30. Forrest CR, Hopper RA. Craniofacial syndromesand surgery. Plast Reconstr Surg. 2013;131:86e–109e.

31. Hopper RA. New trends in cranio-orbital and midface distraction for craniofacial dysostosis. CurrOpin Otolaryngol Head Neck Surg. 2012;20:298–303.

32. Hopper RA, Prucz RB, Iamphongsai S. Achieving differential facial changes with Le Fort III distractionosteogenesis: the use of nasal passenger grafts, cerclage hinges, and segmental movements. Plast Reconstr Surg. 2012;130:1281–8.

33. Swanson JW, Samra F, Bauder A, Mitchell BT, Taylor JA, Bartlett SP. An algorithm for managing syndromic craniosynostosis using posterior vault distraction osteogenesis. Plast Reconstr Surg. 2016;137:829e–41e.

34. Spruijt B, Rijken BF, den Ottelander BK, et al. First vault expansion in Apert and Crouzon-Pfeiffer syndromes: front or back? Plast Reconstr Surg. 2016;137:112e–21e.

35. Mathijssen IM. Guideline for care of patients with the diagnoses of craniosynostosis: working group on craniosynostosis. J Craniofac Surg. 2015;26:1735–807.

36. Meazzini MC, Mazzoleni F, Caronni E, Bozzetti A. Le Fort III advancement osteotomy in the growing child affected by Crouzon's and Apert's syndromes: presurgical and postsurgical growth. J Craniofac Surg. 2005;16:369–77.

37. Shetye PR, Boutros S, Grayson BH, McCarthy JG. Midterm follow-up of midface distraction for syndromic craniosynostosis: a clinical and cephalometric study. Plast Reconstr Surg. 2007;120:1621–32.

38. Bradley JP, Gabbay JS, Taub PJ, et al. Monobloc advancement by distraction osteogenesis decreases morbidity and relapse. Plast Reconstr Surg. 2006;118:1585–97.

39. Hopper RA, Kapadia H, Morton T. Normalizing facial ratios in Apert syndrome patients with Le Fort II midface distraction and simultaneous zygomatic repositioning. Plast Reconstr Surg. 2013;132:129–40.

40. Greig AV, Britto JA, Abela C, et al. Correcting the typical Apert face: Combining bipartition with monobloc distraction. Plast Reconstr Surg. 2013;131:219e–30e.

41. Ponniah AJ, Witherow H, Richards R, Evans R, Hayward R, Dunaway D. Three-dimensional image analysis of facial skeletal changes after monobloc and bipartition distraction. Plast Reconstr Surg. 2008;122:225–31.

42. Dunaway DJ, Hukki JJ, Vuola PMB, et al. Comparison of bipartition distraction with Le Fort II and zygomatic repositioning in Apert Syndrome. Paper presented at: 16th Congress of the International Society of Craniofacial Surgery; September 14–18, 2015; Tokyo, Japan.

43. Lin IC, Slemp AE, Hwang C, Karmacharya J, Gordon AD, Kirschner RE. Immunolocalization of androgen receptor in the developing craniofacial skeleton. J Craniofac Surg. 2004;15:922–7; discussion 928

44. Fearon JA, Munro IR, Bruce DA. Observations on the use of rigid fixation for craniofacial deformities in infants and young children. Plast Reconstr Surg. 1995;95:634–7; discussion 638

45. Persing JA, Posnick J, Magge S, et al. Cranial plate and screw fixation in infancy: an assessment of risk. J Craniofac Surg. 1996;7:267–70.

46. Yu JC, Bartlett SP, Goldberg DS, et al. An experimental study of the effects of craniofacial growth on the longterm positional stability of microfixation. J Craniofac Surg. 1996;7:64–8.

47. Chow I, Purnell CA, Gosain AK. Assessing the impact of blood loss in cranial vault remodeling: a risk assessment model using the 2012 to 2013 Pediatric National Surgical Quality Improvement Program data sets. Plast Reconstr Surg. 2015;136:1249–60.

48. White N, Bayliss S, Moore D. Systematic review of interventions for minimizing perioperative blood transfusion for surgery for craniosynostosis. J Craniofac Surg. 2015;26:26–36.

49. Papay FA, Stein J, Luciano M, Zins JE. The microdissection cautery needle versus the cold scalpel in bicoronal incisions. J Craniofac Surg. 1998;9:344–7.

50. Jimenez DF, Barone CM. Endoscopic craniectomy for early surgical correction of sagittal craniosynostosis. J Neurosurg. 1998;88:77–81.

51. Fearon JA, McLaughlin EB, Kolar JC. Sagittal craniosynostosis: surgical outcomes and long-term growth. Plast Reconstr Surg. 2006;117:532–41.

52. Weinzweig J, Kirschner RE, Farley A, et al. Metopic synostosis: defining the temporal sequence of normal suture fusion and differentiating it from synostosis on the basis of computed tomography images. Plast Reconstr Surg. 2003;112:1211–8.

53. Marchac D, Renier D. The "floating forehead": early treatmentof craniofacial stenosis (in French). Ann Chir Plast. 1979;24:121–6.

54. Selber J, Reid RR, Gershman B, et al. Evolution of operative techniques for the treatment of single-suture metopic synostosis. Ann Plast Surg. 2007;59:6–13.

55. Williams JK, Ellenbogen RG, Gruss JS. State of the art incraniofacial surgery: nonsyndromic craniosynostosis. Cleft Palate Craniofac J. 1999;36:471–85.

56. Selber J, Reid RR, Chike-Obi CJ, et al. The changing epidemiologic spectrum of single-suture synostoses. Plast Reconstr Surg. 2008;122:527–33.

57. Bartlett SP, Whitaker LA, Marchac D. The operative treatment of isolated craniofacial dysostosis (plagiocephaly): a comparison of the unilateral and bilateral techniques. Plast Reconstr Surg. 1990;85:677–83.

58. Fearon JA. Beyond the bandeau: 4 variations on frontoorbital advancements. J Craniofac Surg. 2008;19:1180–2.

59. Tahiri Y, Swanson JW, Taylor JA. Distraction osteogenesis versus conventional fronto-orbital advancement for the treatment of unilateral coronal synostosis: a comparison of perioperative morbidity and short-term outcomes. J Craniofac Surg. 2015;26:1904–8.

60. Kadlub N, Persing JA, da Silva FR, Shin JH. Familial lambdoid craniosynostosis between father and son. J Craniofac Surg. 2008;19:850–4.

61. Ploplys EA, Hopper RA, Muzaffar AR, et al. Comparison of computed tomographic imaging measurements with clinical findings in children with unilateral lambdoid synostosis. Plast Reconstr Surg. 2009;123:300–9.

62. Smartt JM Jr, Reid RR, Singh DJ, Bartlett SP. True lambdoid craniosynostosis: long-term results of surgical and conservative therapy. Plast Reconstr Surg. 2007;120:993–1003.

63. Al-Jabri T, Eccles S. Surgical correction for unilateral lambdoid synostosis: a systematic review. J Craniofac Surg. 2014;25:1266–72.

64. Munro IR, Fearon JA. The coronal incision revisited. Plast Reconstr Surg. 1994;93:185–7.

65. Fearon JA. Rigid fixation of the calvaria in craniosynostosis without using "rigid" fixation. Plast Reconstr Surg. 2003;111:27–38; discussion 39

Innovations in the Management of Temporomandibular Joint Disorders

Aaron D. Figueroa, Joseph W. Ivory, and Rishad Shaikh

Introduction

Temporomandibular joint (TMJ) surgery is one of the more difficult subspecialty fields within oral and maxillofacial surgery. This stems from the complexity of managing difficult patients with multifactorial problems, including chronic pain and the inability to provide curative treatment in most cases. In addition, many previously innovative surgical treatments were found to be unreliable in the long term, and some resulting in Food and Drug Administration (FDA) recall. Innovations have been few in this area, which may stem from the lack of financial reimbursement and a diminishing interest in managing these complex patients outside of large academic centers. Despite this, some of the major innovations in diagnosis and treatment planning have been integrating cone-beam computed tomography (CBCT), intra-oral scanning, and virtual surgical planning (VSP) into daily practice. In addition, computed tomographic angiography (CTA) has been shown to provide useful diagnostic information preoperatively and, combined with interventional radiology procedures, can decrease intra-operative blood loss. Though most non-surgical interventions have remained unchanged, addition of chemodenervation with onabotulinum toxin A or Botox® (Allergan, Madison, New Jersey) has shown some promising results. TMJ arthroscopy has gone through significant innovative changes in the surgical realm, making it an excellent minimally invasive intervention. Advances in open TMJ surgery have included the use of the Mitek anchor (DePuy Synthes, Raynham, Massachusetts) in discopexy procedures and new knowledge in managing discectomy patients when considering grafting materials. Finally, the use of custom alloplastic joint replacements has been widely accepted, along with the integration of CBCT, intra-oral scanning, and VSP. Management of temporomandibular joint dysfunction is a broad topic, and it is the goal of this chapter to help review some of the more recent innovations in diagnosis and management.

Examination and Diagnosis

When managing patients with temporomandibular joint dysfunction (TMD), determining an accurate diagnosis is an important starting point in guiding appropriate treatment. From a diagnostic perspective, CBCT scanning has been one of the most important innovations for oral and maxillofacial surgery practice in recent years. Its application in the management of TMD ranges from its diagnostic value to its integration in treatment planning.

Though CBCT scanning can be an excellent adjunctive diagnostic tool, it is not a replacement for a thorough subjective evaluation and clinical examination. Questionnaires can help draw out subjective information in an organized manner from patients suffering from TMD (Fig. 50.1).

The subjective history and clinical examination should provide enough information for a working diagnosis. This diagnosis can then be confirmed or changed based on imaging findings.

Historically, an orthopantomogram served as an initial screening tool but provides a limited and distorted view of the TMJ complex's bony anatomy. It provides information on the overall shape and cortication of the condyle (Fig. 50.2). The position of the condyle within the glenoid fossa and joint space can also be evaluated. Many oral and maxillofacial surgery offices are equipped with CBCT scanners

A. D. Figueroa
Oral and Maxillofacial Surgery, University of Iowa Hospitals and Clinics, Iowa City, IA, USA
e-mail: aaron-figueroa@uiowa.edu

J. W. Ivory (✉)
Oral and Maxillofacial Surgery, Dwight D. Eisenhower Army Medical Center, Fort Gordon, GA, USA
e-mail: sgtdabney@gmail.com

R. Shaikh
Midwest Oral Maxillofacial Surgery and Implant Center, Saint Louis, MO, USA
e-mail: rshaikh_omfs@icloud.com

Temporomandibular Joint Pain (TMJ) Questionnaire
Department of Oral and Maxillofacial Surgery

1. Do you have pain in your TMJ (jaw joint)?   Y/N
   a. Is the pain on the (circle one):
      Left   **Right**   **Bilateral**
   b. Is the pain:
      Sharp   **Dull**
   c. Is the pain:
      Constant   **Occasional**
   d. Does anything make the pain worse?

      _____

   e. Does anything make the pain better? If so, What?   Y/N

      _____

   f. Are you having pain today?   Y/N
   g. On a scale of 1-10, what would you rate your pain?
   h. When is your TMJ pain the worse?
      Morning   **Afternoon**   **Evening**   **No difference**

2. Do you have joint noise?   Y/N
   a. Is the noise (circle one):

      Clicking   **Popping**   **Grinding**

   b. Is the pain associated with noise in your joint?   Y/N/NA
   c. When does your joint noise occur (circle one)?

      On opening   **On Closing**   **Opening and Closing**

3. Do you get headaches?   Y/N
   a. How bad are your headaches typically?
      Mild   **Moderate**   **Severe**
   b. When do you typically get headaches (cirle one)?
      Morning   **Afternoon**   **Evening**   **No difference**
   c. How many headaches do you get a week?   _____
   d. Where do your headaches typically occur (circle all that apply)?
      Left Forehead   **Right Forehead**   **Left Temple**   **Right Temple**
      Back of Head   **Top of Head**   **Left Eye**   **Right Eye**

4. Do you have pain elsewhere?   Y/N
   a. If so, where?_____
   b. Is the pain
      Mild   **Moderate**   **Severe**

5. Do you clech or grind your teeth?   Y/N
   a. If so, do you clech or grind (circle one)
      Daytime   **Nighttime**   **Both**   **Unsure**

6. Do you get earaches?   Y/N
   a. If so, are they (circle one):
      Mild   **Moderate**   **Severe**
   b. Do they occur (circle one):
      Seldom   **Frequently**   **Constant**
   c. Do you get ringing in your ears?   Y/N
   d. If so, is the ringing (circle one):
      Mild   **Moderate**   **Severe**
   e. Does it occur (circle one)"
      Seldom   **Frequently**   **Constant**

7. Have you tried any nonsurgical therapies for your jaw pain?   Y/N
   a. If so, what were they (meidcations, bite splints, massage therapy, etc...)?
      _____
      _____
      _____

   b. Did they give you any relief?   Y/N

8. Have you had anu surgeries on your TMJ?   Y/N
   a. If so, please indicate how many surgeries you have had on each side:
      Right____   Left____
   b. Did any of these procedures help?   Y/N

9. Do you have problems with other joints in your body?   Y/N
   a. If so, please list which joints are affected below:
      _____
      _____
      _____

10. Do you have depression?   Y/N
    a. If so, are you currently being treated?   Y/N

11. Please list your medications below:
    _____
    _____
    _____

12. Does your TMJ pain affect your quality of life?   Y/N
    a. Does it affect your daily activities?   Y/N
    b. Does it limit your diet?   Y/N
    c. List the foods you are typically unable to eat:
       _____
       _____
       _____

Fig. 50.1 An example TMJ examination questionnaire.

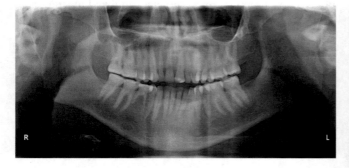

Fig. 50.2 Orthopantomogram showing bilateral severe degenerative joint disease

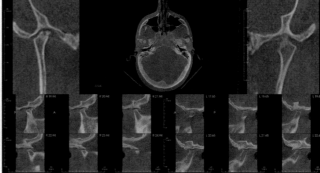

Fig. 50.3 CBCT of the same patient from Fig. 50.2, showing severe degenerative joint disease with coronal and sagittal image reconstruction

making three-dimensional data much more accessible to the surgeon in an office setting [1]. Prior to this, patients would be required to visit a hospital or radiology center to obtain a computed tomography (CT) scan.

The software available for viewing and manipulating the CBCT image data allows for very detailed evaluation and

reconstruction of the images, including creating an orthopantomogram if desired (Fig. 50.3). TMJ viewing windows allow for a detailed view of the condyles in all planes providing much more diagnostic information regarding the cortication of the joint, presence of subchondral cysts, lipping, flattening, and the overall shape of the condyle, fibrous and bony ankylosis, and the presence of bony or cartilaginous pathology among others [2, 3].

Magnetic resonance imaging (MRI) is useful in evaluating soft tissue abnormalities within the joint and has not undergone a significant change but remains a useful tool in diagnosis (Figs. 50.4 and 50.5).

The use of CTA has become helpful in analyzing the vascular anatomy around the joint space and the course of the internal maxillary artery (Fig. 50.6). In some cases, consideration can be placed on embolization of certain vessels that may pose a significant bleeding risk at the time of surgery. This will help keep the surgical field dry and increase the ease of surgery while also lowering the risk of inadvertent vascular compromise for the patient.

Diagnostic nerve blocks and joint injections can be helpful adjuncts in diagnosis but have also been techniques in use for a long time. More recently, TMJ arthroscopy has become an excellent diagnostic tool in evaluating the temporomandibular joint's health.

Integration of standard examination methods with newer imaging and diagnostic protocols can help provide very accurate diagnoses that will help guide appropriate treatment.

Myofascial Pain

Myofascial pain is a condition caused by inflammation of the muscles that control the mandible or myalgia. It is defined by pain at rest, pain on palpation at three or more sites, and at least one palpable painful site on the same side that the patient perceives pain [4]. Many times, it is associated with intra-articular TMD, but it can also be found in isolation. Parafunctional habits like bruxism are commonly seen in patients with myofascial pain. Other contributing factors include hyperfunction, stress, and possibly lack of stable occlusion. Clinically, pain is typically not well localized to the articulation or pre-auricular region but is described as diffuse, involving a whole side of the face, jaw, and temporal regions. Treatments are aimed at reducing parafunction, hyperfunction, stress, and inflammation.

The most recent innovation has been chemodenervation with Botox® (Allergan, Madison, New Jersey). Different approaches have been utilized, but all include injection of varying amounts of Botox® (Allergan, Madison, New Jersey) into the muscles of mastication (Fig. 50.7). When managing myofascial pain, simple injection into the masseter muscles and temporalis muscles seems to be an effective treatment modality. The analgesic effects of Botox® (Allergan, Madison, New Jersey) were first reported by

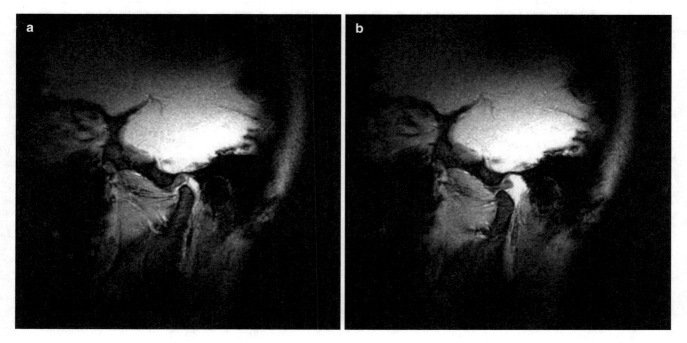

Fig. 50.4 (**a**) TMJ MRI in closed mouth view with normal anatomic position of the articular disc. (**b**) TMJ MRI in open mouth view with normal anatomic relationship between the articular disc, eminence, and condyle

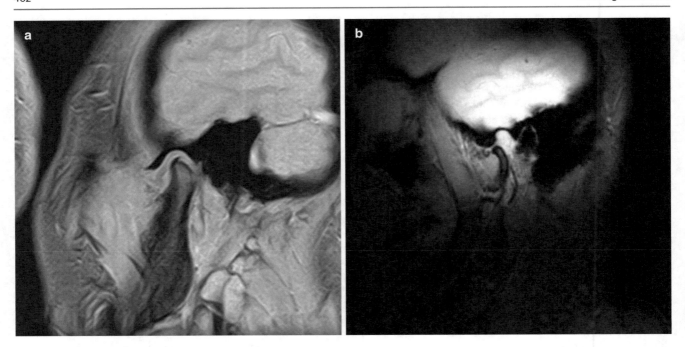

Fig. 50.5 (**a**) TMJ MRI in closed mouth view with anterior disc displacement. (**b**) TMJ MRI in open mouth views with anterior disc displacement without reduction

Binder in 2000, which may relate to the inhibition of the release of substance P and glutamate [5, 6]. Several subsequent studies have demonstrated the analgesic effects of intra-masseteric injections [7–10]. Researchers have reported Botox® (Allergan, Madison, New Jersey) to be superior to trigger point injections with normal saline as well as a local anesthetic with methylprednisolone [11, 12].

However, controversy remains as it has been pointed out that these studies are methodologically diverse, and the sample sizes are typically small. Also, there have been some studies that, though also having a small sample size (and in one case, a 30% dropout rate), failed to show statistically significant pain reductions [13, 14]. Milne reported a case series comparing the results of masseteric Botox® (Allergan, Madison, New Jersey) injections alone with patients receiving masseteric and temporalis injections. He reported that though both groups reported significant and similar reductions in pain scores, those receiving temporalis injections had a slight worsening of their maximum incisal opening (MIO). Therefore, he recommended Botox® (Allergan,

Madison, New Jersey) be relegated to the use in the masseter only [15].

Botox® (Allergan, Madison, New Jersey) remains a promising non-surgical therapy to address myofascial pain. More randomized clinical controlled studies are needed to define the possible benefit further.

Internal Derangements

Internal derangements differ from myofascial pain in that they represent a true intra-articular problem. They are one of the more common problems seen within the TMJ. They occur in many individuals that remain asymptomatic, possibly forever. For some reason, they seem to bring on significant pain and dysfunction in other individuals. Internal derangements arise from a non-anatomic position of the articular disc within the joint capsule at rest and the mandible function. These derangements are divided into anterior disc displacement with reduction and without reduction.

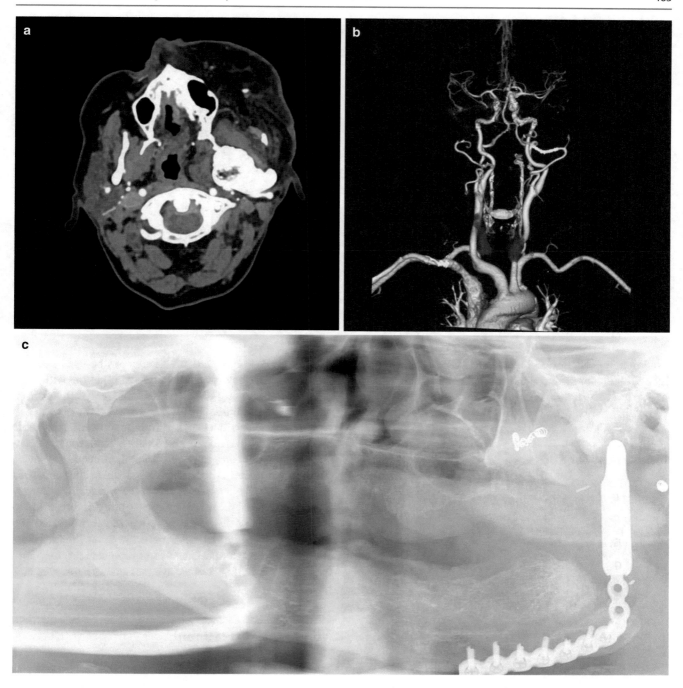

Fig. 50.6 (a) CTA in the axial view with the internal maxillary artery running just posterior to the large ankylotic bony mass. (b) Three-dimensional reconstruction of the vascular anatomy around the ankylo-sis. (c) Post-operative orthopantomogram showing stable position of temporary reconstruction hardware and coils from the pre-operative embolization procedure

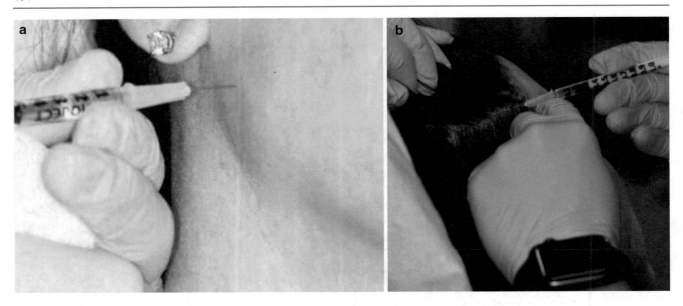

Fig. 50.7 (**a**) Botox® (Allergan, Madison, New Jersey) injection into the masseter muscle. (**b**) Botox® (Allergan, Madison, New Jersey) injection into the temporalis muscle

Traditionally, when speaking of the TMJ's internal derangements, clinicians have used the classification system devised by Wilkes to describe the severity of the derangement (Fig. 50.8).

Indications for Surgery

Absolute	Relative
Pathology	Internal derangements
Synovial chondromatosis	Severe degenerative joint disease
	Idiopathic condylar resorption
Benign/malignant tumors	Juvenile and rheumatoid arthritis
Chondroma	Pain and joint dysfunction refractory to non-surgical measures
Osteochondroma	Hypermobility and dislocation refractory to non-surgical measures
Fibrous and bony ankylosis	
Severe traumatic injuries	

The decision to move forward with surgical intervention to treat TMD should not be taken lightly. All procedures, including those that are minimally invasive, are associated with risks and morbidity and thus must be weighed against the amount of dysfunction and pain. Any TMJ surgery aims to eliminate pathology, decrease pain, and improve function. It should be noted that surgical intervention is unlikely to eliminate all pain in most cases. For this reason, the clinician must be certain of a diagnosis based on clinical exam, diagnostic imaging, and testing with a specific goal in mind before moving forward with surgery. Lysis and lavage procedures can be considered in patients with refractory pain and dysfunction without a definitive underlying cause and lack of improvement from non-surgical modalities.

If pain and dysfunction are improved to an acceptable level with non-surgical measures, a displaced disc or degenerative changes are not of surgical concern. Besides, patients who have failed non-surgical measures and lysis and lavage with no identified intra-articular pathology should not expect the more invasive surgical intervention to yield positive results. Finally, open interventions to the TMJ should be limited. The more the open interventions completed prior to alloplastic joint replacement, the more the chronic pain that should be expected after the final surgical treatment [18].

Non-surgical Treatment

There have been few innovations in non-surgical therapy in the management of TMD. It should be considered as a first-line treatment in most cases, but surgical intervention should not be delayed when clear pathology is present or in cases of severe degenerative joint disease associated with apertognathia, pain, and dysfunction. A study by Suvinen found that out of 37 patients treated conservatively, 81% of patients showed 50% or greater pain severity improvement at follow-up [19]. Most patients will have significant benefits from non-surgical treatment and may therefore not require further surgical intervention.

Stage	Clinical Findings	Radiographic Findings
I	No limitation of opening Painless clicking	Normal disc morphology Mild displacement with early reduction
II	Occasional painful click Intermittent lock	Mild disc deformity Moderate displacement with late reduction
III	Limited opening Frequent painful clicking Joint tenderness	Displaced, nonreducing disc
IV	Limited opening Chronic pain	Severe displacement without reduction Degeneratice bony changes
V	Variable joint pain Joint crepitus	Nonreducing disc with perforation Degenerative bony changes

Fig. 50.8 Wilkes classification of internal derangements [16, 17].

Non-surgical regimens should include splint therapy, pharmacotherapy, diet and habit modification, and physical therapy. Splints are not always benign prostheses, and they can result in worsening symptoms as well as tooth movement and occlusal changes. The goal of these devices is to decrease loading of the TMJ and create a neuromuscular balance that can reduce the reflexive activation of the muscles leading to parafunctional habits.

Flat plane stabilization splints should be the mainstay of treatment. They are permissive and should be fabricated in centric relation. These splints have little chance for significant dental movement and can be used long term. They should be periodically adjusted to ensure that even contact is always achieved [20–24]. Soft splints can also be considered. They are effective and often tolerated in patients who do not tolerate a rigid, flat plane stabilization splint. There is some evidence that they may offer comparable efficacy to that of hard splints in some patients [25, 26]. Regardless of the splint used, regular evaluation should be completed to ensure that no unwanted tooth movement occurs or worsens symptoms and function (Fig. 50.9).

Pharmacotherapy is aimed at controlling inflammation, parafunction, and pain. Typically, this includes the use of NSAIDs, muscle relaxants, and at times corticosteroids [27]. Other medications like tricyclic anti-depressant medications have more recently been shown to benefit from chronic facial pain and bruxism. However, further study is needed as the benefit is not clear [28–32]. Opioid medications are used in the management of acute post-surgical pain. Still, they do not play a role in managing the underlying etiology, and it is the author's opinion that should opioid medications be required for management of pain, it should be deferred to either the primary care provider or a pain specialist.

Concurrent treatment using all modalities may be more beneficial than each on their own. A course of therapy should be completed for at least 1 month before determining its effectiveness and for as long as 3 months.

Surgical Treatment

Innovations in TMJ surgery include the development of diagnostic and therapeutic arthroscopy, Mitek anchors (DePuy Synthes, Raynham, Massachusetts), and custom and stock alloplastic joint replacements. The integration of VSP, CBCT, and intra-oral scans has made planning more accessible and surgery more predictable, safe, and efficient. In addition, CTA, embolization procedures, and the advent of intra-operative CT guidance with systems like Stealth (Medtronic, Minneapolis, Minnesota), have helped to reduce risk and improve results.

TMJ arthroscopy was first described by a Japanese surgeon Ohnishi in 1975 [33]. It was further refined and studied by Murakami, Sanders, and McCain [34, 35]. TMJ arthroscopy has become much more versatile from a diagnostic prospective when compared to arthrocentesis alone. Indications include TMD with lack of improvement from non-surgical measures, continued pain after surgical intervention, internal derangements, and TMJ arthralgia. Contra-indications are TMJ ankylosis or fibrous ankylosis, overlying skin infection, or local factors limiting the success of entering into the joint space. Studies on the benefits of arthroscopy have shown

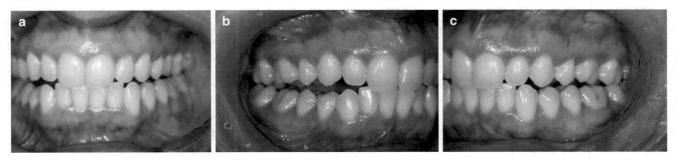

Fig. 50.9 (**a**) Frontal occlusion from chronic long-term use of an anterior repositioning splint resulting in malocclusion. (**b**) Right occlusion view. (**c**) Left occlusion view

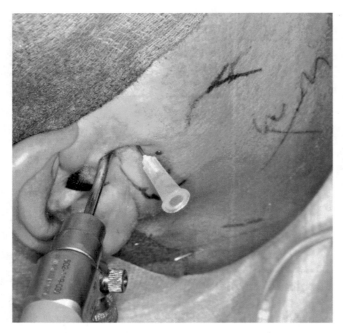

Fig. 50.10 Clinical edits of a 1.9 mm, 30-degree arthroscope (Stryker, Kalamazoo, Michigan) in the superior joint space with a second 20-gauge needle in place for lavage

improvement in pain and function in early- and late-stage diseases [36–38].

TMJ arthroscopy can provide diagnostic and therapeutic value. Typically, it is performed in the operating room under general anesthesia (Fig. 50.10). Zimmer Biomet has more recently come out with a very small arthroscopic camera called the OnePoint™ Scope System (Zimmer Biomet, Jacksonville, Florida) with a diameter of 1.2 mm that can be utilized in the oral and maxillofacial surgery office under intravenous sedation quite safely. This approach can be helpful diagnostically, but it will not offer the more versatile therapeutic interventions available with more standard-sized arthroscopes. Diagnostic evaluation allows visualization of key structures, including the medial synovial drape, pterygoid shadow, retrodiscal tissue, posterior slope of the articu-

lar eminence, articular disc, intermediate zone, and the anterior recess (Fig. 50.11) [35, 39–41].

Therapeutic plans can be made based on the diagnostic information obtained. McCain pioneered the two-puncture arthroscopy technique, which has allowed for introducing instrumentation into the joint, including blunt and sharp instruments, biopsy forceps, rotary instruments, monopolar and bipolar electrocautery, and lasers, among others [35]. Debridement can be completed to address adhesions not managed with lysis and lavage using either motorized instrumentation or electrocautery. Arthroscopic lysis and lavage and surgical arthroscopy are effective in managing internal derangements [42]. Surgical arthroscopy has shown to be successful in managing internal derangements showing significant reduction in pain and improvement in function [36–38, 43, 44]. Though open approaches may achieve similar results, the minimally invasive nature of the arthroscopic approach makes it attractive and innovative [45].

Some have advocated that lysis and lavage alone are adequate, though arthroscopic techniques may yield better results [46, 47]. Arthrocentesis alone does not provide the diagnostic value that arthroscopy does, but it may be technically less demanding and accessible given that it can be completed under local anesthesia with procedural sedation in an office setting. Additionally, it does not require costly arthroscopic equipment. Data suggest that it is also effective in improving pain and dysfunction [47].

Therapeutic medicaments can also be injected into the joint space. Examples have included corticosteroids, hyaluronic acid, morphine, and local anesthetic. More recently, platelet-rich plasma (PRP) injection, platelet-rich growth factor, and platelet-rich fibrin have been newer innovations. A study by Kutuk et al. compared the use of PRP, hyaluronic acid, and corticosteroid and found PRP to be more effective in reducing pain [48]. There have been promising results from other studies as well. However, a clear benefit over current treatments has not been established [49–52].

TMJ arthrotomy and arthroplasty are considered openjoint interventions and have not changed drastically in recent years. Arthrotomy involves surgery within the joint space,

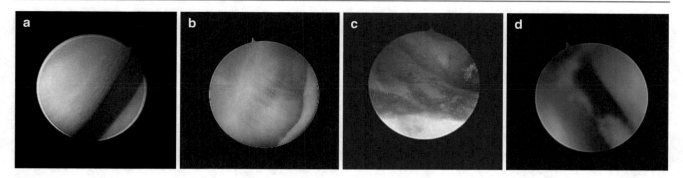

Fig. 50.11 (**a**) Intermediate zone. (**b**) Pterygoid shadow. (**c**) Retrodiscal tissue with creeping synovitis and hyperemia. (**d**) Fibrillation of the fibrocartilage

while arthroplasty will include alteration to the bony anatomy. Disc repositioning and discectomy are the most commonly performed procedures with an open approach. Indications for disc repositioning include anterior disc displacement with or without reduction, failure of conservative therapy, and arthroscopic procedures failure. Indications for discectomy include disc displacement with or without reduction, perforation, and fragmentation. Both procedures are undertaken by either a pre-auricular or endaural surgical approach. The Al-Kayat extension can be considered superior to improve access, though it is usually not necessary [53]. Once the superior joint space is accessed, the disc is then visualized for its position and inspected for perforations or tears. Should it be found to be healthy, then repositioning can be considered.

Wolford pioneered the use of Mitek anchors (DePuy Synthes, Raynham, Massachusetts) in TMJ surgery [54, 55]. The technique involves using a small titanium anchor with nickel-titanium wings that are drilled into the condylar neck and used as a fixation point for posterior and lateral repositioning of the articular disc (Fig. 50.12). In a study by Wolford and Mehra, they provide a description for the procedure and found that out of the 105 patients evaluated, 74% of patients had no pain, 13% of patients had mild pain, 8.5% patients had moderate pain, and 3% of patients still had severe pain at the longest follow-up [54]. Another study by Montgomery et al. showed that although in about 80% of patients the disc position did not seem to change significantly on imaging, pain was improved in 89% of patients [56]. Regardless, the decision to repair or reposition the articular disc should be approached with caution in order to minimize open procedures in the future.

If the disc is found to be damaged, fragmented, or torn, then a discectomy procedure may be more beneficial. Studies have shown that when the disc and/or articular cartilage is removed, there are morphological changes that occur to the condyle [57]. The incidence and severity of condylar remodeling seem to be much more extensive in patients who received additional condylar surgery in addition to discec-

tomy, such as a high condylar shave or debridement of the fibrocartilage [58]. Surgeons have long sought an adequate material to place in the joint space after discectomy procedures. Alloplastic materials like silastic and Proplast-Teflon (Vitek, Inc, Houston, Texas) were used, though they ultimately fell out of favor, with the latter being recalled by the FDA [59]. Various autografts from different anatomic locations such as costal cartilage, auricular cartilage, dermis, fat, dermis–fat, fascia, and temporal muscle have been used with mixed results [60]. While an acceptable technique, auricular cartilage grafting has a high failure rate and does not prevent degenerative changes [61]. While providing adequate tissue in close proximity to the TMJ, the temporalis muscle flap has been shown to result in pain, restricted mouth opening, and cosmetic defects [62]. Of the various autogenous materials available, fat and the dermis-fat grafts are the most promising. Placement of fat within the joint space after discectomy is thought to prevent organized clot formation, leading to ankylosis. Dimitroulis has published several case series on the technique, touting very low rates of ankylosis, significant improvements in quality of life, and the formation of interpositional material between the condyle and the fossa [63–65]. However, there are concerns about donor site morbidity.

Amniotic membranes and amniotic cords have been gaining more and more popularity in oral and maxillofacial surgery. They have been applied to implant surgery, complex intraoral reconstruction, vestibulopathy, and TMJ surgery [66]. A rat model showed that they were biocompatible and prevented adhesion formation in abdominal wall reconstruction [67]. Tuncel showed that they prevented adhesions and osteophytes formation when used as an interpositional arthroplasty material in the treatment of fibrous ankyloses in rabbit models [68]. Akhter presented a case study of 13 patients who were treated for bony ankyloses using a layered amniotic membrane in which all patients demonstrated improved pain and mobility at 1-, 6-, and 12-month intervals [69]. Nardini hypothesized that the antimicrobial, anti-inflammatory, low immunogenicity, and analgesic properties of amnion membranes would make

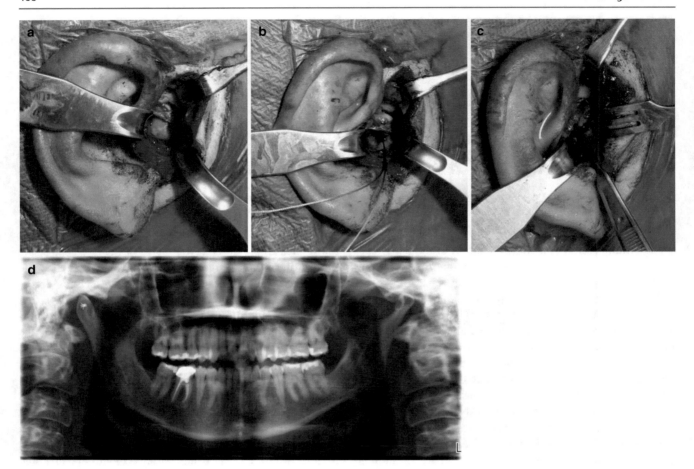

Fig. 50.12 (**a**) Isolation of the articular disc. (**b**) Placement of the Mitek anchor (DePuy Synthes, Raynham, Massachusetts). (**c**) Articular disc repositioned and sutured in place. (**d**) Post-operative orthopantomogram showing the Mitek anchor within the condylar neck

them an ideal interpositional material within the TMJ [70]. Investigators recently presented a case series that involved discectomy followed by implantation of cryopreserved viable osteochondral allograft combined with a viable cryopreserved umbilical cord tissue allograft. The reported outcomes suggest that the interpositional implantation of osteochondral allograft and umbilical cord tissue graft after TMJ discectomy could be a solution for reducing TMJ-related pain and restoring TMJ function, though longer follow-up and prospective multicenter studies are warranted. It should be noted that most patients experienced an improvement in symptoms but decreased MIO [71].

Consideration can also be given to discectomy without replacement (Fig. 50.13). A study by Homlund et al. reports an 83% success rate at 1 year after discectomy procedures [72]. Miloro et al. also showed a success rate of discectomy without replacement of around 83%. They also advocate that given the success rate and reduction in success with multiple operations, discectomy can be considered an initial intervention rather than a procedure of last resort after unsuccessful discopexy procedures [18, 73, 74].

Though both disc repositioning and discectomy are valid surgical interventions that are shown to be successful, care should be taken to decide on which intervention is pursued. The Mitek anchor (DePuy Synthes, Raynham, Massachusetts) may make disc repositioning more predictable in the long term. Discectomy with and without replacement seems to be a safe surgical option in many cases.

Total joint replacement (TJR) has become much more common in the last 20 years due to the emergence of stable long-term results with the prostheses available for use [18, 75–78]. Many different prostheses, such as the Christensen fossa and various TMJ replacement devices were engineered over many years of development and study with various degrees of success. These gave rise to the modern patient-fitted prosthesis from TMJ Concepts (Ventura, California) and the stock prostheses from Walter Lorenz Surgical Inc. now Zimmer Biomet (Jacksonville, Florida) [79, 80]. Indications for TJR include ankylosis, severe degenerative joint disease, pathology, failed previous surgery, failed previous autogenous joint replacement, condylar agenesis, avascular necrosis, developmental abnormalities, and traumatic injury.

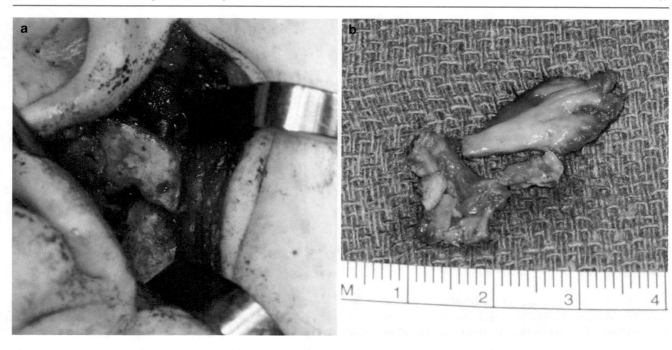

Fig. 50.13 (a) Clinical image of TMJ after disc removal without replacement. (b) Fragmented residual articular disc

Currently, a stock prosthesis is available from Zimmer Biomet (Jasksonville, Florida) as well as a patient-fitted prosthesis from TMJ Concepts (Ventura, California). The indications for use are similar for both. The advantages of the stock device include potentially lower cost and immediate availability. Patients with more severe bony deformities or those requiring concomitant movement of the mandible in a significant manner will be better suited for a patient-fitted prosthesis. The disadvantages of the patient-fitted prosthesis are cost and time required for fabrication.

Both the stock and patient-fitted prostheses have good long-term outcome data supporting their use as safe and effective [76, 77]. It is the author's opinion that the patient-fitted prosthesis may be easier to place if more immediate surgery is not needed. The stock prosthesis is excellent in the management of traumatic injuries [81].

In addition to the advent of these prostheses, the integration of CBCT into planning has been significant innovation in treatment. A patient may no longer require a medical-grade CT scan in the planning stages, which makes obtaining the DICOM data simpler and more cost-effective. In addition, with the use of the TMJ concepts (Ventura, California), patient-fitted prosthesis integration with VSP is more straightforward and accurate. Movahed describes the traditional approach and the computer-assisted approach that allows for complex movement of the mandibular position in combination with maxillary orthognathic procedures [82, 83]. With the advent of intra-oral scanners, the use of stone dental models and impressions is not necessary, and a fully digital workflow can be utilized in contrast to Movahed's initial description.

The authors use a similar workflow described below.

1. CBCT data and intra-oral scan data are sent to both TMJ Concepts (Ventura, California) and KLS Martin (Jacksonville, Florida).
2. Using Individualized Patient Solutions (IPS) software with KLS Martin (Jacksonville, Florida) engineers, the final occlusion is set from the intra-oral scan data (Fig. 50.14).
3. The LeFort procedure and position of the maxilla are determined in all planes (Fig. 50.15).
4. The mandible is set to meet this position based on the final occlusion.
5. Gap arthroplasty and coronoidectomy, if desired, are marked and completed digitally.
6. This planning data is used to create an intermediate and final splint.
7. The data is shared with TMJ Concepts (Ventura, California) to fabricate the patient-fitted prosthesis (Fig. 50.16).

Another added benefit of this workflow is creating cutting guides for planned osteotomies and bone reduction if desired.

This workflow has helped to improve the accuracy of planning and surgical outcomes while decreasing the difficulty of surgery.

When managing large ankylotic bony masses, pathology, or multi-operative joints, bleeding can pose a signifi-

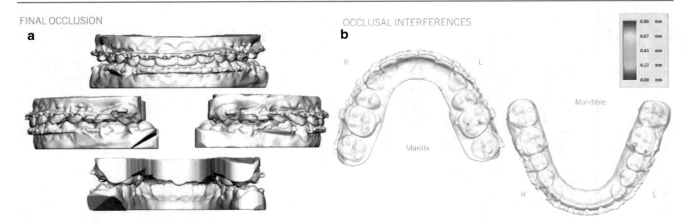

Fig. 50.14 (**a**) Final occlusion set digitally using intra-oral scan data. (**b**) Pressure map revealing points of contact and adjustments for planned final occlusion

cant risk. The use of CTA can be helpful in analyzing the vascular anatomy around the joint space and the course of the internal maxillary artery. In some cases, embolization of the vessels that may pose a significant bleeding risk at the time of surgery should be considered. This will help keep the surgical field dry and increase the ease of surgery while also lowering the risk of inadvertent vascular compromise for the patient. A case series by Susara et al. evaluated five cases of ankylosis and found a decrease in blood loss on the embolized side, and the ease of surgery improved [84]. Hossameldin et al. evaluated 14 patients with ankylosis and found that all patients suffered less than 250 mL of blood loss [85]. Should embolization not be possible, the

anatomic information obtained remains valuable to the surgeon to help avoid vascular compromise and decrease blood loss.

Finally, in cases of pathology or large bony ankylotic masses, intra-operative CT guidance can help avoid complications. These systems offer surgical probes that allow the surgeon to translate the probe's position to an anatomic location on the CT scan, helping the surgeon to avoid damaging anatomic structures which are medial to the surgical field. In cases requiring significant recontouring of the temporal bone, CT guidance can help prevent inadvertent entrance into the middle cranial fossa as well [86, 87].

Fig. 50.15 (**a**) VSP plan including the preoperative state, the intermediate position after digital gap arthroplasty and sagittal split osteotomy, and final position with LeFort I osteotomy and final occlusion. (**b**) Final data showing LeFort I, sagittal split osteotomy, and gap arthroplasty to be shared with TMJ Concepts (Ventura, California)

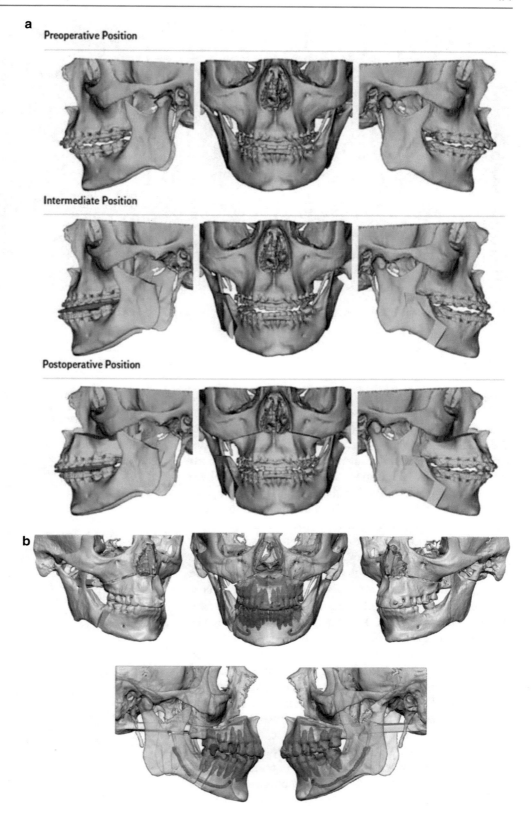

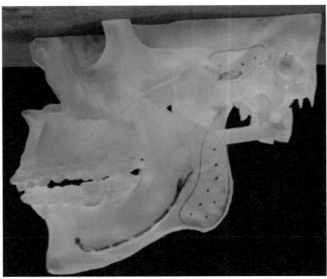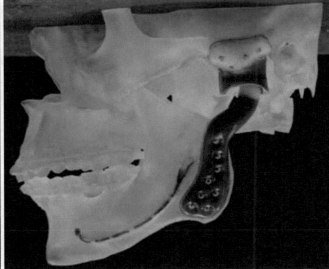

Fig. 50.16 Pre-operative TMJ Concepts (Ventura, California) plan with 3D printed models created from data shared by IPS. (KLS Martin, Jacksonville, Florida)

Conclusion

Patients with TMD can be difficult to manage, but with the integration of recent innovations into management protocols, outcomes can be improved. Integrating CBCT imaging data and diagnostic arthroscopy can help form very accurate diagnoses that will help guide patients and surgeons to appropriate interventions. Innovations in TMJ arthroscopy have helped to provide a minimally invasive management option to many patients and surgeons. This has included the introduction of different therapeutic medications into the joint. Additionally, the use of Botox® (Allergan, Madison, New Jersey) in the management of myofascial pain seems to be showing promising results, though more investigations are needed. Traditional open arthroplasty and arthrotomy procedures have moved toward using adjuncts like the Mitek Anchor (Dupuy Synthes, Raynham, Massachusetts), amniotic membranes, and tissue grafts in discectomy procedures. And finally, one of the most innovative changes in the field has been the stable and predictable use of patient-fitted and stock alloplastic joint replacements. This treatment has been further refined with the integration of digital workflows in planning. Some of the risks have been decreased with the use of intra-operative CT navigation as well as pre-operative CTA and embolization. As we look to the future, tissue engineering may provide a more stable graft in discectomy procedures, and digital platforms will likely continue to evolve rapidly, making surgery more predictable while decreasing risk.

References

1. De Vos W, Casselman J, Swennen GR. Cone-beam computerized tomography (CBCT) imaging of the oral and maxillofacial region: a systematic review of the literature. Int J Oral Maxillofac Surg. 2009;38:609.
2. Barghan S, Tetradis S, Mallya S. Application of cone beam computed tomography for assessment of the temporomandibular joints. Aust Dent J. 2012;57(Suppl 1):109.
3. Zain-Alabdeen EH, Alsadhan RI. A comparative study of accuracy of detection of surface osseous changes in the temporomandibular joint using multidetector CT and cone beam CT. Dentomaxillofac Radiol. 2012;41:185.
4. Fallah HM, Currimbhoy S. Use of botulinum toxin A for treatment of myofascial pain and dysfunction. J Oral Maxillofac Surg. 2012;70:1243.
5. Binder WJ, Brin MF, Blitzer A, Schoenrock LD, Pogoda JM. Botulinum toxin type A (BOTOX) for treatment of migraine headaches: an open-label study. Otolaryngol Head Neck Surg. 2000;123:669.
6. Aoki KR. Review of a proposed mechanism for the antinociceptive action of botulinum toxin type A. Neurotoxicology. 2005;26:785.
7. Acquadro MA, Borodic GE. Treatment of myofascial pain with botulinum A toxin. Anesthesiology. 1994;80:705.
8. Freund B, Schwartz M, Symington JM. The use of botulinum toxin for the treatment of temporomandibular disorders: preliminary findings. J Oral Maxillofac Surg. 1999;57:916.
9. von Lindern JJ, Niederhagen B, Bergé S, Appel T. Type A botulinum toxin in the treatment of chronic facial pain associated with masticatory hyperactivity. J Oral Maxillofac Surg. 2003;61:774.
10. Ali R, Webster K, Kennedy D. A review of treatment outcomes for patients receiving intra-masseteric botulinum toxin-A for the management of facial myofascial pain. Br J Oral Maxillofac Surg. 2017;55:e146.
11. Kurtoglu C, Gur OH, Kurkcu M, Sertdemir Y, Guler-Uysal F, Uysal H. Effect of botulinum toxin-A in myofascial pain patients with

or without functional disc displacement. J Oral Maxillofac Surg. 2008;66:1644.

12. Porta M. A comparative trial of botulinum toxin type A and methylprednisolone for the treatment of myofascial pain syndrome and pain from chronic muscle spasm. Pain. 2000;85:101.

13. Nixdorf DR, Heo G, Major PW. Randomized controlled trial of botulinum toxin A for chronic myogenous orofacial pain. Pain. 2002;99:465.

14. Ernberg M, Hedenberg-Magnusson B, List T, Svensson P. Efficacy of botulinum toxin type A for treatment of persistent myofascial TMD pain: a randomized, controlled, double-blind multicenter study. Pain. 2011;152:1988.

15. Milne S, Carter L, Cooper T. An audit of the efficacy of botulinum toxin for myofascial pain. Br J Oral Maxillofac Surg. 2016;54:e124.

16. Wilkes CH. Internal derangements of the temporomandibular joint. Pathological variations. Arch Otolaryngol Head Neck Surg. 1989;115:469.

17. Wilkes CH. Surgical treatment of internal derangements of the temporomandibular joint. A long-term study. Arch Otolaryngol Head Neck Surg. 1991;117:64.

18. Mercuri LG. Subjective and objective outcomes in patients reconstructed with a custom-fitted alloplastic temporomandibular joint prosthesis. J Oral Maxillofac Surg. 1999;57:1427.

19. Suvinen TI, Hanes KR, Reade PC. Outcome of therapy in the conservative management of temporomandibular pain dysfunction disorder. J Oral Rehabil. 1997;24:718.

20. Carraro JJ, Caffesse RG. Effect of occlusal splints on TMJ symptomatology. J Prosthet Dent. 1978;40:563.

21. Tsuga K, Akagawa Y, Sakaguchi R, Tsuru H. A short-term evaluation of the effectiveness of stabilization-type occlusal splint therapy for specific symptoms of temporomandibular joint dysfunction syndrome. J Prosthet Dent. 1989;61:610.

22. Türp JC, Komine F, Hugger A. Efficacy of stabilization splints for the management of patients with masticatory muscle pain: a qualitative systematic review. Clin Oral Investig. 2004;8:179.

23. Dimitroulis G, Gremillion HA, Dolwick MF, Walter JH. Temporomandibular disorders. 2. Non-surgical treatment. Aust Dent J. 1995;40:372.

24. Greene CS, Menchel HF. The use of oral appliances in the management of temporomandibular disorders. Oral Maxillofac Surg Clin North Am. 2018;30:265.

25. Pettengill CA, Growney MR, Schoff R, Kenworthy CR. A pilot study comparing the efficacy of hard and soft stabilizing appliances in treating patients with temporomandibular disorders. J Prosthet Dent. 1998;79:165.

26. Wright E, Anderson G, Schulte J. A randomized clinical trial of intraoral soft splints and palliative treatment for masticatory muscle pain. J Orofac Pain. 1995;9:192.

27. Heir GM. The efficacy of pharmacologic treatment of temporomandibular disorders. Oral Maxillofac Surg Clin North Am. 2018;30:279.

28. Sharav Y, Singer E, Schmidt E, Dionne RA, Dubner R. The analgesic effect of amitriptyline on chronic facial pain. Pain. 1987;31:199.

29. Plesh O, Curtis D, Levine J, McCall WD. Amitriptyline treatment of chronic pain in patients with temporomandibular disorders. J Oral Rehabil. 2000;27:834.

30. Rizzatti-Barbosa CM, Nogueira MT, de Andrade ED, Ambrosano GM, de Barbosa JR. Clinical evaluation of amitriptyline for the control of chronic pain caused by temporomandibular joint disorders. Cranio. 2003;21:221.

31. Raigrodski AJ, Christensen LV, Mohamed SE, Gardiner DM. The effect of four-week administration of amitriptyline on sleep bruxism. A double-blind crossover clinical study. Cranio. 2001;19:21.

32. Mohamed SE, Christensen LV, Penchas J. A randomized double-blind clinical trial of the effect of amitriptyline on nocturnal masseteric motor activity (sleep bruxism). Cranio. 1997;15:326.

33. Onishi M. Aarthroscopy of the temporomandibular joint (author's transl). Kokubyo Gakkai Zasshi. 1975;42:207.

34. Murakami K. Rationale of arthroscopic surgery of the temporomandibular joint. J Oral Biol Craniofac Res. 2013;3:126.

35. McCain JP. Arthroscopy of the human temporomandibular joint. J Oral Maxillofac Surg. 1988;46:648.

36. Breik O, Devrukhkar V, Dimitroulis G. Temporomandibular joint (TMJ) arthroscopic lysis and lavage: outcomes and rate of progression to open surgery. J Craniomaxillofac Surg. 2016;44:1988.

37. Al-Moraissi EA. Arthroscopy versus arthrocentesis in the management of internal derangement of the temporomandibular joint: a systematic review and meta-analysis. Int J Oral Maxillofac Surg. 2015;44:104.

38. Kaneyama K, Segami N, Sato J, Murakami K, Iizuka T. Outcomes of 152 temporomandibular joints following arthroscopic anterolateral capsular release by holmium: YAG laser or electrocautery. Oral Surg Oral Med Oral Pathol Oral Radiol Endod. 2004;97:546.

39. Holmlund A. Diagnostic TMJ arthroscopy. Oral Surg Oral Diagn. 1992;3:13.

40. Murakami KI, Lizuka T, Matsuki M, Ono T. Diagnostic arthroscopy of the TMJ: differential diagnoses in patients with limited jaw opening. Cranio. 1986;4:117.

41. Murakami K, Ono T. Temporomandibular joint arthroscopy by inferolateral approach. Int J Oral Maxillofac Surg. 1986;15:410.

42. González-García R, Rodríguez-Campo FJ. Arthroscopic lysis and lavage versus operative arthroscopy in the outcome of temporomandibular joint internal derangement: a comparative study based on Wilkes stages. J Oral Maxillofac Surg. 2011;69:2513.

43. McCain JP, Hossameldin RH, Srouji S, Maher A. Arthroscopic discopexy is effective in managing temporomandibular joint internal derangement in patients with Wilkes stage II and III. J Oral Maxillofac Surg. 2015;73:391.

44. McCain JP, Sanders B, Koslin MG, Quinn JH, Peters PB, Indresano AT, Quinn JD. Temporomandibular joint arthroscopy: a 6-year multicenter retrospective study of 4,831 joints. J Oral Maxillofac Surg. 1992;50:926.

45. Al-Moraissi EA. Open versus arthroscopic surgery for the management of internal derangement of the temporomandibular joint: a meta-analysis of the literature. Int J Oral Maxillofac Surg. 2015;44:763.

46. Indresano AT. Surgical arthroscopy as the preferred treatment for internal derangements of the temporomandibular joint. J Oral Maxillofac Surg. 2001;59:308.

47. Nitzan DW, Dolwick MF, Martinez GA. Temporomandibular joint arthrocentesis: a simplified treatment for severe, limited mouth opening. J Oral Maxillofac Surg. 1991;49:1163.

48. Gokçe Kutuk S, Gökçe G, Arslan M, Özkan Y, Kütük M, Kursat Arikan O. Clinical and radiological comparison of effects of platelet-rich plasma, hyaluronic acid, and corticosteroid injections on temporomandibular joint osteoarthritis. J Craniofac Surg. 2019;30:1144.

49. Bousnaki M, Bakopoulou A, Koidis P. Platelet-rich plasma for the therapeutic management of temporomandibular joint disorders: a systematic review. Int J Oral Maxillofac Surg. 2018;47:188.

50. Cömert Kiliç S, Güngörmüş M. Is arthrocentesis plus platelet-rich plasma superior to arthrocentesis plus hyaluronic acid for the treatment of temporomandibular joint osteoarthritis: a randomized clinical trial. Int J Oral Maxillofac Surg. 2016;45:1538.

51. Chung PY, Lin MT, Chang HP. Effectiveness of platelet-rich plasma injection in patients with temporomandibular joint osteoarthritis: a

systematic review and meta-analysis of randomized controlled trials. Oral Surg Oral Med Oral Pathol Oral Radiol. 2019;127:106.

52. Haigler MC, Abdulrehman E, Siddappa S, Kishore R, Padilla M, Enciso R. Use of platelet-rich plasma, platelet-rich growth factor with arthrocentesis or arthroscopy to treat temporomandibular joint osteoarthritis: systematic review with meta-analyses. J Am Dent Assoc. 2018;149:940.

53. Al-Kayat A, Bramley P. A modified pre-auricular approach to the temporomandibular joint and malar arch. Br J Oral Surg. 1979;17:91.

54. Mehra P, Wolford LM. The Mitek mini anchor for TMJ disc repositioning: surgical technique and results. Int J Oral Maxillofac Surg. 2001;30:497.

55. Mehra P, Wolford LM. Use of the Mitek anchor in temporomandibular joint disc-repositioning surgery. Proc (Bayl Univ Med Cent). 2001;14:22.

56. Montgomery MT, Gordon SM, Van Sickels JE, Harms SE. Changes in signs and symptoms following temporomandibular joint disc repositioning surgery. J Oral Maxillofac Surg. 1992;50:320.

57. Abdala-Júnior R, Cortes ARG, Aoki EM, Ferreira S, Luz JGC, Arita ES, de Oliveira JX. Impact of temporomandibular joint discectomy on condyle morphology: an animal study. J Oral Maxillofac Surg. 2018;76:955.e1.

58. Dimitroulis G. Condylar morphology after temporomandibular joint discectomy with interpositional abdominal dermis-fat graft. J Oral Maxillofac Surg. 2011;69:439.

59. McKenna SJ. Discectomy for the treatment of internal derangements of the temporomandibular joint. J Oral Maxillofac Surg. 2001;59:1051.

60. Dimitroulis G. A critical review of interpositional grafts following temporomandibular joint discectomy with an overview of the dermis-fat graft. Int J Oral Maxillofac Surg. 2011;40:561.

61. Ioannides C, Freihofer HP. Replacement of the damaged interarticular disc of the TMJ. J Craniomaxillofac Surg. 1988;16:273.

62. Lam D, Carlson ER. The temporalis muscle flap and temporoparietal fascial flap. Oral Maxillofac Surg Clin North Am. 2014;26:359.

63. Dimitroulis G. The interpositional dermis-fat graft in the management of temporomandibular joint ankylosis. Int J Oral Maxillofac Surg. 2004;33:755.

64. Dimitroulis G, McCullough M, Morrison W. Quality-of-life survey comparing patients before and after discectomy of the temporomandibular joint. J Oral Maxillofac Surg. 2010;68:101.

65. Dimitroulis G, Trost N, Morrison W. The radiological fate of dermis-fat grafts in the human temporomandibular joint using magnetic resonance imaging. Int J Oral Maxillofac Surg. 2008;37:249.

66. Kesting MR, Wolff KD, Nobis CP, Rohleder NH. Amniotic membrane in oral and maxillofacial surgery. Oral Maxillofac Surg. 2014;18:153.

67. Akhter M, Ahmed N, Arefin MR, Sobhan MU, Molla MR, Kamal M. Outcome of amniotic membrane as an interpositional arthroplasty of TMJ ankylosis. Oral Maxillofac Surg. 2016;20:63.

68. Kesting MR, Wolff KD, Mücke T, Demtroeder C, Kreutzer K, Schulte M, Jacobsen F, Hirsch T, Loeffelbein DJ, Steinstraesser L. A bioartificial surgical patch from multilayered human amniotic membrane-in vivo investigations in a rat model. J Biomed Mater Res B Appl Biomater. 2009;90:930.

69. Tuncel U, Ozgenel GY. Use of human amniotic membrane as an interpositional material in treatment of temporomandibular joint ankylosis. J Oral Maxillofac Surg. 2011;69:e58.

70. Guarda-Nardini L, Trojan D, Paolin A, Manfredini D. Management of temporomandibular joint degenerative disorders with human amniotic membrane: hypothesis of action. Med Hypotheses. 2017;104:68.

71. Connelly ST, Silva R, Gupta R, O'Hare M, Danilkovitch A, Tartaglia G. Temporomandibular joint discectomy followed by disc replacement using viable osteochondral and umbilical cord allografts results in improved patient outcomes. J Oral Maxillofac Surg. 2020;78:63.

72. Holmlund A, Lund B, Weiner CK. Discectomy without replacement for the treatment of painful reciprocal clicking or catching and chronic closed lock of the temporomandibular joint: a clinical follow-up audit. Br J Oral Maxillofac Surg. 2013;51:e211.

73. Miloro M, Henriksen B. Discectomy as the primary surgical option for internal derangement of the temporomandibular joint. J Oral Maxillofac Surg. 2010;68:782.

74. Miloro M, McKnight M, Han MD, Markiewicz MR. Discectomy without replacement improves function in patients with internal derangement of the temporomandibular joint. J Craniomaxillofac Surg. 2017;45:1425.

75. Mercuri LG. Alloplastic temporomandibular joint reconstruction. Oral Surg Oral Med Oral Pathol Oral Radiol Endod. 1998;85:631.

76. Wolford LM, Mercuri LG, Schneiderman ED, Movahed R, Allen W. Twenty-year follow-up study on a patient-fitted temporomandibular joint prosthesis: the Techmedica/TMJ concepts device. J Oral Maxillofac Surg. 2015;73:952.

77. Granquist EJ, Bouloux G, Dattilo D, Gonzalez O, Louis PJ, McCain J, Sinn D, Szymela V, Warner M, Quinn PD. Outcomes and survivorship of biomet microfixation total joint replacement system: results from an FDA postmarket study. J Oral Maxillofac Surg. 2020;78:1499.

78. Granquist EJ, Quinn PD. Total reconstruction of the temporomandibular joint with a stock prosthesis. Atlas Oral Maxillofac Surg Clin North Am. 2011;19:221.

79. De Meurechy N, Mommaerts MY. Alloplastic temporomandibular joint replacement systems: a systematic review of their history. Int J Oral Maxillofac Surg. 2018;47:743.

80. Mercuri LG, Wolford LM, Sanders B, White RD, Hurder A, Henderson W. Custom CAD/CAM total temporomandibular joint reconstruction system: preliminary multicenter report. J Oral Maxillofac Surg. 1995;53:106.

81. Giannakopoulos HE, Quinn PD, Granquist E, Chou JC. Posttraumatic temporomandibular joint disorders. Craniomaxillofac Trauma Reconstr. 2009;2:91.

82. Movahed R, Teschke M, Wolford LM. Protocol for concomitant temporomandibular joint custom-fitted total joint reconstruction and orthognathic surgery utilizing computer-assisted surgical simulation. J Oral Maxillofac Surg. 2013;71:2123.

83. Movahed R, Wolford LM. Protocol for concomitant temporomandibular joint custom-fitted total joint reconstruction and orthognathic surgery using computer-assisted surgical simulation. Oral Maxillofac Surg Clin North Am. 2015;27:37.

84. Susarla SM, Peacock ZS, Williams WB, Rabinov JD, Keith DA, Kaban LB. Role of computed tomographic angiography in treatment of patients with temporomandibular joint ankylosis. J Oral Maxillofac Surg. 2014;72:267.

85. Hossameldin RH, McCain JP, Dabus G. Prophylactic embolisation of the internal maxillary artery in patients with ankylosis of the temporomandibular joint. Br J Oral Maxillofac Surg. 2017;55:584.

86. Yu HB, Shen GF, Zhang SL, Wang XD, Wang CT, Lin YP. Navigation-guided gap arthroplasty in the treatment of temporomandibular joint ankylosis. Int J Oral Maxillofac Surg. 2009;38:1030.

87. Gui H, Wu J, Shen SG, Bautista JS, Voss PJ, Zhang S. Navigation-guided lateral gap arthroplasty as the treatment of temporomandibular joint ankylosis. J Oral Maxillofac Surg. 2014;72:128.

Shohreh Ghasemi and Farhad Vahidi

Introduction

Rapid developments in dental pharmacotherapeutics mean that surgeons need to consistently upgrade their expertise concerning modern drugs, applicable changes in therapy, and drug involvement. These drugs play important roles in treating xerostomia, loss of blood during retraction of the gingiva, ulceration, and inflammation. They also contribute to alleviation of dentinal hypersensitivity throughout the tooth setting and to improvement of gingival resilience against disease.

Anesthetics, nonsteroidal anti-inflammatory drugs (NSAIDs), and antibiotics are administered to patients undergoing dental surgery. It is of paramount importance to ascertain the correct dosage, considering these drugs' properties, and to be observant regarding the possibilities of toxic effects or serious side effects [1].

Prescribing is the process of selecting a single drug or multiple drugs to be given to or taken by the patient, the duration of the drug treatment, and its dosage. It is tailored to the individual patient and an ever-changing clinical system. However, the specific properties of drugs are not the only relevant factors; prescribing sequences or methods may also be affected by economic, communal, cultural, and/or marketing factors.

The World Health Organization (WHO) recommends stating the problem that the patient has (detection), identifying the therapeutic purpose of the medication, and then considering various approaches before opting for a treatment that is certified as reliable and successful. Prescribing is a distinctly patient-based procedure. The likelihood of a cure is increased by providing the patient with concise facts and directions. The outcome must be examined in an appropriate time frame. The treatment can be terminated when the ailment is resolved [1–3]. Every phase is repeated if the ailment persists [1].

Dental prescribing of drugs is done only for immediate treatment or particularly for surgical operations. Dentists need drug expertise and must comply with global guidelines for drug prescribing.

Indications for Use of Drugs in Oral Surgery

Drugs are used in oral surgery for the following indications:

- To treat *Candida* infections (antifungals)
- To cure xerostomia (artificial saliva)
- To manage pain (NSAIDs, anesthetics, and analgesics)
- To prevent or cure bacterial infections (antibiotics)
- To alleviate anxiety (muscle relaxants)
- To avoid tooth decay (fluoride)
- To control gingivitis and plaque (mouthwashes)

Antibiotics

Amoxicillin (Amoxil) and penicillin are the antibiotics most commonly utilized to prevent or treat numerous infections that can occur following dental surgery. Dental afflictions include infections that occur following dental surgery, such as heart infections, infections around the wisdom teeth, periapical abscesses, and periodontal infections [4, 5].

One of the purposes of antibiotic use in dentistry is to stop the movement of bacteria (which are always present on tissue surfaces) into the bloodstream. This is particularly important in patients with malfunctioning or artificial heart valves, as blood-borne bacteria can infect the valves and

S. Ghasemi (✉)
Department of Oral and Maxillofacial Surgery, Augusta University, Augusta, GA, USA
e-mail: sghasemi@augusta.edu

F. Vahidi
Department of Prosthodontics, New York University, New York, NY, USA
e-mail: fv1@nyu.edu

cause disease. Antibiotics can be administered intravenously, orally, or intramuscularly. Their use is commonly initiated before dental surgery and continued for a maximum of a few doses or for less than 24 hours in some cases [6].

The American Academy of Orthopedic Surgeons (AAOS) and American Heart Association (AHA) guidelines for antibiotic prophylaxis before dental surgery were amended in 2007 and 2013, respectively, on the basis of lack of proof justifying application of antibiotic prophylaxis to prevent endocarditis and prosthetic joint infections [7–13]. Hence, the AAOS and AHA significantly amended their guidelines for preprocedural infection prophylaxis. The directions for employing antibiotics for infective endocarditis prophylaxis before dental surgery now propose use of antibiotics only in patients with specific heart ailments who are undergoing specific dental surgical procedures [8].

Prophylaxis is suggested for patients with prosthetic heart valves, patients with a history of infective endocarditis, patients with particular congenital cardiac conditions, and heart transplant patients who have cardiac valvulopathy [8].

Prophylaxis is advised for these patients undergoing dental surgery that involves manipulation of gingival tissue or perforation of the oral mucosa (implantations and extractions) or the periapical area of the teeth. In accordance with the American Dental Association (ADA)/AHA guidlines in 2013, and in 2016, the ADA/AAOS advised stopping the practice of prescribing antibiotics for patients with knee and hip prosthetic joint implants undergoing any dental surgery [9–13] with use of local anesthesia.

Previously, most patients undergoing dental surgery were given antibiotics prophylactically. As per the presently accessible valid report, only 8.2% of antibiotic prescriptions for infection prophylaxis were appropriate; most of these were given after the surgery [12, 13].

Excessive prescribing of antibiotics in dentistry can be greatly reduced if the postoperative antibiotic directive for patients undergoing extractions or implantations is changed to just a single dose before the surgery [14].

Instructions out of scope to avoid infective endocarditis and prosthetic joint infections must be improved to give appropriate directions on prophylactic prescribing of antibiotics.

Endeavors to ensure appropriate antimicrobial stewardship (comprising documentation of indications for medication use) in the dental field may optimize prescribing of antibiotics for infection prophylaxis [15].

Microbial resistance to antibiotics is now one of the most severe health problems worldwide [1]. It has been estimated that approximately 30% of antibiotic prescriptions in primary treatment are unnecessary [2, 3].

Only 10% of all antibiotic prescriptions in the community are issued by dentists, whose antibiotic prescribing ranks fourth behind those of family health practitioners, pediatricians, and internists [12–14, 16]. The reason for most dental prescribing of antibiotics is infection prophylaxis [6]. The suitability of dental recommendations for prophylactic antibiotic use before dental surgery is yet to be ascertained in the USA.

According to current reports, use of antibiotics before the majority of dental surgeries confers no definite advantage, and when antibiotics are not used, the risk of infection is actually lower [7].

The incidence of short-term bacteremia during dental procedures has been estimated to be similar to that during regular oral health care [8–11].

Moreover, unnecessary antibiotic prescribing can have severely harmful consequences such as bacterial resistance to antibiotics, allergic reactions, and *Clostridium difficile* infection (CDI). CDI occurs as a result of short-term consumption of antibiotics for prevention of dental infections [6]. In an epidemiological survey of community-associated CDI, one of the main reasons for use of antibiotics was dental antibiotic prophylaxis, followed by treatment of upper respiratory tract infections [12].

When patients have allergic reactions to amoxicillin or penicillin, use of erythromycin (Benzamycin, Emgel, Ery, Ilotycin, Staticin) is usually recommended. Antibiotics such as amoxicillin and penicillin are administered for numerous infections that can occur after dental surgery.

Clindamycin (Cleocin HCl) is mainly given to treat major infections due to susceptible anerobic bacteria. It is therefore used successfully for dental abscesses in soft tissue and bone, which do not recover well when erythromycin or penicillin are used [1–16].

Chlorhexidine (Peridex, PerioChip, PerioGard) is used to regulate gingivitis and plaque in the mouth or in periodontal pockets (the areas between the gums and the teeth) [14]. It is available as a chip (which is utilized as an add-on to root planing and scaling operations performed to minimize the depth of the pockets near the teeth in adult patients with periodontitis) or a wash, which supports antimicrobial control between dental appointments and does not conflict with erythromycin or penicillin.

Periodontal infections can be cured by use of tetracyclines, such as doxycycline (Atridox).

It should be noted that:

- Tooth discoloration, tooth fillings, and use of dentures or other mouth aids are likely outcomes of chlorhexidine use. When tetracycline is utilized during the tooth generation stages (which occur from the last half of gestation until the age of 8 years), it can lead to brown, gray, or yellow staining of the teeth.
- Application of anesthesia is intended only for short-term pain relief; it should not be used for extended periods.

Prescribing Recommendations

The recommendations for prescribing antibiotics are as follows:

Penicillin 500 mg four times daily for 1–2 weeks: This should be taken on an empty stomach 1 hour before or 2 hours after eating.

Clindamycin 150–300 mg three or four times daily for 1–2 weeks: This is a better choice of antibiotic for patients who are allergic to penicillin. The risk of (temporary) secondary pseudomembranous colitis after clindamycin therapy is minimal. Clindamycin is mainly given to treat major infections due to susceptible anerobic bacteria. It is therefore used successfully for dental abscesses in soft tissue and bone, which do not recover well when erythromycin or penicillin are used [1–16].

Clavulanic acid/amoxicillin 500/125 mg or 875/125 mg twice daily for 1–2 weeks: A once-daily dose may be taken for a longer term for jaw osteonecrosis and recurring soft tissue infection.

Metronidazole 250 mg once daily or twice daily for 1–2 weeks: Patients must be instructed not to take this with alcohol.

When patients have allergic reactions to penicillin or amoxicillin, use of erythromycin is usually recommended. Antibiotics such as penicillin and amoxicillin are administered for numerous infections that can occur after dental surgery.

Tetracyclines, such as doxycycline, are administered to cure periodontal infections.

Chlorhexidine is used to regulate gingivitis and plaque in the mouth or in periodontal pockets. It is available as a chip (which is utilized as an add-on to root planing and scaling operations performed to minimize the depth of pockets near the teeth in adult patients with periodontitis) or a wash, which supports antimicrobial control between dental appointments and does not conflict with erythromycin or penicillin. When 0.12% chlorhexidine gluconate mouthwash is used, the patient should clean the mouth with 5.0 ml for 30–60 seconds twice daily and then expectorate. Dark discoloration and a tingling sensation are side effects of inflammatory mucosal infection.

Local Anesthetics

Local anesthetics are drugs that, when administered as a local injection or topical medication, can result in temporary absence of any sensory awareness, particularly awareness of pain; these drugs cause extreme stimulation followed by depression (Bennett, 1984). For successful function, local dental anesthetics have a few criteria, such as rapid onset, extreme innate movements, a sufficient duration of effect (30–60 minutes for regular dental care), a high efficiency-to-toxicity ratio, low systemic toxicity, and negligible risks of serious adverse outcomes [17–19].

Topical Local Anesthetics

Topical local anesthetics are used in the oral cavity to alleviate pain at injection sites and across ulcerations. The availability of lotion, spray, and solution formulations is an added attribute of topical anesthetics. Topical anesthetics are applied to eliminate pain in the surface layer of the mouth's lining. They are administered to lessen discomfort from external irritation in the mouth or to immobilize a region prior to administration of an injectable local anesthetic [19].

At present, benzocaine (Orajel, Anbesol) is the standard topical anesthetic utilized during dental procedures.

Prescribing Recommendations

The recommendations for prescribing topical anesthetics are as follows:

2% viscous lidocaine solution: The mouth should be rinsed with 2–5 ml for 60 seconds. The solution should then be expectorated; it should not be swallowed. Use of viscous lidocaine is especially beneficial for pain relief just before a meal, and it can also be given with various topical treatments if a stinging sensation persists.

Morphine liquid 10 mg/5 ml, administered orally: The mouth should be rinsed with 2–5 ml for 5 minutes. The liquid should then be expectorated; it must not be swallowed. A higher dose (10 mg/ml) can be used but only with caution. It is commonly utilized as a restorative cure to minimize the necessity for large doses of systemic analgesics.

Magic mouthwash: This contains equal measures of lidocaine, diphenhydramine, and bismuth subsalicylate liquids. The mouth should be rinsed with 2–5 ml for 60 seconds. The mouthwash should then be expectorated. A small amount can be swallowed in cases of extreme posterior oropharyngeal discomfort, but this is advised only for adult patients.

Injectable Local Anesthetics

These are introduced into the deeper tissues of the mouth and act by suppressing signals from pain-detecting nerves. They are therefore utilized to minimize pain, particularly in surgeries involving opening and drilling of tissues. The standard local anesthetics used are 2% lidocaine hydrochloride and 2% mepivacaine (Carbocaine) [18–20] (Table 51.1).

Chemically, local anesthetics are categorized as:

Table 51.1 Injectable local anesthetics used in dentistry

Parameters	Lignocaine	Articaine	Bupivacaine	Prilocaine	Mepivacaine
Concentrations					
Local anesthetic	2–3%	4%	0.25–0.5%	3–4%	2–3%
Vasoconstrictor	1:50,000–1:100,000	1:100,000–1:200,000	Without epinephrine	Felypressin 1:1,850,000	Epinephrine 1:66,000–1:100,000
Chemical class	Amide	Amide with ester side chain	Amide	Amide	Amide
Effect					
Onset	Rapid	Rapid	Slow	Slow	Rapid
Duration	120–240 min	140–270 min	4–8 h	90–360 min	120–180 min
Maximum dose	4.5–7mg/kg	4–7mg/kg	2.5–3mg/kg	5–7mg/kg	5–7mg/kg

Table 51.2 Recommended dosages of injectable local anesthetics

Recommendations (Bernett, 1984)	With vasoconstrictor	Without vasoconstrictor
Dosage	500 mg (6.6 mg/kg)	300 mg (4.4 mg/kg)
Maximum number of syringes in healthy patients	12.5	7.5

1. *Amide types:* lignocaine, mepivacaine, bupivacaine, and etidocaine
2. *Esters:* cocaine, procaine, tetracaine, and benzocaine

Caution is required when giving local anesthetics combined with vasoconstrictor agents to patients with cardiac arrhythmias, pheochromocytoma, unstable or uncontrolled angina, congestive cardiac failure, diabetes, or hyperthyroidism (Table 51.2).

In the event of an allergic reaction, an instant antidote is an intravenous injection of epinephrine (adrenaline) 0.01 ml/kg, in addition to an antihistamine, such as chlorpheniramine 10–20 mg, hydroxyzine 50 mg, or promethazine hydrochloride 25 mg.

Standard anesthetics are inhaled and include anxiolytics, such as nitrous oxide, that calm the patient during their dental treatment. Anxiolytics are used frequently, and their use together with local anesthetics is sometimes recommended.

Application of anesthesia is intended only for short-term pain relief; it should not be used for extended periods (Table 51.3).

Antifungals

Antifungals are utilized to cure candidiasis in the oral cavity, denture stomatitis, oral thrush, and abscesses (in combination with antibiotics). Specific antifungals such as nystatin (Mycostatin) are utilized to cure *Candida albicans* infection in the mouth, comprising denture stomatitis and thrush. Nystatin is available as troches/lozenges and as a suspension,

Table 51.3 Complications associated with dental local anesthesia

Complications	Effects
Local block complications	Muscle pain due to local infiltration, paresthesia due to nerve injury, middle ear problems, ophthalmic complications, palpation complications, palpitations, nausea, vomiting
Injection complications	Blood vessel injury, skin blanching, necrosis and ulceration, needle breakage, infection
Adverse reactions	Syncope, vasovagal attack, toxic effects (excitement or depression), allergic reaction (if immediate: targeting the lungs and circulatory system; if delayed: minor-type reaction)

to be taken orally. Patients are directed to take the suspension in two halves, where each dose is applied to different sides of the mouth (left and right) in order to keep the suspension in the mouth for as much time as possible by rinsing the mouth with it before swallowing it [19].

Prescribing Recommendations

The recommendations for prescribing antifungals are as follows:

Nystatin suspension 100,000 U/ml: The mouth should be rinsed with 5.0 ml for 2–3 minutes, then the suspension should be swallowed. It should be used four times daily for 7 days. It can be taken once daily for prophylaxis [15–18].

Triamcinolone and nystatin ointment: The ointment should be spread on the corners of the mouth twice daily to treat angular cheilitis until it is resolved; this treatment can be continued as required.

Depending on the severity and spread of candidiasis, fluconazole 100–200 mg can be taken once daily for 1–2 weeks. A dosage of 100–200 mg once weekly or twice weekly is usually beneficial to prevent recurrence of candidiasis in patients requiring long-term prophylaxis. Occurrence of side effects is highly unlikely but may include nausea, vomiting, and elevations in hepatic enzyme levels [18–20].

Other Dental Medications

Fluorides

Fluorides are an ingredient in toothpaste and are used to avoid tooth decomposition. They are available from most retailers of dental products and can be purchased without a prescription. When prescribed by a physician, a prescription-strength form of fluoride (Acidul) is also obtainable [12–16]. 1.1% sodium fluoride gel is applied by brushing before sleep. The patient should be directed to expectorate the residual gel but to then not rinse the mouth with water. Otherwise, the gel can be applied to the teeth with use of a fluoride tray, which should be kept in the mouth for a minimum of 15 minutes each night.

Antiseptics

Antiseptic mouth rinses are obtainable without a prescription from retailers of dental products. They are utilized to alleviate plaque and gingivitis, and to eradicate germs that cause halitosis.

Saliva Substitutes (Used to Treat Salivary Gland Hypofunction)

Saliva substitutes (Saliva Substitute, Xero-Lube, Moi-Stir, Salix, Optimoist, Salivar, Mouth Kote) are utilized for treating dry mouth, which can occur in association with other illnesses or sometimes as a complication of autoimmune diseases. Saliva substitutes are commonly available as sprays and can be used as required.

Prescribing Recommendations

The recommendations for prescribing saliva substitutes are as follows:

Pilocarpine 5 mg three times daily: This dosage can be increased to 7.5 or 10 mg three times daily, but patients usually find the side effects difficult to tolerate. The standard ones are lacrimation, skin reddening, hyperhidrosis, nausea, and dizziness. Pilocarpine is contraindicated in patients with limited-angle glaucoma or poor asthma control, and it should generally not be used in patients with persistent obstructive pulmonary disease.

Cevimeline 30 mg three times daily: Cevimeline is believed to have distinct affinity for salivary gland muscarinic receptors. The dosage can be increased, but this is known to be associated with harmful side effects [1–6].

Benzodiazepines

Benzodiazepines, such as diazepam (Valium), are administered for temporary relief of patient anxiety. These drugs have a calmative effect on the patient during dental surgeries, such as treatment of temporomandibular joint dysfunction. Diazepam undergoes hepatic metabolism by oxidative reduction, and both the parent molecule and the active metabolites are particularly influenced by old age, hepatic dysfunction, and drug–drug interactions [21–25]. Given these shortcomings, use of diazepam for oral sedation has largely been supplanted by use of more suitable alternatives to benzodiazepines.

There are numerous benzodiazepine formulations with virtually identical safety and sedative efficacy profiles. Individual differences in the onset and duration of the clinical effects are due to differences in these drugs' specific pharmacokinetic profiles. Understanding of these differences will enable the practitioner to select the right drug at the right dose for the right patient and for the right procedure [23].

Diazepam is considered the grandfather of its drug class. It has been available for more than 42 years and is used widely. Its onset of action is rapid (occurring within 20–40 minutes after administration) and its plasma concentration peaks within 1–2 hours after oral administration. In adults, it is used in a dose range of 2–10 mg. Diazepam has a long elimination half-life (20–80 hours) because it has multiple active metabolites (nordazepam [desmethyldiazepam] and oxazepam) [16, 22].

Lorazepam (Ativan)

Lorazepam is considered an intermediate-acting benzodiazepine, given its elimination half-life of approximately 10–20 hours. Lorazepam is therefore less affected by variables such as old age, hepatic dysfunction, and drug–drug interactions. It has oral bioavailability of 83–100%, with the peak plasma concentration being observed 1–2 hours after administration. The onset of action occurs within 60 minutes after oral administration [18, 23].

Triazolam (Halcion)

Triazolam is used widely for short-term treatment of insomnia. Its lack of active metabolites and its rapid onset and short duration of action make it a near-ideal antianxiety medication for dental patients [21]. Its onset of action occurs within 30 minutes after administration [23].

Midazolam (Versed)

Midazolam is rapidly absorbed when it is administered orally either as a premixed syrup or by dilution of the intravenous formulation in a pH-balanced liquid vehicle. Its onset of action occurs within 15–30 minutes after oral administration. It has largely been replaced as a medication for sedation in pediatric patients. In an assessment of its pharmacodynamic effects, an oral dose of triazolam 0.25 mg was found to be equivalent to midazolam 5–8 mg administered orally.

Nonsteroidal Anti-inflammatory Drugs

Management of postsurgical discomfort is the primary requirement in the initial stage of recovery in the majority of patients undergoing dental surgery. The drugs usually recommended for this purpose after minor oral surgery are NSAIDs; thus, it is rarely necessary to resort to use of narcotic drugs. It may be beneficial to prescribe drugs with analgesic anti-inflammatory activity. However, they pose risks in patients with asthma, a history of peptic ulceration, or some other specific conditions; hence, utilization of paracetamol with or without concomitant codeine is more advisable [21].

Some practitioners consider it preferable to administer an analgesic before surgery so there is an adequate amount of the drug in the system when the local anesthetic effects begin to wane. Many patients have determined ideal concentrations of analgesics that have been effective for them [22–24].

Prescribing Recommendations
The recommendations for prescribing NSAIDs are as follows:

20% ketoprofen ointment: A compounding pharmacist must make up this drug or dose to ensure the appropriate dosage. It should be spread on the skin of the infected region between once daily and four times daily. Side effects are very infrequent with topical treatment [24–26].

1% diclofenac sodium gel: It is important to adhere to the directions for usage as stated on the packaging.

Ibuprofen 200–400 mg: This should be taken every 4–6 hours (no more than 3200 mg/day) [26–31]. It should be consumed with care, and the dosage should be amended in patients with impaired renal function. The standard side effects include nausea, stomach ache, diarrhea, vomiting, renal failure, abnormal liver function test results, and skin rash or face breakouts [26].

Steroid Drugs

Steroids are used widely in dentistry for their anti-inflammatory and immunosuppressive properties. Corticosteroids have revolutionized the management of several disabling conditions but are often used in inappropriate dosages. Steroid substances are naturally produced in our bodies [32]. Commonly used steroid drugs include hydrocortisone, dexamethasone, methylprednisolone, and prednisolone. Dental patients with a history of corticosteroid use may require special consideration before receiving any dental treatment. Steroids are sometimes misused or prescribed in excessive doses, and are prescribed even before minor dental procedures. Corticosteroids are regarded as a double-edged sword for patients. Despite their various advantages, they also have severe side effects. These drugs are one of the most misused types of drugs in terms of dosage [33–36].

The risks associated with excess glucocorticoid administration are relatively small. They include electrolyte balance impairment and hypertension [34–36].

The current review emphasizes the uses and guidelines for use of corticosteroids in dentistry. Steroids are used after oral surgical procedures to limit postoperative inflammation. In 1974, Hooley [32] and Hohl elaborated on use of steroids to prevent postoperative edema [34, 37, 38]. Hooley further concluded that topical use of steroids helps to prevent ulceration and excoriation, which result from retraction of the lips and corners of the mouth during surgery. Steroids are also used to treat various diseases such as oral submucous fibrosis, oral lichen planus, erythema multiforme, pemphigus vulgaris, bullous and mucous membrane pemphigoid, Bell's palsy, central giant cell granuloma, postherpetic neuralgia, and Melkersson–Rosenthal syndrome [31–41].

Steroids may exacerbate certain conditions. They are therefore contraindicated [34–41] in patients with:

- Primary bacterial infection
- Hypersensitivity
- Peptic ulceration
- Diabetes mellitus
- Hypertension
- Pregnancy
- Osteoporosis
- Herpes simplex infection
- Psychosis
- Epilepsy
- Congestive heart failure
- Renal failure [42–45]

Conclusion

This overview is intended as a review of medications used in the dental office. It is not meant to replace continuing education provided by experts with advanced training in this area. Appropriate selection of medication and good patient management are of paramount importance to maintain safe practice.

References

1. de Vries TPGM, Henning RH, Hogerzeil HV, Fresle DA. Guide to good prescribing: a practical manual [document reference WHO/DAP/94.11]. Geneva: World Health Organization Action Programme on Essential Drugs, 1994. http://whqlibdoc.who.int/hq/1994/WHO_DAP_94.11.pdf. Accessed 6 Jan 2012.
2. Mendonca JM, Lyra DP Jr, Rabelo JS, et al. Analysis and detection of dental prescribing errors at primary health care units in Brazil. Pharm World Sci. 2010;32:30–5.
3. Cherry WR, Lee JY, Shugars DA, White RP Jr, Vann WF Jr. Antibiotic use for treating dental infections in children: a survey of dentists' prescribing practices. J Am Dent Assoc. 2012;143:31–8.
4. Guzman Alvarez R, Campos Sepulveda AE, Martinez Gonzalez AA. Knowledge about local anesthetics in odontology students. Proc West Pharmacol Soc. 2009;52:118–9.
5. Hupp JR, Ellis III E, Tucker MR: Contemporary Oral And Maxillofacial Surgery (ed 6). St. Louis, MO, Elsevier, 2014.
6. Grassi RF, Pappalardo S, De Benedittis M, Petruzzi M, Giannetti L, Cappello V, Baglio OA. Drugs in oral surgery. Brief guidelines for adult patients. Minerva Stomatol. 2004;53(6):337–44. English, Italian. PMID: 15266288.
7. Grabow L, Hein A, Hendrikx B, Thiel W, Schilling E. Gleichwertigkeit von oraler und intramuskulärer Prämedikation. III. Wirkung der Prämedikation auf Anästhesie und postoperative Schmerzen [Equivalence of oral and intramuscular premedication. III. Effect of premedication on anesthesia and postoperative pain]. Anasth Intensivther Notfallmed. 1986;21(4):181–6. German. PMID: 2875673.
8. Wilson W, Taubert KA, Gewitz M, et al. Prevention of infective endocarditis: guidelines from the American Heart Association: a guideline from the American Heart Association Rheumatic Fever, Endocarditis, and Kawasaki Disease Committee, Council on Cardiovascular Disease in the Young, and the Council on Clinical Cardiology, Council on Cardiovascular Surgery and Anesthesia, and the Quality of Care and Outcomes Research Interdisciplinary Working Group. Circulation. 2007;116:1736–54.
9. Sconyers JR, Crawford JJ, Moriarty JD. Relationship of bacteremia to toothbrushing in patients with periodontitis. J Am Dent Assoc. 1973;87:616–22.
10. Chung A, Kudlick EM, Gregory JE, et al. Toothbrushing and transient bacteremia in patients undergoing orthodontic treatment. Am J Orthod Dentofac Orthop. 1986;90:181–6.
11. Pallasch TJ, Slots J. Antibiotic prophylaxis and the medically compromised patient. Periodontol 2000. 1996;10:107–38.
12. Chitnis AS, Holzbauer SM, Belflower RM, et al. Epidemiology of community-associated *Clostridium difficile* infection, 2009 through 2011. JAMA Intern Med. 2013;173:1359–67.
13. Watters W 3rd, Rethman MP, Hanson NB, et al. Prevention of orthopaedic implant infection in patients undergoing dental procedures. J Am Acad Orthop Surg. 2013;21:180–9.
14. Quinn RH, Murray JN, Pezold R, Sevarino KS, et al. The American Academy of Orthopaedic Surgeons appropriate use criteria for the management of patients with orthopaedic implants undergoing dental procedures. J Bone Joint Surg Am. 2017;99:161–3.
15. Van der Meer JT, Van Wijk W, Thompson J, et al. Efficacy of antibiotic prophylaxis for prevention of native-valve endocarditis. Lancet. 1992;339:135–9.
16. Sollectio TP, Lockhart PB, Truelove E, et al. The use of prophylactic antibiotics prior to dental procedures in patients with prosthetic joints. J Am Dent Assoc. 2015;146:11–6.
17. American Academy of Pediatric Dentistry. Useful medications for oral conditions. In: The reference manual of pediatric dentistry. Chicago: American Academy of Pediatric Dentistry, 2020;

pp 592–598. https://www.aapd.org/globalassets/media/policies_guidelines/r_usefulmeds.pdf. Accessed 14 April 2017.
18. American Dental Association. Medications and oral health. Chicago: American Dental Association. Accessed 14 April 2017.
19. Curtis JW Jr, JB ML, Hutchinson RA. The incidence and severity of complications and pain following periodontal surgery. J Periodontol. 1985;56:597–601.
20. Moore PA, Deuben RR. Oral analgesic drug combinations. Dent Clin North Am. 1984;28:413–22.
21. Hooley JR, Bradley PB, Haines MP. Plasma cortisol levels following short term betamethasone therapy for oral surgery procedures. Trans Int Conf Oral Surg. 1973;4:188–90.
22. Williamson LW, Lorsen EL, Osbon DB. Hypothalamic pituitary–adrenal suppression after short term dexamethasone therapy for oral surgical procedures. J Oral Surg. 1980;38:20–8.
23. Hargreaves KM, Troullos ES, Dionne RA. Pharmacologic rationale for the treatment of acute pain. Dent Clin North Am. 1987;31:675–94.
24. Mense S. Sensitization of group IV muscle receptors to bradykinin by 5-hydroxytryptamine and prostaglandin E2. Brain Res. 1981;225:95–105.
25. Basran GS, Morley J, Paul W, Turner-Warwick M. Evidence in man of synergistic interaction between putative mediators of acute inflammation and asthma. Lancet. 1982;24:935–7.
26. Vane JR. Inhibition of prostaglandin synthesis as a mechanism of action for aspirin-like drugs. Nature. 1971;231:232–5. Scopus (6941)
27. Hepso HU, Lokken P, Bjornson J, Godal HC. Double-blind crossover study of the effect of acetylsalicylic acid on bleeding and postoperative course after bilateral oral surgery. Eur J Clin Pharmacol. 1976;10:217–25. Scopus (43)
28. Skjelbred J, Lokken P. Acetylsalicylic acid vs. paracetamol, effects on post-operative course. Eur J Clin Pharmacol. 1977;12:257–69. Scopus (61)
29. Petersen JK. The analgesic and anti-inflammatory efficacy of diflunisal and codeine after removal of impacted third molars. Curr Med Res Opin. 1978;5:525–35.Scopus (22)
30. Rosenquist JB, Rosenquist KI, Lee PKM. Comparison between lidocaine and bupivacaine as local anesthetics with diflunisal for postoperative pain control after lower third molar surgery. Anesth Prog. 1988;35:1–4.
31. Rosenquist JB, Nystrom E. Long-acting analgesic or long-acting local anesthetic in controlling immediate postoperative pain after lower third molar surgery. Anesth Prog. 1987;34:6–9.
32. Hooley JR, Hohl TH. Use of steroids in the prevention of some complications after traumatic oral surgery. J Oral Surg. 1974;32:864–6.
33. Swingle WW, Remington JW, Drill VS, Kleinberg W. Differences among adrenal steroids with respect to their efficacy in protecting the adrenalectomized dog against circulatory failure. Am J Phys. 1942;136:567–76.
34. Sambandam V, Neelakantan P. Steroids in dentistry—a review. International Journal of Pharmaceutical Sciences Review and Research. 2013;22:240–5.
35. Saravanan T, Subha M, Prem P, Venkatesh A. Corticosteroids—its role in oral mucosal lesions. International Journal of Pharma and Bio Sciences. 2014;5:439–46.
36. Borle RM, Borle SR. Management of oral submucous fibrosis: a conservative approach. J Oral Maxillofac Surg. 1991;49:788–91.
37. Manson SC, Brown RE, Cerulli A, Vidaurre CF. The cumulative burden of oral corticosteroid side effects and the economic implications of steroid use. Respir Med. 2009;103:975–94.
38. Kallali B, Singh K, Thaker V. Corticosteroids in dentistry. JIAOMR. 2011;23:128–31.
39. Bernard P, Charneux J. Bullous pemphigoid: a review. Ann Dermatol Venereol. 2011;138:173–81.

40. Martinez AE, Atherton DJ. High-dose systemic corticosteroids can arrest recurrences of severe mucocutaneous erythema multiforme. Pediatr Dermatol. 2000;17:87–90.

41. Baker PR. Diagnosis and management of Bell's palsy. Oral Maxillofac Surg Clin North Am. 2000;12:303–8.

42. Lokken P, Olsen I, Norman-Pedersen K. Bilateral surgical removal of impacted lower third molar teeth as a model for drug evaluation: a test with ibuprofen. Eur J Clin Pharmacol. 1975;8:209–16. Scopus (97)

43. Sisk AL, Bonnington GJ. Evaluation of methylpredisolone and flurbiprofen for inhibition of the postoperative inflammatory response. Oral Surg Oral Med Oral Pathol. 1985;60:137–45. Scopus (67)

44. DiRosa M, Calignano A, Carnuccio R, Ialenti A, Sautebin L. Multiple control of inflammation by glucocorticoids. Agents Actions. 1985;17:284–9. Eggleston D.J.

45. Nally F. Hazards of systemic corticosteroid therapy. Oral Surg Oral Med Oral Pathol. 1971;31:590–4. Scopus (3)

Future of the Oral Surgery

52

Fargol Mashhadi Akbar Boojar and Heliya Ziaei

Robotic Surgery

Robot-assisted surgery has attracted the attention of surgeons in different specialties during the past two decades. Although there is minimal evidence of its clinical success in oral and maxillofacial surgery, its increasing popularity in head and neck operations is undeniable [1]. It can be labeled as telesurgery, as this procedure can be performed without the surgeon's in-person presence.

The first clinical application of robots in head and neck surgery was introduced in 1999, while previous preclinical tests were conducted in 1994 by Kavanagh [2, 3]. Since 1999, many animals, cadaver, phantom, and clinical studies were conducted in various minor and major oral and maxillofacial surgeries (OMFS) [4].

Critical vital organs in the head and neck area with high neural and vascularized areas complicate the optimal accessibility to the surgical field [5]. Due to the need for a wide dissection area to approach the surgical site with routine transpharyngeal or transcervical approaches, minimally invasive techniques become highly important in OMFS surgeries [4, 6].

Transoral robotic surgery (TORS), which was first introduced and performed by McLeod et al. in 2005, provides suitable and deeper access to the surgical area in minor surgeries and overcome some of the limitations of conventional techniques [7, 8] (Fig. 52.1).

Many robotic systems have been introduced in recent years; one of the most effective robotic technologies is the Da Vinci surgical system. Its manipulators have the most similarity to the human wrist movements and provide a

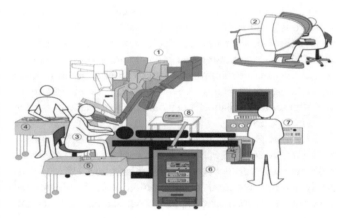

Fig. 52.1 Surgical setting. 1, Da Vinci robot; 2, first surgeon at the console; 3, second surgeon at the patient's head; 4, nurse at the instruments table; 5, second table for Da Vinci robot devices; 6, rack for imaging equipment; 7, anesthetist; 8, monopolar/bipolar cautery. (Reproduced with permission from Lawson et al. [8])

three-dimensional view of the surgical site [1, 9]. Based on a systematic review and meta-analysis, robotic surgery's most clinical application was transoral tumor resection, reconstructive surgeries, neck dissection, and flap harvesting consequently [1]. Still, it shows clinical success in flap harvesting, nerve transferring, reconstructive and cosmetic surgeries, thyroidectomy, and parathyroidectomy [7].

Reducing the operation time, enhancing visualization and precision, and eliminating some of the patients' post-surgical morbidity are among the most significant benefits of robotic surgery compared to conventional techniques, which need more well-designed controlled-trial studies to approve it [10, 11].

There is a lack of evidence regarding the usage of robot-assisted surgery in orthognathic operations, cosmetic surgeries, extensive trauma and fractures, and sleep apnea syndrome; future well-designed pre-clinical and clinical studies are required.

F. Mashhadi Akbar Boojar (✉)
School of Dentistry, Research committee of Golestan Medical University, Gorgan, Iran
e-mail: Fargolfarzan@yahoo.com

H. Ziaei
DDS, Faculty of Dentistry, Tehran University of Medical Sciences, Tehran, Iran

Head and Neck Cancer

Treating oral cancer is a long-term procedure requiring a combination of treatment modalities such as surgical excision, radiotherapy, and chemotherapy [12]. The oral side effects of these procedures may result in lifelong oral rehabilitation, which is challenging for both patients and physicians [12, 13],

Although the main goal of treating oral squamous cell carcinoma (OSCC) as a fatal cancer is the patients' survival, in recent years, surgeons emphasize minimally invasive procedures to reduce post-operative morbidities, maintain oral functions, and improve patients' quality of life (QOL).

One of TORS's principal aims in treating head and neck cancerous lesions is reducing the operation and in-patient time, eliminating invasive approaches, and reducing the side effects [13]. Maintaining speech and swallowing functions, which are usually compromised due to conventional surgical procedures, are crucial for preserving the patients' quality of life after tumor excision. This would be possible with robotic surgery [14, 15].

Moore et al. were pioneers of performing TORS in treating oral cancer in 45 patients with oropharyngeal squamous cell carcinoma followed by neck dissection [15]. In this study, similar to various clinical studies, the oropharyngeal functions were recovered rapidly, visualization and manipulation of the area were enhanced, in-patient time reduced, and transoral laser surgery limitations were resolved [11, 15, 16]. It reduces probable human errors in the head and neck's dense and crucial anatomical structures by tremor filtering and motion scaling technology [4].

Based on a comprehensive cohort study, robotic surgery in early-stage SCC (T1, T2) had superior clinical outcomes such as less positive margins, fewer complications, and long-term survival rates than non-robotic surgery [17]. TORS also resulted in successful oncological and postoperative outcomes in residual or recurrent SCC and can be considered as an alternative for conventional techniques in these patients [17].

Based on recent studies, it has been proposed that TORS can reduce postoperative complications of pharyngeal cancer and can be an alternative to adjuvant therapies such as chemoradiotherapy in some cases. According to a review of the evidence, it has satisfactory glottic and supraglottic pharyngeal cancer, but the clinical findings are controversial in several studies [16]. Although TORS's speed and effectiveness in supraglottic cancer treatment have priorities compared to the conventional techniques, it has its limitations. TORS require more working space in the surgical field. Airways compromises its optimal accessibility from the anatomical aspect; this fact resulted in less precision during the operation and remaining more positive margins after surgery in the robot-assisted surgery group in a pilot study [18, 19].

Therefore, in some patients with special conditions (e.g., trismus, inadequate transoral exposure for optimal manipulation, and vocal cord mobility impairment), TORS is completely contraindicated [18].

Postoperative hemorrhage and aspiration pneumonia are among the most commonly reported disadvantages of TORS in head and neck cancer surgery [13]. Future novel technologies of robots may resolve the limitations of the Da Vinci system. The novel systems should overcome some previous challenges such as providing proper hemostasis, precisely cutting the margins and providing less positive margins, and delivering optimal energy to the target area [20].

All in all, TORS's equal oncological success compared to conventional techniques in cancer patients has been reported in many clinical studies because TORS results in improving QOL with fewer complications [18, 20].

Cleft Lip and Palate

According to the growing popularity of robot-assisted surgeries in the head and neck area, transoral robotic cleft surgery (TORCS) was performed in cadaver studies in the recent decade for approving further clinical applications [21–23]; based on these pilot studies, it is concluded that this technique provides excellent 3D visualization, convenient manipulation, and precise dissection. Subsequent clinical studies confirmed the clinical success of cleft lip and palate surgery with TORCS [23]. Nevertheless, the Da Vinci robotic system manipulators' size and the smaller size of the pediatric airway anatomy in the surgical field are important limitations of this surgical technique [24]. Besides, the duration of robot-assisted cleft surgery was longer compared to conventional surgery [23].

Novel surgical robot technologies with a more delicate design should be performed for enhancing their application in pediatric surgeries. Further comprehensive clinical studies should be conducted to certify the safety and efficacy of TORCS.

The Perspective of Minimally Invasive Surgery (MIS)

Minimally invasive surgery (MIS) can be referred to as endoscopic surgery, minimally invasive surgical arthroscopy, video-assisted surgery, telescopic surgery, and minimal-access surgery. Treatments that may involve an endoscope include laser therapy, which can be used for destroying cancer cells. Photodynamic therapy can destroys tumors by using a laser after injecting it with a light-sensitive substance. Endoscope can use in orthognathic surgery, sialoendoscopy, and temporomandibular joint (TMJ) disorders in oral and maxillofacial surgery [25].

As we mentioned before, speech and swallowing functions usually compromise due to conventional surgery. New approaches like minimally invasive techniques can stop or reduce these results.

Endoscopy has been used for decades as a supportive technique for directing minimally invasive oral surgical procedures and, in recent years, has been used increasingly in endoscopically assisted operative techniques. In the future, we can use these methods in the field of dentistry because we can achieve the best results with a minimal postoperative problems. Three-dimensional planning and navigated surgery will also play a significant role in the future. Navigation allows surgeons to maneuver through the surgical field certainty and to put instruments and implants onto the ideal area with exactness and accuracy [26].

Minimally Invasive Intraoral Approach (MIIA)

We can perform MIIA for treatment of abscess and neck phlegmon with odontogenic origin when the infections spread up to the inferior mandibular margin and no further, so it is better to evaluate the anatomical localization of abscess with CT or MRI, and then we can use the best surgical approach.

The results of one study in 2020 show the achievement of MIIA in comparison with conventional treatments.

Some of the advantages of this procedure are as follows: (1) excellent healing rates, (2) avoidance of injury to nerves and vessels in sensitive conditions, (3) patients not suffering from relapses during follow-up, (4) obtaining a shorter postoperative recovery, and (5) reduction in the length of hospitalization [27].

Dental Implant and Endoscopic Approaches

Complications of dental implantation in the posterior maxilla still occur, including acute and chronic sinusitis, oriental fistula (OAF), and implant dislocation and migration into the paranasal sinuses [28].

With the broad indications for dental implantation, complication rates have increased. Dental implant displacement into the maxillary sinus can occur during the restoration of posterior maxillary teeth, but it is rare.

Displacement of a dental implant to the maxillary sinus can happen preoperatively or postoperatively.

Some of the reasons for preoperative operations are as follows: placement of implants in sites with inadequate bone height and volume, surgical inexperience, improper surgical procedures such as over-preparation of the recipient site,

application of a heavy force during implant insertion, or sinus membrane perforation during the drilling procedure. Focal osteoporotic bone marrow defect (FOBMD) is commonly located in the mandibular edentulous posterior area of a middle-aged female. It is one reason for implant displacement in the mandible.

We can use endoscopic sinus surgery to remove the implant and restore sinus patency. If the implant is displaced to deeper areas (commonly anterior and inferior) of the maxillary sinus, a pre-lacrimal recess approach can provide a panoramic view of the maxillary sinus and is a good alternative Caldwell-Luc operation in terms of mucosal preservation and postoperative complications.

One of the reasons for the migration of dental implant is inadequate bone height. For patients with displacement dental implants, we suggest to remove the foreign body [29].

Endoscopic sinus surgery (ESS) can provide removal of foreign body, treatment of rhinosinusitis, and establishment of a patent maxillary ostium [27].

Endoscopic sinus surgery (ESS) has also been proposed as the preferred procedure for the removal of dislodged dental implants [28].

ESS is an effective and minimally invasive method to remove displaced dental implants and restore sinus health. Computed tomography can be used to localize a foreign body, but it may migrate before the operation. The PLR (pre-lacrimal recess) offers a direct and panoramic view of the maxillary sinus and can assist with the removal of difficult-to-reach foreign bodies. Multi-disciplinary cooperation between otolaryngologists and oral surgeons can improve treatment results [29, 30].

Implant Surgery Using CAD/CAM (Guided Surgery or Static Navigation)

Implant surgery using CAD/CAM surgical templates has become widely used, and now, a new technology, dynamic navigation, is gaining popularity. Conventional free-handed implant placement has evolved into a guided approach, which has led the way into a navigated technique.

Computer-assisted dynamic navigation has been commonly employed in neurosurgery, orthopedics, and ear, nose, and throat surgery for many years. It has recently been implemented for dental implant surgery [33–35].

Dynamic navigation, in its present form, utilizes real-time, motion-tracking, optical technology to track the implant drill and patient during the preparation of the osteotomy and implant placement to match a virtually planned implant position. Two types of motion tracking are available: active tracking system and passive tracking system arrays, which use reflective spheres to reflect infrared light emitted from a light source back to a camera.

Advantage of dynamic navigation method: Implant placement accuracy is predictable with accuracy approximating 0.4 mm with angular deviation approximating 4°. But the rates of failure in dynamic navigation are similar to that in traditional methods [31, 32].

Surgical Navigation for Oral and Maxillofacial Surgery

Navigation allows surgeons to maneuver through the surgical field with confidence and to place instruments and implants on to the desired location with accuracy and precision. The applications of navigation technology in oral and maxillofacial surgery continue to increase. Surgical navigation allows enhancement of both surgical precision and accuracy owing to real-time confirmation of position, without the need to obtain additional intaoperative images which can expose patients to additional radiation, navigation technology may also facilitate surgery when dealing with soft tissue lesions where access is limited by allowing for minimally invasive access compared with traditional open approaches, which may require extensive dissection for exposure. Indications for surgical navigation in OMFS have been described as complex unilateral orbital wall fractures comminuted unilateral fractures of the lateral midface, bony tumors, bony reconstruction of complex 3-dimensional anatomy, and for removal of foreign bodies [36].

Temporomandibular Joint Arthroscopy

TMJ disorder is a multifactorial disease process caused by muscle hyperfunction or parafunction, traumatic injuries, hormonal influences, and articular changes. Physicians have used various types of splints since the eighteenth century for the treatment of TMJ disorders. Today, the use of splints has become one of the most common in-office initial treatments for TMD-associated pain [37].

Treatment of TMJ disorder can be divided into three procedures: noninvasive, minimally invasive, and invasive options. The future of TMJ-MIS may be through regenerative medicine approaches such as tissue engineering [38]. TMJ disorders encompass all age groups; it is generally considered to affect young- to middle-aged adults (20–40 years old) [37].

During the twentieth century, arthroscopic surgery was regarded as one of the three most significant improvements in the treatment of patients with conditions affecting the musculoskeletal system.

In addition to joint replacement and internal fixation of fractures, TMJ arthroscopy could be an effective and minimally invasive form of surgical intervention for treating Wilkes II, III, and IV TMJ disorders in the pediatric population. It is an approach that has been used for more than 40 years to ameliorate pain and restore function. It might play a role in the early identification and treatment of disorders of the TMJ articular disc and synovium. These days, we have the plasma sprayer system for arthroscopy. Plasma is composed of highly ionized particles. These ionized particles can reduce tissue volume by separating molecules from each other. It only causes little damage to surrounding healthy tissues, not the whole tissues. And because of its benefit, it could be key for the next step required in arthroscopy – resection [39].

Laparoscopic Surgery

The history of general laparoscopic surgery dates back to the introduction of appendectomy by Semm in 1980 [40].

In recent years, the da Vinci® system's robotic surgery has attracted attention and a limited number of institutions have reported various results.

The Soloassist® system is a joystick-guided robotic scope holder. Scope holders can reduce the number of participants in surgery and provide a stable surgical field without tremors. Initially, scope holders were only invented to fix the scope [41, 42] (Fig. 52.2).

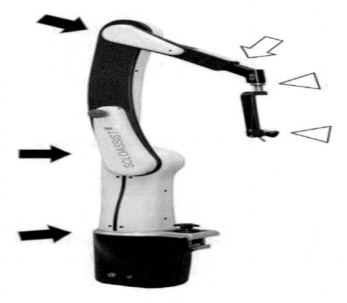

Fig. 52.2 Soloassist II has six joints: three are computer-controlled (black arrows), one can be adjusted manually (white arrow), and two act as a gimbal joint following the movement of the main body (white arrowheads). With minimally invasive procedures, surgeons work with both hands. As a consequence, the Soloassist is controlled by a joystick positioned on the instrument. (This figure is reproduced with permission from Ohmura et al. [42])

Shortly, the development of active scope holders might play an important role in laparoscopic surgery.

Advantages: Full functionality for general surgery, urology, and gynecology. No manual camera guidance is required. A stable and steady image enhances the quality of surgery. The assistant surgeon is now free to do more demanding tasks; it can reduce the trauma to the pitons. The Soloassist is compatible with all commercially available operating tables and endoscopes, thus protecting your investments. Setup and disassembly of the system can be performed in conjunction with your usual preparation procedures and do not add to operating time. The camera-holding system shows a very high velocity for head and neck surgery. This advantages shows that Solloassist has potential to use for surgery in the mandible fracture [43].

Paranasal Sinuses and Skull Base Robot Prototype

Endoscopic approaches to the nose, paranasal sinuses, and anterior skull base continue to expand with modern innovations and improved surgical strategies.

A new dedicated PSSB robot system is in development by a team of engineers and physicians at Vanderbilt University. This robotic system seeks to address the limitations in current instrumentation by utilizing a new concentric tube technology [44, 45].

The small footprint of the PSSB robot will facilitate less crowding at the surgical field, allowing both the scrub nurse/tech and assistants to more easily maneuver near the patient.

Robotic surgical systems for paranasal sinus and skull base surgery are achievable soon [46].

Navigation for Oral and Maxillofacial Surgery

Navigation methods are classified into two types. In the first type, a stereo vision system is employed to conduct a 3D registration. This method is usually suitable for a subject with a clear texture like sinus, but failures can easily occur. In the second type, an endoscope is employed to conduct a 3D registration.

In innovative robotic surgery, surgeons do not create a direct impact on surgical results. But it can help reduce errors that occurs due to the fatigue of a surgeon. In this new technique, the patient lies down on the surgical bed and an oral and maxillofacial surgeon placed close to the patient's head. It can help focus on the teeth or other regions on which the surgeon wants to perform a surgery. With this new technique, surgeons would not be tired during osteotomy as they do not hold the device for a long time to drill or cut in the target bone area. In this new technique, the surgeon starts the operation

and allows the navigation system to guide the robot precisely to complete the operation. Two screens display the VR image and output data in real time. An autonomous OMS robot that can detect a skull's pose and automatically finish an operation under the surveillance of a surgeon was proposed.

But the navigation systems' costs are very high, and the time for preparation for the surgery is longer compared to the conventional technique. The navigation procedure gives more security, particularly in complex cases, and may result in a better clinical outcome for the patient. Further development of software programs may reduce the preoperative planning time and time spent during the operation [47].

Yomi (New Robot in Maxillofacial Surgery)

Yomi is the first and the only FDA-cleared robot-assisted dental surgery system since 2018; the first country to use this system is China. Surgical robotic technology helps dentists to successfully place dental implants. Yomi provides computerized navigation to aid in arranging pre-operative and intra-operative phases of dental implantation surgery. The system offers physical guidance through haptic robotic innovation, which constrains the drill in position, depth, and direction to reduce errors from human sources. The assistive innovation gives the specialist full oversight, which allows for clear visualization of the surgical site. Yomi is intended to empower a minimally invasive flapless methodology, which has been demonstrated to prompt quicker medical procedures, faster recovery, and less pain for the patient. It manages a specialist's hand to the exact point and area for an arranged osteotomy [48].

Conclusion

The purpose of this chapter is to determine some new technologies that may become valuable in maxillofacial surgery or other kinds of treatments in dentistry in the future.

Medical robots are one of the greatest scientific achievements of modern surgery. They can be used in different types of surgery like paranasal sinus surgery or implant surgery. It can also help surgeons become safe from infections like Covid-19, one of the most important diseases these days.

The development of robotic technology is also necessary for the future development of maxillofacial surgery, but it is necessary to consider the most desirable cost-benefit for patients struggling with diseases under limited medical expenses. Naturally, as a surgeon, robotic surgery is very interesting. There is a desire to perform it as a surgeon, but making it universally applicable to various diseases would require immense financial resources, manpower, and a new educational system.

References

1. Nehme J, Neville J, Bahsoun A. The use of robotics in plastic and reconstructive surgery: a systematic review. JPRAS Open. 2017;13:4–5.
2. Kavanagh KT. Applications of image-directed robotics in otolaryngologic surgery. Laryngoscope. 1994;104:283.
3. Lueth TC, Hein A, Albrecht J, Demirtas M, Zachow S, Heissler E, Klein M, Menneking H, Hommel G, Bier J. A surgical robot system for maxillofacial surgery. IECON '98 Proc 24th Annu Conf IEEE Ind Electron Soc (Cat No98CH36200). 1998;4:2470.
4. De Ceulaer J, De Clercq C, Swennen G. Robotic surgery in oral and maxillofacial, craniofacial and head and neck surgery: a systematic review of the literature. Int J Oral Maxillofac Surg. 2012;41:1311.
5. Evans BT, Coombes D, Mahadevan V, Brennan PA. Maxilla and zygoma. InClinical Head and Neck Anatomy for Surgeons. CRC Press. 2015: pp. 162–171.
6. Sukegawa S, Kanno T, Furuki Y. Application of computer-assisted navigation systems in oral and maxillofacial surgery. Jpn Dent Sci Rev. 2018;54:139.
7. Garas G, Arora A. Robotic head and neck surgery: history, technical evolution, and the future. ORL. 2018;80:1.
8. Lawson G, Matar N, Remacle M, et al. Transoral robotic surgery for the management of head and neck tumors: learning curve. Eur Arch Otorhinolaryngol. 2011;268:1795–801.
9. Dwivedi J, Mahgoub I. Robotic surgery: a review on recent advances in surgical robotic systems. InFlorida Conference on Recent Advances in Robotics. 2012: pp. 10–11.
10. Maan ZN, Gibbins N, Al-Jabri T, D'Souza AR. The use of robotics in otolaryngology–head and neck surgery: a systematic review. Am J Otolaryngol. 2012;33:137.
11. Voutyrakou D, Papanastasis T, Chatsikian M, Katrakazas P, Koutsouris D. Transoral robotic surgery (TORS) advantages and disadvantages: a narrative review. J Eng. 2009;1:3–4.
12. Petrovic I, Rosen EB, Matros E, Huryn JM, Shah JP. Oral rehabilitation of the cancer patient: a formidable challenge. J Surg Oncol. 2018;117:1729.
13. Golusiński W. Functional organ preservation surgery in head and neck cancer: transoral robotic surgery and beyond. Front Oncol. 2019;9:2–3.
14. Kalantari F, Rajaeih S, Daneshvar A, Karbasi Z, Salem M. Robotic surgery of head and neck cancers, a narrative review. Eur J Transl Mylo. 2020;30:2–4.
15. Moore EJ, Olsen KD, Kasperbauer JL. Transoral robotic surgery for oropharyngeal squamous cell carcinoma: a prospective study of feasibility and functional outcomes. Laryngoscope. 2009;119:2156.
16. Rinaldi V, Pagani D, Torretta S, Pignataro L. Transoral robotic surgery in the management of head and neck tumors. Ecancermedicalscience. 2013;7:359.
17. Nguyen AT, Luu M, Mallen-St Clair J, Mita AC, Scher KS, Lu DJ, Shiao SL, Ho AS, Zumsteg ZS. Comparison of survival after transoral robotic surgery vs nonrobotic surgery in patients with early-stage oropharyngeal squamous cell carcinoma. JAMA Oncol. 2020;6:1555.
18. Byrd J, Ferris R. Is there a role for robotic surgery in the treatment of head and neck cancer? Curr Treat Options in Oncol. 2016;17:2–4.
19. Ansarin M, Zorzi S, Massaro MA, Tagliabue M, Proh M, Giugliano G, Calabrese L, Chiesa F. Transoral robotic surgery vs transoral laser microsurgery for resection of supraglottic cancer: a pilot surgery. Int J Med Robot. 2014;10:2–3.
20. Ross T, Tolley N, Awad Z. Novel energy devices in head and neck robotic surgery – a narrative review. Robot Surg Res Rev Volume. 2020;7:25.
21. Khan K, Dobbs T, Swan M, Weinstein G, Goodacre T. Trans-oral Robotic Cleft Surgery (TORCS) for palate and posterior pharyngeal wall reconstruction – a feasibility study. J Plast Reconstr Aesthet Surg. 2015;69:2–4.
22. Podolsky D, Fisher D, Riff K, Looi T, Drake J, Forrest C. Infant robotic cleft palate surgery: a feasibility assessment using a realistic cleft palate simulator. Plast Reconstr Surg. 2017;139:455e.
23. Nadjmi N. Transoral robotic cleft palate surgery. Cleft Palate Craniofac J Off Publ Am Cleft Palate-Craniofacial Assoc. 2016;53:326.
24. Al Omran Y, Abdall-Razak A, Ghassemi N, Alomran S, Yang D, Ghanem A. Robotics in cleft surgery: origins, current status and future directions. Robot Surg Res Rev Volume. 2019;6:41.
25. Pedroletti F, Johnson BS, McCain JP. Endoscopic techniques in oral and maxillofacial surgery. Oral Maxillofac Surg Clin. 2010;22(1):169–82.
26. Hakim MA, McCain JP, Ahn DY, Troulis MJ. Minimally invasive endoscopic oral and maxillofacial surgery. Oral Maxillofac Surg Clin. 2019;31(4):561–7.
27. Galli M, Fusconi M, Federici FR, Candelori F, De Vincentiis M, Polimeni A, Testarelli L, Cassese B, Miccoli G, Greco A. Minimally invasive intraoral approach to submandibular lodge. J Clin Med. 2020;9(9):2971.
28. Chiapasco M, Felisati G, Maccari A, Borloni R, Gatti F, Di Leo F. The management of complications following displacement of oral implants in the paranasal sinuses: a multicenter clinical report and proposed treatment protocols. Int J Oral Maxillofac Surg. 2009;38(12):1273–8.
29. Jeong KI, Kim SG, Oh JS, You JS. Implants displaced into the maxillary sinus: a systematic review. Implant Dent. 2016;25(4):547–51.
30. Manor Y, Anavi Y, Gershonovitch R, Lorean A, Mijiritsky E. Complications and management of implants migrated into the maxillary sinus. Int J Periodontics Restorative Dent. 2018;1:38(6).
31. Sgaramella N, Tartaro G, D'Amato S, Santagata M, Colella G. Displacement of dental implants into the maxillary sinus: a retrospective study of twenty-one patients. Clin Implant Dent Relat Res. 2016;18(1):62–72.
32. Chang PH, Chen YW, Huang CC, Fu CH, Huang CC, Lee TJ. Removal of displaced dental implants in the maxillary sinus using endoscopic approaches. Ear Nose Throat J. 2020;0145561320931304:1–4.
33. Ewers R, Schicho K, Truppe M, Seemann R, Reichwein A, Figl M, Wagner A. Computer-aided navigation in dental implantology: 7 years of clinical experience. J Oral Maxillofac Surg. 2004;62(3):329–34.
34. Strong EB, Rafii A, Holhweg-Majert B, Fuller SC, Metzger MC. Comparison of 3 optical navigation systems for computer-aided maxillofacial surgery. Arch Otolaryngol–Head Neck Surg. 2008;134(10):1080–4.
35. Block MS, Emery RW. Static or dynamic navigation for implant placement—choosing the method of guidance. J Oral Maxillofac Surg. 2016;74(2):269–77.
36. Lübbers HT, Jacobsen C, Matthews F, Grätz KW, Kruse A, Obwegeser JA. Surgical navigation in craniomaxillofacial surgery: expensive toy or useful tool? A classification of different indications. J Oral Maxillofac Surg. 2011;69(1):300–8.
37. Klasser GD, Greene CS. Oral appliances in the management of temporomandibular disorders. Oral Surg Oral Med Oral Pathol Oral Radiol Endodontol. 2009;107(2):212–23.
38. Liu F, Steinkeler A. Epidemiology, diagnosis, and treatment of temporomandibular disorders. Dental Clins. 2013;57(3):465–79.
39. Monje F. Future of minimally invasive surgery in temporomandibular joint pathology. Stomatol Dis Sci. 2020;30:4.

40. Semm K. Endoscopic appendectomy. Endoscopy. 1983;15(02):59–64.
41. Arezzo A, Schurr MO, Braun A, Buess GF. Experimental assessment of a new mechanical endoscopic solosurgery system: Endofreeze. Surg Endosc Other Interv Tech. 2005;19(4):581–8.
42. Ohmura Y, Suzuki H, Kotani K, Teramoto A. Laparoscopic inguinal hernia repair with a joystick-guided robotic scope holder (Soloassist II®): retrospective comparative study with human assistant. Langenbeck's Arch Surg. 2019;404(4):495–503.
43. Kristin J, Geiger R, Knapp FB, Schipper J, Klenzner T. Use of a mechatronic robotic camera holding system in head and neck surgery. HNO. 2011;59(6):575–81.
44. Rucker DC, Jones BA, Webster RJ III. A geometrically exact model for externally loaded concentric-tube continuum robots. IEEE Trans Robot. 2010;26(5):769–80.
45. Burgner J, Swaney PJ, Rucker DC, Gilbert HB, Nill ST, Russell PT, Weaver KD, Webster RJ. A bimanual teleoperated system for endonasal skull base surgery. In: 2011 IEEE/RSJ international conference on intelligent robots and systems. IEEE; 2011. p. 2517–23.
46. Nimsky C, Rachinger J, Iro H, Fahlbusch R. Adaptation of a hexapod-based robotic system for extended endoscope-assisted transsphenoidal skull base surgery. min-Minim Invasive Neurosurg. 2004 Feb;47(01):41–6.
47. Ma Q, Kobayashi E, Suenaga H, Hara K, Wang J, Nakagawa K, Sakuma I, Masamune K. Autonomous surgical robot with camera-based markerless navigation for oral and maxillofacial surgery. IEEE/ASME Transact Mechatron. 2020;25(2):1084–94.
48. Nayyar N, Ojcius DM, Dugoni AA. The role of medicine and technology in shaping the future of oral health. J Calif Dent Assoc. 2020;48(3):127.

Index

Printed in the United States
by Baker & Taylor Publisher Services